Comprehensive
HEALTH

Catherine A. Sanderson, PhD
Professor of Psychology
Amherst College
Amherst, Massachusetts

Mark Zelman, PhD
Associate Professor of Biology
Aurora University
Aurora, Illinois

Pedagogy Developers

Melanie Lynch, M.Ed.
Health Education Specialist
State College Area High School North
State College, Pennsylvania

Melissa Munsell
Instructional Specialist
Physical Education and Health Department
North East Independent School District
San Antonio, Texas

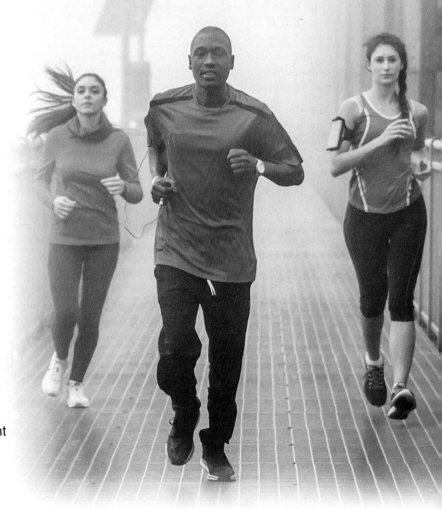

Publisher
The Goodheart-Willcox Company, Inc.
Tinley Park, Illinois
www.g-w.com

About the Authors

Catherine A. Sanderson is the Manwell Family Professor of Life Sciences (Psychology) at Amherst College. She received a bachelor's degree in psychology, with a specialization in Health and Development, from Stanford University, and received both master's and doctoral degrees in psychology from Princeton University. Professor Sanderson's research examines how personality and social variables influence health-related behaviors such as safer sex and disordered eating, the development of persuasive messages and interventions to prevent unhealthy behavior, and the predictors of relationship satisfaction. This research has received grant funding from the National Science Foundation and the National Institute of Health. Professor Sanderson has published over 25 journal articles and book chapters in addition to four college textbooks, a high school health textbook, and a popular press book on parenting. In 2012, she was named one of the country's top 300 professors by the Princeton Review.

Mark Zelman is an Associate Professor of Biology at Aurora University, Aurora, Illinois. He received a bachelor's degree in biology at Rockford College, with minors in chemistry and psychology. He received a PhD in microbiology and immunology at Loyola University of Chicago, where he studied the molecular and cellular mechanisms of autoimmune disease. During his postdoctoral research at the University of Chicago, he studied aspects of cell physiology pertaining to cell growth and cancer. Dr. Zelman supervises undergraduate research on streptococcal and staphylococcal infections, and mechanisms of antibiotic resistance. He also teaches in the science education graduate program for biology and chemistry high school teachers. He has published articles on microbiology, infectious disease, autoimmune disease, and biotechnology, and he has written two college texts on human diseases and infection control. Dr. Zelman is an officer of the Illinois State Academy of Sciences.

Pedagogy Developers

Melanie Lynch is past-president of Health Education for Pennsylvania State Association for Health, Physical Education, Recreation and Dance (PSAHPERD) and has been a health education specialist at State College Area High School, State College, Pennsylvania, for the past 21 years. She attended Penn State University and received a bachelor's degree in exercise and sport science with a teaching emphasis and a master of education. In 2004, Melanie received Pennsylvania's Health Teacher of the Year Award from PSAHPERD. She is also the recipient of the Eastern District Health Teacher of the Year Award from the Society of Health and Physical Educators (SHAPE America), which was formerly AAHPERD, and Pennsylvania's Professional Honor Award from PSAHPERD. She was also recognized as National Health Teacher of the Year by SHAPE America in 2016. Melanie has trained hundreds of teachers as a Health Education Assessment Project (HEAP) trainer for the state of Pennsylvania.

Melissa Munsell is an instructional specialist in the Physical Education and Health Department at North East Independent School District, in San Antonio, Texas, and serves as the K-12 Health Education Lead for the district. Melissa received a bachelor's degree in kinesiology from The University of Texas at Austin and is certified to teach Physical Education K–12 and Health Education 6–12, among other endorsements, in the state of Texas. She has 23 years of teaching and administrative experience, with six of those years teaching health education at the high school level. She has also served as vice president of the Health Division of the Texas Association for Health, Physical Education, Recreation, and Dance (TAHPERD), and presents workshops and lectures on various health topics locally and statewide.

Contributors and Reviewers

Contributors

Goodheart-Willcox Publisher would like to thank the following classroom instructors who contributed to the development of the *Before You Read*, *Warm-Up Activity*, *Lesson Review* questions and activities, and the *Chapter Review and Assessments*.

Michael A. Cleffi II
Health and Physical
  Education Teacher
Bethlehem Area School District
  (Freedom High School
  and Liberty High School)
Bethlehem, Pennsylvania

Kathryn Smith, MAT
Family and Consumer
  Sciences Teacher
Issaquah High School
Issaquah, Washington

Reviewers

Goodheart-Willcox Publisher and the authors would also like to thank the following instructors who reviewed selected manuscript chapters and provided valuable input into the development of this textbook program.

Laura Abbott
Health Education Teacher
Cabot Junior High North
Cabot, Arkansas

Karen Asbell
Health Teacher
St. Charles High School
St. Charles, Missouri

Tempe Beall
Health Educator
Centennial High School
Ellicott City, Maryland

Heather Bowen
Health Educator
Springfield Central High School
Springfield, Massachusetts

Hannah Brewer
Assistant Professor of Health
  Education
Slippery Rock University
Slippery Rock, Pennsylvania

Sandra Bricker
Health Education Teacher
Rocky River High School
Rocky River, Ohio

Kelly Brown
Health Teacher
Marriotts Ridge High
  School
Marriottsville, Maryland

Siobhan Carey
Health Educator
Sachem North High School
Lake Ronkonkoma,
  New York

Mike Cleffi
Health and Physical
  Education Teacher
Freedom High School &
  Liberty High School
Bethlehem, Pennsylvania

Denise Coats
Health Teacher
Lake Highlands High School
Dallas, Texas

Toni Cochrane
Teen Pregnancy Prevention
  Program Coordinator
Fort Dodge High School
Fort Dodge, Iowa

Sarah Coleman
Health Teacher
Fulton County Schools
East Point, Georgia

Lynne Conchieri
Health Teacher
High School of Commerce
Springfield, Massachusetts

Kim Cooke
Health and Physical
  Education Specialist
Charlotte-Mecklenburg Schools
Charlotte, North Carolina

Janet Daniels
Health Teacher
Thomasville Middle School
Thomasville, North Carolina

Sonji Davis
Health Educator
Waukegan High School
Waukegan, Illinois

Ann DeBoer
Health Teacher
Seaholm High School
Birmingham, Michigan

Lauren DeViney
Health Science Teacher
Waltham High School
Waltham, Massachusetts

Jennifer Evetts
Lifetime Wellness Teacher
Glencliff High School
Nashville, Tennessee

Julia Feldman
Health Science Specialist
Oakland Unified School
District
Oakland, California

Amanda Forcucci
PreK-12 Curriculum Director,
Physical Education and
Health
Hamden Public Schools
Hamden, Connecticut

Judy Gawlinski
Family and Consumer
Sciences Educator
Union City High School
Union City, Pennsylvania

Laura Gilpin
Health Science Educator
Cumberland County
High School
Crossville, Tennessee

Frith Gladdis
Health Teacher
Del Campo High School
Fair Oaks, California

Nikki Guerra
Health and Physical
Education Teacher
Freedom High School
Bethlehem, Pennsylvania

Joseph Halowich
Health Teacher
Parkside High School
Salisbury, Maryland

Lori Harper
Physical Education Teacher
Springfield Public Schools
Springfield, Massachusetts

Amy Hawk
Health Teacher
Greene County Schools
Greeneville, Tennessee

Lori Hewlett
Chairperson for Health
Education
Sachem Central School
District
Lake Ronkonkoma,
New York

Danielle Hill
Health and Physical
Education Teacher
Chicopee High School
Chicopee, Massachusetts

Marcy Horn
Health Teacher
Rochester Early College
International High
School
Rochester, New York

Kellie Danna Hurst
Health Teacher
Westminster High School
Westminster, Maryland

Michelle Ifill-Roseau
Health Teacher
White Plains High School
White Plains, New York

Ed Jones
Health & Physical
Education Department
Chairman
Houston ISD-Lee
High School
Houston, Texas

Leslie Karp
Health Teacher
Chavez High School
Houston, Texas

Jen Lohmeyer
Health and Physical
Education Teacher
Oakwood High School
Dayton, Ohio

Lori Mediate
Health Education
Coordinator
Fairfield Public Schools
Fairfield, Connecticut

Diane C. Miller
Health Educator
Sachem North High School
Lake Ronkonkoma,
New York

Susan Nash
Health Educator
Groves High School
Birmingham, Michigan

Judith R. Peters, MBA, HHSA
Office of Health, Safety, and
Physical Education
The School District of
Philadelphia
Philadelphia, Pennsylvania

Erin Phelps
Health Education Teacher
St. Petersburg High School
St. Petersburg, Florida

Michelle Scarpulla
Assistant Professor
Temple University
Philadelphia, Pennsylvania

Linda Schrader
Health and Physical
Education Teacher
Mishawaka High School
Mishawaka, Indiana

Jim Smith
HPE Department Head
Northmont High School
Clayton, Ohio

Kathryn Smith
Family and Consumer
Sciences Teacher
Issaquah High School
Issaquah, Washington

Mark Temons
Science Teacher, retired
Muncy High School
Muncy, Pennsylvania

Brief Contents

Contents

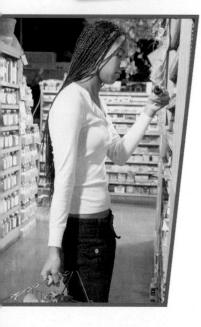

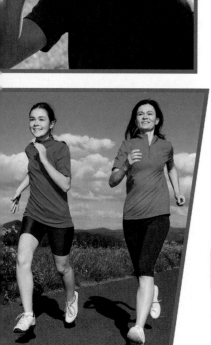

Unit 4   Understanding and Avoiding Hazardous Substances

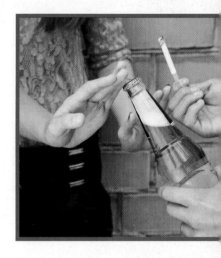

Unit 5   Diseases and Disorders

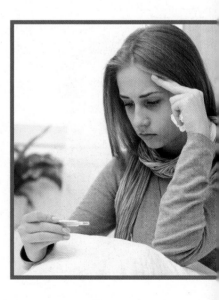

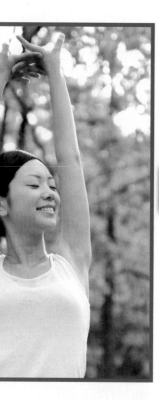

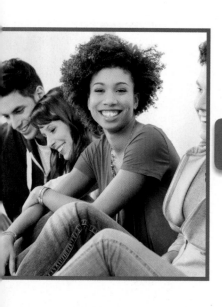

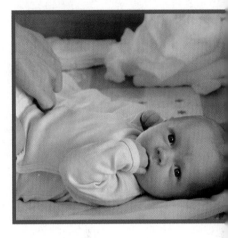

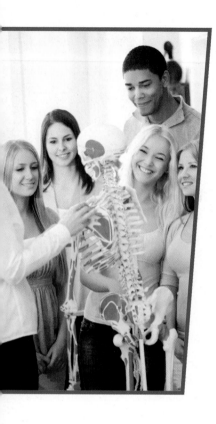

Special Features

What's Your Health and Wellness IQ?

Research in Action

CASE STUDY

SKILLS FOR HEALTH AND WELLNESS

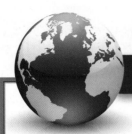

Local and Global Health

Personal Profile

Health across the Life Span

Spotlight on / Health and Wellness Careers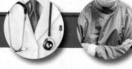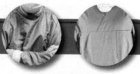

To the Student

We wrote this exciting new textbook for high school health and wellness classes based on our experiences as professors of psychology (Catherine Sanderson) and biology (Mark Zelman), and as the accomplished authors of college-level textbooks. Our combined backgrounds give us a deep well of knowledge of the most current scientific theory and research to draw from.

Perhaps the most valuable experience we had in preparing to write this book is our roles as parents to a combined total of seven children, ages 8 through 22. After all, in writing this book, we both reflected frequently on our experiences as parents and our goal of ensuring that our own children maintain excellent physical, emotional, intellectual, and social health.

This book includes all of the standard topics found in high school health and wellness books—including nutrition, physical fitness, substance use and abuse (including alcohol and tobacco), stress management, disease prevention, and healthy relationships. Additionally we also included essential material not often found in such books. This material includes chapters discussing the impact of sleep on psychological and physical well-being and strategies for maintaining a positive body image (even in the face of media pressure to achieve unrealistic body shapes and sizes). You'll also read how health can change across a person's life span, including during adolescence.

We wanted our book to give high school students the most current health information, presented in an engaging writing style so students would enjoy reading the book. We also filled the book with practical skills teenagers can use in their own lives.

Finally, as the authors of successful college-level textbooks, we felt confident in our research and writing abilities, but felt that the pedagogy was better left to master teachers. We would like to thank Health Education Specialist Melanie Lynch, of State College Area High School North, State College, Pennsylvania, and Instructional Specialist Melissa Munsell, of North East Independent School District, San Antonio, Texas, for developing the questions and activities that are a vital part of this course. We hope you are delighted with the final product, and wish all readers of this book a lifetime of good health.

Cath A. Sanderson

Mark Zelman

Unit 1 Introduction to Health and Wellness

Big Ideas

- Each dimension of health—physical, emotional, intellectual, and social—impacts your total wellness.

- You can raise your level of health and wellness by acquiring knowledge and skills that can help you make healthful choices.

- Having risk factors increases a person's chance of developing a disease or disorder, or experiencing an injury.

- Many risk factors can be controlled or eliminated.

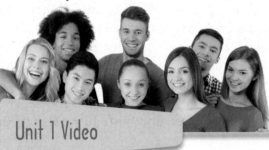

Unit 1 Video

Making the Right Choices Videos

The choices you make every day about the foods you eat, the people you hang out with, and the way you spend your time affect your health. Making the right choices, however, isn't always easy for people. In this video, some teenagers make choices that negatively impact their health.

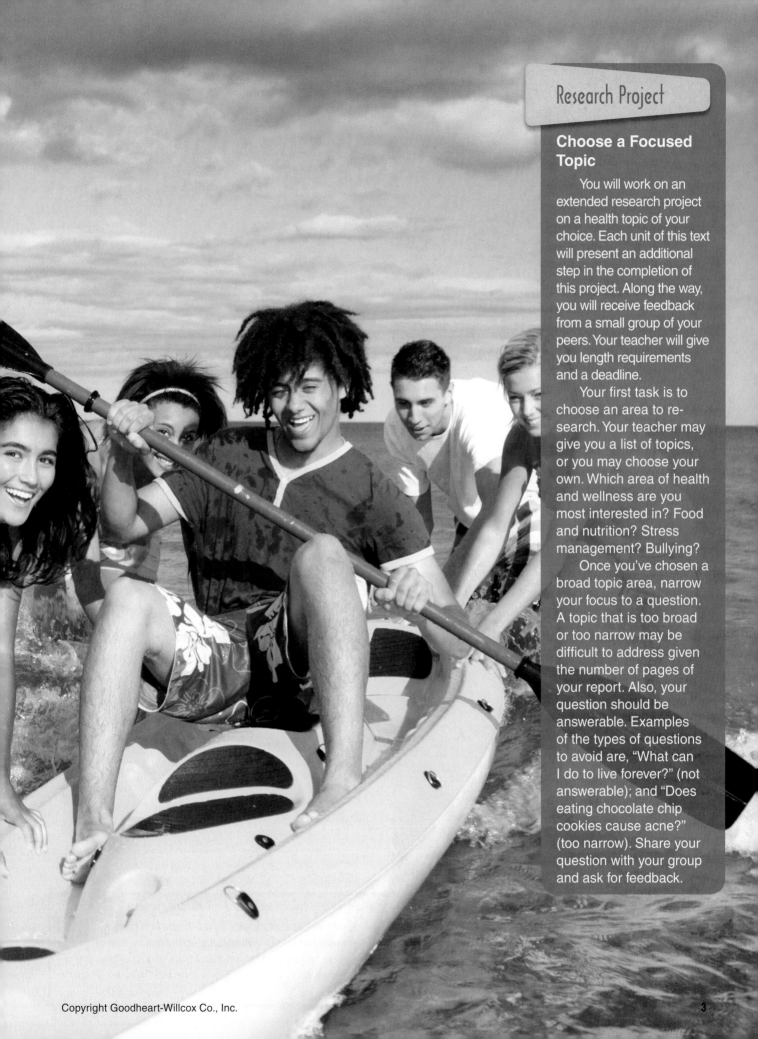

Choose a Focused Topic

You will work on an extended research project on a health topic of your choice. Each unit of this text will present an additional step in the completion of this project. Along the way, you will receive feedback from a small group of your peers. Your teacher will give you length requirements and a deadline.

Your first task is to choose an area to research. Your teacher may give you a list of topics, or you may choose your own. Which area of health and wellness are you most interested in? Food and nutrition? Stress management? Bullying?

Once you've chosen a broad topic area, narrow your focus to a question. A topic that is too broad or too narrow may be difficult to address given the number of pages of your report. Also, your question should be answerable. Examples of the types of questions to avoid are, "What can I do to live forever?" (not answerable); and "Does eating chocolate chip cookies cause acne?" (too narrow). Share your question with your group and ask for feedback.

Chapter 1

Understanding Your Health and Wellness

Lesson 1.1

Defining Health and Wellness

Lesson 1.2

Health and Wellness Knowledge

Lesson 1.3

Personal Skills for Health and Wellness

Lesson 1.4

Our Healthcare System

While studying this chapter, look for the activity icon ⬀ to:
- **review** vocabulary with e-flash cards and games;
- **assess** learning with quizzes and online exercises;
- **expand** knowledge with animations and activities; and
- **listen** to pronunciation of key terms in the audio glossary.

G-WLEARNING.com

www.g-wlearning.com/health/

What's Your Health and Wellness IQ?

Take this quiz to see what you do *and* do not *know about health and wellness. If you cannot answer a question, pay extra attention to that topic as you study this chapter.*

1. *Identify each statement as* True, False, *or* It Depends. *Choose* It Depends *if a statement is true in some cases, but false in others.*
2. *Revise each* False *statement to make it true.*
3. *Explain the circumstances in which each* It Depends *statement is true and when it is false.*

Health and Wellness IQ Assess

1. Diseases and disorders are the same.	True	False	It Depends
2. Good friendships and family relationships make you healthy.	True	False	It Depends
3. Mental illness can affect your social health.	True	False	It Depends
4. Goals are not an important part of your health.	True	False	It Depends
5. You don't have to be sick to be unhealthy.	True	False	It Depends
6. You can change behaviors that make you unhealthy.	True	False	It Depends
7. You don't need annual check-ups with your doctor.	True	False	It Depends
8. A person's workplace can affect his or her well-being.	True	False	It Depends
9. You cannot find reliable health information on the Internet.	True	False	It Depends
10. Intellectually healthy people do not care about school.	True	False	It Depends

Setting the Scene

When you were a young child, you didn't choose what you ate—your parents and guardians did. When you exercised, it wasn't because you thought it was good for you, but because it was fun. Still, you had limited choices in the matter—the adults in your life took you to parks and introduced you to jump ropes, scooters, and bikes. They also worked hard to keep you safe and injury free.

Now that you're an adolescent you make many of your own choices, including choices that affect your health. For example, if your school cafeteria offers pizza and a salad bar, you make the choice between the two. You also decide whether or not you will be physically active, or sit in front of a TV or computer screen much of the day. And you decide whether or not to take risks, such as riding in a car driven by an intoxicated friend, or lighting a first cigarette and taking a puff.

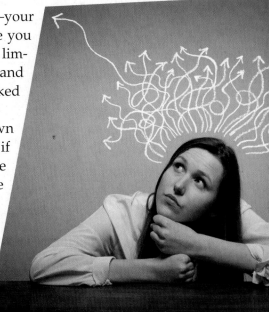

Many of the choices you make today will impact your health and quality of life in either a positive or negative way. Why not learn how to make choices that will positively impact your life—today and for years to come? This textbook will help you develop a foundation of knowledge, skills, and resources on which to build a healthy, fulfilling life.

Defining Health and Wellness

Key Terms E-Flash Cards

In this lesson, you will learn the meanings of the following key terms.

acute diseases
chronic diseases
disease
disorder
emotional health
intellectual health
optimal health
physical health
social health
well-being
wellness

Before You Read

Brainstorming Health and Wellness

Write Health and Wellness *in the center of a chart then* add *physical, emotional, intellectual, and* social *as offshoots. Brainstorm and record your ideas about these four areas of health before you read the lesson.*

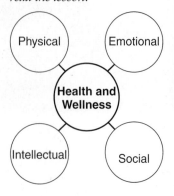

Physical — Emotional

Health and Wellness

Intellectual — Social

Lesson Objectives

After studying this lesson, you will be able to

- define wellness and understand the four main aspects of well-being;
- analyze how physical, emotional, intellectual, and social aspects of wellness are interrelated;
- explain the status of health as it relates to a continuum;
- differentiate between disease and disorder; and
- evaluate the four main causes of disease and how they impact wellness.

Warm-Up Activity

Making Health-Related Choices
Think about some of the choices you have made over the last week. Make a list of choices that had a positive impact on your health and choices that were risky to, or maybe had a negative impact on, your health. Cross out each risky choice and replace it with a positive, healthier choice that you could have made.

Choice	Was my choice *positive* or *negative* for my health?	If *negative*, a positive choice I could have made instead would be:

According to her doctor, 16-year-old Janine is the picture of health. She recently passed a physical exam with flying colors. But when she is under stress—which is often—Janine is so anxious that she can't sleep or focus on her schoolwork. She is frequently tired and eats on the go. She dropped soccer and took up smoking with her boyfriend and his friends. Janine avoids making decisions and planning for her future. Instead, she prefers to "go with the flow."

Nathan, also 16, was born with a respiratory problem that makes running and playing most sports difficult. He, however, manages his illness by making sure to follow his doctor's instructions and by taking the medicine prescribed for his condition. He also makes sure to eat well, get plenty of sleep, and get a moderate amount of exercise. He does not smoke or drink. His optimistic and upbeat attitude attracts other people to him, so he has many friends. He sets goals for his future, and is confident that he will succeed if he works hard.

Who do you think is healthier—Janine or Nathan? In the past, many people would say that Janine is healthier. In many Western societies, including the United States, health was defined in purely medical terms as the absence of physical illness and disease. According to this view, Janine would be considered healthier than Nathan, who has a chronic illness, even if it is well managed.

Many public health experts and medical professionals now embrace a broader definition of health and may conclude that Nathan is the healthier one. For example, although Janine is able-bodied, she smokes. This puts her at risk of someday becoming one of the 440,000 people in the United States who die prematurely from a smoking-related disease each year. Janine also doesn't get the sleep and exercise her body needs. While Nathan is confident and optimistic, Janine is often anxious and lacks the skills needed to set goals and make decisions that impact her health and well-being in a positive way.

Well-being is a state of health and wellness. What do you associate with well-being? Scientists took this question to people of all ages and from many cultures. They found that people associated well-being with a number of characteristics. They said people in a state of well-being

- generally feel good about their present condition;
- have a sense of fulfillment and a positive mood;
- enjoy a long life;
- engage in behaviors that promote health and prevent mental and physical illness;
- do not have mental and physical illnesses;
- are socially connected, have relationships, and participate in social activities;
- are productive at school, work, and home;
- have a sense of purpose;
- have access to basic resources to meet their basic needs; and
- have a safe physical and social environment, including a safe home and work environment.

It's clear that, for people around the world, being healthy is associated with more than just the absence of disease.

"Health is not only the absence of infirmity and disease, but also a state of physical, mental, and social well-being." —World Health Organization

well-being
a state of health and wellness in which one feels safe, fulfilled, and productive, and looks forward to enjoying a long life

Dimensions of Health and Wellness

wellness

a healthy balance of physical, emotional, intellectual, and social health

Health and wellness involve the *whole* person—not just a person's physical health, how much the body weighs, or how many push-ups and laps around the track someone can do.

Wellness is a balance of physical, emotional, intellectual, and social health (Figure 1.1). What are the characteristics of these different dimensions of health?

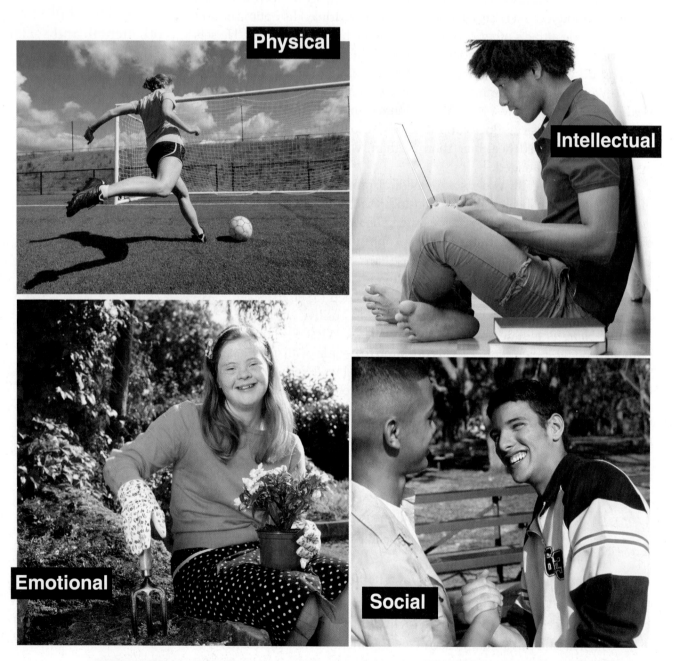

Physical

Intellectual

Emotional

Social

Figure 1.1   There are four dimensions of health and wellness—the physical, emotional, intellectual, and social dimensions. *Give an example of how a problem in one dimension of health can impact another dimension.*

Physical Health

Physical health is the dimension of health that refers to how well your body functions. If you have a physically healthy body, you are not slowed by disease. Your body functions well and allows you to participate in the activities of daily life. You can also cope with the stresses of disease, injury, aging, and an active lifestyle. In other words, being physically healthy enables you to do more than walk to school or lift a bag of books—you can recover from a sprained ankle, fight off the flu, and have the energy to cope with daily stresses.

physical health
a dimension of health that involves your body, including physical fitness and the ability to cope with everyday physical tasks

Emotional Health

A state of well-being also requires emotional, or *mental*, health. Your emotions, your mood, how you feel about yourself, and how you view the world are all parts of your **emotional health**. People who have good emotional health are not affected by mental illness. They express their thoughts and feelings clearly and cope well with stress. They also maintain mature relationships, respecting and valuing others and themselves.

Many teens experience problems with their emotional health but may not realize it. For example, persistent feelings of sadness or worry are not healthy. These feelings can keep you from doing well in school or participating in your favorite activities. Poor emotional health can also interfere with your sleep, diet, and exercise, and prevent you from forming friendships. The good news is that treatment can help you feel better.

emotional health
a dimension of health that involves your emotions, mood, outlook on life, and beliefs about yourself

Intellectual Health

Related to emotional health is the idea of **intellectual health**. Intellectually healthy people have a positive attitude about learning new topics. They can think clearly and critically, and face challenging problems with optimism. With these skills and attitudes, they can enjoy exploring exciting new ideas. In an ever-changing world, people who are intellectually healthy have an advantage over others because they are able to adapt, learn, and grow.

intellectual health
a dimension of health that involves your ability to think clearly and critically, learn, and solve problems

Social Health

Can you imagine your life with no human interaction? It is unhealthy for humans to live in isolation because humans are social animals who must interact and communicate with one another. Social health is another dimension of well-being. *Social health* refers to how well you get along with other people.

Your relationships with family, friends, boyfriends, or girlfriends should be enjoyable and supportive (Figure 1.2). These relationships should not make you feel bad about yourself. You should never be physically harmed or threatened by friends or family. Trust and honest communication are important parts of healthy relationships. Social skills and healthy relationships give people the support they need to enjoy life and meet its challenges. Healthy relationships are among your most valuable resources.

social health
a dimension of health that involves your communication skills, relationships, and ability to interact with others

Figure 1.2

Hanging out with friends has health benefits as long as the friendships are honest and supportive. *In what ways do your friends have a positive impact on your health?*

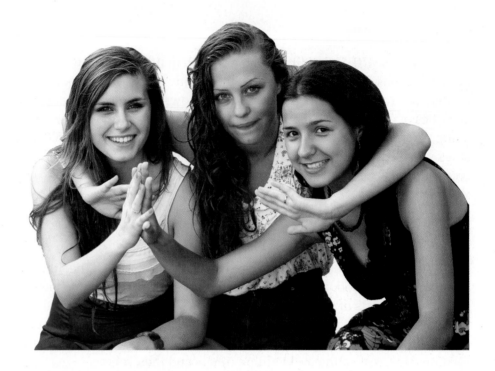

Interaction of Wellness Dimensions

The physical, emotional, intellectual, and social dimensions of health interact with and affect each other. A disturbance in one dimension of health may lead to a disturbance in another. Likewise, an improvement in one dimension may lead to improvements in others.

For example, suppose someone who is physically fit and eats well develops the mental illness known as *depression*. When people are depressed, their emotional health suffers, but the illness can eventually impact other dimensions of health. People who are depressed may be less motivated to eat properly (physical health), have difficulty concentrating (intellectual health), and pull back from their friends and family (social health).

A Continuum of Health

People often think of well-being as a dichotomy (one or the other)—you are either healthy or you are not. This is not, however, an accurate description of health. A person's health status normally lies somewhere between the extremes of poor and excellent. This range in health status is described as a *continuum* (Figure 1.3). Most people experience one or more problems that put their health status in the center of the wellness continuum.

Optimal health lies at one end of the continuum. Optimal health is not just the absence of disease. Optimal health is a state of superb health and wellness—excellent physical, emotional, intellectual, and social health. People want their health status to be at or near this end of the continuum.

At the other end of the continuum lies disease and premature death. The term *disease* describes an overall poor state of health in which people cannot function normally. As you'll learn, there are many types of diseases and disorders that can affect the body and the mind.

optimal health
a state of excellent health and wellness in all areas of your life

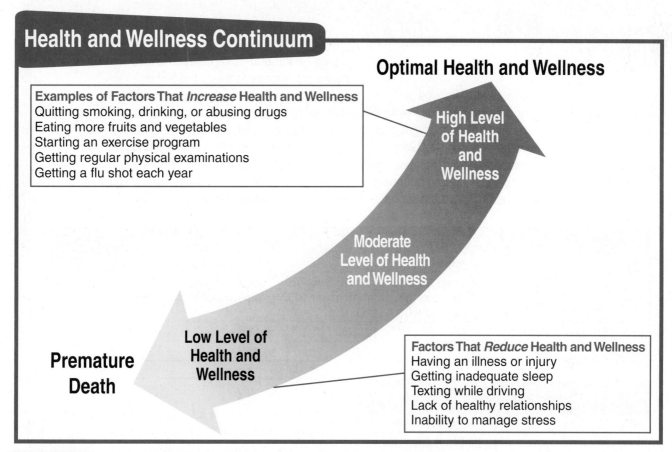

Health and Wellness Continuum

Optimal Health and Wellness

Examples of Factors That *Increase* Health and Wellness
Quitting smoking, drinking, or abusing drugs
Eating more fruits and vegetables
Starting an exercise program
Getting regular physical examinations
Getting a flu shot each year

High Level of Health and Wellness

Moderate Level of Health and Wellness

Low Level of Health and Wellness

Premature Death

Factors That *Reduce* Health and Wellness
Having an illness or injury
Getting inadequate sleep
Texting while driving
Lack of healthy relationships
Inability to manage stress

Figure 1.3 Your level of health and wellness can be plotted on a continuum. The choices you make largely determine where you are on the continuum. *Where would you plot your health status on this continuum today? Explain.*

Diseases and Disorders

Disease is an impairment of the normal function of the body or one of its parts. Diseases directly affect a person's health. You are probably familiar with the effects of diseases such as the common cold and allergies. You may also know about the impact of serious diseases such as cancer.

Some diseases happen quickly and go away in a short time. These are known as *acute diseases*. Common acute diseases include the flu and chicken pox. Other diseases—called *chronic diseases*—last many years or even a lifetime. Diabetes, cancer, and heart disease are chronic diseases.

A disease can be recognized by a set of specific signs and symptoms. Signs are outward indicators of disease that can be detected and measured by others. Examples of signs include a rash, fever, uncoordinated movement, or unconsciousness.

A symptom is a disease indicator that is sensed by the sick person. Examples of symptoms include pain, confusion, depressed mood, or nausea. Symptoms of the flu include exhaustion and muscle aches and pains.

Like a disease, a *disorder* is an abnormal physical or mental condition, but disorder is often used when no single cause can be identified. For that reason, mental illnesses such as anxiety or depression are often called *mental disorders*.

disease
a poor state of health and wellness in various areas of your life

acute diseases
diseases that occur and resolve quickly

chronic diseases
diseases that occur for many years, even for a lifetime

disorder
an abnormal physical or mental condition with no single, identifiable cause

Research in Action

Income and Education Affect Health

Most people living in poverty lack basic nourishment, shelter, and other resources available to people with higher incomes. So you might expect that people living below the poverty level also have less access to educational opportunities and healthcare. Do you think people without adequate nutrition, education, and healthcare experience worse health and more disease than people with adequate access to these resources?

Research shows that, from the poorest country to the wealthiest, income and education are related to quality of health. The Centers for Disease Control and Prevention (CDC) reports the following results of an ongoing study of income, education, and health among children and adults in the United States.

Percentage of US Adults 18 Years of Age and over Contracting Certain Diseases					
	Income		**Education**		
Disease	**Poverty**	**Highest income (four times the poverty level)**	**No high school diploma or GED**	**High school diploma or GED**	**College degree or higher**
Heart disease	13.8%	9.3%	13.7%	12.1%	11.3%
Stroke	4.7%	1.5%	4.5%	3.1%	2.4%

Percentage of US Children under 18 Years of Age Contracting Certain Diseases		
	Income	
Disease	**Poverty**	**Highest income (four times the poverty level)**
Asthma	12.4%	6.7%
Ear infections (3 or more)	7.3%	4.8%

Thinking Critically

1. Are asthma and ear infections more common among poor children or among wealthy children? Explain your answer.
2. Compared to people earning the highest incomes, are people living in poverty three, four, or five times more likely to have a stroke?
3. Does education level affect the risk for stroke and heart disease? Explain your answer.

Lesson 1.1 Review

Know and Understand

1. Define *wellness*. What are the four types of health that relate to wellness?
2. Describe several characteristics of a physically healthy body.
3. Why is social health important to overall wellness?
4. Explain what is meant by the phrase "continuum of health."

Analyze and Apply

5. How are emotional and intellectual health related?

Real World Health

Self-Analysis Draw and label a continuum of health. Make a list of both positive and negative decisions you make that affect your health. Place these decisions or actions onto your health continuum. After labeling your health continuum, circle where you fall—optimal health, some impairment, or disease—on the health continuum. Below your health continuum, list some decisions or actions that you can make in the future to improve your health or keep it at or near optimal health.

Health and Wellness Knowledge

Lesson Objectives

After studying this lesson, you will be able to

- understand the importance of health literacy;
- understand criteria used to determine whether or not information should be accepted as scientific knowledge;
- determine the credibility of sources offering health-related information;
- describe how health promotion relates to safety and impacts the life span; and
- evaluate the importance of lifelong learning as it relates to health and wellness.

Key Terms E-Flash Cards

In this lesson, you will learn the meanings of the following key terms.

health literacy
health promotion
lifelong learning
pseudoscience
science
scientific knowledge

Warm-Up Activity

Being a Knowledgeable Consumer
Think about purchases you've made over the last week and list two to four products that you or a family member have purchased. These products can be food items, hygiene products, recreational or exercise items, or any other types of items. Next to each item, answer the following questions, then write a paragraph commenting on whether you were a smart or not-so-smart consumer.

1. *Was the purchase of this product health-related?*
2. *Did advertising play a role in the purchase of this item?*
3. *Was this purchase positive or negative to your health?*

Product purchased:	
Was this purchase health-related?	
Did advertising play a role?	
Was this purchase positive or negative to my health?	

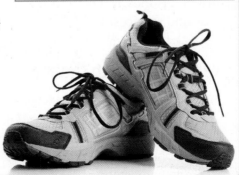

Before You Read

3,2,1

While you are reading this lesson, think about things you discover, things you find interesting, and things you still question. After you finish reading, fill in a chart like the one below.

Discovered
1.
2.
3.
Found Interesting
1.
2.
Question
1.

K nowledge is power. Health knowledge gives you the power to prevent disease and promote your well-being. For example, nearly 45% of high school students have smoked cigarettes. Health knowledge, however, tells us that smoking is addictive, which means the body develops a physical and psychological need for smoking. Also, smoking damages the lungs, heart, and blood vessels. Smokers often develop heart disease, high blood pressure, and lung cancer.

With that knowledge in hand, you can understand why you should avoid cigarette smoking. With the right skills and resources you can apply that knowledge and successfully avoid cigarettes. In this section, you'll learn the kind of knowledge you need to maintain and promote your wellness. These topics will be covered in depth in following chapters.

Health Literacy

health literacy
the ability to locate, interpret, and apply information pertaining to your health

What's the best way to control asthma, muscle cramps, or acne? What can you do to better manage the stress in your life? How can you help a friend with an eating disorder?

Do you know how you would find answers to these questions—good, reliable answers? You wouldn't want answers based on rumors or unreliable sources of information.

As you become familiar with health-related terms, concepts, and facts, you'll develop health literacy. *Health literacy* is the ability to locate, interpret, and apply information pertaining to your health.

Your health literacy builds on basic facts and concepts you learn at home and in school. Knowledge allows you to make informed decisions and healthy choices. Your health and wellness also depends on your ability to access and use reliable information. Doing so involves various skills. These *health literacy skills* include the ability to locate, evaluate, understand, and communicate health-related information (Figure 1.4).

Consumer Literacy and Health

A *consumer* is someone who purchases goods and services. You are a consumer. As you read this text, you will learn how to become an *informed* consumer so that you can make informed, healthy purchases and choices. You will also learn where to find and how to evaluate healthcare-related goods and services.

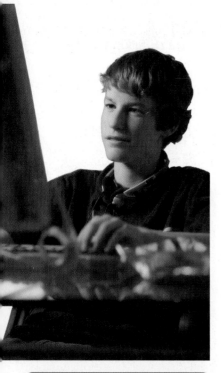

Figure 1.4

Many people go online for answers to questions about their health and wellness. *When was the last time you searched for health information online? What did you find?*

Evaluating Health Claims

"Get six-pack abs in two weeks!"
"You'll catch a cold if you go outside with wet hair."
"The bumps on your skull reveal your character."
"Cell phones cause brain cancer."
"Caffeinated energy drinks will make you perform better on exams."

These are some examples of thousands of health claims you can find in magazines, on websites, and in advertisements. None of these claims are supported by science. What's at stake if you believe these claims? You can waste money and time, and you can harm your health.

Health and wellness are science-based disciplines based on scientific methods. Your health and wellness depend on reliable information (Figure 1.5). You need to be able to distinguish information grounded in science from health claims based on rumor, folk stories, and pseudoscience.

Science or Pseudoscience?

Science is a body of knowledge regarding the natural world, which is based on observation and experimentation. Science poses questions about the natural world—including the human body, human health, and diseases. *Scientific knowledge* is

- *based on experimentation and observation*. Health claims should be backed by a significant amount of scientific research.

- *peer-reviewed*. Reliable scientific information is published in scientific journals following careful scrutiny by qualified scientists.

- *repeatable*. If a discovery has merit and seems to explain an aspect of human health, other scientists should be able to find the same results when performing the same experiment.

In contrast, *pseudoscience* refers to theories and health claims that are described as science-based when they are not. Pseudoscience is characterized by information that is

- not based on repeated experimentation;

- not verifiable by other scientists;

- not published in scientific journals;

- not peer-reviewed; and

- too good to be true!

Self-Advocacy and Interpreting Media

Health-related knowledge will enable you to make healthful purchases and choices. You will be able to resist and avoid the influences from the media, your peers, and questionable pseudoscientific sources. Websites, newspapers, magazines, television, and radio often present health-related information. Some of this information is too good to be true, inaccurate, or misleading.

Agencies, Websites, and Other Media

When using the Internet, you will see several websites when you type in a question about your health. How do you decide which source you should trust? In general, reliable information can be found with agencies or organizations whose primary mission is education, research, or providing

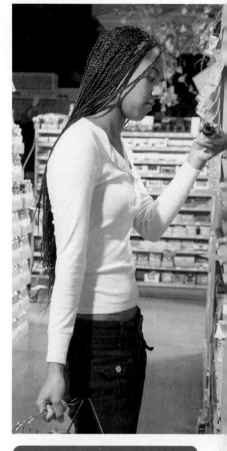

Figure 1.5

As a consumer, you need to know how to gather information from product labels and other sources.

science
a collection of and the pursuit of knowledge about the natural world drawn from observation and experimentation

scientific knowledge
conclusions about the natural world that have been obtained through peer-reviewed, repeatable observation and experimentation

pseudoscience
theories and health claims that are described as being based in science when they are not

direct healthcare. URL stems that are generally considered safe or reliable include .gov, .edu, and .org. Some sources of reliable health information are listed in Figure 1.6.

Websites of businesses that earn profits from the healthcare industry are often not trustworthy. The main goal of a business is to earn profits by selling the product or service it provides. The information a business provides may play up the benefits of what it is selling and play down or omit any negative information.

When searching for information, you should begin with a reliable, general source such as one of those agencies or websites listed in Figure 1.6. You will find some tips for evaluating websites in Figure 1.7 on pages 18 and 19.

Reliable Print Media

When in doubt, ask your school librarian or doctor about a reliable media source. You should be confident that the information you're researching is correct and applicable to your situation. The size or popularity of a newspaper or magazine is not a good indicator of reliable information.

Figure 1.6 Health and Safety Information

Sources of Information	URLs
Centers for Diseases Control and Prevention	www.cdc.gov
MedlinePlus® (U.S. National Library of Medicine, National Institutes of Health)	www.nlm.nih.gov/medlineplus/
U.S. Department of Health and Human Services	www.healthfinder.gov
Office of the Surgeon General	www.surgeongeneral.gov
National Institute of Mental Health	www.nimh.nih.gov
U.S. Food and Drug Administration	www.fda.gov
United States Consumer Products Safety Commission	www.cpsc.gov
National Highway Traffic Safety Administration	www.nhtsa.gov
United States Department of Agriculture	www.choosemyplate.gov
Academy of Nutrition and Dietetics	www.eatright.org
Mayo Clinic	www.mayoclinic.org
American Academy of Pediatrics	www.aap.org
American Cancer Society	www.cancer.org
American Heart Association	www.heart.org
Institute of Medicine of the National Academies	www.iom.edu
Tufts University Health & Nutrition Letter	www.nutritionletter.tufts.edu
National Institute on Drug Abuse	www.drugabuse.gov
World Health Organization	www.who.int
American Red Cross	www.redcross.org

Manny, 15, drags himself out of bed most mornings. He finds it hard to stay alert during classes. During baseball practice, Manny complains about his fatigue to his friends. They tell him that they down energy drinks to give them the spark they need when they are tired in the morning, before baseball practice, and when tackling homework in the evening. Manny wants to learn more and decides to read the label on a popular energy drink.

Thinking Critically

1. How can Manny locate credible, reliable sources of information about energy drinks?

2. Who can he turn to for good information about these drinks?

3. Why is it important to have accurate information about energy drinks?

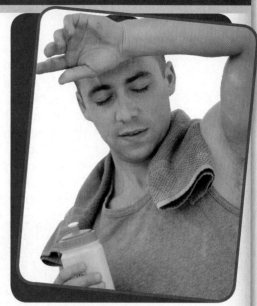

Can energy drinks give Manny the pep he needs to get through his day?

How do you decide if the information is reliable? Here are some indicators:

- The information is included in a news story, not in an opinion piece or editorial.
- The story refers to research published by medical scientists.
- The story gives the names of the researchers and the journal in which the original work is published.
- You can find other stories with the same results.
- The newspaper or magazine is not produced by a company that manufactures or sells medicines or medical devices.

Use your library to find information about health and wellness. Librarians specialize in finding and evaluating sources, so you can rely on their advice should questions arise.

Health Promotion

Health and wellness require your active attention. There is a cause and effect between some of your actions and your health. For example, ignoring your diet will result in poor nutrition. Likewise, if you do not exercise, you will gain weight and increase your risk for heart disease as an adult. You can reverse these effects with the simple acts of eating more healthfully and exercising more often. **Health promotion** means taking charge of your health and wellness. You can do this in many ways. The most important of these is to make responsible, well-informed decisions about your health. To do so, you need to take responsibility to learn as much as you can.

health promotion
a process in which you take charge of your own health and wellness by making responsible and well-informed decisions

How to Evaluate Websites

1. *Who is paying for the site and what is their goal in creating the site?*

Website A: The Physicians Academy for Better Health created this site. When you click on "About Us," you find out that it's a group of medical professionals. The address and phone number for the group is provided—a good sign.

Website B: The Institute for a Healthier Heart created this site. You can click on "About this Site" to learn more about them. But the plug for a new drug and the online store should lead you to suspect the site is run by a business. The information may be slanted to persuade you to buy the company's products.

Website A

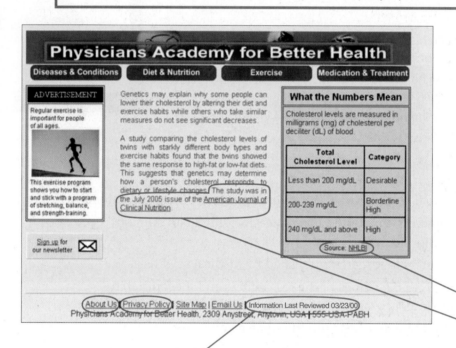

2. *Is the information given up-to-date?*

Website A: This web page lists the date when the information was last reviewed. This allows you to check whether the information is current or out-of-date. You want the most current information you can find.

Website B: Gives no information about the date the information was provided or updated. You should search the site for more clues. If it isn't given, you cannot trust that the information is up-to-date.

Figure 1.7A & B

These fictitious websites are part of a tutorial, "Evaluating Internet Health Information," created by the National Library of Medicine of the National Institutes of Health. You can learn more about evaluating health websites at their website.

3. If there are ads on the website, are they clearly identified as ads?

Website A: The ad for the exercise program is clearly labeled as an advertisement.

Website B: The ad for the new drug is not labeled as an advertisement. If it's hard to distinguish between ads and content, this may be done intentionally to confuse you and to get you to purchase something.

Website B

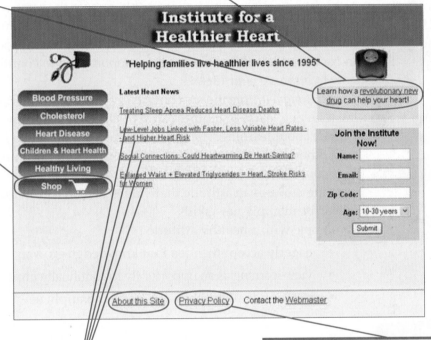

5. Does the site ask you for personal information? If so, why?

Both sites contain a link to a privacy policy which should tell you how the information you type in will be used by the group. You may not want your information sold or used by other advertisers or other parties.

4. Are sources of statistics and information cited?

Website A: On the home page alone, descriptions about studies and statistics are followed by citations for the sources.

Website B: The sources are not given on the home page. This is a bad sign. Without citations you cannot evaluate the credibility of the information.

lifelong learning
a continuing pursuit of learning and studying that carries through your entire life; a key component of your ability to take charge of your own health

Understanding Wellness across the Life Span

As you pass through the stages of life, different wellness issues will become important. Early life events and health habits can set the stage for either a healthful adulthood or for disease. In addition, each stage of life presents its own challenges (Figure 1.8). This textbook, especially Unit VIII, *The Human Life Cycle*, will help you understand many elements of wellness across the life span.

Lifelong Learning

Researchers are constantly uncovering new information about the human body and its health. The core principles regarding physical, mental, and social health will probably remain the same over time, but specific elements are likely to evolve along with our understanding. This should not deter you from keeping up with this fast-growing body of knowledge. In contrast, view this as an ongoing opportunity to continually learn about how to improve your life.

Lifelong learning means continually learning and studying throughout life. Lifelong learning requires an *aptitude* for health knowledge and a good *attitude* about learning. *Aptitude* refers to your ability to learn and increase your knowledge. Your *attitude* refers to a frame of mind when learning new concepts and facts, which is just as important as your ability. Lifelong learning requires an attitude that values personal growth and an eagerness to learn and apply new skills.

People with a healthy attitude

- eagerly accept the idea that knowledge grows;
- view learning as an opportunity to continually improve themselves;
- are confident that they can learn and apply new knowledge.

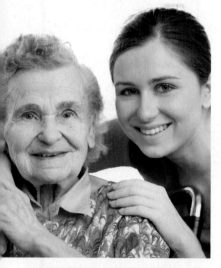

Figure 1.8

Each stage of life presents unique health challenges. *Which health challenges are the older woman and the teenage granddaughter likely to face because of their ages?*

Lesson 1.2 Review

Know and Understand Assess

1. What is a consumer?
2. List the three criteria that information must meet to be considered scientific knowledge.
3. Identify four traits that characterize information as pseudoscience.
4. Describe the term *health promotion*.
5. How do aptitude and attitude relate to lifelong learning?

Analyze and Apply

6. How are knowledge, skills, and resources interrelated and dependent on each other?

7. Why is the ability to determine the credibility of a health-related source of information important?

Real World Health

Using Reliable Websites Compare two websites that feature a health-promotion strategy of your choice. For example, you may want to research dieting, exercise plans, or energy drinks. Compare one website that is supported by a reliable organization—a government, professional, or educational organization—to a website that is sponsored by a for-profit company. How do these websites differ? Which website is more reliable? Do you notice any claims of pseudoscience? When you have researched the two websites thoroughly, write a brief summary analyzing the reliability of each website.

Personal Skills for Health and Wellness

Lesson Objectives

After studying this lesson, you will be able to

- use a decision-making model to make healthy choices;
- develop a plan to achieve long- and short-term goals;
- learn refusal skills to stand up to peer pressure; and
- identify sources of social support pertaining to your well-being.

Key Terms 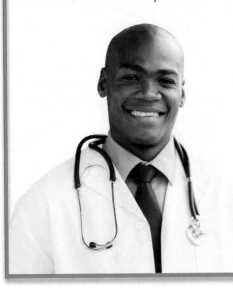 E-Flash Cards

In this lesson, you will learn the meanings of the following key terms.

decision-making skills
goals
interpersonal skills
refusal skills

Warm-Up Activity

Annual Physical Exam
One way to practice prevention and health maintenance is to have an annual physical exam. List some reasons why you should have an annual exam and explain why it would be important to know your family's health history for this type of exam. If you were having an annual exam today, what are three questions related to your present health and well-being that you would want to ask the doctor? List these three questions.

My Reasons

heart trouble in family

I've been overly tired

better to be safe than sorry

My Questions

How often should I have an exam?

How long have you been practicing?

If I have a hidden problem, will you find it?

Before You Read

Chalk Talk

Before you read the lesson, your teacher will have the main lesson headings—Decision-Making and Goal-Setting Skills and Standing Up to Pressure—written around the room. Without talking, move around the room and briefly write what you think you know about each lesson heading under the heading. You may add to other students' ideas by connecting a line from your comment to theirs. After reading the lesson, add new information that you have learned.

I n the previous lesson, you learned that maintaining and promoting your health requires knowledge. But sometimes knowledge alone is not enough—you also need the skills to put that knowledge to work. This section will introduce you to the health and wellness skills you need to achieve and maintain your physical, emotional, and social wellness.

Decision-Making and Goal-Setting Skills

decision-making skills
your ability to make choices about your health and wellness

Decision-making skills are tools you can use to make choices about your health and wellness. Decision-making and goal-setting skills will help you move closer to and maintain optimal health and wellness. These skills will serve you well in all aspects of your life.

Making Good Decisions

You make decisions each day that affect your health and wellness. For instance, should you stay up late playing video games, or should you get a good night's sleep? Should you exercise on a painful knee? Should you eat that second piece of pie? You may need to make decisions about friendships, dating, alcohol and drug use, smoking, and sexual activity.

How you approach making a decision is important. It may be advantageous to seek advice when making some decisions. In some cases, decisions will be collaborative. In other cases, they will need to be made individually by you. Making good decisions involves skill. You can use the following decision-making process as a guide.

Step 1: Define the problem.
Step 2: Explore alternatives.
Step 3: Select the best alternative.
Step 4: Act on your decision.
Step 5: Evaluate your decision.

Setting and Reaching Goals

goals
a short-term or long-term plan of action that will guide you to the state of wellness you hope to reach

Goals are important for many aspects of life, including your health. It's important to set and work toward goals, and the skills to do so can be learned. A *goal* is a specific endpoint that signifies the state of wellness you hope to reach. Do you have goals regarding your physical, mental, or social wellness?

Goals can be short- or long-term. A short-term goal is a goal you want to accomplish in the near future, or within days or weeks. A long-term goal requires more time—months or years—to achieve. Reaching a long-term goal may involve achieving a series of short-term goals.

Effective goals are SMART. This means that they are

- **Specific**—set out exactly what achieving the goal would look like;
- **Measurable**—have results that can be quantified;
- **Action oriented**—describe the action that will be taken;
- **Realistic**—are achievable; and
- **Timely**—are achievable within a reasonable period of time.

Personal Profile

Do Your Skills Need Improvement?

I regularly set goals. **yes no**

I consider the impact of my decisions on others. **yes no**

I set deadlines. **yes no**

I break long-term goals into short-term goals. **yes no**

I do not let others force me to do what I don't want to do. **yes no**

I communicate my feelings honestly to others. **yes no**

I work well with others. **yes no**

I can identify reliable sources of information. **yes no**

I can disagree with someone and remain friends. **yes no**

Add the number of yes answers to assess the skills you need to make healthy choices. The more yes answers, the better your skills.

How to Set a SMART Goal

Step 1. Assess the situation. What is important to you? What needs improvement? Try to think of all the ways in which you could improve.

Step 2. Identify a specific and realistic goal. Write down the specific goal you want to achieve within a few days or weeks. A goal should be measurable so that you know when you have reached it. A goal should also be achievable.

Step 3. Define the steps or actions you must take to achieve your goal. You may need to break big goals into smaller, more achievable steps. These are your short-term goals, which lead to your long-term goals.

Step 4. Set a reasonable timeline. Take out a calendar and pick a realistic date for the completion of your goal. If you have a series of short-term goals, set dates for their completion. Write down the dates on your calendar.

Step 5. Act on your goal. Follow your plan for achieving your goal.

Step 6. Monitor your progress. Keep track of your progress. If you are not making progress in reaching your goal, determine what is getting in your way and what you can do to surmount these roadblocks.

Step 7. Reward yourself. Identify something you want and treat yourself when you reach your goal. Giving yourself a reward when you achieve a goal can keep you motivated.

Remember that not all goals are appropriate for all people. Before you set a goal, it's important to determine your values, or what is important to you, and to assess your current situation.

Mastering goal-setting skills will enable you to continually grow and improve yourself, your health, and your overall well-being.

Standing Up to Pressure

You are in charge of your behaviors, decisions, health, and well-being. Others can, however, exert a powerful influence on your behavior or decisions. In several chapters of this text, you'll learn how people—such as your family and peers—can influence you in both positive and negative ways. You'll also learn how the messages you receive from the media and from society can shape your behavior and choices, and impact your wellness.

Abstinence and Refusal Skills

Refusal skills can help you respond to peer influences and conflicting messages without compromising your own goals, values, and health. These skills will help when you are confronted with offers and pressures to engage in activities that you feel are inappropriate or unhealthy (Figure 1.9). With these skills, you can make independent, informed decisions despite the hindering messages you receive from peers and society.

For example, you might be pressured to use drugs, cigarettes, or alcohol. You could be pressured to engage in sexual activity or an activity that is illegal, inappropriate, or unhealthy. Strong peer pressure can make refusal difficult. This book will help you learn and apply refusal skills to these situations.

Pressure to engage in sexual activity can seem intense, especially if you believe that everyone else is engaging in these activities. But the truth is that many teens are not sexually active. Instead, they have made the decision to abstain from sex. *Abstinence* is the decision not to engage in sexual activity.

refusal skills
your ability to stand up to pressures and influences that hinder your progress toward wellness

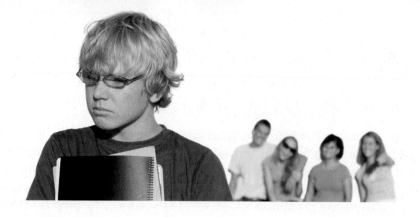

Figure 1.9

Being responsible for your health and wellness requires that you resist pressure from others to do things that can endanger your health. *In what types of situations do teenagers encounter pressure from their peers to do things that may endanger their health?*

Abstinence is the only strategy for preventing pregnancy that is 100% effective. Abstinence is also the only strategy that is 100% effective in preventing infection with sexually transmitted infections, including HIV/AIDS. This book will discuss abstinence and related skills for maintaining abstinence.

Getting Along with Others

interpersonal skills
your ability to interact positively with those around you

Interpersonal skills include the ability to communicate and relate positively and constructively with other people. Healthy relationships are important for health and wellness, especially for social wellness. For example, it is well known that people in unhealthy or abusive relationships experience more physical, mental, and emotional problems than others. The ability to cope with mental and physical illness depends on a person's social support system.

People with serious illnesses depend on others in many ways. For example, people handle depression better and recover faster with support from family and friends. Depressed people need encouragement and help getting to their doctor or therapist for treatment. Without social support, a person's depression may remain untreated and become worse.

People who have strong interpersonal skills can often cultivate and maintain healthy relationships. Good interpersonal skills rely on effective communication, negotiation, collaboration, and the ability to resolve conflicts. Assertiveness, respect, trust, self-esteem, and honesty are also important.

Lesson 1.3 Review

Know and Understand Assess

1. Identify the five steps in the decision-making process.
2. What is a SMART goal?
3. Define *refusal skills*.
4. List four examples of interpersonal skills.

Analyze and Apply

5. Choose one decision you need to make and analyze what barriers might hinder you. What would be the advantage of seeking advice? Should you make the decision collaboratively or individually?

Real World Health

Making Decisions Using Health-Related Skills
Imagine these two scenarios: (1) possibly riding to a football game with a friend who texts and drives, and (2) going to a friend's house for a party after the basketball game and discovering his parents are out of town. You don't want to be involved in either of these situations, but you don't want to upset your friend. What should you do? Write a narrative or draw a comic strip outlining how the conversation with your friend might go, and what you could say or do to exclude yourself from either of these situations.

Our Healthcare System

Lesson Objectives

After studying this lesson, you will be able to

- explain the role of a physician in your health;

- give examples of various medical specialists in the healthcare industry;

- outline differences among available healthcare settings;

- deconstruct how the US healthcare system functions, including services, insurance, and the role of the government; and

- assess the importance of prevention and health maintenance.

Warm-Up Activity

Learning New Terms

Find a current events article relating to healthcare in the United States. As you read the article, highlight any unfamiliar terms and write each term in a chart similar to the one below. While reading this lesson, write a definition next to each term in your chart as you come across the term in the text. You may need to consult a dictionary for terms not mentioned in this lesson. Reread your article with these new terms in mind and summarize your findings to the class.

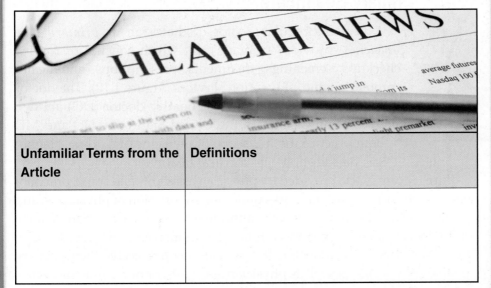

Unfamiliar Terms from the Article	Definitions

Key Terms 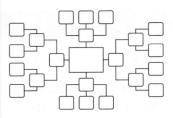 E-Flash Cards

In this lesson, you will learn the meanings of the following key terms.

Affordable Care Act
deductible
generic drug
inpatient facility
outpatient facility
Patient's Bill of Rights
premium
primary care physician
specialist

Before You Read

Healthcare Mindmap

Write the term healthcare *in the middle of the mindmap below. As you read this lesson, fill in topics related to healthcare in each bubble. Continue to identify and explain related topics to complete the map as you read.*

The modern healthcare system can be overwhelming and difficult for consumers to navigate. In the United States, healthcare comes in many forms and is delivered in different settings by many types of professionals.

The healthcare industry has shifted its focus from treatment to prevention, an approach intended to promote a healthier population and less expensive healthcare. This lesson is an introduction to the healthcare system in the United States. You will learn how you, as a healthcare consumer, can use the system to promote your health and wellness.

Healthcare Services

The healthcare field employs more people than any other type of business in the United States. The field is diverse and includes many types of professions and healthcare services. Some professions provide highly specialized services. Following is a list of the types of services the healthcare industry performs:

- diagnosis—the identification of a disease, disorder, or disability
- treatment—the use of medicine, surgery, counseling, or other therapy to deal with a condition
- rehabilitation—the recovery of function following surgery, disease, or injury
- prevention—services for reducing potential causes of diseases, disorders, and injuries
- education—the teaching of self-care, health promotion, first aid, and disease prevention
- research—the scientific study of the causes, treatments, and prevention of diseases and disorders

Primary Healthcare

A person's regular doctor (pediatrician or ***primary care physician***) provides primary care, which consists of routine checkups, screenings, treatments, prescriptions, and health promotion and prevention services (Figure 1.10). The doctor of medicine (MD) and the osteopathic doctor (DO) are two types of physicians. In the United States, the DO and MD both practice the full scope of medicine, including diagnosis, prescription, and medical treatment.

Primary care is also provided by physician assistants and nurse practitioners. The physician assistant works under the supervision of physicians, and usually provides the same types of healthcare services as a physician. A nurse practitioner possesses an advanced nursing education and can provide many of the same services as a doctor. Today many people receive their primary care from physicians, as well as physician assistants, or nurse practitioners.

primary care physician
a regular doctor who provides checkups, screenings, treatments, and prescriptions

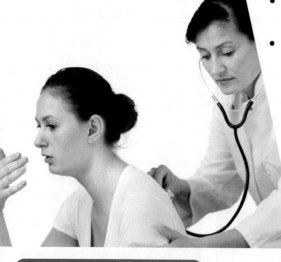

Figure 1.10

A primary care physician is the doctor you will see for most of your healthcare needs. This doctor will refer you to a specialist when necessary.

Medical Specialists

Primary care physicians refer their patients to *specialists*, who possess extra training and experience with certain types of diseases and disorders. The common types of specialists and the care that they provide are listed in Figure 1.11.

Healthcare Settings

Healthcare professionals work in diverse settings. *Inpatient facilities* are hospitals where patients reside while they receive comprehensive diagnosis, treatment, surgery, therapy, and rehabilitation (Figure 1.12). *Outpatient facilities* treat patients who reside in the community and who don't require a hospital. Most healthcare in the United States is delivered in outpatient settings. These settings include

- doctors' offices and private healthcare clinics that provide check-ups, physical therapy, day surgery, counseling, addiction treatment, rehabilitation, eye and dental care;
- hospital emergency rooms;
- urgent care or walk-in clinics;
- health clinics and counseling centers located in high schools and colleges; and
- county public health clinics.

Government's Role

The unit within the United States government responsible for providing leadership, funding, and oversight of the healthcare system is the Public Health Service of the United States Department of Health and Human Services. The United States government itself does not provide healthcare services, with three exceptions: the Veterans Administration provides healthcare for military veterans, the Military Health System provides healthcare for all active and retired military personnel and their families, and the Indian Health Service provides healthcare for Native American Indians.

Health Insurance

How do people pay for healthcare? A three-day hospital stay costs an average of $30,000! It costs about $7,500 to fix a broken leg. One medicine may cost more than $100 each month, and a counselor can cost more than $100 for one hour each week. Healthcare is expensive, and most people cannot afford to pay the full cost of services such as diagnosis, treatment, counseling, or therapy.

Instead, most people buy insurance to help pay for healthcare costs. Most people get this insurance through their employer. Employers offer health insurance to full-time employees as a benefit. Most employers split the cost of an insurance plan with their employees.

specialist
medical providers who are extensively trained in one or two areas of health; a physician may refer you to a specialist to seek specific treatments

inpatient facility
a hospital where patients reside overnight while receiving diagnosis, treatment, surgery, therapy, and rehabilitation

outpatient facility
a healthcare establishment where patients receive diagnosis or treatment, but do not reside overnight

Figure 1.11 Physician Specialists

Cardiologist: heart disease

Gastroenterologist: diseases and disorders of the digestive system

Neurologist: diseases and disorders of the brain, nerves, spinal cord

Oncologist: cancer specialist

Orthopedist: bones, joints, and muscles

Pediatrician: children from infancy through adolescence

Psychiatrist: mental illnesses and disorders

Surgeon: surgical treatment of diseases and disorders

Figure 1.12

Hospitals are a type of inpatient facility where patients receive medical testing and treatment, including surgery. *How is an inpatient facility different from an outpatient facility?*

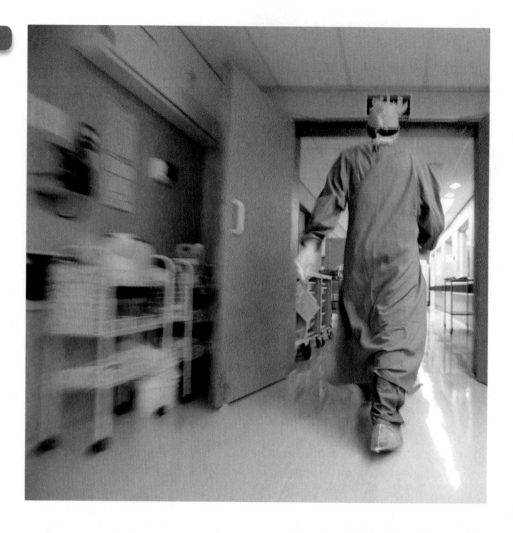

premium
a regular fee paid in exchange for insurance services

deductible
the amount you pay for healthcare services each year before your insurance company begins to take on the cost

Insurance helps people afford medical costs in different ways. People pay their insurance company a regular fee called a ***premium***, usually each month. The company collects premiums from many customers and pools this money to pay for the healthcare costs of its customers. The customers pay the regular monthly premium even if they do not get medical care during that month (Figure 1.13).

Insurance companies usually require customers to pay an amount called a ***deductible***. The deductible is the amount a person pays for healthcare services each year before the insurance company begins to pay for an agreed upon portion of healthcare costs. Many insurance plans also require their customers to make co-payments, a fixed amount for medical services such as a doctor's office visit. For example, you might need to pay $20 for a visit to the doctor when you get an annual checkup.

The two main types of insurance are the health maintenance organization (HMO) and the preferred provider organization (PPO). An HMO pays for costs of the basic healthcare services and many other specialized services. In this plan, a person must use doctors, hospitals, clinics, and services that are members of the HMO network. A PPO pays for costs of healthcare provided by a group of doctors and healthcare providers, or a hospital. The PPO allows people more flexibility in choosing their healthcare providers than an HMO, but the PPO is more expensive.

Medicare and Medicaid

The US government funds some types of health insurance, such as Medicare. Medicare is insurance made available for people 65 years of age and older. During their working years, people pay a tax that is removed from their paychecks. This money is pooled to pay for the healthcare costs of elderly people. Through this system, healthcare insurance is provided for older people who have retired from work and have no other form of health insurance.

Medicare is also available for people younger than 65 who are disabled and unable to work. People who have worked but are no longer able to work due to a disability can receive benefits from the Social Security Administration of the United States.

Medicaid is a form of health insurance funded by the individual states and the US government. Medicaid pays for healthcare costs of people living in poverty, who have no way to pay for insurance or medical expenses.

Affordable Care Act

The Patient Protection and Affordable Care Act, also called the *Affordable Care Act*, was signed into law on March 23, 2010 to address rising insurance costs and barriers to obtaining health insurance. The Affordable Care Act makes insurance available to all eligible Americans and eliminates some of the problems that made affordable health insurance so difficult to obtain. Four key elements of the Affordable Care Act are expanded access to insurance, cost reduction and affordability, improved healthcare, and the Patient's Bill of Rights.

Expanded Access to Insurance. The Affordable Care Act expands access to health insurance in the following ways:

- Insurance companies must provide insurance even if you have a serious disease at the time you want to purchase their insurance. These diseases are called "pre-existing conditions." In the past, an insurance company could refuse to sell you insurance if you had a serious disease such as cancer or diabetes.

- Young adults can be covered through age 26 by their parent's health insurance.

- Insurance companies cannot stop insuring customers for no apparent reason. This is important because, in the past, insurance companies could decide to stop providing insurance for minor reasons or no reason at all.

- Many businesses are now required to provide health insurance for their employees.

Cost Reduction and Affordability. Some aspects of the Affordable Care Act attempt to reduce costs:

- Insurance companies cannot suddenly increase the costs of premiums without publicly explaining their decision.

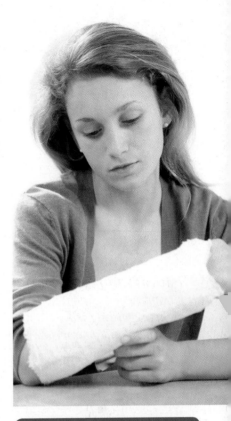

Figure 1.13

Medical care, including treatment for a broken arm, is often very costly.

Affordable Care Act
law passed in 2010 to expand access to insurance, address cost reduction and affordability, improve the quality of healthcare, and introduce the Patient's Bill of Rights

- People and businesses can shop for the best insurance plans for their needs in a system called an "Open Marketplace." This system publishes products and costs from all insurance companies, hopefully helping to drive down costs.
- Insurance companies cannot stop providing insurance to an individual after he or she reaches the "lifetime limit."

Improved Healthcare. The Affordable Care Act also attempts to improve the quality of healthcare:

- Preventive healthcare is covered at no cost to the patients.
- You can get emergency healthcare anywhere, no matter what kind of health insurance you have.

The Patient's Bill of Rights. The Affordable Care Act also introduced the *Patient's Bill of Rights* (Figure 1.14). It is anticipated that changes will be made to the Affordable Care Act after the 2016 federal and local elections.

Controlling Your Healthcare Costs

You can take control of your healthcare costs. Prevention is the single most important action you can take to reduce your healthcare costs. Additionally, many, but not all, medicines are available as brand-name or generic medicines. *Brand-name medicines* are protected by a patent, which guarantees the manufacturer the sole legal right to make and sell the drug. A patent lasts many years and rewards a business for its ingenuity and the investments it made to produce the drug. Since no one else can make or sell a patented brand-name drug, the company can charge more for it. For that reason, brand-name drugs cost more than generic drugs.

A *generic drug* contains exactly the same active ingredient found in the corresponding brand-name drug. Generic drugs are made by several companies after a patent expires. For that reason, generic drugs cost much less

Patient's Bill of Rights
summary of a patient's rights regarding fair treatment and appropriate information

generic drug
a medication that can be made by many different companies; costs less than brand-name medicines but may be just as effective

Figure 1.14 Patient's Bill of Rights
• Right to informed consent. The healthcare provider must obtain permission from a patient before performing medical procedures. The patient must be informed of the purpose and risks involved with these procedures.
• Right to receive information about their diagnosis and treatment.
• Right to receive all information about the fees for their healthcare.
• Right to receive continuity of care. If a doctor is absent or leaves, the doctor or institution must ensure that another doctor will be available to continue appropriate healthcare.
• Right to refuse treatment or other procedures.
• Right to privacy of their medical information.
• Right to seek a second opinion about medical conditions and treatments.
• Right to change doctors if not satisfied with the healthcare.

than brand-name drugs. You can save money by requesting and purchasing the generic version of your medications, if there is one.

Once you enter the working world, you'll have other options to save money. For example, you can compare premium and deductible costs of various insurance programs, and choose the most beneficial for you. You can also choose to have some of your paycheck deducted and saved in a health savings account or flexible spending account. When you buy certain healthcare products or services, you can get paid for your costs from this account.

Regular Checkups and Screening

You should have an annual physical exam. Tell your doctor about any problems or questions you may have. Together you might be able to spot a problem and prevent it from becoming worse (Figure 1.15).

If a certain disease is common among family members, you and your doctor can discuss lifestyle changes and behaviors that will reduce your risk for developing that disease or disorder. During a regular physical exam, your doctor will record basic health information such as height, weight, heart rate, and blood pressure. Your doctor will also examine your body physically to detect signs of any abnormalities. All of this health information can be tracked over time, allowing you and your doctor to note any changes.

Be prepared to make the most of your doctor visit. Write a list of questions in case you get nervous or forgetful. Begin by telling your doctor what has been bothering you and how long it has been an issue. Ask questions about any medicines prescribed, when you can expect to feel better, and how you can prevent this problem in the future.

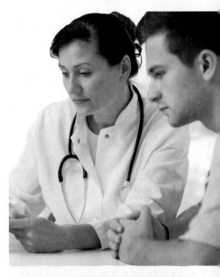

Figure 1.15

During an annual physical exam, your doctor should give you an opportunity to voice questions and concerns you have about your health and development.

Lesson 1.4 Review

Know and Understand
Assess

1. What role does a physician play in your health?
2. List four physician specialists and briefly describe the specialties of each.
3. Name three types of outpatient facilities.
4. Summarize the Affordable Care Act and the four key elements of the Act.
5. What basic health information will your doctor record during a regular physical exam?

Analyze and Apply

6. What is the difference between a physician and a medical specialist?

7. Compare the terms *premium*, *deductible*, and *co-payment*.

Real World Health

Healthcare Accessibility Health-related policies developed by the government seek to make healthcare accessible to all. In small groups, research how health-related policies are developed in the United States. How do culture and the availability and cost of healthcare affect people's health? What barriers do people face in accessing healthcare, and how can they overcome these barriers? How have advances in health information management affected healthcare accessibility? Share your thoughts in a class discussion.

Chapter 1 — Review and Assessment

Lesson 1.1 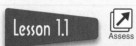 Assess

Defining Health and Wellness

Key Terms

acute diseases
chronic diseases
disease
disorder
emotional health
intellectual health

optimal health
physical health
social health
well-being
wellness

Key Points

- Wellness is a balance of physical, emotional, intellectual, and social health. Each aspect of health impacts the total wellness of an individual.
- The physical, emotional, intellectual, and social dimensions of health interact with and affect each other.
- Health can be described as a continuum that ranges from optimal health to disease. Most people's health status lie somewhere in the middle.
- A disease can be recognized by a specific set of signs and symptoms. A disorder is the term used when no single cause can be identified.

Check Your Understanding

1. The condition of the body, which includes the body's functions and abilities, is called _____ health.
   A. physical
   B. intellectual
   C. emotional
   D. social
2. _____ health is characterized by meaningful, fulfilling, and honest relationships.
   A. Physical
   B. Intellectual
   C. Emotional
   D. Social
3. A person with positive _____ health has a positive attitude toward learning new things.
4. What factors characterize a healthy relationship that contributes to positive social well-being?
5. What is the difference between disease and disorder?
6. What is the difference between signs and symptoms of a disease?
7. **Critical Thinking.** Explain how one dimension of health can affect another.

Lesson 1.2 Assess

Health and Wellness Knowledge

Key Terms

health literacy
health promotion
lifelong learning

pseudoscience
science
scientific knowledge

Key Points

- Health literacy skills include the ability to locate, evaluate, understand, and communicate health-related information.
- To qualify as scientific knowledge, information must be based on experimentation and observation, peer-reviewed, and repeatable.
- Pseudoscience is information presented as science, but cannot be proven as true.
- Reliable sources of online information include URL stems ending in .gov, .edu, and .org.
- Health promotion includes engaging in positive, beneficial activities to improve or maintain your health.

Check Your Understanding

8. Define *health literacy*.
9. Which four skills are needed for health literacy?
10. When information is *not* based on repeated experimentation, verified by other scientists, or peer reviewed, it is considered _____.
    A. science
    B. scientific knowledge
    C. pseudoscience
    D. scientific truth
11. List four signs that indicate information found in print media is reliable.
12. *True or false?* Health-related information is often trustworthy when found on websites of businesses that earn profits from the healthcare industry.
13. *True or false?* Health promotion means taking charge of your health and wellness.
14. Define the term *lifelong learning*.
15. **Critical Thinking.** To be considered scientific knowledge, material must be based on experimentation and observation, peer reviewed, and repeatable. Explain why a new concept must meet all three of these factors to be accepted.

Lesson 1.3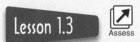

Personal Skills for Health and Wellness

Key Terms

decision-making skills   interpersonal skills
goals   refusal skills

Key Points

- The five steps for decision-making include defining the problem, exploring alternatives, selecting the best alternative, acting on your decision, and evaluating your decision.
- Mastering goal-setting skills enables you to continually grow and improve yourself, your health, and your overall well-being.
- Refusal skills can help you avoid situations in which you feel uncomfortable or unsafe.
- Interpersonal skills can help you effectively communicate your values, preferences, and ideas to others.

Check Your Understanding

16. *True or false?* The final step of the decision-making process is to act on your decisions.

17. A _____ is a specific endpoint that signifies the state of wellness you hope to achieve.

18. Which of the following is the first step in the goal-setting process?
    A. Identify a specific and realistic goal.
    B. Assess the situation.
    C. Reward yourself.
    D. Set a reasonable timeline.

19. Skills that enable you to stand up to pressures and influences that hinder your progress toward wellness are called _____ skills.
    A. refusal
    B. intrapersonal
    C. decision-making
    D. goal-setting

20. The ability to communicate and relate positively and constructively with other people is called _____ skills.

21. **Critical Thinking.** How do your values impact your goals and decisions?

Lesson 1.4

Our Healthcare System

Key Terms

Affordable Care Act   Patient's Bill of Rights
deductible   premium
generic drug   primary care physician
inpatient facility   specialist
outpatient facility

Key Points

- Primary care physicians provide regular, general care for patients. Medical specialists possess extra training and experience with certain types of diseases and disorders.
- US citizens have three main options for obtaining health insurance: purchasing insurance through their employer, qualifying for Medicare or Medicaid, or applying for health insurance under the Affordable Care Act.
- Methods of controlling healthcare costs include promoting your health and wellness through prevention, using generic drugs instead of brand-name drugs, and comparison shopping.
- Attending regular health checkups and screenings and being an informed consumer of health services can help you maintain and promote your health.

Check Your Understanding

22. Your regular doctor is called a primary care _____.
    A. psychiatrist   C. physician
    B. medical specialist   D. psychologist

23. What is the difference between an inpatient facility and an outpatient facility?

24. What are the two main types of insurance offered in the United States.

25. *True or false?* According to the Patient's Bill of Rights, patients have legal rights when receiving healthcare.

26. Why do physicians recommend an annual visit to the doctor's office?

27. **Critical Thinking.** What role does the United States government play in the healthcare industry?

Health and Wellness Skills

28. **Communicate with Others** Imagine that you have a health issue that you need help with. Who would you go to for help? Write a story about why and how you would go to this person for help.

29. **Set Goals** Create a chart for setting goals. Within your chart, include the six goal-setting steps that were outlined in Lesson 2. Decide what health-related goals you want to achieve and fill in your chart accordingly.

30. **Analyze Influences** Think about your day-to-day surroundings and the situations that have either a positive or a negative influence on you. Create a poster that reflects these situations. You may draw your poster by hand or use pictures that you have cut from magazines.

31. **Access Information** Research the leading causes of death among teenagers (ages 15-24) and adults (ages 45-54). The Centers for Disease Control and Prevention (CDC) is a credible source to consult. Compare and contrast your findings, focusing on the top three causes of death in each age group. What information does your research show that would explain the different causes of death in each age group?

Hands-On Activity: Family Health History

This activity will allow you to trace your family health history and become familiar with diseases or disorders that might be prevalent in your family.

Steps for this Activity

1. Open a discussion about this assignment with your parents or guardians, and decide, as a family, if you will complete this assignment on paper or on a website. The United States Surgeon General and the CDC offer a web-based tool called "My Family Health Portrait." This can be used to collect and organize family information, which can be printed out upon completion.

2. You will be trying to gather as much health information as possible from your relatives including parents, siblings, grandparents, uncles and aunts, nieces and nephews, half-brothers and half-sisters, great uncles and great aunts, and cousins. Be sure to gather information on chronic illnesses, pregnancy complications, developmental disabilities, and other genetic disorders. Examples might include, but are not limited to, cancer, diabetes, heart disease, high blood pressure, stroke, vision problems, depression, Alzheimer's disease, and alcoholism.

3. An individual's health information is personal and private. You may have family members who do not want to discuss this topic or share information, and this should be respected.

4. Once you have gathered as much family health information as possible, complete "My Family Health Portrait."

5. After you have completed your family health portrait, write a letter to a family member. In your letter, share health information that you have become more aware of, habits that you will change in your life based on your findings, and how this knowledge has helped you make better decisions for your future.

6. If you were adopted, ask your adoptive parents if they were given medical information about your biological parents. If you are unable to gather any family health history for any reason, consult with your family physician and do the best that you can to complete the assignment.

7. If you and your family make the decision not to complete a family health portrait, substitute a discussion with your family, or with one family member, about your health history. Then complete the letter to a family member, as outlined in Step 5.

Core Skills

Math Practice

The healthcare industry employs millions of people in the United States. The healthcare industry can be broken down into several different categories of occupations. Review the table below, which shows five occupational categories of the healthcare industry and the number of people employed in each category. Then answer the questions that follow. Round your answers to the nearest whole number.

Healthcare Practitioners and Technical Occupations	
Category	Number of Job Holders in Industry
General Medical and Surgical Hospitals	2,863,320
Offices of Physicians	994,810
Nursing Care Facilities	418,310
Health and Personal Care Stores	348,470
Home Healthcare Services	297,820
Total	4,922,730

32. Of the occupations shown, what percentage of people is employed in general medical and surgical hospitals?
    A. 12 percent
    B. 35 percent
    C. 58 percent
    D. 65 percent

33. What percentage of people is employed in home healthcare services?
    A. 2 percent
    B. 4 percent
    C. 6 percent
    D. 18 percent

34. What percentage of people is employed in nursing care facilities and offices of physicians?
    A. 48 percent
    B. 38 percent
    C. 28 percent
    D. 29 percent

Reading and Writing Practice

Read the passage below and then answer the following questions.

A person's regular doctor (pediatrician *or* primary care physician) *provides primary care, which consists of routine checkups, screenings, treatments, prescriptions, and health promotion and prevention services. The doctor of medicine (MD) and the osteopathic doctor (DO) are two types of physicians. In the United States, the DO and MD both practice the full scope of medicine, including diagnosis, prescription, and medical treatment.*

35. What is the main topic the author is describing in this paragraph?
    A. healthcare services
    B. physicians
    C. doctors of medicine
    D. osteopathic doctors

36. What is another term for *regular doctor*?
    A. doctor of medicine
    B. osteopathic doctor
    C. psychologist
    D. primary care physician

37. Based on the context, what is the meaning of the word *scope*?
    A. range
    B. scoop
    C. healthcare services
    D. limit

38. Which of the following services does a primary care physician offer?
    A. routine checkups, screenings, treatments, and prescriptions
    B. health promotion and prevention services
    C. Both A and B.
    D. The text does not say.

39. According to the text, what do an MD and DO have in common?
    A. They are both types of physicians.
    B. They are both types of psychologists.
    C. Neither an MD nor a DO provides medical treatment.
    D. The text does not say.

40. Based on the information provided, write two or three sentences that describe situations in which you would need to visit your primary care physician.

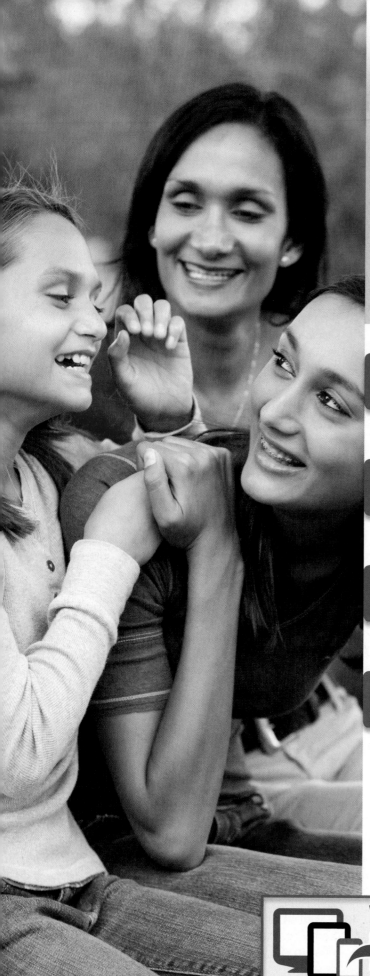

Chapter 2

Risk Factors: Behavior, Genes, Environment

While studying this chapter, look for the activity icon to:
- **review** vocabulary with e-flash cards and games;
- **assess** learning with quizzes and online exercises;
- **expand** knowledge with animations and activities; and
- **listen** to pronunciation of key terms in the audio glossary.

G-WLEARNING.com

www.g-wlearning.com/health/

Take this quiz to see what you do *and* do not *know about how behavior, genes, and the environment affect health and wellness. If you cannot answer a question, pay extra attention to that topic as you study this chapter.*

1. *Identify each statement as* True, False, *or* It Depends. *Choose* It Depends *if a statement is true in some cases, but false in others.*
2. *Revise each* False *statement to make it true.*
3. *Explain the circumstances in which each* It Depends *statement is true and when it is false.*

Health and Wellness IQ 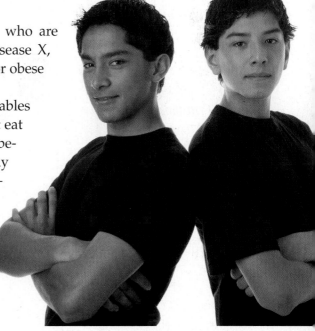 Assess

1. All diseases have one cause.	True	False	It Depends
2. If you inherit a gene for a health problem, you will get that health problem.	True	False	It Depends
3. Car crashes kill thousands of teenagers each year.	True	False	It Depends
4. Smoking does not cause any health problems.	True	False	It Depends
5. Obesity is inherited.	True	False	It Depends
6. A nutritious diet protects a person from many types of diseases.	True	False	It Depends
7. The leading cause of death in the United States is heart disease.	True	False	It Depends
8. A person's workplace and type of work affects their health and wellness.	True	False	It Depends
9. A person's level of education has no effect on their health and wellness.	True	False	It Depends
10. Many health problems can be prevented by changing behavior.	True	False	It Depends

Setting the Scene

Suppose there are two young men, Todd and Randy, who are brothers. Their parents and several grandparents have Disease X, which tends to run in families. People who are overweight or obese also have a greater risk of developing Disease X.

Todd eats a healthful diet—plenty of fruits and vegetables and lean meats—and he exercises regularly. Randy does not eat healthfully or exercise regularly. Not surprisingly, Randy becomes overweight, while Todd's weight remains in a healthy range. Who has a greater chance of developing Disease X—Randy or Todd?

This example illustrates how health and wellness result from the interplay of many factors. These factors include the genes you inherited from your parents and your lifestyle choices. Your living and working environments, your education, and other social influences contribute as well. In this chapter you will learn how all of these factors, individually and in combination with each other, can affect your health and wellness.

Factors Affecting Health and Wellness

Key Terms E-Flash Cards

In this lesson, you will learn the meanings of the following key terms.

life expectancy

life span

morbidity

mortality

quality of life

risk factors

Before You Read

Health and Wellness Factors

In a mindmap like the one shown below, identify the different factors that affect the health and wellness of an individual. Write, "factors that affect health & wellness" in the middle oval. In the surrounding circles, write the different factors that affect people's health and wellness.

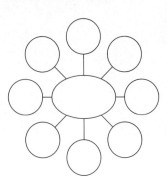

Lesson Objectives

After studying this lesson, you will be able to

- explain the relationship between health and life expectancy;
- relate the morbidity of a disease to its effect on a population;
- summarize how scientists monitor mortality to determine the severity of a condition;
- determine how health and wellness relate to quality of life; and
- describe three categories of risk factors.

Warm-Up Activity

Family Life Spans

Create timelines, like the ones shown, below that illustrate the life spans of all the people in your family. Your timelines should include as many generations as possible.

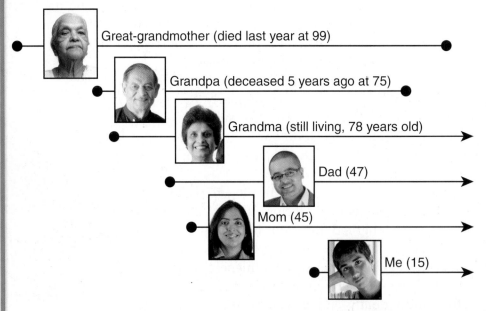

Great-grandmother (died last year at 99)

Grandpa (deceased 5 years ago at 75)

Grandma (still living, 78 years old)

Dad (47)

Mom (45)

Me (15)

I n Japan, women born today are expected to live to 86 years of age. In Kenya, women are expected to live to 61 years of age. Are Japanese women healthier than Kenyan women?

In the United States, children die before five years of age at twice the rate of children in Germany. Are German children healthier than American children?

How long people are expected to live is just one of many ways to describe health.

How Scientists Describe Health

Before we look at the factors affecting health, let's look at how scientists describe human health. Medical scientists monitor a few key characteristics of people and populations that reveal information about the health of those people and populations. These key characteristics include life expectancy, life span, morbidity, mortality, and quality of life.

Life Expectancy

Life expectancy is an estimate of how long a person is likely to live. Each year, life expectancy is typically reported for the average person born in that year. Life expectancy can, however, be calculated for any group of people at any age.

For example, the life expectancy for all Americans born in 2014 is 78.8 years. The females in this group have a longer life expectancy—81.2 years, compared with 76.4 years for males. The average life expectancy has increased significantly, as shown in Figure 2.1.

As the health of a population improves, so will its life expectancy. What factors do you think might be responsible for the increased life expectancy of Americans?

life expectancy
an average estimate of how long a person will live

Figure 2.1
Life Expectancy

	1960	2014
All (male and female)	69.77	78.8
Female	73.1	81.2
Male	66.66	76.4

Life Span

Life span is the actual number of years a person lives. A person's life span may be greater or less than the life expectancy for all people born in the same year. A person's life span is affected by his or her health, which in turn is influenced by several factors to be discussed in this chapter. Obviously, a person's life span is affected most by the presence of diseases and disorders.

life span
the average length of a person's life measured in years

Morbidity

The term *morbidity* describes the presence of a disease, disorder, injury, or other condition that affects the health of a population. A disease with high morbidity means that many people have the condition. The presence of just a few cases indicates low morbidity in the population.

morbidity
the prevalence of a disease, disorder, condition, or injury in a population

Medical scientists are interested in the morbidity associated with a certain condition because it tells them how big an impact that condition has on a population. For example, scientists studied the morbidity of acquired immune deficiency syndrome (AIDS) in different age groups. They learned that most new cases of AIDS occur in adolescents and young adults 15 to 24 years of age. This knowledge can impact what kinds of programs are created to combat the spread of AIDS.

The morbidity of a disease can decrease or increase over time. For example, most cases of influenza (the flu) occur from November to March each year in the United States. Doctors use this information to prevent influenza by giving vaccinations (the flu shot) before the "flu season" begins (Figure 2.2).

Mortality

Mortality describes the number of deaths caused by a disease, disorder, injury, or other condition in a population. By comparing the mortality of different conditions, scientists can determine how serious a particular condition is for a population, as compared to other conditions. For example, studies of mortality show that heart disease and cancer combined cause nearly half of all deaths in the United States.

The study of mortality in different age groups reveals which conditions are the biggest problems for each group. For example, a review of mortality among children and adolescents reveals that car crashes and unintentional injuries are the leading causes of death for those age groups.

Monitoring mortality in a population over time can reveal useful information. For example, during the years between 2000 and 2009, the number of people in the United States who died from heart disease decreased by 28%. At the same time, cancer deaths decreased by 12%. This suggests that progress was made in the prevention, diagnosis, and treatment of heart disease and cancer.

During the same years, though, deaths from drug poisoning nearly doubled. As a result, doctors, teachers, medical scientists, and government officials are trying to learn why more people are dying in this way. Educational and prevention programs are being developed to reduce the number of accidental poisonings.

Quality of Life

Another way to assess a person's health and wellness is to look at his or her *quality of life*. This is a person's level of satisfaction with various aspects of his or her life. Remember that health and wellness is not just the absence of disease and death. Thus, a person who seems physically well can have a poor quality of life. For example, a physically fit person with no outer signs of disease may be exhausted, sleepless, and depressed from the stress of holding down three jobs.

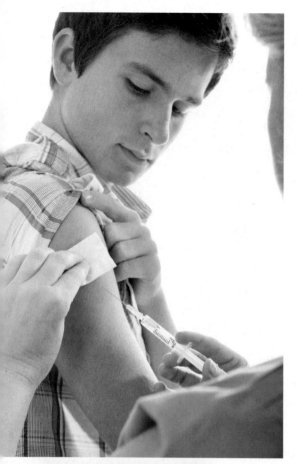

Figure 2.2

The best way to protect yourself against the flu is to be vaccinated each year prior to flu season. *Do you get your flu shot every year? If not, why not?*

mortality
the number of deaths caused by a disease, disorder, condition, or injury in a population

quality of life
a person's level of satisfaction with his or her life

Local and Global Health
Infant and Maternal Mortality

You may already know that people have different health outcomes depending on where they live in the world. However, you may not be aware of how vast these differences can be. Following are some comparisons of mortality statistics for infants and mothers in different countries.

Infant mortality describes the number of infants who die among all live births. How many babies die per 1,000 births in different areas of the world?

- Iceland: 2 infants
- Mozambique: 67 infants

Maternal mortality describes the number of mothers who die shortly after giving birth. How many mothers die shortly after giving birth in different areas of the world?

- Sweden: 4 mothers per 100,000 births
- Afghanistan: 396 mothers per 100,000 births

In addition, health inequalities occur among people within the same country. For example, infant mortality in Bolivia is related to the mother's level of education: How many infants die after being born to educated women versus uneducated women?

- No education: 100 infants die per 1000 births
- At least a high school education: 40 infants die per 1000 births

Household income is also associated with mortality of children under 5 years of age in all countries. Mortality among children under 5 years of age is highest among households with the lowest income. Mortality is lowest among households with the highest income in nearly every country.

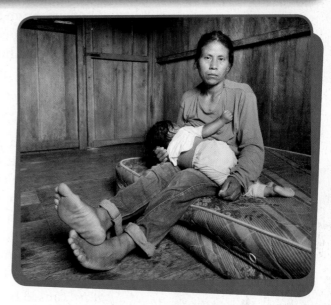

Thinking Critically

1. Why does a mother's level of education affect her infant's chance of survival?

2. Why does the amount of money a person makes affect his or her chance of living a long, healthy life?

3. Health inequalities occur in the United States, too. Research these inequalities and answer the following questions. How are income and poverty related to health in the United States? How is educational level related to health in the United States? How can these health inequalities be corrected?

Consider two people with the same disease, such as arthritis. One person has access to good healthcare, medicine, and physical therapy. This person remains independent, is relatively free from pain, is employed, and enjoys hobbies. In contrast, the other person does not get medical care for her arthritis and, as a result, the arthritis gets worse. This person cannot move around independently; suffers from joint pain; and cannot drive, work, or enjoy recreational activities. These two individuals have the same disease but experience a very different quality of life.

There are several methods for measuring a person's quality of life. For example, the *Ferrans and Powers Quality of Life Index (QLI)* was developed by researchers Carol Estwing Ferrans and Marjorie Powers. The QLI measures people's quality of life in four areas: health and functioning, psychological and spiritual, social and economic, and family. Most methods assess the same four areas of health and wellness. To begin, people fill out the QLI questionnaire. From the answers provided, researchers can assess each person's ability to fully engage in activities of daily living and the level of satisfaction with his or her personal and social life.

What Causes Disease?

If you had a health problem, and you knew the specific cause, you could address the cause and fix the problem. Better still, you could avoid the cause and avoid the disease altogether.

Unfortunately, the connection between any single cause of disease and the disease itself is neither clear nor simple. Determining the cause of a disease is a complicated and difficult process (Figure 2.4). A disease, disorder, injury, or other condition usually results from several causes, or an interaction among causes. These causes fall into the following categories:

- *genetic*: caused by faulty genes
- *nutritional*: caused by lack of a key nutrient or dietary excess
- *infectious*: caused by microscopic living things such as bacteria and viruses
- *traumatic*: caused by physical damage to the body
- *environmental*: caused by exposure to harmful aspects of the environment
- *behavioral*: caused by behaviors or choices a person makes

Multiple causes are related to many diseases. For example, people who suffer from depression often have a relative with the condition, giving the disorder a genetic cause. Researchers have also identified environmental factors that people with depression tend to share. Type 2 diabetes has its roots in genetic, behavioral, nutritional, and environmental factors. You will learn that in many cases a single cause is not responsible for health and wellness problems.

Risk Factors

Risk factors are aspects of people's lives that increase the chances they will develop a disease or disorder, or experience an injury. For example, consider the risk factors for heart disease. They include having family members with heart disease, especially parents, brothers, and sisters. This is known as a *family history* of heart disease.

Additional heart disease risk factors arise from behavior or other diseases. For example, smoking and an inactive lifestyle both increase a person's chances of developing heart disease. Diseases such as diabetes and high blood pressure also greatly increase that risk.

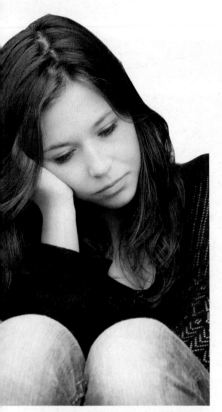

Figure 2.3

Quality of life is a key factor in determining health and wellness. *Why might this girl's quality of life be low even if she is physically fit and free of disease?*

risk factors
aspects of a person's life that increase the likelihood he or she will develop a disease or infection, or experience an injury

Having a risk factor for a disease, disorder, or an injury does not mean that a person is guaranteed to develop that health problem. Compared with someone who does not have the risk factor, however, the person with a risk factor has a greater chance of developing the disease, disorder, or injury.

For example, having a close relative who has high blood pressure does not mean you are destined to develop this condition. Taking steps to improve your health and wellness, such as eating healthy food and exercising regularly can decrease your chances of developing high blood pressure. This genetic risk factor does, however, increase the likelihood that you will develop the condition if you are not careful.

The more risk factors for a particular disease or disorder that a person has, the greater the chance that he or she will develop the disease or disorder. Therefore, it makes sense to remove as many risk factors as possible. In the case of heart disease, some risk factors are controllable. For example, you can avoid smoking, exercise regularly, and lower your blood pressure with diet and exercise.

As shown in Figure 2.5 on the next page, risk factors fall into three basic categories—behavioral, environmental, and genetic.

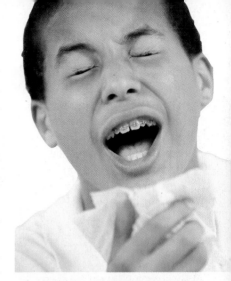

Figure 2.4

What do you think might be the cause, or causes, of this boy's coughing and sneezing?

Research in Action

The Human Genome Project and Human Disease

The human genome consists of all the genes in the human body. The goal of the Human Genome Project was to read the complete sequence of the building blocks comprising human DNA. In April 2003 the work was complete and, for the first time, the human genome could be read.

This project has yielded information about 1,800 disease genes. The information is being used by researchers to create tests that permit doctors to screen people for genetic diseases and risk factors for disease.

Many exciting projects have come from this research. One area of study concerns medicines. Having information about people's genes may help doctors fine-tune the medicines they prescribe for their patients. By analyzing the genes in a cancer cell, doctors can select the medicine that works best against that cancer.

By the time you are an adult, chances are that this research will have helped create additional treatments that may prevent genetic diseases and cancer.

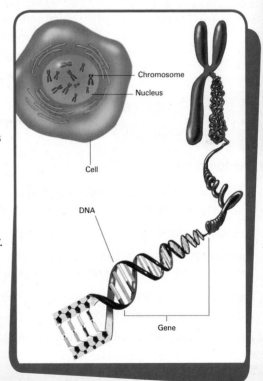

The long, stringy DNA that makes up genes is spooled within chromosomes inside the nucleus of a cell.

Thinking Critically

1. What are some advantages of being able to screen people genetically for disease risk factors? Are there disadvantages to this ability?

2. What one disease would you most like to see eliminated through this research? Why?

Figure 2.5

Many health and wellness experts divide risk factors into three basic categories: behavioral, environmental, and genetic. *Which type of risk factor is represented by each of these photos?*

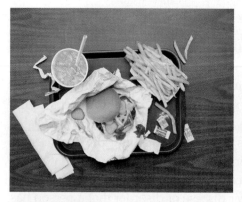
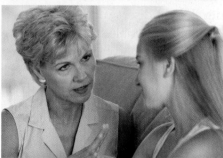
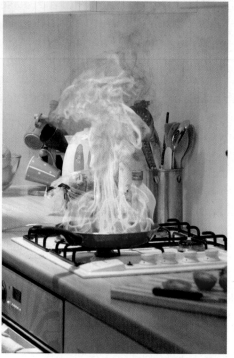

Additionally, risk factors can be categorized as modifiable or non-modifiable. *Modifiable risk factors* can be controlled, reduced, or eliminated. Many behavioral and lifestyle risk factors are modifiable. As mentioned earlier, a person can quit smoking and remove that risk factor for heart disease.

Non-modifiable risk factors cannot be changed or eliminated. Age, gender, and genetic risk factors are typically non-modifiable. The remainder of this chapter will explore many types of behavioral, genetic, and environmental risk factors.

Lesson 2.1 Review

Know and Understand

1. List three characteristics of a population that scientists monitor for information about health.
2. Explain how life expectancy differs from life span.
3. Explain what scientists can determine by comparing the mortality of different conditions.
4. Describe how a person who seems physically well can have a poor quality of life.
5. List the three basic categories of risk factors.

Analyze and Apply

6. What factors might be responsible for the increase in life expectancy over time?

7. How can two people with the same disease have different qualities of life?

Real World Health

Interview individuals from each side of your family to gather information about your ancestors. After you have learned as much as possible, write the names of your ancestors and what caused their deaths. Some of your family members may have died from disease, while others may have died because of an accident. Find out the age of death, cause of death, and risk factors present in that person's life for each individual.

Behavioral Risk Factors

Lesson Objectives

After studying this lesson, you will be able to

- explain the effect of behaviors on health;
- relate risky behaviors to accidents; and
- describe behaviors that can affect health.

Warm-Up Activity

Assessing Your Health

Consider and write your answer to the following question: What behaviors and activities do you engage in that might jeopardize your health or your life? In a table like the one shown below, list your answers:

Behavior or Activity	How might this jeopardize my health?

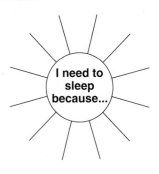

Key Terms ▱ E-Flash Cards

In this lesson, you will learn the meanings of the following key terms.

behavioral risk factors
distracted driving behaviors
physical fitness
sexual activity

Before You Read

The Importance of Sleep

In a mindmap like the one shown below, write five to six statements about the importance of sleep to your health.

I need to sleep because...

D riving a car under normal conditions can be risky. Would you do something that makes driving even more hazardous? You may not personally endanger yourself, but research shows that one in four teenagers has ridden in a car when the driver had been drinking alcohol. The decision to get into a car with someone drunk at the wheel puts you at risk for injury. You may even be in this situation without knowing your friend has been drinking.

Behavioral (lifestyle) risk factors are choices and behaviors that increase a person's chance of developing a disease, unhealthy condition, or injury. Many of these behaviors begin during childhood and adolescence, continue into adulthood, and can affect a person's health for years to come. For example, children with an inactive lifestyle are more likely to become physically inactive adults. Inactive adults have a higher risk for developing obesity, hypertension, and heart disease.

Some behaviors have an immediate impact on health. Other behaviors have both short-term and long-term effects (Figure 2.6).

behavioral risk factors
choices a person makes that increase his or her chances of developing diseases, disorders, or injuries

Figure 2.6

This girl's decision to order a soft drink may seem like a minor decision, but it will impact her health and wellness. *What will the short-term effects be? the long-term effects?*

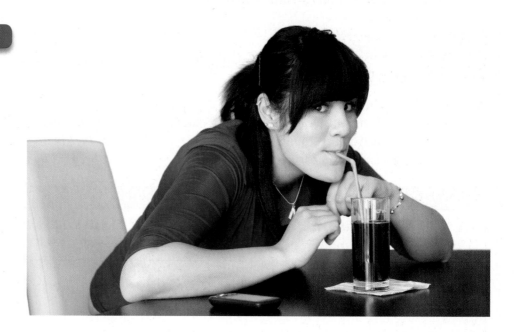

Unintended Injuries

Accidents are the leading cause of death among children and adolescents in the United States and worldwide. Public health officials and doctors refer to "accidental" deaths and injuries as *unintended injuries*. The word *accident* suggests that these injuries are not controllable, that they "just happen" to people, and therefore cannot be prevented. However, you can prevent injuries by reducing the risk factors that lead to injuries.

Car Crashes

Car crashes cause most of the injury-related deaths on record. Thousands of teenagers are killed in car crashes each year; hundreds of thousands are injured. Per mile driven, drivers 16 to 19 years of age are three times more likely to be in fatal car accidents than older drivers.

Extensive research has been done to find out why teenagers are more prone to car crashes than other age demographics. Researchers found that teenagers engage in several types of behavior that increase their risk of having accidents. For example, when teenage drivers were surveyed, about one in three said they had texted or e-mailed while driving. Texting significantly increases the risk for a car crash, as do other **distracted driving behaviors** such as driving with more than one passenger under 18 years of age. Research also shows that more than half of drivers who are 16-24 years of age do not use seat belts.

Other Injuries

Injuries can also arise from risky behaviors other than driving. For example, head injuries occur more frequently when people do not wear a helmet while bicycling, skateboarding, or snowboarding. Despite this evidence, many teens still make the choice not to wear helmets when engaging in these activities (Figure 2.7).

Other outdoor activities, such as canoeing, can be risky if proper safety measures are not taken. You can prevent accidental drowning by wearing a personal flotation device while canoeing. If you are caught outdoors during a thunderstorm or other severe weather situation, you can avoid serious injury by simply going indoors and taking precautions.

Tobacco, Alcohol, and Drug Use

One behavior can raise your blood pressure, harden your arteries, and greatly increase your chance for a heart attack or stroke. Smoking cigarettes will do all of that.

Tobacco, alcohol, and drug use greatly increase the risk for many diseases and injuries. Use of these substances is a modifiable risk factor because people can choose not to smoke, drink alcohol, or take drugs. You will learn more about these risk factors in chapters 9, 10, and 11.

Sexual Activity

Research shows that teen **sexual activity** tends to be fairly risky. According to most studies, over 40 percent of teens have had sexual intercourse, and many of those teens have failed to use any type of birth control. As you probably already know, engaging in unprotected sex is a risk factor for contracting sexually transmitted infections, including HIV/AIDS. You will learn more about these risk factors in chapter 13.

Nutrition and Physical Activity

Your health is influenced by what you eat, how much you eat, and your level of physical activity. Nutritional excesses or deficiencies are risk factors for many health problems. For example, diets low in fiber and high in red meat increase a person's risk for developing cancer of the *colon* (large

distracted driving behaviors
risky driving actions typically taken by teenagers; include texting, talking on the phone, and driving with one or more passengers under 18 years of age

sexual activity
behavior related to sexual intercourse; considered a risk factor for teenagers

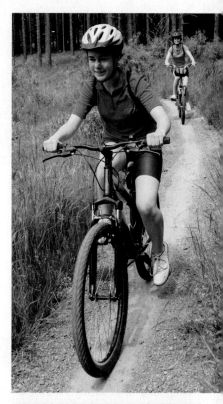

Figure 2.7

Some teens, such as those in this photo, have a tendency to minimize their risk factors; other teens do not. *To which group do you tend to belong?*

physical fitness
the state of being fit; attained by maintaining a healthful diet and exercise regimen

intestine). Diets high in calories, salt, and fat can lead to heart disease, high blood pressure, stroke, cancer, and obesity.

The combination of excess calories and physical inactivity leads to obesity. Obesity is a risk factor for many serious diseases, such as heart disease, diabetes, stroke, high blood pressure, cancer, arthritis, and other health problems. You will learn more about obesity and other nutrition-related risk factors in chapter 4.

Doctors are concerned about the dietary and exercise habits of children and adolescents because these habits tend to persist into adulthood. Research suggests that today's adolescents need to improve their dietary and exercise habits. Nearly 30% of high school students get less than one hour of physical activity per day, with half of these students not exercising at all. Over half of high school students do not attend physical education classes, where they could get regular exercise and learn about *physical fitness* (Figure 2.8).

Media and Technology

Scientists have examined the impact of television, the Internet, movies, and computer games on health and wellness. These are some of the interesting findings:

- The more hours people watch television, the more likely they are to be overweight or obese.
- The more hours people play video games, the more likely they are to be obese.
- A poor body image and the risk for eating disorders have been attributed to viewing media images of men and women.

Based on these findings, do you think limiting your media exposure to a more moderate level would benefit your health? How much or how little you use the various media and technology outlets is a modifiable risk factor. You can choose to switch off the computer or TV at any time.

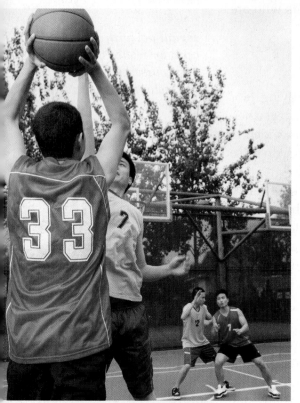

Figure 2.8

These boys probably decided to play basketball because they enjoy it. *Do you think this decision will have a negative or positive effect on their long-term health?*

SKILLS FOR HEALTH AND WELLNESS

Put Knowledge to Work

The skills listed below are ones that can help you live a healthy adolescent life:

- Understand how to refuse alcohol, tobacco, unwanted sexual activity, or other risky behaviors.
- Understand the causes of disease so you can reduce your risk for developing disease.

- Practice abstinence to avoid unwanted pregnancy and sexually transmitted infections.
- Learn safety and first aid to reduce your risk for severe injuries.
- Choose healthful, nutritious food.
- Maintain an active lifestyle and get regular exercise.

Sun Exposure

Scientific studies have shown that sun exposure is the leading risk factor for skin cancer and the premature aging of skin (Figure 2.9). Tanning beds also expose you to dangerous ultraviolet radiation and can cause skin cancer. People with light-colored skin and eyes are especially at risk for skin cancer.

Sleep

The lack of sleep is associated with poor health. It reduces a person's resistance to disease and impairs his or her driving skills. It also increases the risk for the mental health problems such as depression and anxiety.

Teenagers need at least nine hours of sleep each night and sometimes require more to stay alert and active during the day. However, fewer than one out of three high school students get eight hours of sleep on school nights. You will learn more about sleep in chapter 7.

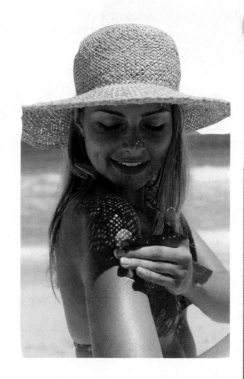

Personal Profile

Are You Active?

These questions will help you assess your commitment to physical activity.

Do you use the stairs instead of the elevator? **yes no**

Do you ride your bike or walk to school, if possible? **yes no**

If you drive to school or work, do you park far from the building so that you get a good walk to and from your car? **yes no**

Do you wake up 45 minutes earlier to jog, walk, or bike before going to school or work? **yes no**

Add up the number of yes answers to assess your degree of physical activity. The more yes answers you have, the higher your rate of physical activity.

Lesson 2.2 Review

Know and Understand ⬀ Assess

1. Why do people who start smoking at a young age and continue into adulthood have a higher risk for related diseases?
2. Name five diseases for which obesity is a risk factor.
3. Why does watching television or playing video games contribute to obesity?
4. List two effects of sun exposure.

Analyze and Apply

5. Give an example of one short-term and one long-term behavioral impact on health.
6. Why might lack of sleep increase risk factors for depression and anxiety?

Real World | Health

Using the Internet, research the following causes of death. Then list how many deaths in the United States in the past year can be attributed to each cause.
- car accidents (specify how many of these were connected to alcohol use, speeding, distracted driving, or the influence of illegal substances)
- alcohol
- illegal drug use
- legal drug use (medications and over-the-counter drugs)
- sexual activity (diseases or other sexual behaviors that led to death)
- nutrition
- extreme sports

Write a short paragraph detailing your findings.

Genetic Risk Factors

Key Terms 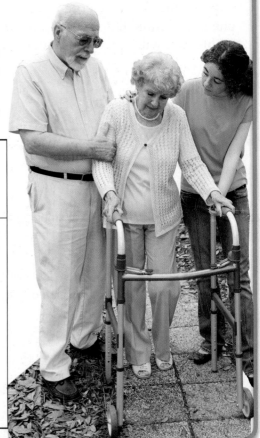 E-Flash Cards

In this lesson, you will learn the meanings of the following key terms.

blood cholesterol

family history

genes

immune system

inherited disease

pathogens

Lesson Objectives

After studying this lesson, you will be able to

- define and describe genes;

- explain the ways in which genes are involved in the inheritance of characteristics;

- give examples of diseases that are influenced by genes; and

- summarize ways to reduce or eliminate risk factors for genetically linked diseases.

Before You Read

KWL Chart: Genetic Disorders

Create a KWL chart like the one below. Before reading this lesson, write what you know and what you want to know about genetic disorders in the appropriate columns. After studying the lesson, write what you have learned.

K What you <u>K</u>now	W What you <u>W</u>ant to know	L What you have <u>L</u>earned

Warm-Up Activity

Family History
What genetic disorders are prevalent in your family? In a table like the one below, list any genetic disorders in your family and the names of your family members who were affected by it.

Genetic Disorders:	Family Members Affected:

You physically resemble your biological parents and you even share some of their behaviors, abilities, likes, and dislikes. Your nose might be shaped like your mother's. If your father does not like the taste of cheese, you may not either. You may never make the basketball team because you are as uncoordinated as your mother. Maybe you are allergic to pollen like your father. These characteristics are partly shaped by your genes (Figure 2.10).

Genes contain the blueprint for the structure and function of your cells. Your genes direct how you grow and develop, influence your personality, and affect your health. Humans have 20,000 to 25,000 genes, which are composed of deoxyribonucleic acid, a chemical often referred to as *DNA*.

Genes are bundled in packages called *chromosomes*. Chromosomes are located in the nucleus, a specialized compartment of each cell. Humans inherit half of their chromosomes from each parent. The unique combination of genes from your parents determines many of your body's characteristics.

Your genes do not act alone. Some of your characteristics are strongly influenced by your genes, but others result from the interactions between genes and other factors. For example, your height is determined by genes, but the height you actually achieve can be altered by diet or disease.

Genes and Disease

The role of genes in disease development varies from one disease to another. Infectious diseases are caused by microscopic living things called *pathogens*, which include bacteria, viruses, and parasites. Genes influence your resistance to diseases by specifying how your immune system is built. The *immune system* consists of cells and chemicals that fight infections. Everyone's immune system differs in its ability to fight infections. In this way, genes have some influence over whether you will contract certain infectious diseases.

In rare cases, a disease is described as an *inherited disease*. An example is sickle cell anemia. People who have sickle cell anemia inherit a single

genes
segments of DNA that determine the structure and function of your cells and affect your development, personality, and health

pathogens
microscopic living things that may cause infections or other illnesses

immune system
the body's mechanism for fighting infections and diseases

inherited disease
a disease caused by defective genes passed down from an ancestral line

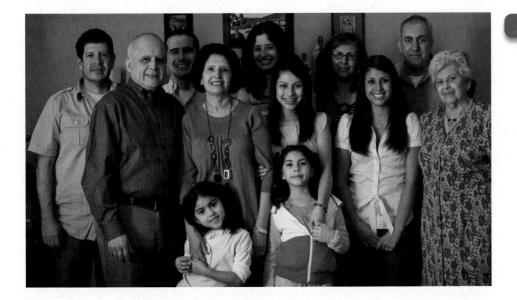

Figure 2.10

What causes family members to resemble each other in different ways?

Carol's mother has skin cancer. Both Carol and her mother have fair eyes, hair, and skin. Carol read that cancer is a genetic disease and she is concerned that she will also get skin cancer no matter what she does.

Thinking Critically

1. Why should Carol be concerned about getting skin cancer?

2. Explain how other risk factors affect Carol's chances of getting skin cancer.

3. How can Carol reduce her chances of getting skin cancer?

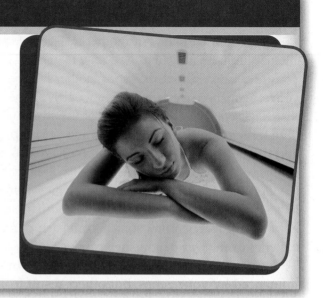

defective gene from each parent, which affects the shape of red blood cells. The defective genes cause red blood cells to be formed abnormally, which reduces the blood's ability to carry oxygen.

In researching the causes of disease, scientists have found that the role of genes is much more complex than the sickle cell anemia example described above. Some diseases are thought to be caused by several genes. Other diseases are likely caused by interactions among genes. In some cases, genes might cause disease only under certain environmental conditions. The following are some examples of how genes influence but do not cause disease themselves. For more general information about these diseases, see chapter 14.

Heart Disease, Cancer, and Genes

Heart disease is the leading cause of death in the United States. Doctors have long recognized that the risk for heart disease runs in families, meaning that the causes of heart disease include genetic factors.

Heart disease is probably caused by several genes. For that reason, doctors study a person's *family history*—the record of disease within a family—to determine a person's genetic risk for heart disease. Having a close relative, such as a father, mother, brother, or sister, with heart disease suggests that a person may have inherited a tendency toward developing heart disease.

A genetic disorder called *familial hypercholesterolemia* is associated with heart disease. People who have this disorder develop extremely high levels of **blood cholesterol**, a fatty substance that blocks arteries and causes heart disease (Figure 2.11). Other than this, no *specific* genes have been linked to heart disease.

Inheriting genes called *BRCA1* and *BRCA2* increases a woman's risk of developing some types of breast or ovarian cancer. Inheriting these genes is not, however, a sufficient reason on its own for someone to develop breast cancer. Damage to other genes must also occur, and environmental factors may be responsible for triggering this damage. In fact, most of the women who develop breast cancer do not have the *BRCA1* and *BRCA2* genes. This suggests that other genes are involved, or that lifestyle and environmental

family history
the record of a disease's presence and impact within a family

blood cholesterol
a fatty substance that resides in the blood and can block arteries if a healthy level is not maintained

factors are also important for determining the cause of breast cancer.

Some types of colon cancer are strongly associated with the inheritance of certain genes. For example, colon cancer affects many people with the condition known as *familial polyposis*. This condition causes the growth of abnormal masses, called *polyps*, in the colon. These polyps are a well-known risk factor for colon cancer.

People who have a close relative with this condition should take precautions and begin screening for colon cancer as a young adult. When caught early, polyps can be removed and colon cancer can be prevented.

The causes of most cases of colon cancer are not yet understood. They appear to arise from complex interactions among other genes or from lifestyle and behavioral factors. These factors include being overweight or physically inactive, smoking, and heavy alcohol use.

Exposure to the sun's ultraviolet radiation is the main cause of skin cancer. It is clear, however, that genes play a role in a person's susceptibility to developing melanoma. For example, a person whose parent or sibling has melanoma is at greater risk for developing this type of cancer.

In addition, melanoma occurs more often in people with fair skin and light-colored eyes and hair, characteristics which are determined by genes. People with these characteristics, or with a family history of melanoma, should take precautions such as wearing a high SPF sunscreen when outdoors. These precautions reduce the chances of getting skin cancer, even if a person has a family history with the disease.

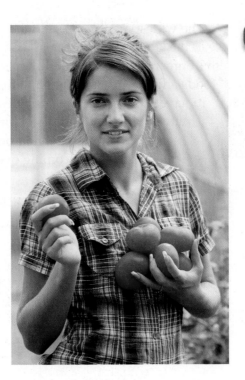

Although genes can put people at risk for certain diseases, people can reduce their risks by eating healthfully.

Mental Illness and Genes

Mental illness includes several serious disorders such as depression, anxiety, bipolar disorder, and schizophrenia. Studies of families and identical twins have shown that genes are involved in the development of these disorders. As with so many other diseases and disorders, however, genes are only part of the story. Research suggests that a person's environment also influences the risk for developing mental disorders.

Weight and Genes

Scientific studies show that the tendency to become overweight and obese is rooted in genetics. In most cases, multiple genes are responsible. These genes affect a person's ability to burn calories, store fat, and burn fat. Genes also influence a person's appetite and levels of physical activity.

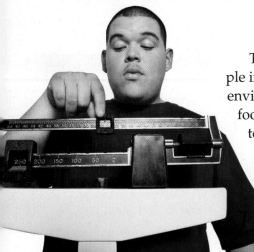

The widespread increase in the number of overweight and obese people in the United States is most likely caused by additional behavioral and environmental factors. These factors include easy access to high-calorie foods and drinks. Compared with people in the past, people today tend to have more sedentary lifestyles and jobs with decreased physical activity (Figure 2.12). People with genetic risk factors are exposed to several environmental and behavioral risk factors, which increases the chances of becoming overweight and obese.

Diabetes and Genes

Type 2 diabetes mellitus, also called *adult-onset diabetes*, is a disorder resulting in a high blood sugar level.

The genetic risk factors for diabetes include having a family history of the disorder. People whose ancestry is African-American, Hispanic, or Native American have a higher risk for diabetes. Certain groups of Asian Americans and Pacific Islanders also have a higher risk for diabetes. People with these genetic risks must avoid other known risk factors for type 2 diabetes, such as obesity, physical inactivity, and high-calorie diets.

What You Can Do

Although you are "stuck" with the genes you receive, there are actions you can take to help prevent genetically linked diseases and disorders. First, you should learn about your family's history for diseases. Ask your biological relatives for information. Then learn about the risk factors associated with the diseases that run in your family.

Once you have this information, you can try to eliminate or reduce your risk factors for these diseases. By eliminating extra risk factors for a certain disease, you can hopefully lower your chances of getting that disease. Reducing these risk factors is just another way you can maintain your health and wellness.

Figure 2.12

Research shows that your genes play a key role in determining your weight. Yet more people are obese today than in years past. *Why do you think obesity is increasing?*

Lesson 2.3 Review

Know and Understand
Assess

1. What causes infectious diseases?
2. What role do genes play in infectious diseases?
3. Explain why doctors study a patient's family history.
4. List a type of cancer that has genetic risk factors.

Analyze and Apply

5. Give an example of how genetic, environmental, and behavioral factors can contribute to obesity.
6. How might identical twins who were separated at birth be helpful in determining the role of genes in mental illness?

Real World (Health

This chapter includes several examples of diseases and disorders that run in families, or in which genes play a role. Working with two or three classmates, choose one of these diseases or disorders and develop a short presentation that answers the following question: *Should someone without a family history of this disease feel confident that he or she will not develop it?* Use the Internet to research the disease or disorder and find evidence that supports your answer. Include information about the evidence you found, such as who did the research and where and when it was published. Summarize the conclusions of the study and present your findings to the class.

Environmental and Socioeconomic Risk Factors

Lesson Objectives

After studying this lesson, you will be able to

- recognize environmental and socioeconomic risk factors;
- explain how environmental and socioeconomic risk factors affect health; and
- summarize ways to reduce or eliminate environmental and socioeconomic risk factors for diseases.

Key Terms E-Flash Cards

In this lesson, you will learn the meanings of the following key terms.

climate
environment
environmental risk factors
geography
hazard
socioeconomic risk factors

Warm-Up Activity

Daily Health

Write the schedule of your typical day on a piece of paper, including choices you make regarding nutrition, exercise, and entertainment. In a chart like the one shown below, list your activities and then write one or two sentences about how you think each activity will affect your risk of injury or illness.

Activity	How does this activity affect my risk of injury or illness?

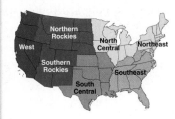

Before You Read

Geographic Risks

Using the map below, identify risk factors specific to each geographical region. List these risk factors and compare your answers with your classmates' answers.

Mike is a construction worker in the Midwest. He spends time outdoors year-round while building roads and bridges. Sandy works for the same construction company as Mike, but is an engineer. She designs building plans on the computer in her office. Mike is exposed to the weather and various work environment **hazards**, but he is physically active most of the day. Sandy is not exposed to weather extremes or construction hazards but, compared to Mike, she is physically inactive at work.

Since Mike and Sandy experience different work environments and hazards, they have different risk factors for injury and disease. **Environmental risk factors** are characteristics of your surroundings, such as regional climate and the weather, which may cause you injury or disease. Your workplace and home environments may include hazards that place your health in jeopardy. **Socioeconomic risk factors** involve a person's level of education, type of work, income level, and access to healthcare. Socioeconomic risk factors can also affect your health and well-being.

In this section you will learn to recognize environmental and socioeconomic risk factors. You will also learn how they can affect your health and what you can do about them.

Environmental Risk Factors

Your **environment** includes the circumstances, objects, or conditions that surround you in your everyday life. The climate in which you live, the kind of workplace where you spend your time, and your home are all part of your environment. In general, your environment is probably a safe place. Every environment has its risk factors that can create the opportunity for disease, injury, or other conditions. Let's look at several different environmental risk factors.

Climate and Geography

Climate is a region's overall pattern of temperature, precipitation, wind, and weather conditions. **Geography** refers to features of the land and any bodies of water that are present in an area. Both climate and geography influence living conditions and present different kinds of risk factors for injury and disease (Figure 2.13). No matter where you live, there are risk factors involved with both your climate and geography.

hazard
an aspect of your environment that puts you at risk for disease or injury

environmental risk factors
characteristics of your surroundings that may expose you to injury or disease

socioeconomic risk factors
characteristics of your status in society that may expose you to injury or disease

environment
the circumstances, objects, and conditions of your surroundings

climate
the overall environmental weather pattern of a region

geography
the features of the land

Figure 2.13

What might be some hazards to your health if you lived in each of these regions?

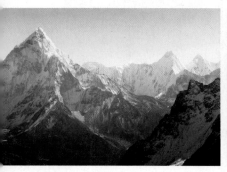 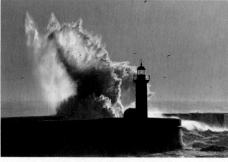 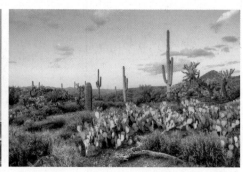

Hazardous Substances and Work Conditions

Exposure to dangerous substances or hazardous conditions increases the chance for an injury or illness. Hazards may be encountered anywhere, including work, school, in the community, or at home. As a person's exposure to hazards increases, the person is more likely to become injured or sick.

Workplace Hazards. Hazards differ from workplace to workplace. When present, such hazards must be eliminated or reduced to remove the risk of illness and injury for employees. Examples of workplace hazards and associated injuries or diseases include the following:

- *loud noise*: hearing loss
- *flying debris*: vision damage or bodily injury
- *hazardous chemicals*: burns, poisoning, nerve damage, respiratory disease, asthma
- *power tools*: trauma, cuts, burns
- *computer use*: eye strain, repetitive use injuries to hands and wrists

Workplaces present several types of risk factors that can be identified and avoided (Figure 2.14).

Physical Activity in the Workplace. Jobs differ in their physical demands. Some types of work require regular and sometimes vigorous activity, while other jobs entail almost no physical activity. Studies of different occupations have found considerable differences in physical activity.

The level of physical activity is reflected in the number of *calories*—units of energy—used to perform that activity. For example, compare the physical activity levels of three average men who weigh 155 pounds. The first man, a website designer, works mainly at a desk and uses about 102 calories per hour. The second man, a carpenter, uses about 260 calories each hour as he lifts heavy objects and runs errands. The third man, a firefighter, carries a heavy pack and works in extreme conditions. He uses about 892 calories per hour.

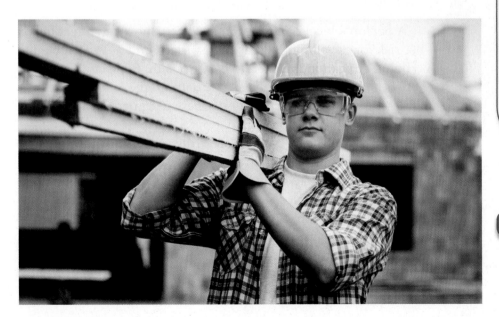

Figure 2.14

How is this worker protecting himself against potential risks to his health?

What if these three men never exercised outside of the workplace? In particular, if the website designer does not get regular physical activity outside of work, he leads a sedentary, inactive lifestyle. This type of lifestyle can lead to weight gain and cardiovascular disease.

The total amount of physical activity in your day affects your health. That is why it is important for students to get physical activity outside of school, where they spend most of their time sitting. People whose work requires them to be inactive most of the day should also plan physical activity outside of work. Your level of activity at school or work is not a modifiable risk factor, but you control your level of physical activity at home. Simple changes such as waking up early to jog, walk, or bike can increase your level of physical activity and improve your health.

Hazards in the Home. What hazards can be found around the home? The greater the exposure to these hazards, the greater the risk for health problems or injuries caused by them. It is important to recognize that such hazards exist as soon as possible. Examples of hazards in the home and associated health problems include

- *lead*: poisoning, brain damage, learning disabilities;
- *asbestos*: lung damage and lung cancer;
- *radon gas*: lung cancer; and
- *fire*: burns, smoke inhalation, injury, and death.

Socioeconomic Risk Factors

Socioeconomic factors include level of education, income, and status in society. Whether you have graduated college, how much money you earn, and what neighborhood you live in are all encompassed in socioeconomic factors. These factors might also influence a person's access to healthcare. Scientists have studied how these social factors influence health and wellness.

Education

A person's level of education has been shown to affect his or her risk for developing diseases, disorders, and health problems. Higher education is linked to better health. For example, scientists have found that college graduates in the United States are less likely to be overweight or obese than people with a high school education or less.

The reason for this correlation between education and health is not clear. It may be that people with more education have access to more information about nutrition and physical activity. Perhaps people with more education earn more money, and therefore have access to better medical care. With more information and medical care, these people can better avoid health problems like obesity.

The relationship between education and health has been proven worldwide and in many different areas. It has been found that better-educated women tend to have healthier babies than their less-educated peers (Figure 2.15). Infant mortality is lower in better-educated populations across the globe.

Figure 2.15

The more education this young mother has, the more likely it is that her baby will be healthy.

People with more education also tend to have a higher life expectancy than others no matter their geographic location.

Economic Factors

Income level is also related to a person's health. People with a higher income tend to have better health than people with a lower income (Figure 2.16). Exactly how this works is unclear, but scientists have linked lower income to poor health-related behaviors and risk factors. For example, people from low-income households are more likely to

- smoke cigarettes;
- be physically inactive;
- live in neighborhoods with fewer health resources, fewer clinics, and less access to healthy groceries;
- live in low-income neighborhoods with less opportunity to be physically active outdoors;
- have fewer opportunities to prevent or treat developing health problems;
- not get screened for diseases such as colon cancer and breast cancer; and
- suffer from depression.

In addition, children from low-income families tend to spend more time each day watching television and playing video and computer games. They are also less likely to have all of their required vaccinations, making them more prone to certain diseases.

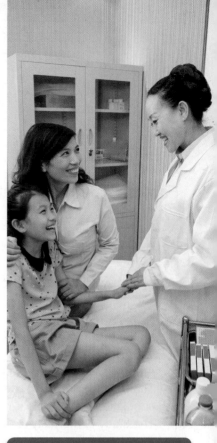

Figure 2.16

The quality and availability of healthcare can vary based on a person's income level.

Lesson 2.4 Review

Know and Understand Assess

1. List three examples of socioeconomic factors.
2. Describe five types of workplace hazards and examples of associated injuries.
3. List three ways to build more physical activity into your day.
4. What are four types of hazards found in the home and their associated health risks?

Analyze and Apply

5. Choose two careers and compare and contrast their physical demands and risk factors, as well as the life spans of people in these careers. Describe which career you would prefer.

Real World Health

Environmental Responsibility Environmental issues, such as air and water pollution, impact the risk factors you encounter. Consider your environment and write a journal entry answering the following questions: How can you stay informed about environmental issues? How do air and water pollution affect the environment, and how can you reduce your risk related to them? What modes of active transport (for example, walking) could you use to reduce pollution? What environmental protection programs exist worldwide and in your community? Make an action plan for yourself to spread word about reducing pollution and improving the environment.

Chapter 2   Review and Assessment

 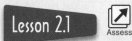
Factors Affecting Health and Wellness

Key Terms

life expectancy   mortality
life span   quality of life
morbidity   risk factors

Key Points

- As the health of a population improves, so will its life expectancy.
- A person's life span is affected by his or her health.
- The morbidity of a disease describes its effect on a population.
- The study of mortality in different age groups reveals which conditions are the biggest problems for each group.
- A person's health can affect his or her quality of life.

Check Your Understanding

1. *True or false?* Females have a longer life expectancy than males.

2. A disease with high morbidity means _____.
   A. few people have the condition
   B. many people have the condition
   C. the condition has caused many deaths
   D. the condition has caused few deaths

3. Risk factors_____.
   A. ensure the development of a problem
   B. are only caused by genes
   C. increase the chances of developing a disease
   D. are only caused by environment

4. *True or false?* Life span is another term for life expectancy.

5. Which of the following terms describes the level of satisfaction people have with various aspects of their lives?
   A. life expectancy
   B. mortality
   C. quality of life
   D. morbidity

6. Risk factors fall into three basic categories: _____, genetic, and environmental.

7. **Critical Thinking.** Give three examples of causes of disease and explain which category each belongs in.

Behavioral Risk Factors

Key Terms

behavioral risk factors   physical fitness
distracted driving   sexual activity
behaviors

Key Points

- Behavioral factors may have short-term and long-term effects on health.
- Behavioral risks can cause accidents and injuries.
- Risky behaviors include tobacco, alcohol, and drug use and unsafe sexual activity.
- Physical activity, limited sun exposure, and adequate sleep can all help reduce risk for illness and disease.

Check Your Understanding

8. _____ result in unintentional injuries.

9. *True or false?* Smoking is a modifiable risk factor.

10. _____ contributes to obesity.
    A. Watching television
    B. Sun exposure
    C. Bicycling
    D. Jogging

11. Driving while texting and interacting with multiple passengers while driving are examples of _____ driving behaviors, which can cause accidents.

12. *True or false?* Teenagers need at least nine hours of sleep each night.

13. Per mile driven, drivers between the ages of 16 and 19 are _____ times more likely to be in fatal car accidents than older drivers.
    A. ten
    B. two
    C. five
    D. three

14. *True or false?* Tanning in a tanning bed is a way to lower your risk of developing skin cancer.

15. **Critical Thinking.** Why do people start smoking despite widespread knowledge of the health risks?

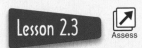

Genetic Risk Factors

Key Terms

blood cholesterol
family history
genes

immune system
inherited disease
pathogens

Key Points

- Genes may cause an inherited disease or influence a person's resistance to disease.
- Family members may share risk factors for heart disease and stroke.
- Some common cancers have genetic risk factors.
- Obesity and overweight are caused by hereditary, behavioral, and environmental factors.

Check Your Understanding

16. *True or false?* Physical characteristics of humans are determined by genes alone.

17. Bacteria and viruses that cause disease are called _____.

18. _____ is a fatty substance that blocks arteries and causes heart disease.
    A. A gene
    B. Blood cholesterol
    C. A stroke
    D. A polyp

19. *True or false?* Environment influences the risk of mental illness, but genetics do not.

20. Which body system consists of cells and chemicals that fight infection?
    A. nervous system
    B. immune system
    C. cardiovascular system
    D. digestive system

21. *True or false?* Some diseases are thought to be caused by more than one gene.

22. **Critical Thinking.** What are some ways you can prevent development of genetically linked diseases that run in your family?

Environmental and Socioeconomic Risk Factors

Key Terms

climate
environment
environmental risk factors

geography
hazard
socioeconomic risk factors

Key Points

- Socioeconomic risk factors affect well-being.
- Climate and geography present risk factors for injury and disease.
- Health hazards can be found in the workplace and the home.
- Education, economic status, and access to healthcare resources are all socioeconomic factors.

Check Your Understanding

23. A(n) _____ is a unit of energy used to perform physical activities.

24. Which of the following home hazards can result in poisoning and brain damage?
    A. lead
    B. asbestos
    C. radon gas
    D. fire

25. *True or false?* People with lower incomes tend to have better health than people who have more money.

26. Which of the following is *not* an environmental risk factor?
    A. weather
    B. geography
    C. hazardous substances
    D. family history

27. *True or false?* Workers whose jobs consist of typing on computers are not at risk of developing injuries due to workplace hazards.

28. **Critical Thinking.** Why might a person's level of education be linked to his or her health?

Health and Wellness Skills

29. **Practice Healthy Behaviors and Reduce Health Risks.** Using the information you have about your family history, go to your doctor and talk to him or her about what diseases you may be predisposed to. Have your doctor perform a complete health screening on you, and then talk with your doctor about what behaviors you could change to increase your overall health and delay the possible onset of genetic illnesses.

30. **Set Goals.** Design a plan to delay or prevent the onset of the illnesses that run in your family. Identify one or two behaviors you want to change, and then outline a few SMART goals that will motivate you to engage in a healthier lifestyle.

31. **Communicate with Others.** Sometimes nothing matters more than family. Assess your family members' lifestyles and environment. Have a discussion with your parents about how they maintain their health and environment. What environmental protection programs can help your family maintain their environment and health?

32. **Advocate for Health.** Plan a fitness walk that will raise money for health facilities that treat those with lifestyle-related and genetic diseases. Set a monetary goal and ask companies, family, and friends to donate. In addition, ask different organizations that deal with nutrition, obesity, and disease prevention to be present at your fitness walk and help raise awareness.

Hands-On Activity

Identifying Risk Factors in My Environment

You read about different types of risk factors throughout chapter 2 and focused on *Environmental Risk Factors* in lesson 2.4. Follow the steps below to identify risk factors that may be present in your own environment.

Materials Needed

- smartphone capable of taking pictures, or camera
- poster board (alternative to poster board, markers, and tape: connect to classroom computer for digital presentation)
- markers
- tape

Steps for This Activity

1. Your first task is to identify as many potential risk factors as possible in your personal environment—in your home, in your neighborhood, at school, and in your community. Since many of your risk factors may be the same as those identified by your classmates, focus closely on your own home; your job, if you have one; places that your family

visits regularly; and any other aspects of your environment that make it unique.

2. Take pictures of objects, conditions, and people engaged in activities that represent each risk factor that you identified. Be creative in determining the best possible photo to represent or symbolize a particular risk factor.

3. After collecting this information, design a 'plan of attack' for how you will keep yourself as healthy as possible while confronting one or two of the most threatening risk factors you found.

4. Present your plan, along with the corresponding photos, to your class using a poster or a digital presentation as a visual aid.

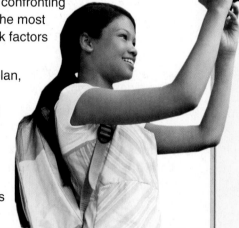

Core Skills

Math Practice

The following graph shows mortality rates among adolescents 15–19 years of age by leading cause and sex. Study the graph and then answer the questions.

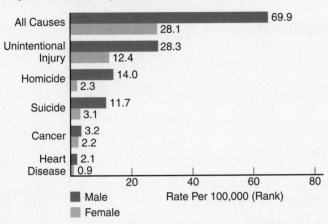

Mortality Rates Among Adolescents Aged 15-19 Years, by Selected Leading Cause and Sex

- All Causes: Male 69.9, Female 28.1
- Unintentional Injury: Male 28.3, Female 12.4
- Homicide: Male 14.0, Female 2.3
- Suicide: Male 11.7, Female 3.1
- Cancer: Male 3.2, Female 2.2
- Heart Disease: Male 2.1, Female 0.9

Rate Per 100,000 (Rank)

■ Male
■ Female

33. How many deaths per 100,000 occurred due to all causes for males and females combined?
    A. 69.9
    B. 28.1
    C. 98.0
    D. 100,000

34. How many more males than females died from unintentional injury?
    A. 15.9 per 100,000
    B. 28.3 per 100,000
    C. 12.4 per 100,000
    D. 25 per 100,000

35. What percentage of the females died from heart disease?
    A. 0.9%
    B. 3%
    C. 10%
    D. 13%

36. In a group of one million randomly selected adolescent males, how many are likely to die of homicide?
    A. 14
    B. 23
    C. 140
    D. 28

Reading and Writing Practice

Read the passage below and then answer the questions.

Some behaviors have an immediate impact on health. For example, wearing a helmet while bicycling reduces the chances of a severe head injury, but 88% of high school teens never wear a helmet while bicycling. Other behaviors have both short-term and long-term effects. Smoking cigarettes reduces your lungs' ability to use oxygen, and makes you susceptible to respiratory infections. Smoking is known to cause lung cancer and increase the risk for heart disease in adulthood. Even so, nearly one in five high school students currently smoke cigarettes. Because smoking is addictive, it is likely that these teens will become adult smokers.

37. What is the author's main idea in this passage?
    A. Smoking is addictive.
    B. Too many teens smoke cigarettes.
    C. Teens do not need to wear biking helmets unless they race competitively.
    D. Behaviors can have immediate, short-term, and long-term health effects.

38. Why is it likely that teen smokers will become adult smokers?
    A. Smoking is known to have an immediate impact on health.
    B. Smoking is addictive.
    C. A smoker is susceptible to respiratory infections.
    D. Smoking raises the risk for heart disease for people with a family history of heart disease.

39. What is *not* a short-term effect of smoking?
    A. heart disease
    B. a reduction in the lungs' ability to use oxygen
    C. susceptibility to respiratory infections
    D. addiction to tobacco products

40. Write a paragraph about behaviors other than those mentioned in the passage above that have an immediate effect on your health. Share your paragraphs in class.

Unit 2 Nutrition and Food Choices

Big Ideas

- What you eat determines whether or not your body will have the nutrients it needs to stay healthy.

- Maintaining a healthy weight is an important part of wellness.

- A healthy weight for one person may not be a healthy weight for someone else.

- Having a distorted body image can lead some people to develop eating disorders.

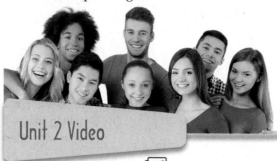

Unit 2 Video

Dining Dilemma Videos

Teenage friends try to order meals at a diner from an uncooperative waiter. The waiter has the scoop on hidden ingredients in their favorite foods. Will the friends find healthy choices on the menu to satisfy their hunger?

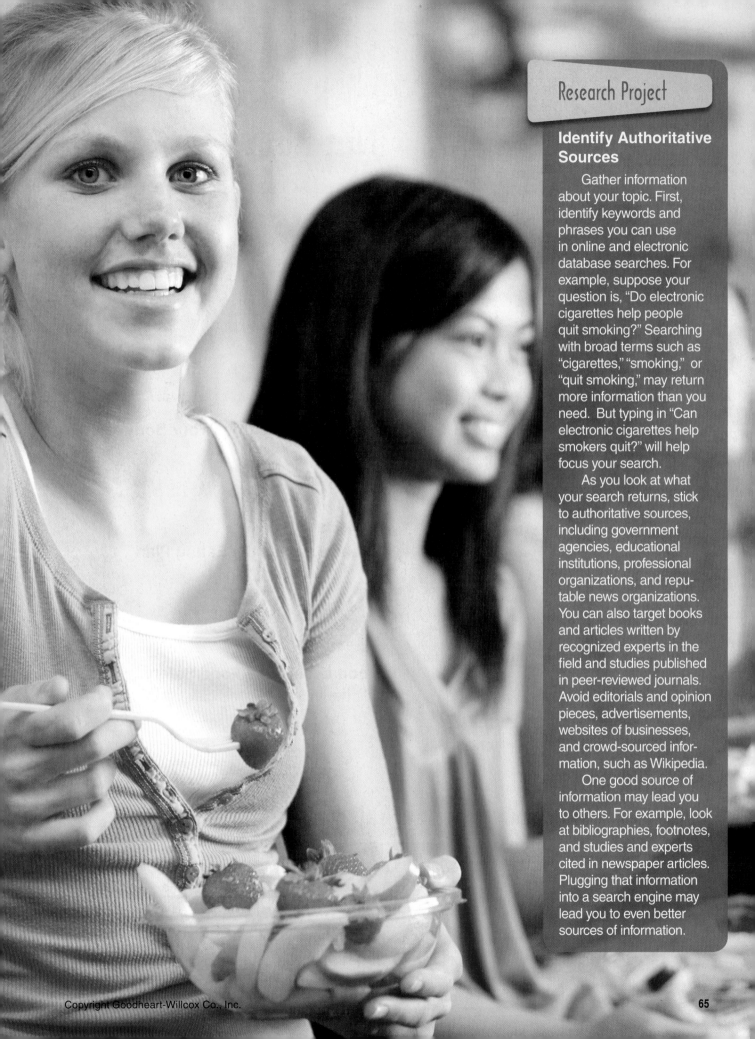

Identify Authoritative Sources

Gather information about your topic. First, identify keywords and phrases you can use in online and electronic database searches. For example, suppose your question is, "Do electronic cigarettes help people quit smoking?" Searching with broad terms such as "cigarettes," "smoking," or "quit smoking," may return more information than you need. But typing in "Can electronic cigarettes help smokers quit?" will help focus your search.

As you look at what your search returns, stick to authoritative sources, including government agencies, educational institutions, professional organizations, and reputable news organizations. You can also target books and articles written by recognized experts in the field and studies published in peer-reviewed journals. Avoid editorials and opinion pieces, advertisements, websites of businesses, and crowd-sourced information, such as Wikipedia.

One good source of information may lead you to others. For example, look at bibliographies, footnotes, and studies and experts cited in newspaper articles. Plugging that information into a search engine may lead you to even better sources of information.

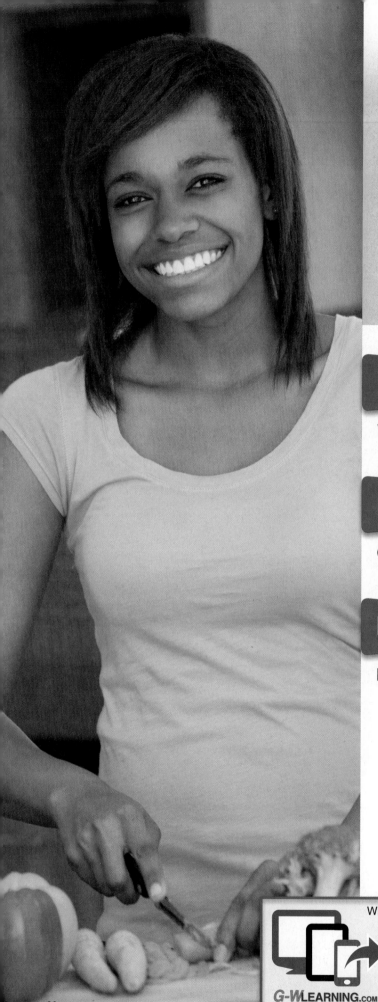

Chapter 3
Nutrition

While studying this chapter, look for the activity icon ↗ to:
- **review** vocabulary with e-flash cards and games;
- **assess** learning with quizzes and online exercises;
- **expand** knowledge with animations and activities; and
- **listen** to pronunciation of key terms in the audio glossary.

G-WLEARNING.com

www.g-wlearning.com/health/

Take this quiz to see what you do and do not know about nutrition. If you cannot answer a question, pay extra attention to that topic as you study this chapter.

1. *Identify each statement as* True, False, *or* It Depends. *Choose* It Depends *if a statement is true in some cases, but false in others.*

2. *Revise each* False *statement to make it true.*

3. *Explain the circumstances in which each* It Depends *statement is true and when it is false.*

Health and Wellness IQ [Assess]

	True	False	It Depends
1. Fiber is a good source of energy.	True	False	It Depends
2. Essential amino acids are produced by your body.	True	False	It Depends
3. Unsaturated fats are better for your health than saturated fats.	True	False	It Depends
4. Drinking 8½ to 11½ glasses of fluids a day is a good strategy for maintaining good health.	True	False	It Depends
5. Taking regular supplements of vitamins and minerals is a good strategy for improving your overall health.	True	False	It Depends
6. Fruit juices and whole fruits provide approximately the same level of nutrients to your body.	True	False	It Depends
7. Eating a candy bar or drinking a sugary soda is a healthful strategy for boosting your energy level.	True	False	It Depends
8. Keeping cold foods cold and hot foods hot is a good strategy for preventing food poisoning.	True	False	It Depends
9. Proteins, carbohydrates, and fats all have the same number of calories per gram.	True	False	It Depends
10. No cure exists for food allergies.	True	False	It Depends

Setting the Scene

What have you eaten today? Did you eat a nutritious breakfast such as whole-grain cereal with milk? Or did you grab a piece of toast as you raced out the door? Or did you skip breakfast completely?

Now think about what you ate for lunch. Did you choose a well-balanced meal from the school cafeteria, or did you eat a sandwich and yogurt that you brought from home? Did you skip lunch, planning to grab fast food after school?

Although you may not have thought much about the food choices you've made today, what you eat has a major impact on your overall health. This chapter examines nutrition, the processes by which an organism—you—takes in and uses food. You'll learn about different types of nutrients your body needs, how nutrients help your body stay healthy, and strategies for making healthful and safe food choices.

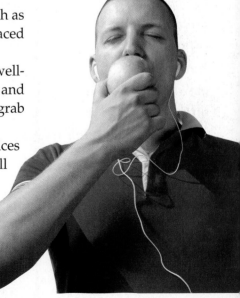

What Nutrients Does Your Body Need?

Key Terms 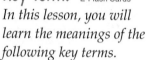 E-Flash Cards

In this lesson, you will learn the meanings of the following key terms.

amino acid
anemia
carbohydrate
cholesterol
dehydration
fat
fat-soluble vitamin
fiber
glucose
glycogen
hormone
mineral
nutrient
osteoporosis
protein
saturated fat
trans fat
unsaturated fat
vitamin
water-soluble vitamin

Before You Read

Favorite Food Nutrients

List the 10 foods that you eat most frequently. Next to each food, write many or few nutrients. Check your guesses after you read this lesson.

Lesson Objectives

After studying this lesson, you will be able to

- identify the six types of nutrients;
- understand the role of each nutrient in the body;
- identify sources of each nutrient;
- evaluate the importance of water; and
- recognize the conditions under which the body's supply of water needs to increase.

Warm-Up Activity

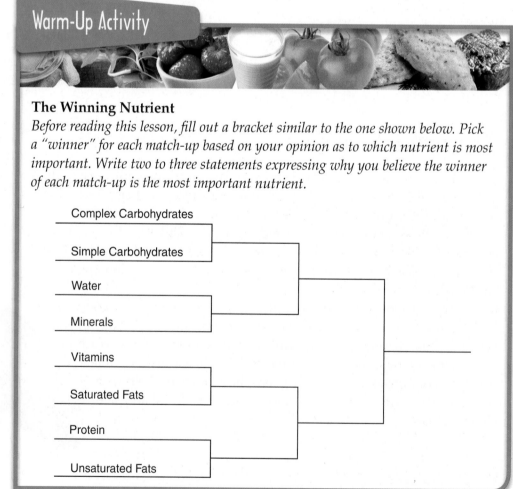

The Winning Nutrient
Before reading this lesson, fill out a bracket similar to the one shown below. Pick a "winner" for each match-up based on your opinion as to which nutrient is most important. Write two to three statements expressing why you believe the winner of each match-up is the most important nutrient.

Complex Carbohydrates
Simple Carbohydrates
Water
Minerals
Vitamins
Saturated Fats
Protein
Unsaturated Fats

Do you know that the foods and beverages you eat and drink impact virtually all aspects of your wellness, including how tall you are, how much you weigh, the strength of your muscles, and the complexion of your skin? Food contains *nutrients*, which are chemical substances that give your body what it needs to grow and function properly.

There are six general types of nutrients:

- carbohydrates
- fats
- protein
- minerals
- vitamins
- water

nutrient
a chemical substance that gives your body what it needs to grow and function properly

Some of these nutrients provide the energy your body needs for daily activities such as playing sports, dancing, and riding a bicycle. The body also needs this energy to perform many important internal functions. These functions include maintaining a stable body temperature, providing energy to the brain and nervous system, and building body tissues.

Other nutrients enable certain critical bodily functions to occur. For example, the body needs vitamins and minerals to build new cells, strengthen its bones, and carry oxygen to its tissues. Nutrients also regulate crucial physiological processes in your body, such as breathing and digesting (Figure 3.1).

In this lesson, you will learn about the three types of nutrients—carbohydrates, proteins, and fats—that provide energy to your body. You will also read about three types of nutrients—vitamins, minerals, and water—that serve other functions in your body.

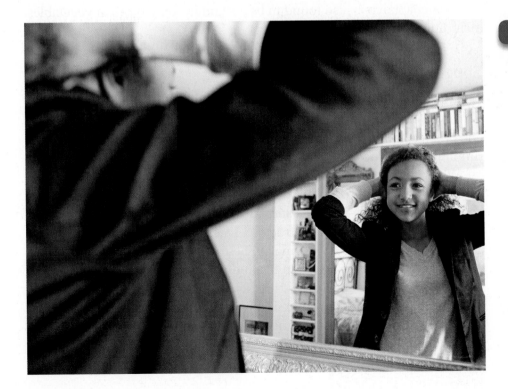

Figure 3.1

What do you notice about this teen's appearance that suggests she eats nutritious meals on a regular basis?

Carbohydrates

carbohydrate
a nutrient and major source of energy for the body

Carbohydrates, a major source of energy for the body, are found in fruits, vegetables, grains, and milk products. Carbohydrates are also known as *saccharides*, or *sugar and starch molecules*. These molecules serve as a source of chemical energy that the body can utilize quickly. Carbohydrates can be described as either simple or complex. There are three distinct types of carbohydrates: sugar, starch, and fiber.

Sugars

Sugars such as fructose, glucose, sucrose, and lactose, are classified as *simple carbohydrates*. These simple sugar compounds occur naturally in some foods, including fruits, maple syrup, and dairy products.

glucose
a type of carbohydrate and the preferred source of energy for the brain and central nervous system

Glucose is the preferred source of energy for your brain and central nervous system. It is glucose that powers your brain, enabling you to concentrate and pay attention in class.

The table sugar people add to their coffee or use in baking is *sucrose*, which has been extracted from sugarcane or sugar beets. When sugar appears in the ingredient list of a processed food, the product contains sucrose. It is common for processed foods such as cereals, breads, desserts, and sugar-sweetened beverages to contain added sugars such as sucrose.

Starches

Starches, which are chains of glucose linked together, are called *complex carbohydrates*. During digestion, your body breaks down starches into smaller glucose units, making the glucose available for use as energy. Products made from grains, such as bread, cereal, rice, and pasta, are rich sources of starch. Starch is also found in beans and in some types of vegetables, including potatoes, peas, and corn.

Supplying Energy

Your body breaks down carbohydrates into glucose to obtain energy. Have you ever skipped breakfast and then had trouble concentrating in one of your early morning classes? This difficulty is caused by your body running out of glucose.

When it is in need of energy, the body can use glucose immediately. This is why having a candy bar or soft drink, both loaded with sugar, can give you a quick "pick-me-up." The sucrose in these snacks is quickly and easily broken down into glucose and fructose. Later in this chapter, you will learn about the disadvantages of relying on these types of foods for energy.

glycogen
a stored version of glucose located in the muscles and liver; supplies energy between meals

Glucose can also be stored in the liver and muscles for later use. When glucose is stored in these areas, it is known as **glycogen**. However, after enough glycogen has been stored, any extra glucose is converted by the liver into fat, which is stored in the fat tissue. The body uses glycogen from the muscles and liver, or the fat stored in the fat tissue, when it needs energy between meals or to fuel activity.

Fiber

Fiber is a tough complex carbohydrate that the body is unable to digest. This type of carbohydrate is found only in plant-based foods, including fruits, most vegetables, whole grains (such as whole-wheat bread or brown rice), and nuts.

Although fiber does not provide the body with energy, it does have important health benefits:

- **Lowers cholesterol.** Fiber attaches to cholesterol and carries it out of the body during digestion. *Cholesterol* is a type of fat made by the body that is also present in some foods. Having too much cholesterol in the body increases a person's risk of developing heart disease, high blood pressure, and stroke.

- **Balances level of glucose.** By balancing the level of glucose in the blood, fiber can help control some types of diabetes.

- **Adds bulk to stools.** Fiber maintains the healthy functioning of the digestive system by adding bulk to stools, which helps prevent problems such as constipation (hard stools) and hemorrhoids. Hemorrhoids are swollen, painful veins in the rectum that are caused from straining to pass hard stools.

- **Can prevent overeating.** Because high-fiber foods take longer to chew than many other types of food, people eating a high-fiber meal are inclined to eat less than they would otherwise. Fiber also slows the movement of food out of your stomach and into your intestines (Figure 3.2). This means that you feel full faster, which helps prevent overeating and obesity.

Protein

Protein is a nutrient the body uses to build and maintain all of its cells and tissues, including muscles, bones, skin, hair, fingernails, and organs. Protein also provides energy when carbohydrates and fats are lacking in the diet.

Your body uses up and loses protein every day. Certain activities result in cell loss, which also means protein loss. You lose protein when you

- brush your hair—the hair left in the brush contains protein;

- shower—the skin cells that slough off during showering contain protein;

- trim your fingernails—the nail clippings contain protein;

- sweat—the skin cells that are lost when sweating contain protein; and

- urinate—protein is lost through urination.

fiber
a complex carbohydrate that the body is unable to digest

cholesterol
a type of fat made by the body that is also present in some foods

protein
a nutrient the body uses to build and maintain all types of cells; can provide energy in the absence of fat and carbohydrates

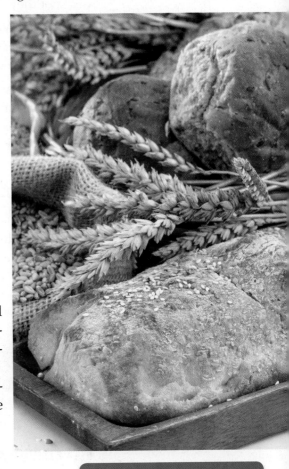

Figure 3.2

High-fiber carbohydrates like whole-grain breads, rice, and pastas make you feel full faster. *How do you think feeling full faster helps prevent obesity?*

You need to take in protein to replace what is lost every day. Fortunately, in the United States, many foods that people eat on a regular basis contain protein. If you're like most Americans, you eat more protein than you need.

Types of Proteins

amino acid
a small chemical unit that makes up proteins

hormone
a chemical substance in your body that influences many basic processes

All proteins are made up of smaller chemical units called ***amino acids*** (Figure 3.3). Twenty different amino acids join in various combinations to make all types of protein. Some of these amino acids are produced in the body. These are called *nonessential amino acids*.

Other types of amino acids are *not* produced by the body; you can only get them by eating particular foods. This type of amino acid is called an *essential amino acid* because it is essential that your diet includes this type of nutrient.

Protein sources are divided into two types, depending on whether or not they include all of the essential amino acids:

- A *complete protein* source contains all nine of the essential amino acids. This type of protein is found in animal-based foods such as meat, poultry, eggs, fish, and dairy products (milk and cheese).
- An *incomplete protein* source lacks one or more of the essential amino acids. This type of protein is found in legumes (dry beans and peas), tofu, nuts and seeds, grains, some vegetables, and some fruits.

Figure 3.3

Steak is a complete protein, meaning it contains all nine essential amino acids. *Do you consider complete protein foods like steak to be "healthy"? Why or why not?*

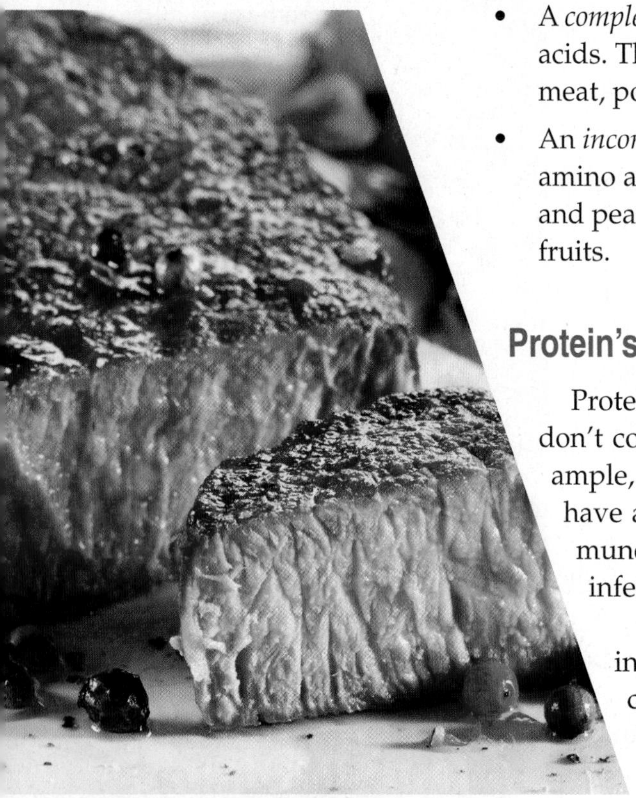

Protein's Role in the Body

Protein is required for the body to function properly. People who don't consume enough protein risk serious consequences. For example, since immune cells are made of protein, individuals who have a protein deficiency are more likely to have weakened immune systems, which make it more likely for them to develop infections and diseases.

Protein plays other important roles in the body, including acting as enzymes and hormones. ***Hormones*** are chemical messengers that influence many basic processes in your body. Protein also serves as a transporter in the body and is involved in fluid and pH balance.

Protein and Vegetarians

Because some vegetarians avoid eating all (or most) foods from animal sources, they must rely on plant-based sources of protein to meet their protein needs. With some planning, a vegetarian diet can easily meet the recommended protein needs of adults and children. People who eat a vegetarian diet need to take in different types of food that can work together to provide all of the essential amino acids.

No single plant source contains all of the essential amino acids. You must eat multiple types of protein-rich plants to obtain all of the amino acids. For this reason, vegetarians must ensure they are including complementary proteins in their diet. *Complementary proteins* are two or more incomplete protein sources that together provide adequate amounts of all the essential amino acids.

For example, rice contains low amounts of certain essential amino acids; however, these same essential amino acids are found in greater amounts in dry beans. Similarly, dry beans contain lower amounts of other essential amino acids that are found in larger amounts in rice. Together, rice and beans provide adequate amounts of all the essential amino acids (Figure 3.4).

In the past, it was thought that complementary proteins needed to be eaten at the same meal for the body to use them together. Now studies show that the body can combine complementary proteins that are eaten at different times during the day, as long as they are eaten within the same day.

Fats

Fats are a type of nutrient that is largely made up of fatty acids, which provide a valuable source of energy. Fatty acids are a particularly important source of energy for muscles. Common fats in the diet include saturated fats, unsaturated fats, trans fats, and cholesterol.

Saturated Fats

Saturated fats are found primarily in animal-based foods, such as meat and dairy products. These are called *saturated* fats because the carbon atoms in these fats have *all* the hydrogen atoms they can hold. Saturated fats are typically solid at room temperature.

Unsaturated Fats

Unsaturated fats are found in plant-based foods such as vegetable oils, some peanut butters and margarines, olives, salad dressing, nuts, and seeds (Figure 3.5 on the next page). As you might guess, unsaturated fats do *not* have all the hydrogen atoms they could hold. They have at least one double bond to which an additional hydrogen atom can be added. Unsaturated fats are liquid at room temperature.

Trans Fats

Trans fats are created by a process known as *hydrogenation*, which bombards an unsaturated fat with hydrogen atoms and changes double bonds to single bonds. This makes the fat more saturated and, therefore, more solid. This

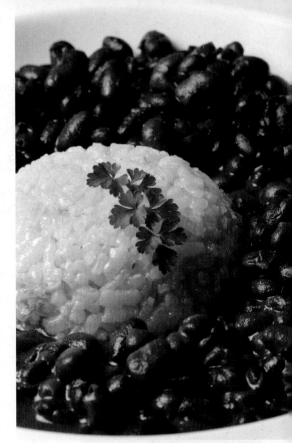

Figure 3.4

Eating enough of the right complementary proteins can provide your body with all nine essential amino acids in a day. *What are some meals you eat that might combine complementary proteins?*

fat
a type of nutrient, composed of fatty acids, that is a valuable source of energy, especially for muscles

saturated fat
a type of fat found primarily in animal-based foods that is solid at room temperature

unsaturated fat
a type of fat that is liquid at room temperature and is found in plant-based foods

trans fat
a type of fat that is created by hydrogenation; poses health risks acknowledged by the FDA

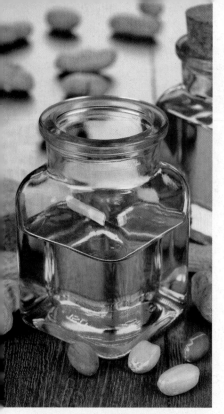

Oils and nuts both contain unsaturated fats.

type of fat is found in many processed foods, such as packaged cookies, chips, doughnuts, and crackers. You may see trans fats listed as *partially hydrogenated oils* on ingredient lists. Some trans fats occur naturally and are found in food from animals, such as cows and goats.

Cholesterol

Cholesterol is a waxy, fatlike substance that is found in foods from animal sources, but is also produced by the body. Too much cholesterol can cause health problems.

Fats: Positives and Negatives

Your body stores excess dietary fats present in the foods you eat as body fat. Despite the negative publicity that body fat gets, it is important to your body's health. Body fat

- supplies energy to the body when food is unavailable;
- acts as a cushion to protect internal organs; and
- provides a layer of insulation to help regulate body temperature so you don't get too hot or too cold.

Likewise, the dietary fats you consume play an important role in the absorption and transport of certain types of vitamins through the bloodstream. These fats also help absorb and transport other nutrients during digestion. As a bonus, dietary fats enhance the flavor and texture of foods. Eating unsaturated fats may reduce the risk of heart disease.

Although fats are important for the body to function, some fats may be better for you than others. Saturated fats tend to be associated with elevated levels of cholesterol in the blood. Diets that are high in this type of fat may cause many long-term health problems, including cardiovascular disease, stroke, some types of cancer, and diabetes. Recent studies suggest, however, that highly refined carbohydrates may have a greater effect on heart disease than saturated fat.

Some scientists believe trans fats pose worse health risks than saturated fats. Many cities and states have required restaurants to limit their use of trans fats. In 2015, the United States Food and Drug Administration (FDA) declared that trans fats were not "generally recognized as safe" (GRAS). The FDA gave food companies a period of three years to remove artificial trans fats from their food products.

Vitamins

vitamins
organic substances derived from plants or animals, which are necessary for normal growth and development

Vitamins are organic substances, meaning they are derived from plants or animals and contain carbon. Like other nutrients, vitamins are necessary for normal growth and development. They help regulate various body processes, such as blood clotting, immune system functions, and the maintenance of healthy skin. They also help the body release the energy found in proteins, fats, and carbohydrates. Different vitamins have distinct functions in the body (Figure 3.6).

Figure 3.6 Types and Functions of Vitamins

Vitamin	Function	Sources
Fat-Soluble Vitamins		
Vitamin A	helps fight infection and improve immune function, promotes bone health, supports reproduction, maintains the health of the retina	some vegetables (carrots, kale, broccoli), dairy products, meat
Vitamin K	helps with blood coagulation and blood clotting	liver, cereals, cabbage
Vitamin D	helps the body absorb calcium, which leads to strong teeth and bones; involved in regulation of cell growth, immune and neuromuscular function, and reduction of inflammation	fish, egg yolks, fortified dairy products, cereals, sunlight
Vitamin E	protects red blood cells from oxidation	whole grains, leafy greens, nuts
Water-Soluble Vitamins		
Vitamin B$_1$ (Thiamin)	helps the body change carbohydrates into energy	pork, legumes, enriched or whole-grain products, ready-to-eat cereals
Vitamin B$_2$ (Riboflavin)	involved in metabolism	milk, cheese, leafy vegetables, liver, kidneys, legumes, tomatoes, mushrooms, almonds
Vitamin B$_3$ (Niacin)	helps maintain healthy skin and nerves, and improves circulation	eggs, lean meats, nuts, poultry, legumes, avocado, potatoes
Vitamin B$_5$ (Pantothenic acid)	helps the body use nutrients for energy	beef and chicken liver, potatoes, sunflower seeds, cooked mushrooms, yogurt
Vitamin B$_6$ (Pyridoxine)	involved in the reactions that generate energy from food; is required for proper development of the brain, nerves, and skin	avocado, banana, meat, nuts, poultry, whole grains
Vitamin B$_7$ (Biotin)	assists with metabolism and the production of hormones and cholesterol	milk, nuts, pork, egg yolk, chocolate
Vitamin B$_9$ (Folic Acid)	essential to numerous bodily functions, including cell division and the growth and production of healthy red blood cells	leafy vegetables, fortified cereals, bread
Vitamin B$_{12}$ (Cyanocobalamin)	helps form red blood cells, maintain the central nervous system, and regulate metabolism	meat, eggs, milk and milk products, poultry, shellfish
Vitamin C	promotes healing within the body; is essential for healthy teeth and gums and the production of collagen	citrus fruits, many vegetables (broccoli, cabbage, spinach, and tomatoes)

Your body requires sufficient amounts of 13 different vitamins. Your body is unable to create these vitamins, so you need to absorb them from the foods you eat. Unlike carbohydrates, protein, and fat, your body requires only very small amounts of these nutrients to function properly.

Types of Vitamins

Vitamins can be divided into two distinct types—water-soluble and fat-soluble. Whether a vitamin is fat soluble or water soluble determines how it is stored and transported throughout the body.

water-soluble vitamin
a type of vitamin that dissolves in water and passes into the bloodstream

fat-soluble vitamin
a type of vitamin that dissolves in the body's fat, where it is stored for later use

Water-soluble vitamins dissolve in water, pass into the bloodstream during digestion, and are either used immediately by the body or are removed by the kidneys during urination. For this reason, these vitamins should be included in your meals every day. There are nine water-soluble vitamins—vitamin C and the B vitamins.

Fat-soluble vitamins dissolve in the body's fats and are stored in the body for later use. Because fat-soluble vitamins are stored by the body for longer periods, excessive intake may result in toxic levels. There are four fat-soluble vitamins—vitamins A, D, E, and K.

Sources of Vitamins

Where should you get your vitamins? Can't you just pop a multivitamin pill? Eating a balanced diet that contains a variety of foods can easily provide you with the appropriate amounts of all the vitamins you need.

Obtaining vitamins from your daily diet is preferable to taking vitamin supplements for several reasons. First, vitamin supplements do not contain all of the nutrients and other substances that your body needs and which are contained in foods. Some of these substances contained in food, but not in supplements, may even help your body better utilize the vitamins. Furthermore, some supplements provide larger-than-needed doses of vitamins, which may cause unhealthy levels in the body. A lesser problem with large doses of vitamins is waste—the unneeded amounts do not stay in the body and are simply excreted in the urine.

When deciding whether or not to take a vitamin supplement, you should consult your healthcare provider. People at certain life stages—such as pregnant women, infants, and older adults—and individuals who are ill may benefit from vitamin supplements. However, their healthcare providers should recommend the amount and type of supplements to take.

Minerals

mineral
inorganic elements found in soil and water; ingested by the body after being absorbed into plants

Minerals are inorganic elements that come from the earth, and which are found in soil and water. Minerals are absorbed by plants from the soil and water. You then absorb minerals from the plants you eat, the water you drink, or from animal food sources that have absorbed the minerals.

Your body needs a total of 20 different minerals (Figure 3.7). These minerals are divided into two distinct types—macrominerals and trace minerals. *Macrominerals* are those minerals your body needs in quantities greater than 100 milligrams a day to maintain good health. *Trace minerals* are those minerals your body needs in very small amounts—less than 100 milligrams daily—to stay healthy. Although only small amounts are needed, trace minerals are very important.

Your body needs minerals to grow and develop normally. People who fail to take in enough of a particular mineral experience serious health consequences, such as

osteoporosis
a dangerous condition in which bones are fragile and may break easily; can be caused by a lack of calcium during childhood and adolescence

- **osteoporosis**, a condition in which bones become fragile and may break easily, which can be caused by a lack of calcium during childhood and adolescence;

Figure 3.7 Types and Functions of Minerals

Mineral	Function	Sources
Macrominerals		
Calcium	necessary for muscle, heart, and digestive system health; builds bone and supports the synthesis and function of blood cells	dairy products, eggs, canned fish with bones (salmon, sardines), green leafy vegetables, nuts, seeds, tofu
Phosphorus	present in bones and cells; assists with energy processing and other functions	red meat, dairy foods, fish, poultry, bread, rice, oats
Magnesium	contributes to bone health; required for physiological processes in the body	raw nuts, soy beans, spinach, chard, tomatoes, beans
Sulfur	promotes metabolism and communication between nerve cells; helps the body resist bacteria and protect against toxic substances	meats, fish, poultry, eggs, milk, legumes
Sodium	helps maintain normal blood pressure; regulates the body's fluid balance	table salt (sodium chloride), milk, spinach
Chloride	assists with maintaining proper amount of bodily fluids	table salt
Potassium	assists with heart function, skeletal and muscle contraction, and digestive function	legumes, potato skin, tomatoes, bananas, papayas, lentils, dry beans, whole grains, yams, soybeans
Trace Minerals		
Iron	carries oxygen from the lungs to the tissues	red meat, leafy green vegetables, fish (tuna, salmon), eggs, dried fruits, beans, whole grains, enriched grains
Zinc	assists with immune function, reproduction, and nervous system functions	beef, pork, lamb, nuts, whole grains
Iodine	assists with making thyroid hormones	table salt, some types of fish (cod, sea bass, perch, haddock), dairy products
Selenium	protects cells from damage and regulates thyroid hormone action and other processes	vegetables, fish, red meat, grains, eggs, chicken
Copper	assists with metabolism and red blood cell formation; helps with the production of energy for cells	shellfish, whole grains, beans, nuts, potatoes, dried fruits, cocoa
Manganese	assists with bone formation, metabolism, and wound healing	nuts, legumes, seeds, whole grains, tea, leafy green vegetables
Fluoride	prevents dental cavities and stimulates new bone formation	fluoridated water, most seafood, tea, gelatin
Chromium	helps maintain normal blood sugar (glucose) levels	beef, liver, eggs, chicken, apples, bananas, spinach, green peppers
Molybdenum	helps the body process proteins and other substances	legumes, grains, leafy vegetables, liver, nuts

- *anemia*, a condition that causes weakness, fatigue, and headaches, which occurs when people do not take in enough iron; and

- *cretinism*, a severe birth defect that is caused by a lack of iodine during pregnancy.

As with vitamins, eating a nutritious and balanced diet generally provides all of the minerals your body needs.

anemia
a condition causing weakness, tiredness, and headaches; results from decrease in red blood cells or insufficient hemoglobin

Jessica is 15 years old and a sophomore in high school. She is very busy with many activities—performing in the choir, volunteering with Big Brothers/Big Sisters, and playing on the junior varsity softball team. She often finds herself eating in the car as she races from one activity to another. Because Jessica is a vegetarian, she typically eats lots of carbohydrates (such as breads and pasta), vegetables, and fruits.

Over the last few months, Jessica has found herself feeling very tired and out of breath during softball practice. She even finds herself struggling to climb a flight of stairs. She is also having regular headaches.

Jessica's parents took her to the doctor to figure out what was causing her to feel so tired. Blood work revealed that Jessica is showing signs of anemia, which is caused by a deficiency of iron in her blood. She is now making changes to her diet in an effort to take in more iron in the foods she eats. Jessica is also taking an iron supplement.

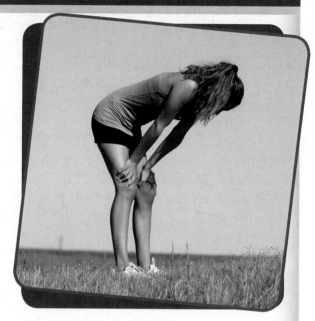

Thinking Critically

1. What do you think are the primary factors that led Jessica to become anemic?

2. What are some strategies that you think could help Jessica eat more nutritious foods, including more foods that are high in iron?

3. What advice would you give other teenagers who find themselves in the same situation as Jessica to help prevent them from adopting unhealthy eating habits?

Water

Water is necessary for most bodily functions. In fact, although people can live for several weeks, and even months, without taking in any other type of nutrients, they can survive only a few days without water.

Water helps your body in a number of ways, including

- maintaining a normal temperature;
- cushioning and lubricating your joints;
- protecting your spinal cord and other sensitive tissues;
- getting rid of wastes (through urination, perspiration, and bowel movements); and
- moving oxygen, nutrients, wastes, and other materials throughout the body.

dehydration
a condition in which the body's tissues lose too much water

Because your body loses water every day through urination, sweat, and even exhaling breath, you need to ingest water to replace what your body loses and prevent dehydration. *Dehydration* is a dangerous condition in which the body's tissues lose too much water. Without enough water, the body cannot cool itself, and blood pressure can drop dangerously low as water leaves the blood.

Individuals should drink 8½ to 11½ cups of fluids per day to maintain adequate water in the body. Most of your water needs are met through the water and other beverages you drink. However, you can also get some fluid through the foods you eat. For example, eating broth soups and other foods that have high water content is a great way to replenish a depleted water supply. Foods such as celery, tomatoes, apples, oranges, and melons have high water content.

Fluid needs can change. For instance, women who are pregnant or lactating have increased fluid requirements. Infants also have a greater need for fluids. Although older adults may experience a decreased sensation of thirst, their fluid needs are the same as when they were younger.

Under normal conditions, most people can maintain appropriate amounts of water in their body simply by drinking when they are thirsty and when they are eating a meal. Some conditions, however, may require additional fluids to maintain hydration. Specifically, your body needs more water when you are

- outside in hot weather for a long period of time,

- engaging in vigorous physical activity (Figure 3.8),

- running a fever, or

- experiencing diarrhea or vomiting.

Feeling thirsty is a signal that your body needs more water. If possible, drink enough water to prevent the experience of feeling thirsty.

Figure 3.8

Drinking water even before you are thirsty will keep your body hydrated. *What tools could you use to remind yourself to drink water before your body feels thirsty?*

Lesson 3.1 Review

Know and Understand Assess

1. Name the six types of nutrients.
2. Explain the difference between glucose and glycogen.
3. Describe the role of protein in the body.
4. List three functions of body fat.
5. How are minerals categorized as either *macro* or *trace*?
6. List at least four conditions in which the body needs more than the usual amount of water.

Analyze and Apply

7. Compare and contrast saturated fats and unsaturated fats.
8. Analyze the importance of fiber in the diet.

Real World Health

Revisit the Before You Read activity at the beginning of this lesson. For any of your favorite foods that have few nutrients, suggest two healthier options that you can eat instead. Explain why each option is healthier using information from the lesson, or do your own research to justify your response.

Lesson 3.2

Creating a Healthy Eating Plan

Key Terms E-Flash Cards

In this lesson, you will learn the meanings of the following key terms.

calorie

metabolism

nutrient-dense food

overnutrition

undernutrition

Lesson Objectives

After studying this lesson, you will be able to

- interpret the key concepts from the *Dietary Guidelines for Americans*;
- summarize recommendations from the MyPlate food guidance system; and
- analyze the hazards of poor nutrition.

Before You Read

Healthy Choices Mindmap

Place the phrase healthy food choices *in the middle of a mindmap similar to the one shown here. Brainstorm to create a mindmap about this important phrase. What phrases, key terms, or bodily functions are related to the foods that you choose to eat?*

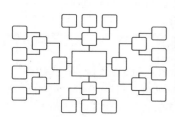

Warm-Up Activity

Food Influences
Using a graphic organizer similar to the one shown here, list six factors that influence your food choices and six benefits of a healthy diet.

FACTORS	BENEFITS
1. _____	1. _____
2. _____	2. _____
3. _____	3. _____
4. _____	4. _____
5. _____	5. _____
6. _____	6. _____

When you eat nutritious foods today, you lower your risk of developing diseases later in life. People who follow a healthy eating plan and maintain a healthy body weight are less likely to develop serious illnesses such as heart disease, high blood pressure, diabetes, stroke, and cancer. Eating a nutritious diet also prevents health problems such as obesity, cavities, iron deficiency, and osteoporosis.

Overall, the body needs about 45 different nutrients per day. This is why eating a varied diet full of nutritious foods is important for maintaining good health.

A healthy eating plan includes foods that supply the amounts and types of nutrients your body needs to be healthy. In this section, you will learn how to make smart food choices and how to create a balanced diet. You will also learn about the hazards of poor nutrition.

Dietary Guidelines

The United States Departments of Agriculture (USDA) and Health and Human Services (HHS) publish the *Dietary Guidelines for Americans*, which is revised every five years. The *Dietary Guidelines* provides recommendations for establishing eating patterns to promote health. The guidelines promote five key concepts:

- Follow a healthy eating pattern across the life span.
- Focus on variety, nutrient density, and amount.
- Limit calories from added sugars and saturated fats and reduce sodium intake.
- Shift to healthier food and beverage choices.
- Support healthy eating patterns for all.

Meet Needs Within Calorie Limits

As you learned earlier in this chapter, nutrients provide the body with the energy it needs to function. The energy provided by food is measured in a unit called a *calorie*. Foods that provide larger amounts of energy are higher in calories than foods that provide smaller amounts of energy.

calorie
a unit of measurement for energy provided by food

Some types of nutrients provide more calories than others (Figure 3.9 on the next page). Carbohydrates and protein each provide 4 calories per gram. Fats provide 9 calories per gram, more than any other source.

Your calorie balance in a given day is determined by two factors:

- the number of calories you consume through eating and drinking (this is energy *in* to your body)
- the number of calories you burn through the work of your *metabolism* and your daily physical activities (this is energy *out* of your body)

metabolism
the rate at which the body uses energy

Your body burns calories to perform the many functions of your metabolism that keep you alive, such as eating, sleeping, and breathing. You also burn calories in the course of daily life—while walking to class, lifting a heavy backpack, and cleaning your room.

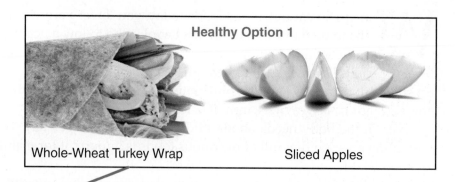

Healthy Option 1

Whole-Wheat Turkey Wrap   Sliced Apples

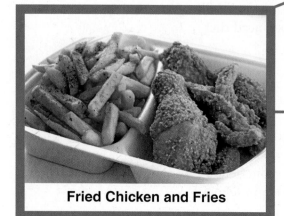

Fried Chicken and Fries

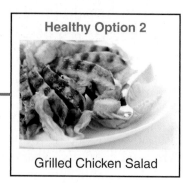

Healthy Option 2

Grilled Chicken Salad

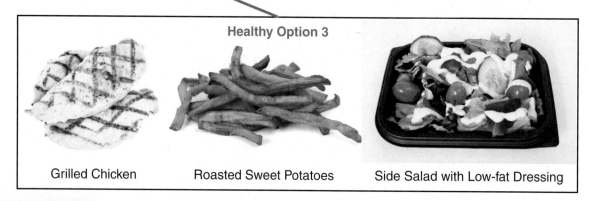

Healthy Option 3

Grilled Chicken   Roasted Sweet Potatoes   Side Salad with Low-fat Dressing

---

Figure 3.9

You can use your new knowledge of nutrition to "make over" meals and eat healthier.

Maintaining Weight. You can maintain your weight by balancing calories consumed with calories burned throughout the day.

Calories in = Calories burned

Gaining Weight. When you consume more calories than your body burns, an energy imbalance occurs. The number of calories you take in and burn doesn't have to balance each day. If you take in more calories than you burn over time, however, you will gain weight. Those extra calories are stored in the body (mostly as fat).

Calories in > Calories burned

Losing Weight. An energy imbalance also occurs if, over time, you burn more calories than you take in. As you can probably guess, if you burn more than you consume, you will lose weight.

Calories in < Calories burned

Factors That Influence Your Calorie Needs. The number of calories you need to take in each day depends on different factors, including age, gender, height, weight, and level of physical activity (Figure 3.10). For example, older people typically don't need to consume as many calories as younger people, men have greater calorie needs than women, and people who are physically active burn more calories than those who are less active.

Shift to Nutrient-Dense Foods

Calorie balance is only part of the equation. A healthy diet requires that the foods you choose are nutrient dense. The *Dietary Guidelines* defines **nutrient-dense foods** as foods that provide vitamins, minerals, and other substances that contribute to adequate nutrient intakes or may have positive health effects, with little or no solid fats and added sugars, refined starches, and sodium.

In addition to focusing on nutrient-dense foods, you should also avoid or limit intake of foods that contain solid fats, added sugars, refined grains, and sodium.

Consider the following examples of ways to consume approximately 100 calories:

- A medium-sized apple contains about 100 calories. These calories mostly come from naturally occurring sugars in the apple. In addition to calories, the apple supplies your body with fiber, vitamins, and minerals.

- An 8-ounce glass of a sugary soda (about two-thirds of a can) also contains about 100 calories. These calories come from the added sugars in this drink—there are 10 teaspoons of sugar in a 12-ounce can of soda. However, there is little to no nutrient value in this soda.

Your body benefits more in terms of nutrients when you eat an apple than when you drink a soda, even though both choices provide 100 calories.

Avoid "Empty Calories." The added sugars and solid fats found in some foods are called "empty calories." These sugars and fats are called *empty calories* because they supply few, if any, nutrients to a person's diet.

Calories from added sugars and solid fats contribute up to 40% of daily calories for children and teenagers (2 to 18 years of age). Approximately half of those calories come from six sources: soda, fruit drinks, dairy desserts (such as cheesecake or ice cream), grain desserts (such as cookies or cake), pizza (with meat), and whole milk.

The most common pizza choices and whole milk supply needed nutrients such as calcium and vitamins, but they also contain many "empty calories" from solid fats. More nutrient-dense options are veggie pizza with whole-grain crust and nonfat milk.

Figure 3.10 Recommended Daily Calorie Intake

Age	Male/ Moderately Active	Female/ Moderately Active
	Calories	
10	1,800	1,800
11	2,000	1,800
12	2,200	2,000
13	2,200	2,000
14	2,400	2,000
15	2,600	2,000
16	2,800	2,000
17	2,800	2,000
18	2,800	2,000
19–20	2,800	2,200
21–25	2,800	2,200
26–30	2,600	2,000
31–35	2,600	2,000
36–40	2,600	2,000
41–45	2,600	2,000
46–50	2,400	2,000
51–55	2,400	1,800
56–60	2,400	1,800
61–65	2,400	1,800

nutrient-dense food
a relatively low-calorie food that provides vitamins, minerals, and other healthful substances

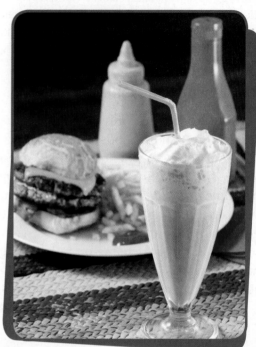

In a recent study, researchers wanted to examine the effects of food logos and packaging on children's taste preferences. The study sought to discover if children believe that food from McDonald's tastes better than the same food from a grocery store.

Researchers asked 63 children (from 3 and 5 years of age) to taste five different foods: chicken nuggets, a hamburger, French fries, baby carrots, and milk. The chicken nuggets, hamburger, and French fries were all from McDonald's. The carrots and milk were from a grocery store.

Each type of food was divided into two portions. One portion was wrapped in a McDonald's wrapper or placed in a McDonald's bag. The second portion was given to the children in a wrapper or bag without the McDonald's logo. Therefore, the children tasted each of the five types of foods twice—once in McDonald's packaging and once with generic packaging.

Can you guess what these researchers found? Overall, children preferred the taste of foods and drinks they thought were from McDonald's. After taste-testing, the children said the chicken nuggets, fries, carrots, and milk wrapped in the McDonald's logo tasted better than the foods in grocery store packaging, even though the foods were exactly the same.

Thinking Critically

1. What factors do you think contribute to children's belief that food from McDonald's tastes better? What role is played by family, society, and the media in the formation of this belief?

2. The children in this study were very young. Do you think researchers would find the same results with older children and teenagers? Why or why not?

3. What are the consequences of the children's beliefs about McDonald's food? Can you think of strategies for changing such beliefs? Do you think such efforts could be effective?

Consider How Food Is Prepared. The way food is prepared also influences the number of calories it contains. Fried foods, for example, have more calories than baked or raw foods because the fried food absorbs oil or butter while frying. A grilled chicken leg has 60 calories whereas a fried chicken leg has 130 calories. Something as simple as the method of food preparation can cause the food's calories to double.

Food can also provide different nutrients depending on how it is served. For example, apples with their skins on have more fiber than peeled apples. This is one reason why eating an apple is better for you than eating applesauce or drinking apple juice. By peeling and processing fruits and vegetables, you are removing some of their nutrients. Leaving the skin or peel on gives you a much more nutritious option (Figure 3.11).

Chips (fried in oil)	Mashed (with whole milk and butter)	Baked (without butter or sour cream)
Fiber	5%*	13%	18%
Total Fat	16%	14%	0

* percentages are daily recommended amounts

Figure 3.11

Potatoes can be prepared many different ways, including mashing, baking, and frying. *Which of these potato options is the most nutritious? the least nutritious? Why?*

Healthy Eating Patterns

Healthy eating patterns must be supported in all settings, including the home, school, work, and community. There are a number of guides available to help individuals implement healthy eating patterns. For example, the USDA food patterns discussed in the *Dietary Guidelines* can help people trying to maintain calorie balance and focus on nutrient-dense foods. The USDA food patterns serve as the basis for the MyPlate food guidance system.

MyPlate Food Guidance System

In 2011, the USDA created the MyPlate food guidance system to help individuals put the *Dietary Guidelines* into practice (Figure 3.12). The MyPlate graphic is designed to remind people about the proportion of different foods they should eat at a meal.

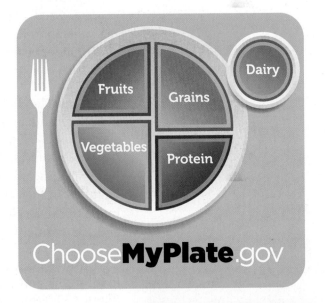

Food Groups

The MyPlate diagram includes the five food groups: fruits, vegetables, grains, protein foods, and dairy. Oils are not included on the MyPlate graphic because they are not considered a food group. Oils are, however, a necessary part of a healthful diet as well.

Figure 3.12

MyPlate illustrates the recommended proportions of the different food groups that people should eat in a day. *How much does your daily diet align with these suggestions? What food groups should you eat more of? less of?*

Fruits. Foods in the fruit group are often good sources of nutrients many diets are lacking, such as potassium, fiber, vitamin C, and folic acid. Fresh, frozen, canned, and dried fruits, as well as fruit juices, are included in this group. Fruit juices, however, lack the fiber found in whole fruits, and are not as nutrient dense as whole fruits. For this reason, whole fruits should be selected more often than juice.

Grains. This group includes foods made from wheat, rice, oats, cornmeal, barley, or other cereal grains. Foods in the grains group are classified as either whole grains or refined grains.

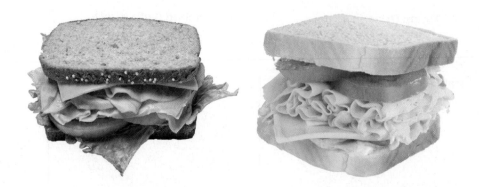

Figure 3.13

These two turkey and cheese sandwiches look very similar, but one is healthier than the other. Why?

A food is considered *whole grain* if it contains the entire grain kernel—the bran, germ, and endosperm (Figure 3.13). *Refined grains* have been processed to produce a finer texture and improved shelf life, and no longer contain the whole kernel.

Examples of whole grains include brown rice, oatmeal, whole-wheat bread, and wild rice. Examples of refined grains include couscous, crackers, and white bread.

Vegetables. Most foods in the vegetables group are naturally low in fat and calories, and are important sources of many nutrients, including potassium, fiber, folic acid, and vitamins A and C. By definition, this means vegetables are often very nutrient dense. Vegetables may be fresh, frozen, canned, dried, raw, cooked, whole, cut up, or juiced.

Vegetables are divided into five subgroups—dark green, starchy, red and orange, beans and peas, and other. You should consume vegetables from each of these groups every week.

Dairy. The dairy group includes many foods that are high in calcium, including milk and foods made from milk such as cheese and yogurt. You should choose foods in this group that are low fat or fat free.

Foods such as cream and butter, which are made from milk, but contain little calcium, are not included in this group. Calcium-fortified soy milk is included in this dairy group as an option for individuals who are lactose intolerant. Dairy foods are often good sources of potassium and protein, and are frequently fortified with vitamin D.

Protein Foods. The protein foods group includes meat, poultry, seafood, beans and peas, eggs, processed soy products, and nuts and seeds (Figure 3.14). Including a variety of protein foods in your meal plan each

Figure 3.14 Protein Content of Various Foods	
Food Type	**Grams of Protein**
1 cup of milk	8
1 cup of cooked dry beans	16
3-ounce piece of meat	21
8-ounce container of yogurt	11

Figure 3.15 Recommended Protein Dietary Allowance by Age

Age (in years)	Grams of Protein Needed Daily
children ages 1–3	13
children ages 4–8	19
children ages 9–13	34
girls ages 14–18	46
boys ages 14–18	52
women ages 19–70+	46
men ages 19–70+	56

week improves your nutrient intake and supplies health benefits. The *Dietary Guidelines* recommend that you include at least eight ounces of cooked seafood in your meal plan each week (Figure 3.15).

In addition to protein, foods in this group may supply niacin, thiamin, riboflavin, B_6, vitamin E, iron, zinc, and magnesium. Some seafood contains fats believed to reduce the risk of heart disease. Plant-based proteins are often rich in fiber.

Some animal-based proteins are high in saturated fats and cholesterol, which may increase the risk for heart disease. For this reason, you should select cuts of meat and poultry that are lean or low fat more often.

Women who are pregnant or breastfeeding should avoid seafood that is high in mercury such as shark, swordfish, tilefish, and King mackerel, and limit canned white tuna (albacore) to less than six ounces per week.

Oils. Oils are not considered a food group, but do provide essential nutrients and must be included in your diet. Oils are naturally present in many plants and fish. Often the oil is extracted from a food source and sold as liquid oil. For instance, olive oil is extracted from olives. Other examples of oils include corn oil and canola oil. Avocados, nuts, and some fish are common sources of oils that are typically included in the diet.

Oils are unsaturated fats and are, as you read earlier, typically liquid at room temperature. Saturated fats, however, are not oils and come from animal sources. Saturated fats commonly found in the diet include butter, milk fat, beef fat, pork fat, and poultry fat. Saturated fat in the diet may contribute to chronic health conditions such as heart disease.

Recommended Amounts

The MyPlate food guidance system provides tools to help you develop a personalized food plan. This daily food plan outlines the amounts you should consume from each food group and provides information for making nutrient-dense choices.

The amount of food you need from each of the food groups is affected by the factors discussed earlier—age, gender, height, weight, and level of physical activity. Other factors such as health conditions, pregnancy, and lactation can affect your nutrient needs as well.

Personal Profile

Are You at Risk of Poor Nutrition?

These questions will help you assess how much you are putting your own health at risk by practicing poor eating habits.

I rarely drink soda and sugar-sweetened drinks. **yes no**

I limit how often I eat foods that are high in salt. **yes no**

I drink skim or low-fat milk every day. **yes no**

I drink at least 8½ to 11½ cups of water or other fluids a day. **yes no**

I limit or avoid saturated fats such as butter, cream, and cheese. **yes no**

I eat at least 2½ cups of fruits and vegetables each day. **yes no**

I eat foods that are high in whole grains—such as brown rice, oatmeal, and whole-wheat bread—at least once a day. **yes no**

I choose meats that are leaner cuts and trim away the fat and skin. **yes no**

I eat at least 8 ounces of fish or seafood each week. **yes no**

I choose beans or peas (legumes) as a main dish at least once a week. **yes no**

Add up the number of yes answers to assess your eating habits. The more yes answers, the lower your risk for poor nutrition.

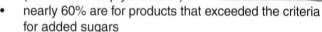

Health in the Media

Advertisements for Unhealthy Foods

The average child watching children's television programming sees an estimated 10,000 TV commercials for food products in a year. Unfortunately, most of these advertisements are for foods with poor nutritional content.

- about 91% are for foods or beverages that are high in fat, sodium, or added sugars (foods with "empty calories")
- nearly 60% are for products that exceeded the criteria for added sugars
- about 20% exceeded other guidelines, including those for total fat, saturated plus trans fat, and sodium
- none of the advertisements are for beverages that meet nutritional guidelines

Not surprisingly, children who see advertisements for unhealthy food on TV are more likely to want to eat high-fat and high-sugar foods. Researchers in one study showed children an episode of a popular cartoon. Some children saw five minutes of commercials for toys before the cartoon, while another group saw five minutes of commercials for snacks and fast food.

After watching the cartoon, researchers gave the children a list of various food items and asked them to choose which ones they would like to eat. The children who saw the food commercials were more likely to pick unhealthy foods than children who saw the toy commercials.

Thinking Critically

1. Present a convincing argument for reducing the number of unhealthy food advertisements shown on television. Cite evidence from the study mentioned above and this chapter. Incorporate your argument into a letter to your congressperson asking him or her to support these efforts.

2. Generate a list of strategies that could be used to avoid the influence of these advertisements.

undernutrition
a condition in which the body takes in too few nutrients for health and growth

overnutrition
a condition in which the body takes in too much of some nutrients or too many calories

Poor Nutrition

Healthy eating plans identify the amounts and types of food individuals should consume to obtain the nutrients needed for good health. These plans have been developed to help individuals avoid the problems associated with poor nutrition, or malnutrition, which includes both undernutrition and overnutrition.

Undernutrition

When people do not receive the needed nutrients from the food they eat, they experience *undernutrition.* This means they take in too few nutrients for health and growth.

Healthy eating is especially important for children and teenagers, since the body undergoes considerable growth and development during these life stages. Undernutrition can lead to growth problems; children who don't receive enough nutrients may never reach their full height. Undernutrition can also lead to serious and even life-threatening problems, including brain damage, impaired vision and blindness, and bone deformities.

Undernutrition during pregnancy affects the health of the fetus. When a woman who is pregnant doesn't consume sufficient nutrients, the growing fetus may not receive enough nutrients to develop properly.

Overnutrition

Although many people think about poor health in terms of not getting *enough* nutrients, poor health can also be caused by consuming *too much* of some nutrients. This type of *overnutrition* is often caused by people eating too many foods that contain high amounts of added sugar, solid fat, sodium, or refined carbohydrates, or simply too many calories.

Foods high in solid fats, added sugars, refined grains, and sodium are believed to contribute to a variety of health conditions. For instance, evidence suggests that as an individual's sodium intake decreases, so does his or her blood pressure. Maintaining a normal blood pressure reduces the risk of heart and kidney diseases.

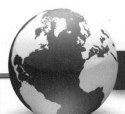

Local and Global Health
Nutrition

Good nutrition is essential for normal health and development. Children who eat well-balanced diets do better in school, have fewer illnesses, and are more likely to become healthy adults.

Sadly, an estimated 93 million children under five years of age are undernourished worldwide. Undernutrition is defined as both a lack of calories and an inadequate amount of nutrition.

Undernutrition is caused by a number of different factors, including

- poverty, which leads to a lack of money to buy food;
- disease, which can cause a problem absorbing nutrients;
- food shortages, which can be caused by agricultural productivity issues; and
- dietary practices, such as an overreliance on a single food source (for example, corn or rice).

Undernourished children have a lowered resistance to infection and are more likely to die from common childhood illnesses, such as diarrhea and respiratory infections. More than a third of child deaths worldwide are caused by a lack of nourishment, with approximately 6 million children dying of hunger each year.

Percentage of Child Underweight in Selected Countries			
Country	Percentage	Country	Percentage
Bangladesh	32.6	Rwanda	9.3
Pakistan	31.6	China	3.4
India	29.4	Morocco	3.1
Ethiopia	25.2	Peru	3.1
Afghanistan	25	Mexico	2.8
Cambodia	23.9	Germany	1.1
Kenya	11	United States	0.5

Thinking Critically

1. What do you believe are the primary causes of the widely different rates of undernutrition in different countries? Explain your answer.
2. How do you think the rates of undernutrition in different countries will change over time? What are some factors that might cause rates of undernutrition to increase in a given country? to decrease?
3. What strategies could the US government or other governments take to decrease the rate of childhood undernutrition in their countries and worldwide? Which strategies would you support? Which would you oppose?

Lesson 3.2 Review

Know and Understand Assess

1. What are the five key concepts communicated in the *Dietary Guidelines*?
2. List five factors that affect the number of calories needed by an individual.
3. List the five vegetable subgroups and provide an example of your favorite vegetable for each subgroup.
4. Describe how undernutrition during pregnancy affects the fetus.

Analyze and Apply

5. Analyze a typical meal that you eat using the recommendations from the MyPlate food guidance system. How does your meal rate?

6. Evaluate why an individual must select nutrient-dense foods to consume a healthy diet.

Real World Health

Now that you have learned about nutritional recommendations, use the MyPlate website to evaluate your own nutritional and energy needs. How much of each food group should you eat per day? How does this compare to your current eating habits? Analyze how your nutrition can affect your total wellness, including all dimensions of your health.

Food Labels and Food Safety

Key Terms E-Flash Cards

In this lesson, you will learn the meanings of the following key terms.

Daily Values
food additives
food allergy
Food and Drug Admin-
   istration (FDA)
food intolerance
foodborne illness
foodborne infection
foodborne intoxication
generally recognized as
   safe (GRAS)
gluten
organic food

Before You Read

Healthy Food Decisions

List the five facts that you think are most important for a person to look for on a food label when deciding whether or not to eat that particular food. Based on food labels that you have read, do you think there are foods that we should never eat? Why or why not?

Lesson Objectives

After studying this lesson, you will be able to

- analyze a Nutrition Facts label to identify the nutritional value of a food product;
- describe how the order of ingredients is determined on a food label;
- understand the use of claims on food labels;
- describe the consequences of unsafe food handling;
- differentiate between the different types of foodborne illnesses;
- recognize steps to prevent foodborne illnesses; and
- distinguish between food intolerances and food allergies.

Warm-Up Activity

Portion Sizes

Many of us underestimate the amount of food that we eat in a given meal. Analyze the difference between serving sizes and portion sizes, such as those shown in the samples below. Then, identify three strategies to reduce portion sizes to the actual recommended serving sizes.

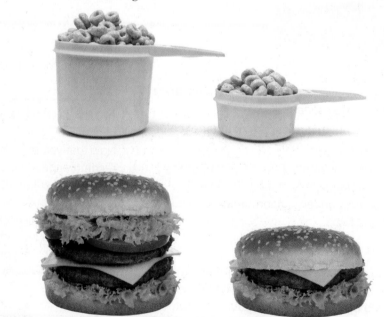

The goal of making good food choices is to provide the right amount of nutrients for your body. Another goal is to make sure the foods and beverages you put into your body are safe.

One of the most helpful strategies for making good food choices is to carefully read the information provided on a packaged food label. These labels contain valuable information about that food, such as how long it will remain fresh, how it should be stored, and the type of nutrients it provides. This section will focus on the important information provided on food labels and how you can avoid becoming ill from the foods you eat.

Daily Values
the recommended amounts of nutrients that a person should consume each day

Understanding Nutrition Facts Labels

To help consumers make good choices about what they eat, the FDA requires any food sold in a package to include a Nutrition Facts label (Figure 3.16). Certain pieces of information are required to be printed on the Nutrition Facts label, including

- serving size (the volume or weight of a single serving of the food);
- number of servings in a package;
- number of calories in each serving;
- amount of different nutrients (including fat, cholesterol, sodium, carbohydrates, fibers, sugars, protein, and some vitamins and minerals) in a serving; and
- percent of daily values for the different nutrients provided in a serving.

The Nutrition Facts label was updated, effective July 2018, to reflect revised serving sizes and include amounts of added sugars, vitamin D, and potassium.

Daily Values

Daily Values are the recommended intake amounts for specific nutrients. The Daily Values for a 2,000-calorie diet are used to calculate the Percent (%) Daily Values for the nutrients on the Nutrition Facts panel. These percentages, therefore, could be higher or lower depending on an individual's daily calorie needs.

The % Daily Value signals whether a serving of food contributes a lot or a little of a particular nutrient to your total daily diet. For example, suppose a food item's % Daily Value for calcium is 20. That means one serving of the food supplies 20% of the daily requirement for calcium for an individual on a 2,000-calorie diet.

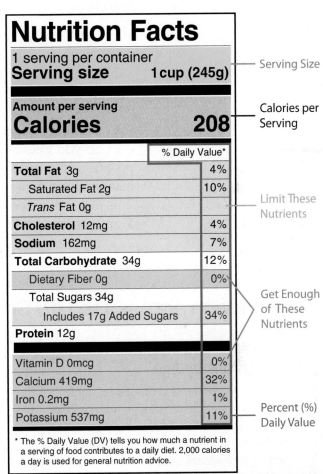

Figure 3.16

Effective July 2018, this new Nutrition Facts label lists added sugars, vitamin D, and potassium. *How does this Nutrition Facts label compare to labels printed before July 2018?*

The % Daily Values can be used to evaluate the overall nutritional quality of a food. Some of the nutrients listed on the label, such as dietary fiber and calcium, are beneficial. Greater % Daily Values for these beneficial nutrients indicate better nutritional value of the food. Other nutrients, such as saturated fat and sodium, should be limited so lower % Daily Values are desirable. Use the following guidelines to interpret % Daily Values:

- 5% or less is low—aim for this when eating total fat, saturated fat, trans fat, cholesterol, and sodium
- 20% or more is high—aim for this when eating dietary fiber, calcium, iron, vitamin D, and potassium

Servings

When you are reading Nutrition Facts labels, remember to check the number of servings provided in the container first. The amount and % Daily Value of nutrients are based on a single serving size, but people may consume more than just a single serving. For example, if the package contains two servings and you consume the entire package, then you have consumed twice the number of calories and nutrients reported in the Nutrition Facts label.

Can you guess how many servings are in a pint of ice cream? Many people would guess one 2-cup serving or two 1-cup servings. Ice cream manufacturers, however, describe a pint of ice cream as three ⅔-cup servings. This means that the calories listed for a single serving of ice cream from a 1-pint container reflect only one-third of the container.

Health across the Life Span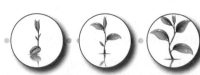

Recommended Macronutrient Proportions by Age

The recommended ranges (at right) for the percentage of calories from protein, carbohydrates, and fat in a diet were established by the Institutes of Medicine. Total calories vary among individuals based on a number of factors including age, gender, height, weight, and level of physical activity.

Analyzing Data

1. According to this table, which age group has the highest recommended percentage of calories from protein?

2. Based on these recommendations, do two-year-olds need the same number of calories per day from carbohydrates as 19-year-olds? Explain your answer.

Age Group	Total Calories		
	% Carbohydrate	% Protein	% Fat
young children (1 to 3 years of age)	45–65%	5–20%	30–40%
older children and adolescents (4 to 18 years of age)	45–65%	10–30%	25–35%
adults (19 years of age and older)	45–65%	10–35%	20–35%

Ingredients in Foods

The information on a food label also includes all the ingredients that were used to make that food. These ingredients are listed in the order in which they contribute weight to a given product. Ingredients that are listed first make up a greater amount of the final product by weight than ingredients that appear near the end of the list. In other words, the closer the ingredient appears to the top of the list, the more of that ingredient in the food (Figure 3.17).

Ingredient Names. Food manufacturers often list ingredients in somewhat confusing ways. This makes it harder to determine exactly what foods are in the product. For example, many different ingredients can add sugar to a food product. All of the following terms can be used to describe sugar that has been added to a food: *corn syrup, corn sweetener, fructose, dextrose, high fructose corn syrup, lactose, maltose, sucrose, malt syrup, molasses, honey, glucose,* and *fruit juice concentrate.* If you see any of these in the ingredient list, you know the food contains added sugars.

Let's take a real-world example to illustrate how different terms for sugar can be used in describing ingredients in a given product. One of the best-selling cereals in the United States lists the following five ingredients first on its nutrition label:

- whole-grain oats
- sugar
- modified corn starch
- honey
- brown sugar syrup

As you can see from this list, four of the top five ingredients are a type of sugar. Can you guess what the sixth ingredient is? Salt. Do you think you might be able to find a more nutrient-dense cereal?

Food Additives. Often food manufacturers add sugar, salt, or other ingredients to extend their product's shelf life, improve its flavor, and for other reasons. Substances that are added to food products to cause desired changes are called *food additives*.

The government regulates food additives and maintains a list of food additives that have proven to be safe. Additives on this list are *generally recognized as safe (GRAS)*. Food manufacturers must obtain approval from the *Food and Drug Administration (FDA)* to use substances that do not appear on the GRAS list.

Food additives must be included in the product's ingredient list. If your goal is to avoid specific food additives, you can find them on the ingredient lists on food labels.

Claims on Labels

Sometimes food labels describe a particular food using a specific claim about its health benefits. For example, a label might describe a food as "low

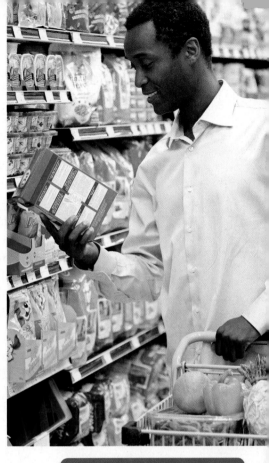

Figure 3.17

Food labels contain a great deal of information. *Do you take advantage of having this information at your fingertips? Why or why not?*

food additives
substances added to food products to cause desired changes

generally recognized as safe (GRAS)
food additives that have been studied and are considered harmless by the government

Food and Drug Administration (FDA)
a government agency that regulates medications, biological products, medical devices, food supply, cosmetics, and radiation-emitting products

fat" or "reduced calories." If these terms are being used, the food must meet certain criteria established by the FDA.

For example, a food described as "low fat" must not contain more than three grams of fat in a single serving. Similarly, the FDA allows manufacturers to state on the label that a food may reduce the risk of heart disease if that food is made up of at least 51% whole-grain ingredients and is low in total fat, saturated fat, and cholesterol.

It is important to understand that even low-fat versions of some foods contain a fair amount of fat. For example, a cup of plain yogurt made with whole milk has 7 grams of fat, whereas a cup made with low-fat milk has 4 grams of fat. Obviously 4 grams of fat is better than 7, but a cup of plain yogurt made from skim milk contains 0 grams of fat. Sometimes ingredients can make all the difference when choosing a more healthful snack option (Figure 3.18).

A food that is described on the label as "organic" also must meet certain criteria. *Organic food* must consist of at least 95% organically produced ingredients. Organic foods must be grown without using any fertilizers or pesticides made from manufactured chemicals, sewage sludge, bioengineering, or high-energy radiation. The United States Department of Agriculture (USDA) created the standards that must be met for food products to be labeled "organic."

Individuals may purchase organic foods for a variety of reasons. Some people are trying to avoid consuming pesticides, hormones, or other substances that are used in the production of nonorganic foods. Others may choose organic foods because they believe these foods are more nutritious; however, research has not yet confirmed this notion.

organic food
a type of food that is produced without pesticides, bioengineering, or high-energy radiation

Figure 3.18 Making More Healthful Food Choices

Less Healthful Choice	More Healthful Alternative
whole milk	low-fat (1%), reduced-fat (2%), or fat-free (skim) milk
ice cream	sorbet, sherbet, fruit smoothie, low-fat ice cream, or fat-free frozen yogurt
pasta with white or cheese sauce	whole-grain pasta with red sauce (marinara) or vegetables (primavera)
cream soups	broth-based soups
donuts, muffins, scones, or pastries	whole-grain English muffins or bagels
cheese	reduced-fat or fat-free cheese
white bread or hamburger bun	whole-grain bread or bun
sour cream	plain, low-fat Greek yogurt
bacon or sausage	Canadian bacon or lean ham
potato chips	popcorn (air-popped or light microwaved), roasted chickpeas, fruits, vegetables
regular ground beef	extra-lean ground beef such as ground round, or ground turkey breast
butter or margarine on toast or bread	fruit spread, jam, or honey on whole-grain bread or toast
frozen breaded fish or fried fish	unbreaded fish or shellfish poached, steamed, or broiled
regular margarine or butter	light spread margarines or olive oil
granola or sweetened breakfast cereal	bran flakes, crispy rice, grits, oatmeal, or reduced-fat granola
deep-dish pepperoni pizza	thin, whole-grain crust veggie pizza
sugar-sweetened soda	seltzer with lime wedge

Improving the Nutrition in Your Diet

The strategies listed below can help you increase the level of nutrition in your own diet.

- Vary your fruit choices to benefit from a wider array of nutrients.

- Select potassium-rich vegetables such as sweet potatoes, tomato products, lentils, and kidney beans often.

- Try to eat two vegetables (choose dark green, red, or orange vegetables often) with your evening meal.

- Make a meal around dried beans or peas (legumes) instead of meat. Substitute pinto or black beans for meat in chili and tacos.

- Include low-fat or nonfat milk or calcium-fortified soy milk as a beverage with meals.

- Substitute whole-grain flour for up to half of the flour called for in pancake, waffle, and other recipes.

- Drink water instead of sugar-sweetened beverages.

- Have a piece of fruit for dessert and skip desserts with added sugar.

- Choose leaner cuts of red meat that include "round" or "loin" in the name and trim away any fat you can see. For chicken and turkey, remove the skin to reduce fat.

- Include fish or seafood high in omega-3 fatty acids such as salmon, trout, or herring in your diet each week.

- Choose whole-grain, unsweetened, ready-to-eat cereals or oatmeal for breakfast.

When Food Causes Illness

Foodborne illness, or *food poisoning*, refers to illnesses that are transmitted by foods. Foodborne illnesses are a common, yet preventable, public health problem. An estimated 48 million people—or 1 in 6 Americans—get sick from consuming foods or beverages each year. About 128,000 of these people are hospitalized, and 3,000 die of foodborne diseases. Most foodborne illness can be prevented by practicing safe food handling.

Foodborne illnesses aren't especially harmful for most people. Many people experience only a brief period of illness and make a full recovery without medical care. However, these illnesses can be dangerous for people who are very old or very young, as well as pregnant women. People who are already in bad health, or have weakened immune systems, can become extremely sick, and can even die from foodborne illnesses.

foodborne illness
a disease that is transmitted by food; food poisoning

Foodborne Illness Caused by Infection

Some foodborne illnesses are caused by agents, such as bacteria, viruses, or parasites. This type of illness is called a *foodborne infection*. Many different disease-causing organisms can contaminate foods—more than 250 different foodborne infections have been discovered. When food is handled improperly, these organisms rapidly multiply to dangerous levels at which foodborne illness becomes more likely.

The most common foodborne illnesses are caused by four agents:

- *Norovirus* (or the Norwalk-like virus) is an extremely common cause of foodborne illness, which causes an acute gastrointestinal illness, including vomiting and diarrhea. This virus spreads primarily from one infected person to another, often through contaminated food, water, or environmental surfaces.

foodborne infection
an illness caused by a bacterium, virus, or parasite that has contaminated a food

- *Salmonella* is a bacterium that is common in the intestines of birds, reptiles, and mammals. It can spread to humans through various foods such as milk products, undercooked eggs, meat, poultry, peanut butter, and cantaloupe.

- *Clostridium perfringens* is a bacterium commonly found on raw meat and poultry, which produces a toxin that causes illness.

- *Campylobacter*, the most commonly identified bacterial cause of diarrheal illness in the world, is an organism that is present in undercooked chicken or another food that has been contaminated with juices from raw chicken (Figure 3.19).

Because these different diseases have many different symptoms, it can be difficult to determine whether a particular illness is caused by something you ate. Nausea, vomiting, abdominal cramps, and diarrhea are, however, common symptoms of many foodborne diseases.

Foodborne Illness Caused by Intoxication

Other types of food poisoning are caused by toxins in the food. These toxins are produced by an organism present in the food. This type of foodborne illness is called **foodborne intoxication**. Three common causes of foodborne intoxication are

foodborne intoxication
an illness caused by toxins that an organism has produced in a food; toxins may also be produced by chemicals, heavy metals, or other substances

- *Escherichia coli (E. coli)*, a bacterium that lives in the digestive tracts of humans and animals and can cause diarrhea, anemia, and kidney failure; although some strains of this bacterium are harmless, other strains can make a toxin that causes infection and disease;

- *Staphylococcus aureus*, a bacterium that can grow in some foods and produce a toxin that causes intense vomiting; and

- *Clostridium botulinum*, a bacterium that grows and produces a powerful paralytic toxin in foods, causing the rare but deadly disease known as *botulism*.

Toxins can be present in food for other reasons. Toxins may be the result of contamination from chemicals, heavy metals, or other substances.

Figure 3.19

Preparing raw meat and vegetables on the same cutting board can cause cross-contamination. *How many cutting boards do you have in your house? How does your family prevent cross-contamination?*

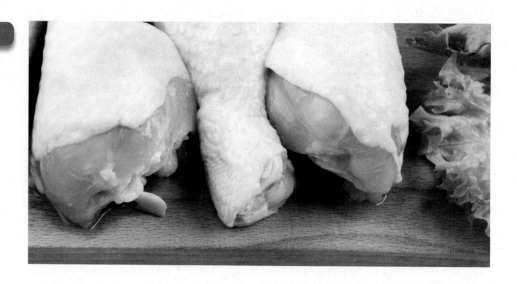

People can become ill if a pesticide is accidentally added to a food, or if naturally poisonous substances are used to prepare a meal. For example, every year people become ill after eating poisonous mushrooms that they mistake for edible mushrooms. Fish may have toxins in their flesh as a result of living in polluted waters.

Preventing Foodborne Illness

Fortunately, there are several effective strategies for preventing foodborne illness. These strategies include the following:

- wash your hands with hot, soapy water for at least 20 seconds before cooking and eating, and after handling uncooked meat (Figure 3.20)
- cook foods to the appropriate temperature
- keep hot foods hot—above 140 degrees Fahrenheit—since microbes die at this temperature
- keep cold foods cold—below 40 degrees Fahrenheit—since microbes divide and produce toxins very slowly at this temperature
- refrigerate and freeze perishable food and leftovers promptly
- wash counters, tables, dishes, and eating utensils with hot, soapy water
- avoid nonpasteurized juice, apple cider, and milk
- wash fruits and vegetables before preparing them
- throw away cans that are leaking or bulging at the top (these are clear signs of botulism)

These strategies can help reduce your risk of getting foodborne illnesses.

Food Sensitivities

Some people experience negative reactions after eating particular types of foods. Food sensitivities are often the cause of these negative reactions. Food sensitivities are categorized as either food intolerances or food allergies. Depending on the type of sensitivity, these reactions can range from mild discomfort to life threatening.

Food Intolerance. *Food intolerances* occur when a person's body can't properly digest a particular type of food. These intolerances often occur gradually, after eating large quantities of a particular type of food or eating a particular food very frequently. For instance, people who are lactose intolerant have difficulty digesting the lactose found in milk and many dairy products because their bodies do not produce the substance required to help digest the lactose. These people may become ill after eating ice cream.

Symptoms caused by food intolerances can include gas, cramps, bloating, heartburn, headaches, and irritability or nervousness. Although these symptoms can be unpleasant, they are not usually life threatening.

People with food intolerances may be able to avoid unpleasant symptoms simply by consuming smaller amounts of the food that makes them ill. In some cases, drugs or dietary supplements may be used to help a person tolerate particular types of food. For example, people who are lactose

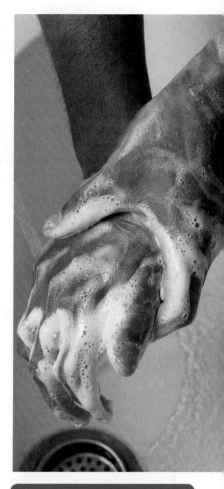

Figure 3.20

Washing your hands can help you avoid foodborne illnesses. *Do you make a point of washing your hands thoroughly before and after you handle foods?*

food intolerance
a condition in which a person cannot properly digest a certain type of food

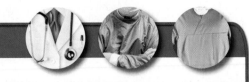

Nutrition

Described below are just a few of the many careers related to nutrition.

Career	Typical Education and Training	Typical Job Duties and Demands	Career Resources
Nutritionist or Dietitian	four-year college degree; some states also require licensing	Nutritionists and dietitians counsel people on how to lead healthier lives by improving their eating habits. They may work to assess a client's nutritional needs, develop meal plans, and achieve health-related goals such as lowering cholesterol levels.	Academy of Nutrition and Dietetics; Commission on Dietetic Registration
Food Science Researcher	four-year college degree, and often a graduate degree	Food science researchers study the chemical composition of food to determine the vitamin, fat, sugar, and protein levels in the food. They also work to make sure food is packaged, stored, and distributed safely.	American Registry of Professional Animal Scientists
Food Service Manager	high school diploma	Food service managers oversee daily restaurant or cafeteria operations. They make sure all health regulations are followed, monitor food preparation activities, and oversee budgets, payroll, and food inventory.	National Restaurant Association; Society for Foodservice Management
Pediatric Dietitian	four-year college degree; most states also require licensing as a Registered Dietitian	Pediatric Dietitians provide nutritional counseling to families and children. They may work with overweight children to help them develop a healthier diet or decrease the risk of health problems developing later on.	Academy of Nutrition and Dietetics; Commission on Dietetic Registration

Exploring Careers

1. Think about your interests, strengths, and weaknesses. Which career appeals most to you? Which career does not interest you?

2. Do you know anyone who works in one of these careers? If so, ask this person why he chose this career and what he likes most and least about the work.

---

gluten
a protein found in wheat, rye, oats, and barley

intolerant can take a dietary supplement called *lactase* that provides the enzyme they need to digest lactose.

Some people have gluten intolerance. **Gluten** is the protein found in wheat, rye, oats, and barley. You may have heard about celiac disease, which causes an inability to process the gluten protein. These people must avoid eating many grain-based products, such as bread, pasta, and cookies. Celiac disease is not a type of food intolerance, however, but rather an autoimmune disease caused by a person's genetics. People can have gluten intolerance without having celiac disease.

Fortunately, many gluten-free food products are now available. These products are suitable for individuals with either celiac disease or gluten intolerance.

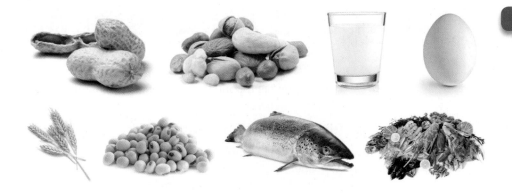

Figure 3.21

A small selection of foods, including the foods pictured at the left, are responsible for the majority of allergic reactions. *What extra precautions do you think people with food allergies have to take when preparing food or eating at a restaurant?*

Food Allergy. A *food allergy* is an immune response to a certain food that the body reacts to as if it were harmful. In contrast to food intolerances, symptoms of a food allergy typically occur very suddenly and can be caused even by tiny amounts of a particular food. People who are highly allergic to a particular food may even experience a reaction if they are exposed to the food on their skin or in the air. Symptoms of an allergic reaction to food can vary widely. Some of the most common reactions include hives or a rash, swelling in the tongue and throat, difficulty breathing, and abdominal cramps (Figure 3.21).

Currently no cure exists for food allergies. Given the more serious reactions associated with food allergies, the best way to manage these allergies is to simply avoid all contact with food that might trigger a reaction.

This is not always as easy as it sounds. Some foods that normally would not contain allergens are manufactured in factories that process other foods containing allergens. For example, an oatmeal cookie that does not contain peanuts may pick up traces of peanut from the peanut butter cookies manufactured at the same factory. The manufacturer must indicate on the package of oatmeal cookies that peanut butter cookies are manufactured in the same facility. This is one more reason people should read food labels.

food allergy
an immune response in which the body reacts to a certain type of food as though the food were a harmful substance; may manifest itself in rashes, swelling, difficulty breathing, indigestion, or dizziness

Lesson 3.3 Review

Know and Understand Assess

1. Identify and describe the components of a food label.
2. Explain how ingredients are listed on a food label.
3. List strategies for preventing foodborne illnesses.
4. Explain the difference between a food allergy and a food intolerance.

Analyze and Apply

5. Analyze the food label provided on page 91 and assess the product's nutritional value.
6. Evaluate the importance of learning to read food labels.

7. Compare and contrast foodborne infection and foodborne intoxication.

Real World (Health

Because you are such a food guru now, write a letter to the food director of your school. This person is responsible for everything served in the cafeteria. In this letter, advocate on behalf of yourself and all your classmates for tools to make healthful food choices. Request that each food served have a large food label beside it so students can make more educated decisions in the lunchroom. Don't forget to list the reasons why this new system would be beneficial to the health of the students.

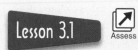
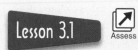

Lesson 3.1
Assess

What Nutrients Does Your Body Need?

Key Terms

amino acid
anemia
carbohydrate
cholesterol
dehydration
fat
fat-soluble vitamin
fiber
glucose
glycogen

hormone
mineral
nutrient
osteoporosis
protein
saturated fat
trans fat
unsaturated fat
vitamins
water-soluble vitamin

Key Points

- There are six main types of nutrients. These are including carbohydrates, protein, fat, vitamins, minerals, and water.
- Carbohydrates can be simple or complex and are a major source of energy for the body.
- Protein is used to build and maintain the body's cells and tissues.
- Common dietary fats are saturated, unsaturated, or trans.
- Vitamins and minerals are involved in many processes throughout the body.
- Water is necessary for most body functions.

Check Your Understanding

1. _____ are chemical substances found in foods that your body needs to grow and function properly.

2. Which of the following is a complex carbohydrate?
   A. starch
   B. glucose
   C. fiber
   D. both A and C

3. *True or false?* Protein is made up of smaller units called *incomplete proteins*.

4. _____ are organic substances required by the body in small amounts.
   A. Minerals
   B. Vitamins
   C. Trans fats
   D. Amino acids

5. Anemia is a condition resulting from insufficient _____.

6. What amount is recommended for daily fluid intake?

7. Which of the following statements is true about fiber?
   A. Fiber is found only in plant-based foods.
   B. Fiber is a good source of energy for the body.
   C. Fiber binds cholesterol and prevents it from leaving the body.
   D. Fiber is a form of protein.

8. _____ are inorganic elements needed by your body in quantities of less than 100 milligrams daily.
   A. Water-soluble vitamins
   B. Amino acids
   C. Trace minerals
   D. Saccharides

9. **Critical Thinking.** If you were trying to determine whether a fat was saturated or unsaturated, what criteria could you use?

Lesson 3.2
Assess

Creating a Healthy Eating Plan

Key Terms

calorie
metabolism
nutrient-dense food

overnutrition
undernutrition

Key Points

- Choose foods and beverages that are healthful.
- Be physically active on a daily basis.
- The MyPlate food guidance system is a guide for healthful eating.
- Both undernutrition and overnutrition can result in poor health.

Check Your Understanding

10. What factors determine an individual's daily calorie needs?

11. *True or false?* Whole fruit is more nutrient-dense than fruit juice.

12. Which of the following is a recommendation of the MyPlate food guidance system?
    A. Make at least half of the grains you eat whole grains.
    B. Make half your plate protein.
    C. Avoid frozen and canned vegetables.
    D. Include at least eight ounces of cooked seafood in your meal plan each week.

13. What types of foods are common sources of oils?

14. Why is undernutrition a concern during childhood and adolescence?

15. Which of the following is likely to result in weight gain?
    A. Calories in = Calories burned
    B. Calories in > Calories burned
    C. Calories in < Calories burned
    D. None of the above.

16. Indicate whether each of the following is an example of a whole grain (WG) or refined grain (RG).
    A. Brown rice
    B. Oatmeal
    C. Couscous
    D. Whole-wheat bread

17. **Critical Thinking.** Explain why nutrient-dense foods do not contain much, if any, added sugar, solid fat, refined grains, or sodium.

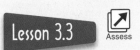
Lesson 3.3 Assess

Food Labels and Food Safety

Key Terms

Daily Values
food additives
food allergy
Food and Drug
   Administration (FDA)
food intolerance
foodborne illness
foodborne infection
foodborne intoxication
generally recognized as
   safe (GRAS)
gluten
organic food

Key Points

- Nutrition Facts labels contain information to help consumers make healthful food choices.
- Understanding how ingredients are listed on food labels can provide you with more information to help you make good food choices.
- Claims made on food labels are regulated by the government.
- Foodborne illness can be prevented by handling food safely.
- Foodborne illness is the result of disease-causing organisms in the food, or by toxins introduced into the food.
- Food allergies differ from food intolerances.

Check Your Understanding

18. *True or false?* The Nutrition Facts label states the number of calories in the entire package of food.

19. A can of tomato soup lists ingredients as follows: tomato puree, water, high fructose corn syrup, wheat flour, salt, potassium chloride, citric acid, ascorbic acid. Does this product contain added sugar? If so, how is it identified on this label?

20. Norovirus, *salmonella*, Clostridium perfringens, and *Campylobacter* are the top four causes of _____.

21. The body's inability to digest milk is an example of _____.
    A. an immune system response
    B. a food allergy
    C. celiac disease
    D. a food intolerance

22. Who establishes the criteria for claims made on food labels?
    A. food manufacturers
    B. Food and Drug Administration
    C. Academy of Nutrition and Dietetics
    D. Department of Health and Human Services

23. *True or false?* Individuals who are highly allergic to a certain food may experience a reaction if they are exposed to the food on their skin or in the air.

24. **Critical Thinking.** Explain why a high % Daily Value is not always an indication of a healthful food choice.

25. **Critical Thinking.** How does temperature play such an important role in preventing foodborne illness?

Health and Wellness Skills

26. **Reduce Health Risks.** Exercise, along with eating healthy, is one of the key factors in obesity prevention. Getting 30–60 minutes of exercise a day can greatly decrease your risk of obesity and other diseases, put you in a better mood, and just be fun! So don't sit, get fit! For each day of the week, write one or two activities you can do to get moving. After each day, make a note regarding what you accomplished toward your exercise goal.

27. **Practice Healthy Behaviors and Reduce Health Risks.** Imagine that you have been elected to a Healthy High School Vending Machine committee, and it is your job to determine which foods your high school's vending machines will include. List at least five healthy criteria that foods must pass to be in the machines. Write a paragraph explaining how the new options will enhance student health.

28. **Comprehend Concepts.** Create six superhero cartoon characters to represent each of the six nutrients. Draw each character and give him or her a creative name. Underneath each drawing, write the following information about each character: What are this character's "super powers" (what he or she does for the body)? How did this character get his or her super powers? Where is this character found? Include at least three foods that provide each nutrient.

29. **Comprehend Concepts.** Label a piece of paper from A to Z. For each letter, write a word or phrase that starts with that letter and pertains to nutrition in some way. Next, write a paragraph about what you learned from this chapter using as many of the words or phrases from your list as possible. You must use at least 10 of the terms, but your goal is to use them all.

30. **Access Information.** Create a menu that includes all of your favorite foods and their nutrition information. Divide your favorite foods into five categories: appetizers (4 items), main courses (6 items), side dishes (5 items), desserts (at least 2 items), and beverages (at least 2 items). Once you have listed your favorite foods by category, research the nutrition information of all the items on your menu. Finally, create a visually pleasing menu with your foods listed by category, their nutrition information, your restaurant name, and pictures. Print your menu to show to the class. At whose "restaurant" would you want to eat?

Hands-On Activity
Healthy Tip of the Day Calendar

Create a 30-day calendar of healthy eating tips. Write a catchy title for your calendar and include a different healthy eating tip for each day. Include at least five pieces of art and verify that all of your tips enhance health. When you are done with your calendar, distribute it to a few of your friends to encourage their healthy eating habits.

Example:

Eating Your Way to Good Health

Sunday	Monday	Tuesday	Wednesday	Thursday	Friday	Saturday
21 Wait for 15 minutes to go for seconds; you may find you are already full.	**22** Trade in that sugary soda for a glass of low-fat or fat-free milk.	**23** Record everything that you eat today. You might be surprised to see how much you're eating.	**24** Substitute fruit for a sugary snack.	**25** Don't skip meals. Skipping a meal can lower your metabolism by five percent, enough to gain a pound every month.	**26** Sample a new nutritious food today.	**27** Sit down with your parents and help plan a week of healthy meals.

Core Skills

Math Practice

Use the information below and on the Nutrition Facts label shown here to answer the questions.

- Proteins supply 4 calories/gram
- Carbohydrates supply 4 calories/gram
- Fats supply 9 calories/gram

Nutrition Facts		
1 serving per container		
Serving size	**1 cup (245g)**	
Amount per serving		
Calories		**208**
		% Daily Value*
Total Fat 3g		4%
Saturated Fat 2g		10%
Trans Fat 0g		
Cholesterol 12mg		4%
Sodium 162mg		7%
Total Carbohydrate 34g		12%
Dietary Fiber 0g		0%
Total Sugars 34g		
Includes 17g Added Sugars		34%
Protein 12g		
Vitamin D 0mcg		0%
Calcium 419mg		32%
Iron 0.2mg		1%
Potassium 537mg		11%

* The % Daily Value (DV) tells you how much a nutrient in a serving of food contributes to a daily diet. 2,000 calories a day is used for general nutrition advice.

31. How many servings are in one container of this food?
    A. two servings
    B. one serving
    C. one-half serving
    D. three servings

32. What is the % Daily Value for saturated fat in this food?
    A. 12%
    B. 18%
    C. 10%
    D. 11%

33. If the entire container of food is eaten, what is the % Daily Value of carbohydrates in this food?
    A. 12%
    B. 10%
    C. 17%
    D. 50%

Reading and Writing Practice

Read the passage below and then answer the questions.

Your body breaks down carbohydrates into the sugar known as glucose, *which is your brain and central nervous system's preferred source of energy. Glucose powers your brain, enabling you to concentrate and pay attention. Have you ever skipped breakfast and then had trouble concentrating in one of your early morning classes? This difficulty is caused by your body running out of glucose.*

When your body needs more energy, it can use glucose immediately. This is why having a candy bar or soft drink, both loaded with sugar, can give you a quick "pick-me-up." The sucrose in these snacks is quickly and easily broken down into glucose and fructose.

When glucose is stored in the muscles and liver for later use, it is known as glycogen. After enough glycogen has been stored, any extra glucose is converted by the liver into fat, which is stored in fat tissue. The body uses glycogen *from the muscles and liver, or the stored fat, when it needs energy between meals or to fuel activity.*

34. What is an important function of glucose?
    A. Maintains the health of the digestive tract.
    B. Acts as an energy source for the brain and central nervous system.
    C. Breaks down nutrients in the small intestine.
    D. Is used by the body to convert carbohydrates into energy.

35. How are glucose and glycogen related?
    A. They are the same substance.
    B. Glucose is needed to digest glycogen.
    C. When glucose is stored in the liver and muscles, it is called *glycogen*.
    D. Glycogen turns into glucose when protein is synthesized in the body.

36. Based on the passage you just read, write two or three sentences about the importance of breakfast.

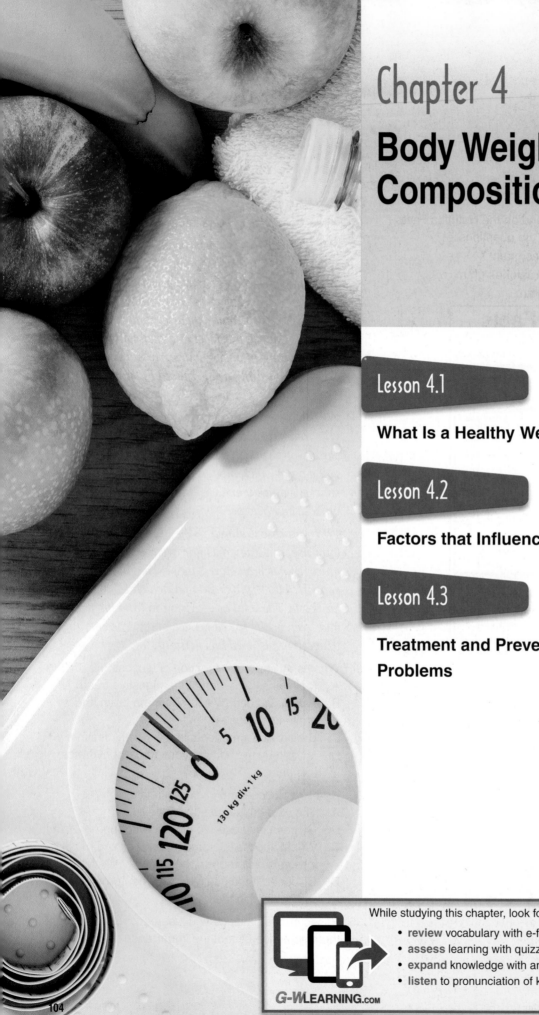

Chapter 4

Body Weight and Composition

Lesson 4.1

What Is a Healthy Weight?

Lesson 4.2

Factors that Influence Weight

Lesson 4.3

Treatment and Prevention of Weight Problems

While studying this chapter, look for the activity icon to:
- **review** vocabulary with e-flash cards and games;
- **assess** learning with quizzes and online exercises;
- **expand** knowledge with animations and activities; and
- **listen** to pronunciation of key terms in the audio glossary.

G-WLEARNING.com   www.g-wlearning.com/health/

Take this quiz to see what you do and do not *know* about body weight and composition. If you cannot answer a question, pay extra attention to that topic as you study this chapter.

1. Identify each statement as True, False, or It Depends. *Choose* It Depends *if a statement is true in some cases, but false in others.*
2. Revise each False *statement to make it true.*
3. Explain the circumstances in which each It Depends *statement is true and when it is false.*

Health and Wellness IQ ⬈ Assess

	True	False	It Depends
1. Calculating body mass index, or *BMI*, is the best way to assess whether or not someone is at a healthy weight.	True	False	It Depends
2. A person who stores fat around the hips and thighs will tend to have more serious health problems than someone who stores fat around the waist or stomach.	True	False	It Depends
3. People who are obese are more at risk of getting diabetes than people who are not obese.	True	False	It Depends
4. The weight of adopted children is more similar to the weight of their biological parents than to the weight of their adoptive parents.	True	False	It Depends
5. People eat more when they are at home than when they are at a restaurant.	True	False	It Depends
6. People eat more when food is served in a large bowl or plate than a smaller one.	True	False	It Depends
7. A person's culture influences the types of tastes and foods they prefer eating.	True	False	It Depends
8. Drugs taken to help with weight loss, such as appetite suppressants and diuretics, can have serious side effects and lead to health complications.	True	False	It Depends
9. Dividing foods into "good foods" and "bad foods" and then attempting to only eat "good foods" is an effective strategy for losing weight.	True	False	It Depends
10. Most food advertising on television focuses on fast food, sugar-based cereals, and soft drinks.	True	False	It Depends

Setting the Scene

Many Americans have difficulty controlling their weight. Among adults 20 years of age and older, seven out of ten are overweight. From 1980 to 2008, rates of obesity in the United States doubled for adults and tripled for children. Approximately 36% of adults and 17% of children and adolescents, from 2 to 19 years of age, are obese.

In a country in which fast food is readily available and people don't get as much exercise as they should, being overweight or obese is common. As you learn more about this topic, you will understand that weight management is a complex and sensitive issue. It is important to remember that all people deserve understanding, support, and respect.

This chapter examines the issues of body weight and composition, which are some of the most important health-related topics in the United States. You will learn how doctors determine where people fall on the weight spectrum. This chapter also covers the health problems caused by being overweight and obese, and various factors that lead to obesity. Finally, you'll learn specific strategies for preventing obesity and maintaining your weight over time.

Lesson 4.1

What Is a Healthy Weight?

Key Terms E-Flash Cards

In this lesson, you will learn the meanings of the following key terms.

body composition

body mass index (BMI)

obesity

overweight

skinfold test

underweight

Lesson Objectives

After studying this lesson, you will be able to

- summarize factors that determine body weight;

- describe strategies for determining healthy weight; and

- recognize health consequences associated with unhealthy weight status.

Warm-Up Activity

Healthy Weight

You have probably noticed that high school students come in a variety of shapes and sizes. There is no right or wrong shape or size for teenagers, but regarding size and weight, some teens are healthier than others.

How would you assess your current weight? Is it a healthy weight for you? Does it fluctuate much from month to month? Before reading this lesson, write a self-assessment of your weight, being as specific as possible about your reasoning. You need not share your assessment with anyone unless you want someone else's opinion about your conclusions.

Before You Read

Body Composition

Read the definition of body composition *on the next page. Then create a diagram similar to the one below. For each category, write as many descriptive words as you can think of in the appropriate circle. If a word describes more than one category, write it in the overlapping area.*

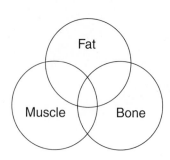

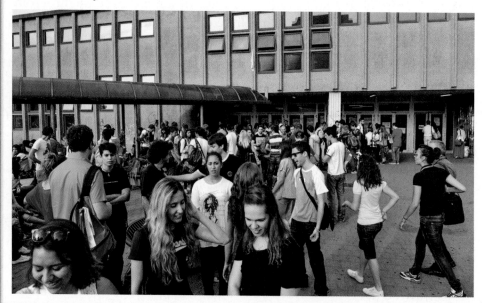

D o you ever wish you weighed more or less than you actually do? Do you ever compare your weight to the weight of someone else? Sometimes people's beliefs about how much they should weigh are influenced by comparisons they make with other people. Perhaps you want to weigh what a friend weighs, or what your favorite celebrity or sports figure weighs. Comparing your weight to the weight of another person, however, is a bad idea. Your ideal weight is a weight at which *your* body is healthy.

Weight and Body Composition

Factors that determine what you should weigh include your age, height, body composition, and gender. Your **body composition** is the ratio of the various components—fat, bone, and muscle—that make up your body. The size and shape of two people who weigh the same, but differ in body composition, can be very different.

Weight is assessed differently for children and teens than for adults because children and teens are still growing. Additionally, as you grow and become taller, your healthy weight range increases.

To better understand the concept of body composition, try to envision what one pound of metal looks like in comparison to one pound of Styrofoam™. It shouldn't be hard to imagine that the Styrofoam will take up much more space than the metal. In the same way, a person who weighs 160 pounds, with a body composition that includes a higher ratio of fat to bone and muscle, will be larger than a 160-pound individual with a lower ratio of fat to bone and muscle.

Your body composition is an important factor in your weight. Muscle and bone weigh more than fat. A person may weigh more than someone else because she is more muscular, not because she is overweight. Athletes often train for long hours, which builds muscle and increases bone density. It should not be a surprise, therefore, that athletes often have considerably lower body fat averages than nonathletes (Figure 4.1).

Gender affects body composition and, therefore, body weight. Male bodies tend to have more muscle than those of females, and female bodies have a greater proportion of fat. On average, adult males have a body-fat percentage of 15% and adult females have a body-fat percentage of 25%. Women have a higher percentage of body fat than men to support their role in reproduction.

Determining a Healthy Weight

For many years, the most common way to determine what people should weigh was to consult a height-weight table that listed various heights

body composition
the ratio of fat, bone, and muscle that naturally make up a person's body

Figure 4.1

Athletic training builds muscles and increases bone density, resulting in a lower percentage of body fat. *Do some types of athletic training build muscles faster than others? Explain.*

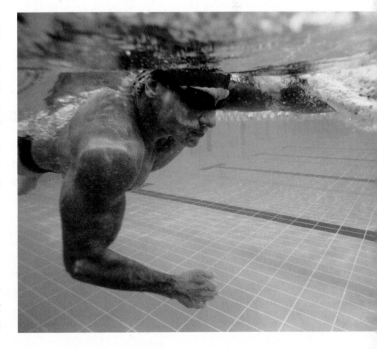

and corresponding weight ranges. More recently, body mass index has been used along with other measures to assess body composition and fat distribution. Although these measures are harder to use than the height-weight charts, they provide more accurate readings.

Body Mass Index (BMI)

body mass index (BMI)
a number calculated from a person's height and weight; an indicator of excess body fat

$$BMI = \frac{Weight\ (lbs.)}{Height\ (in.)^2} \times 703$$

Body mass index (BMI) is a tool used when assessing an individual's weight status. BMI is calculated to determine whether or not a person is a healthy weight for his height. This index is calculated by dividing a person's weight in pounds by his height in inches squared. The quotient is then multiplied by a factor of 703.

Although BMI is calculated in the same way for children, teenagers, and adults, the resulting number is interpreted differently for different age groups. Because children and teens are still growing, their BMI values are plotted on growth charts based on their age and sex. The BMI percentile for children and teenagers indicates the relative position of the person's BMI compared with others of the same sex and age. These charts are found at the back of this text.

overweight
a condition characterized by having excess body weight for a particular height; can be due to fat, bone, muscle, or water

obesity
a condition characterized by having excess body fat; for adults, a BMI of 30 or higher

For children and teens, the Centers for Disease Control and Prevention (CDC) define *overweight* as having, for a particular height, excess body weight from fat, bone, muscle, water, or a combination of these factors. The CDC defines *obesity* as having excess body fat. For adults, the definition is based on specific BMI values. Adults with a BMI between 25 and 29.9 are considered overweight. Adults with a BMI of 30 or higher are considered obese. In simpler terms, to be overweight is to have moderately more body fat than recommended. To be obese is to be even *more* overweight or excessively overweight.

BMI calculation is an easy method for assessing weight status, but it is not perfect. For some individuals, BMI is not an accurate indication of body composition. Because muscle and bone weigh more than fat, some highly fit or muscular people can have a high BMI, which incorrectly places them in the overweight category. Likewise, an individual may have a body weight in the acceptable range, but a high percentage of body fat to muscle. This person's BMI would inaccurately place them in the healthy range.

Other Body Composition Measures

Other methods can be used to measure body composition. These methods vary in their accuracy, cost, and accessibility. A more accurate idea of an individual's health can be determined when one of these methods is used in combination with BMI.

skinfold test
a method of measuring body composition in which a person uses a skinfold caliper to measure the thickness of a fold of fat

The *skinfold test* is a reliable measure of body composition when performed correctly. The person administering the test uses a *skinfold caliper*, which is a device that measures the thickness of a fold of fat. She pinches the skin in specific parts of the body to measure the thickness of the folds of fat there (Figure 4.2 on the next page). These measurements are then added together to calculate an overall percentage of body fat.

Additional methods for measuring body composition include DXA scans, underwater weighing, air displacement, and bioelectrical impedance. Accuracy, availability, time, and cost are factors in determining which methods are used.

Body Fat Distribution

The location of the fat deposits on your body can be as important, if not more important, to your health as how much fat you have. Waist circumference and waist-to-hip ratio are two methods used to assess body fat distribution.

Waist Circumference. Waist circumference measures your waist size. This measurement is simple to obtain and can be an indicator of excess abdominal fat. You can also use this measurement to monitor your progress toward meeting weight management goals you set for yourself.

Waist-to-Hip Ratio. Some people tend to store extra fat around their waist, or abdomen, and chest. These people are said to have apple-shaped figures. Other people tend to store extra fat in their lower bodies—around their hips, seat, and legs. These people are said to have pear-shaped figures.

The waist-to-hip ratio helps identify a person's fat distribution, or where extra fat is stored. This measurement is recommended for use with adults over 20 years of age. Waist-to-hip ratio is not used for children and teens because they are continuing to grow and the shape of their bodies is evolving.

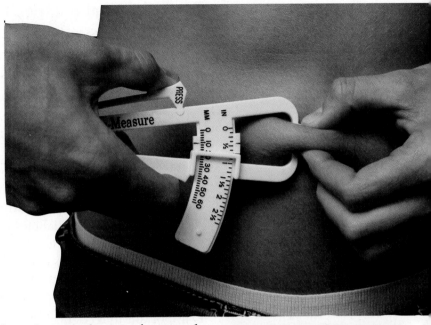

Figure 4.2

A skinfold caliper is used to measure the thickness of a fold of fat. *Why do you think the skinfold test is a good measure of body fat?*

Health Consequences of Under- and Overweight

Regardless of how it is measured and assessed, a person's weight clearly has an impact on his or her health. Being *underweight*, overweight, or obese can cause a variety of negative health consequences.

Underweight and Your Health

Many more people in the United States are overweight than underweight, so this chapter focuses on understanding, preventing, and treating overweight and obesity. Some people do, however, struggle with being underweight.

Causes for being underweight include medical conditions such as cancer, alcohol or drug abuse, genetics, and psychological problems such as depression or an eating disorder. The most common cause of being underweight, however, is a lack of access to food. This is typically caused by poverty. An estimated 13 million American children—one out of every five—live in homes in which sufficient nutritious food is sometimes lacking. Chronic insufficient nutrient intake results in poor health. Deficiency diseases are caused by inadequate intake of various nutrients.

underweight
a condition characterized by having too little body weight for a particular height

Overweight and Your Health

Being overweight contributes to a range of health issues. Overweight individuals are at an increased risk of death, especially death caused by heart disease. They are also at greater risk for developing hypertension (high blood pressure), hyperlipidemia (high cholesterol and high triglycerides), liver and gallbladder disease, and many types of cancer. Cancers of the breast, colon, kidney, pancreas, cervix, and prostate are associated with overweight and obesity.

One of the most common health problems associated with obesity is type 2 diabetes, a disorder in which the body is unable to utilize blood glucose properly. About 80% of adults who have diabetes are also obese. You will learn more about diabetes in chapter 14.

Being overweight is also associated with other, less severe, but disruptive physical consequences. People who are overweight and obese are more likely to experience respiratory, sleep, and joint problems. Obese women are more likely to have trouble getting pregnant. Additionally, it is important to recognize that malnutrition is not unique to underweight individuals. Individuals who are overweight or obese may be consuming too many calories, but may not be receiving all the nutrients needed for health.

Interestingly, the distribution of weight on a body is often a better predictor of the physical consequences of overweight than a person's weight, BMI, or total body fat. Men and women who have metabolic syndrome—which includes storing extra fat around the waist as well as increased blood pressure, high blood sugar, and high cholesterol levels—are at greater risk of developing heart disease, stroke, and diabetes. Men are more likely than women to store fat in the abdomen, which is one factor that leads men to have higher rates of cardiovascular disease than women.

Lesson 4.1 Review

Know and Understand

1. List four factors that determine a person's healthy body weight.

2. Why must we evaluate an adult's weight differently than we would a teenager's?

3. Define *body mass index*.

4. List five reasons underweight occurs.

5. Identify five health risks associated with overweight.

Analyze and Apply

6. Compare and contrast body composition with body fat distribution.

7. What do you think is the best strategy or strategies for assessing healthy weight?

Cite information from the text to support your conclusion.

8. Create and describe two imaginary characters of the same sex, age, and height. One character weighs more than the other but is healthier. Your descriptions should make it clear why the heavier person is healthier.

Real World Health

Using the BMI formula for calculating body composition, identify your BMI. Where are you on the BMI chart? On a separate piece of paper, write a short paragraph explaining what you learned about your body composition.

Factors that Influence Weight

Lesson Objectives

After studying this lesson, you will be able to

- summarize genetic influences on weight;
- understand how social and psychological factors may affect weight;
- explain how cultural factors may affect weight; and
- summarize the effect of socioeconomic status on weight.

Key Terms E-Flash Cards

In this lesson, you will learn the meanings of the following key terms.

culture
ghrelin
leptin
physiological need
portion size
psychological desire

Warm-Up Activity

Favorite Foods

Make a list of your favorite foods and write why each of these foods appeals to you. Read the nutrition labels or research the nutrition information for these foods. Identify whether each food is helpful for losing, maintaining, or gaining weight. Explain your answers.

Favorite food and why I like it	Impact on weight (check one):			Explanation
	Lose	**Maintain**	**Gain**	

Before You Read

My Weight Mindmap

Using a mindmap similar to the one below, identify the different factors that influence your weight. Write Factors that influence my weight *in the middle oval. In the surrounding circles, write all the factors that you can think of. Then, branching off of each circle, draw a square and explain how each factor influences your weight.*

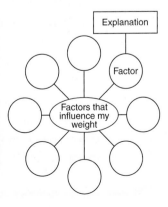

E vidence increasingly suggests that a person's weight is influenced by a number of factors rather than one cause. More is being learned every day about the influence of a person's genetic makeup on weight. The social, psychological, cultural, and socioeconomic factors of everyday life play major roles.

The Influence of Genetics

One factor that influences how much people weigh is their genetic makeup. People who are obese are likely to have family members who are also overweight or obese.

Although obese parents are more likely to have obese children, this association does not necessarily mean that genetic factors alone cause obesity. For example, parents who are overweight might simply serve more high-fat foods to their children, encourage more snacking, or discourage more exercise. Genetic factors do, however, appear to be a significant predictor of a person's BMI.

Twin and Adoption Studies

To examine the influence of genetic factors as opposed to environmental factors on weight, researchers studied a group of identical and fraternal twins. Identical twins share all of their genes, whereas fraternal twins share about half of their genes. Identical twins also tend to share their BMIs more often than same-sex fraternal twins. Researchers found that the BMIs of identical twins were very similar whether the twins grew up together in the same home or apart in different homes. This suggests that the environment has less of an impact on BMI than genetics.

Health across the Life Span

Rates of Obesity by Age

The rate of obesity in the United States varies considerably across the life span. Specifically

- 9% of 2- to 5-year-old children are obese;
- 17% of 6- to 11-year-old children are obese;
- 20% of 12- to 19-year-old adolescents are obese;
- 32% of adults 20 to 39 years of age are obese;
- 40% of adults 40 to 59 years of age are obese; and
- 37% of adults 60 years of age and older are obese.

Why does the rate of obesity increase with age? One major reason is that the body's metabolism, or the rate at which it expends energy (calories), slows down as people age. Even if what you eat—and how much you eat—stays the same over time, you may still gain weight.

Analyzing Data

1. This data is from the United States. What do you think data from other countries would show about rates of obesity at different ages? Would this data look the same or would it change? Why?

2. One explanation for the increase in obesity with age is a change in metabolism. Can you think of other explanations for this increase? What data would you need to test your hypothesis?

Another way to examine the link between genes and weight is to look at children who were adopted. These children are raised by people who are not their biological parents. Studies have shown that the weights of the adopted children were much more similar to the weights of their biological parents than to the weights of their adoptive parents. This finding further suggests that genes have a stronger influence on weight than environment.

How Genes Impact Weight

There are many ways in which the traits you inherit from your biological parents may influence your weight. Researchers have found 32 different genes that may influence weight, including recent evidence that suggests genes may influence obesity. Genetic factors predict a person's height and appear to predict about 40–70% of a person's BMI. Combined, these genes can have a great impact on a person's body composition. Genes also appear to influence peoples' food preferences, their metabolism, and the levels of various hormones in the body.

Genes and Food Preferences. Different people tend to have different preferences for particular types of food, and research shows that genes may influence those preferences. Some people prefer to eat foods that are high in fats, such as chocolate, doughnuts, and ice cream. Other people prefer to eat salty foods such as pretzels, French fries, and potato chips (Figure 4.3).

Genes and Hormone Levels. The levels of various hormones in your body may also be influenced by your genetic makeup. Certain hormones may influence how hungry or full you feel. For example, the hormone *leptin* is an appetite suppressant, meaning high levels of this hormone in your body leave you feeling full. Another hormone, *ghrelin*, makes you feel hungry.

Genes and Metabolism. Genes may also influence your metabolism, or the rate at which your body uses energy to carry out basic physiological processes such as breathing, digesting, and growing. Some people have a high metabolism, and their bodies use more energy to carry out these processes. As a result, they burn more calories each day. Other people have a lower metabolism, so their bodies do not burn as many calories to perform their daily activities.

leptin
a hormone that suppresses appetite and leads to feeling full

ghrelin
a hormone that increases appetite and leads to hunger

Figure 4.3

While genes do not always control your food choices, they may influence your food preferences. *What sorts of foods do the members of your family prefer? Do you also prefer these foods?*

The Limits of Genes

Although genes appear to play a significant role in people being overweight or obese, genes are clearly not the sole factor influencing a person's weight. In the United States, rates of obesity have increased dramatically in recent years. Although peoples' genes are very similar to the genes of their parents and grandparents, the percentage of American adults who are obese has doubled since 1980. If genetics were the only factor influencing weight, rates of obesity would remain steady over time.

The psychological desire for food can stem from a desire to enjoy time with friends and can be a positive thing as long as a person doesn't overeat.

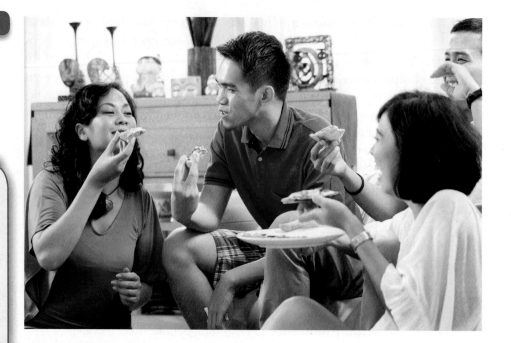

Do You Engage in Mindless Eating?

These questions will help you assess how much you engage in mindless eating.

If there's good food at a party, I'll continue eating even after I'm full. **yes no**

If there are leftovers that I like, I take a second helping even though I'm full. **yes no**

I have trouble not eating ice cream, cookies, or chips if they're around the house. **yes no**

I snack without noticing I'm eating. **yes no**

When I'm sad, I eat to feel better. **yes no**

I think about things I need to do while I'm eating. **yes no**

When I eat at "all you can eat" buffets, I tend to overeat. **yes no**

When I'm eating one of my favorite foods, I don't recognize when I've had enough. **yes no**

Add up the number of yes answers to assess your degree of mindless eating. The more yes answers you have, the higher your rate of mindless eating.

psychological desire
the body's yearning for something; something wanted but not needed

physiological need
the body's requirement for something; necessary

Social and Psychological Factors

Can you think of a time when you ate something, but you weren't actually hungry? What and when people eat is often not influenced by hunger—meaning the *physiological need* for food—but rather, by other factors.

Eating can be triggered by a **psychological desire** for food rather than a **physiological need** for food (Figure 4.4). Social and psychological factors such as your mood, the environment, and even the portion size you are served can influence what and how much you eat.

Mood and Food

Many people eat in response to how they feel. For many people, eating is a big part of celebrating joyous occasions, such as graduations, birthdays, or holidays. Similarly, you might go out with friends for ice cream to celebrate victory after an athletic event or your performance in a school concert.

People also use food to improve their mood when they are feeling anxious, angry, or sad. This tendency to eat more when nervous seems to be more common in women and girls than in men and boys. A study of college students found that 62% of female students reported eating more when they were depressed, but only 29% of male students reported doing so.

People experiencing bad moods tend to gravitate toward comfort foods. Comfort foods, such as ice cream and candy make them "feel better." The sugar in these foods triggers the release of chemicals that contribute to a pleasing sensation and improved mood. Chocolate, another common ingredient in these foods, increases production of hormones that generate feelings of happiness.

Does Feeling Sad Make You Eat Popcorn?

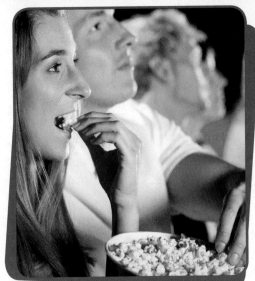

Researchers created a clever study to test whether or not our moods influence how much we eat. They began by creating different moods in different people. To create these moods, they showed people one of two movies:

- a romantic comedy designed to create a happy mood
- a movie in which one of the lead characters dies at a young age, designed to create a sad mood

While watching their assigned movie, people were given a large bucket of hot, buttered, salted popcorn. They were also given water or a diet soda to drink. The researchers then measured how much people ate during each of the two movies.

Can you guess what they found? As predicted, people who watched the sad movie ate 28% more popcorn than the people who watched the happy movie. This study provides evidence suggesting that people eat in part to try to make themselves feel better.

Thinking Critically

1. Why do you think people eat more popcorn when watching a sad movie than when watching a happy movie? Is this difference a reflection of biological, social, or psychological factors?
2. What do you think researchers would find if they gave people a large tray of celery and carrots instead of a large bucket of popcorn? Would people eat more vegetables during the sad movie than the happy movie? Defend your belief.

Environment

Your environment influences your eating in a number of ways. Research shows that people eat more when dining with others than when they are alone. People are particularly likely to consume more when eating with family and friends. The presence of others creates an enjoyable environment, which causes people to linger over the meal longer and eat more. This may explain why people often overeat at long holiday dinners with family and friends.

People also eat more when a variety of foods is available. It's easy to tire of eating the same thing, so more options often encourage greater consumption. This may explain why people are more likely to overeat at all-you-can-eat buffets, or why college students who eat in dining halls sometimes gain weight.

Portion Size

Another factor that contributes to overweight and obesity is the *portion size* in which food is served. Portion sizes served at restaurants in the United States have become much larger over time, which often leads people to overeat. For example, the original glass Coke bottles, manufactured in the 1930s, held 6 ½ ounces. The current "single-size" plastic Coke bottle holds 20 ounces, which is three times as much!

portion size
the amount of food served for a single person

A series of fascinating studies demonstrates that even very subtle environmental factors, such as the size of a serving dish, influence how much people eat. In one study, guests attending an ice cream party were given either a large or small bowl. They were also given either a large or small ice cream scoop to serve themselves. Those who received the large bowl served themselves 31% more ice cream. Similarly, those who scooped their ice cream using the large spoons served themselves 14% more ice cream.

Cultural Factors

culture
the beliefs, values, customs, and arts of a group of people

Culture refers to a group's beliefs, values, customs, and arts. Cultural factors that may affect a person's weight include food and taste preferences, eating patterns, and belonging to certain ethnic groups.

Food and Taste Preferences

People in different cultures prefer different types of foods and tastes. For example, most Americans would not want to eat spiders, snails, and guinea pigs. These foods, however, are considered delicacies in some cultures.

People's food preferences are also shaped by the flavors commonly used in their culture's cooking. For example, spices such as cardamom are common in Indian dishes, while cumin is a staple in Mexican cooking. Some research indicates that taste preferences are shaped before people are born. Babies who are exposed to particular flavors while in their mothers' wombs later show a stronger preference for this flavor. This influences their taste preferences for the rest of their lives.

Eating Patterns

Cultural factors include more than which foods you choose to eat. Your culture also influences how and where you eat, as well as the portion sizes that are considered appropriate. Unfortunately, cultural factors such as the availability and amount of food may also contribute to obesity.

The United States has some of the highest rates of obesity in the world, and also an abundance of fast-food restaurants that feature inexpensive, fatty foods. People often eat on the run, grabbing quick, mass-produced meals. Until recently, even school cafeterias in the United States were serving fast food and soda (Figure 4.5).

The abundance of food and prevalence of large portion sizes in American culture help to explain why immigrants who move to the United States tend to become heavier over time. According to one study, only 8% of immigrants who have lived in the United States for less than a year are obese, whereas 19% of immigrants who have lived in the United States for at least 15 years are obese. These findings suggest that exposure to American culture increases the risk of obesity.

Ethnic Groups

Obesity is more likely to occur among members of certain ethnic groups. It is important to remember, however, that people are individuals.

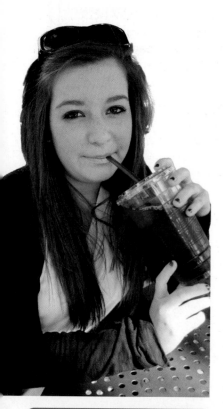

Figure 4.5

Soda is a source of empty calories and a contributor to obesity in the United States.

Local and Global Health
Worldwide Rates of Obesity

During the past 20 years there has been a dramatic increase in obesity in the United States, and rates remain high. In a recent study, every state had a prevalence of obesity greater than 20%. A prevalence in obesity of 30% or more was found in 25 states and four had a prevalence of 35% or more. In Louisiana, the state with the highest rate of obesity, 36% of adults are considered obese. In contrast, in Colorado, the state with the lowest rate of obesity, 20% of adults are considered obese.

This increase in obesity is also seen in other countries. In fact, worldwide obesity has more than doubled since 1980. Here are some of the most recent statistics:

- An estimated 1.9 billion adults 18 years of age and older are overweight.
- An estimated 600 million men and women are obese.
- Nearly 41 million children under five years of age are overweight.

For a long time, health problems caused by being overweight or obese occurred primarily in high-income countries, such as the United States. These problems are now on the rise in low- and middle-income countries as well. Most of the world's population lives in countries where more people die from being overweight and obese than from being underweight.

However, there are still countries where many people, especially children, are unable to get adequate amounts of nutritious foods. An estimated 460 million people worldwide are underweight, which includes people who are malnourished and starving.

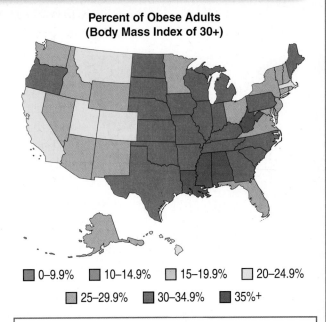

Percent of Obese Adults
(Body Mass Index of 30+)

■ 0–9.9% ■ 10–14.9% ■ 15–19.9% ☐ 20–24.9%
■ 25–29.9% ■ 30–34.9% ■ 35%+

Thinking Critically

1. Given this worldwide increase in obesity, how would you expect the rate of obesity to change over the next 20 years? Should it increase or decrease? Should this change be the same in the United States as it is worldwide, or different? Explain your answer.

2. What factors do you think explain the different rates of obesity and overweight in different states? What are some factors that might lead these rates to increase even more? What would lead them to decrease?

3. What strategies could governments take to decrease the rates of overweight and obesity in their countries? Which strategies would you support? Which would you oppose?

Not everyone in a particular ethnic group has the same habits and preferences. Although there is great variation among the people in each group, these groups tend to have cultural traditions and values that can influence the lifestyles of their members. For example, ethnic groups have traditional dishes based on types of foods available in their countries of origin. This may contribute to people in various groups developing preferences for those foods.

Different groups in society may also have different values and preferences when it comes to ideal weight and appearance. For example, researchers have found that the ideal body weight and shape preferred by African-Americans as a group tends to be heavier and larger than the ideal preferred by European Americans as a group.

Socioeconomic Status

Finally, socioeconomic status plays a role in the prevalence of obesity. Research reveals that children who grow up in low-income neighborhoods are 28% more likely to be obese than children who grow up in wealthier environments. How does growing up in a low-income neighborhood contribute to obesity?

First, this statistic stems from the types of food that lower-income families purchase. These families have fewer dollars to spend on food than higher-income families. To get the most food for their money, lower-income families may purchase lower-cost foods that are high in calories and low in nutritional value.

There are also fewer options for healthy food in lower-income neighborhoods. According to the United States Department of Agriculture, economically depressed neighborhoods often lack grocery stores and farmers' markets where people can buy fresh fruits and vegetables at reasonable prices. Additionally, residents may not own cars to take them to grocery stores. Instead, they have to shop at corner stores and fast-food restaurants, which are more accessible. These stores and restaurants primarily sell processed foods that are high in fat, sugar, and other unhealthy ingredients.

Low-income neighborhoods also offer fewer opportunities for physical activity. Neighborhoods that have sidewalks, bike lanes, and safe parks for play and exercise encourage residents to be physically active. A study found that only 8% of children who lived in these more physically active neighborhoods were obese. The same study found that nearly 16% of children who lived in neighborhoods that did not encourage physical activity were obese. Some families in low-income communities plagued by crime and gang activity may keep their children indoors (Figure 4.6).

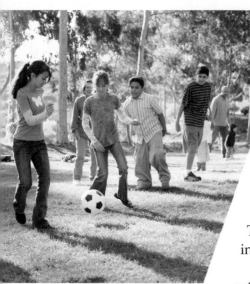

Figure 4.6

Low-income neighborhoods often have no space for children to play and be physically active.

Lesson 4.2 Review

Know and Understand Assess

1. Explain how twin and adoption studies support the theory that genetics plays a role in overweight and obesity.
2. List three social and psychological factors that influence how much and when people eat.
3. What American cultural factor is responsible for an eating pattern that may contribute to weight problems?
4. Identify common obstacles to physical activity in low-income neighborhoods.

Analyze and Apply

5. Evaluate the possibility that genes are solely responsible for an individual's weight. Cite examples from the text to support your analysis.
6. Organize evidence to explain why overweight and obesity are prevalent in the United States.

Real World Health

Select a factor that can influence a person's weight and then research its impact. In your research, answer the following questions:

How does this factor influence weight gain?
How does it influence weight loss?
How many people are affected by this factor?
How does a person know if his or her weight is being influenced by this factor?
How can a person use or address this factor to achieve or maintain a desired weight?

Once you have compiled your research, write a short paper describing the factor you chose.

Treatment and Prevention of Weight Problems

Lesson Objectives

After studying this lesson, you will be able to

- summarize healthy weight-loss strategies;
- recognize unhealthy weight-loss strategies; and
- recall strategies for healthy weight gain.

Warm-Up Activity

Weight Loss Methods

What can a person do to lose weight? In a table similar to the one below, list and briefly explain all of the different methods of weight loss that you can think of. Interview adults you know to identify additional methods. Put an asterisk next to the method or methods you believe are most effective. Then put a check mark next to the method or methods you believe are most healthful. Are there any methods you chose as both effective and healthful? If not, explain why a method you consider effective is not healthful?

Method of Weight Loss	Explanation

Key Terms E-Flash Cards

In this lesson, you will learn the meanings of the following key terms.

all-or-nothing mindset
diuretic
fad diets
fasting
food diary

Before You Read

True or False?

Decide whether the following statements are true or false. After you have read the chapter, check your answers against what you have learned.

_____ 1. *Individuals who are extremely underweight are susceptible to as many health problems as people who are extremely overweight.*

_____ 2. *There are 2000 calories in one pound of fat.*

_____ 3. *The skin caliper test is a method used to measure the amount of fat under a person's skin.*

_____ 4. *Diuretics are supplements that cause the body to lose water weight.*

_____ 5. *It is more important to replenish your body with food than with water.*

A s mentioned earlier, the rate of obesity in the United States is increasing. This means that the major health consequences of obesity are also becoming more prevalent. What can be done to slow the rate of obesity?

One of the most important ways to reduce the number of overweight and obese adults is to help children develop healthy eating habits. Establishing healthy habits at a young age makes it that much easier to avoid obesity later in life. Adults who are overweight were often overweight as children. For example, a study of seven-year-olds found that 40% of the children who were obese became overweight adults. Only 10% of normal-weight children became overweight adults. This lesson discusses steps you can take to prevent overweight and obesity as an individual and as a member of society.

Strategies for Healthy Weight Loss

Making long-term changes to your weight requires a permanent, life-long change in your eating and exercise habits. To maintain your current weight, you must balance calories you consume with calories used during physical activity. Weight loss occurs when you eat fewer calories than are needed for physical activity.

To successfully lose or maintain weight, you must create a healthy eating and exercise plan that is compatible with your daily life. Several strategies follow that can help people lose and maintain their weight.

CASE STUDY   The Challenge of Avoiding Obesity

Jack is 14 and a freshman in high school. At his physical exam last summer, he was surprised to learn that his weight put him in the overweight category. His doctor recommended that he lose some weight. Jack played on soccer and baseball teams in elementary school, but he stopped playing these sports in seventh grade. After school, Jack sometimes rides his bike to a friend's house. Usually, though, he comes home and plays video games or watches television until his parents get home from work. He often snacks on cookies and chips while he watches television.

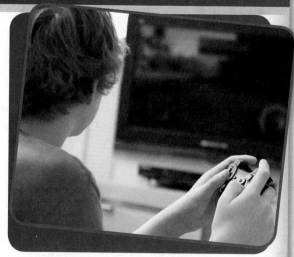

Thinking Critically

1. What do you think are the primary factors that led Jack to become overweight?

2. What are some strategies that could help Jack lose some weight?

3. What advice would you give teenagers in Jack's situation to help them from becoming overweight or obese?

Set and Reward Realistic Goals

One effective strategy for losing weight is to set realistic, short-term goals regarding eating and exercise. For example, you could decide to

- stop snacking between meals;
- eat an apple instead of chips as a mid-morning pick-me-up; or
- go for a walk with a friend instead of watching television after school.

This short-term approach allows you to experience some success and inspires confidence that you can achieve your weight-loss goal. Effective weight-loss techniques focus on gradual weight loss of one to two pounds a week.

This approach can be especially useful if you reward yourself for changing your eating habits, losing weight, or starting to exercise. For example, after successfully losing five pounds or running three miles, reward yourself with a new pair of sunglasses or a trip to the movies with a friend. Obviously, it's better to not use food as a reward!

Monitor Eating

Monitoring exactly when and what you eat is another effective strategy for losing weight. It is easy to forget about some of the calories you consume each day, especially if those calories aren't consumed in a regular meal. For example, you might eat potato chips while you study or have a candy bar as a quick after-school snack, but forget to count those calories as part of your daily total. People often overeat at parties because they aren't conscious of how much they are eating while busy socializing. Individuals who keep a *food diary*, or daily record of what they eat are more successful at managing their weight (Figure 4.7).

Recording what you eat each day will help you become more aware of what triggers you to overeat. After you have determined those triggers, you can try to eliminate them or substitute another type of food.

food diary
a record of what a person eats in each day

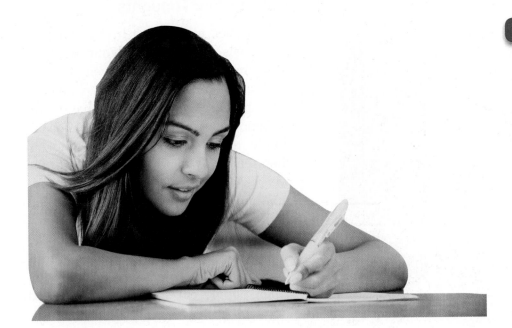

Figure 4.7

Keeping a food diary can help you keep track of what you eat each day, which will help you manage your weight. *Why do you think keeping track of what you eat is so important to weight management?*

Figure 4.8

If you have only healthy options available when you feel like a snack, you are more likely to avoid the sweet or fatty empty calorie snacks.

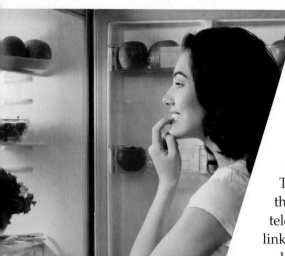

You can follow through on changes to your eating and drinking behavior by keeping only healthy foods and drinks nearby. Do not buy foods that will tempt you. In this way, when you are hungry, you will be grabbing a healthy snack instead of an unhealthy one (Figure 4.8).

Limit Screen Time

Studies have shown that people who spend many hours watching television or playing video games are more likely to be overweight or obese than those who spend less time in front of screens. In a study involving 369 children, researchers examined body composition, including level of body fat and waist size. They also noted hours of daily television viewing and whether televisions were located in bedrooms. Not surprisingly, the children and teenagers who reported having a television in their bedroom watched more TV each day. They were also more than twice as likely to show the highest levels of body fat and waist circumference. Having a television in the bedroom may also lead to decreased sleep, which is linked to obesity (Figure 4.9).

Watching television also increases exposure to commercials for unhealthy foods and beverages. In the United States, food and beverage companies spend billions of dollars a year in advertising, much of it aimed at children and teenagers. More than half of the commercials seen by children and teens are related to food. The majority of these commercials are for fast foods, snack foods, and sugar-sweetened drinks. Predictably, viewing these advertisements increases children's interest in such products. One study estimated that a ban on fast-food advertising during children's television programs could reduce the number of overweight children by 18% and the number of overweight adolescents by 14%.

all-or-nothing mindset
a way of thinking in which a person has to do it "all" right or he or she has done "nothing" right

Figure 4.9

Teens who watch many hours of television, and especially teens who have televisions in their bedrooms, are more likely to be obese. *How many hours of television do you watch each day?*

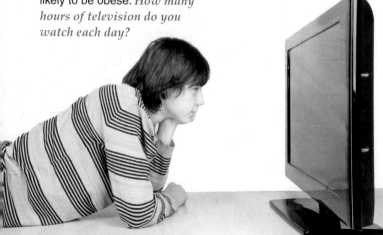

Change Your Thoughts

Another way to reach your weight-loss goals is to change your negative thoughts about eating and weight. Some people give up on their goals very quickly, often because they have negative or unrealistic views about weight loss. For example, these people continually think to themselves "I will never be able to lose the weight." These negative views are common among people who have struggled with weight management for some time.

Adopting an *"all-or-nothing" mindset* about eating can also undermine weight-loss efforts. This type of thinking occurs when people eat something prohibited

Sticking with Your Weight Loss Plans

The strategies listed below can help people stick with their weight-loss plans.

- Make small but healthy changes. This includes switching from sugary soft drinks to water, taking smaller portions of food, and reducing late-night eating.

- Get rid of the unhealthy foods around you. Stop buying foods that are high in fat, sugar, and sodium. Lobby your principal and school nurse to get rid of unhealthy foods from the school cafeteria and vending machines.

- Enlist the support of others. Tell friends and family members about your weight-loss goal, and ask them to support or join in your efforts.

- Develop new strategies for coping with mood-related factors. Many people snack when they feel anxious or sad. If this happens to you, go for a walk, call a friend, or listen to music instead.

- Eat healthier foods when you eat out. Order a salad instead of a hamburger, or ask for a half-portion of your favorite entree. If you really need to order a dessert, split it with a friend (or two).

- Stay focused and positive. Remind yourself of the benefits of losing weight—a longer life span, more spending money, and feeling better physically.

- Build rewards into your weight-loss plan. When you meet a goal, buy some new music, clothing, or something else you've been wanting.

- Don't let one lapse lead to a return of your old eating habits. If you slip up and eat a food you are trying to avoid, or eat too much, quickly refocus on your weight-loss plan.

by their eating plan and, because they believe they have failed, give up on the plan. For example, a dieter may eat one brownie and think, "Well, I've blown it now," and proceed to eat the entire tray.

Creating a distinction between "good foods" and "bad foods," and then permanently avoiding all bad foods will set you up for failure. Instead, it is best to eat desired foods in moderation.

What are positive ways to think about losing weight? First, remember that losing weight takes time, so you shouldn't expect instant success. Losing weight gradually through permanent lifestyle changes is more likely to help you achieve long-term weight loss. Second, remember that everyone who is trying to create new eating and exercise habits experiences slip-ups or lapses. The important thing is to keep these lapses brief and return to the new habits you are trying to adopt as quickly as possible.

Enlist the Support of Friends and Family

Changing eating and exercise behaviors is difficult, so it is helpful to have support from those around you. Simply having a friend who will go to the gym or go for walks with you can help.

Some people participate in formal groups to lose weight. Group approaches are especially effective because they provide social support as well as healthy competition. Interventions designed to decrease obesity in children are especially effective if parents are involved and supportive. The best results occur when parents change their own habits and provide healthier foods for their children. Having children assist with cooking is also a good strategy (Figure 4.10 on the next page).

Speak with a Healthcare Professional

Consulting with a healthcare professional is always recommended when you are struggling with weight management. These professionals can help you determine the weight-loss strategy that is best for your health.

Unhealthy Weight-Loss Strategies

As many as 45 million adults in America diet each year. Americans spend a tremendous amount of money—an estimated $33 billion each year—on weight-loss programs and products. Although these programs and products are highly profitable for the people who sell them, they often promise more than they can deliver.

The amount of weight people lose on any of these programs tends to be small and temporary. As a result, most people who participate in weight-loss programs regain about one-third of any weight lost within one year and return to their initial weight within three to five years.

Fad Diets

Many people try to lose weight using **fad diets**. These diets often forbid eating certain types of food groups (such as carbohydrates) and may require the purchase of special, and often expensive, prepared meals. One example of a fad diet is **fasting**, which means not eating any food or drink except water for an entire day. Another example is a *juice cleanse diet*, in which a person consumes only juice and water for several days.

The goal of these fad diets is to lose a significant amount of weight in a short time. Unfortunately, these types of diets can result in muscle loss and nutritional deficits, which is dangerous to your health. In addition, any weight that is lost in this type of diet is almost always quickly regained because the habits that led to the initial weight gain persist.

Drugs

People may also try different types of drugs, such as appetite suppressants and diuretics, to help with weight loss. Appetite suppressants trick the body into believing that it is not hungry, or that the stomach is full. These drugs work by increasing levels of chemicals in the brain that affect mood and appetite. **Diuretics**, or *water pills*, help the body eliminate salt (sodium) and water, mostly through increased urination. The loss of water causes a drop in weight.

fad diet
a diet that is extremely popular for a certain time period; often unhealthy

fasting
the practice of not eating or drinking anything except water for a set period of time

diuretic
a supplement that causes a person to lose fluids

Figure 4.10

By encouraging your caregivers to eat healthy foods and by helping your caregivers cook, you can better manage the foods you consume. *What meals could you offer to prepare with your family?*

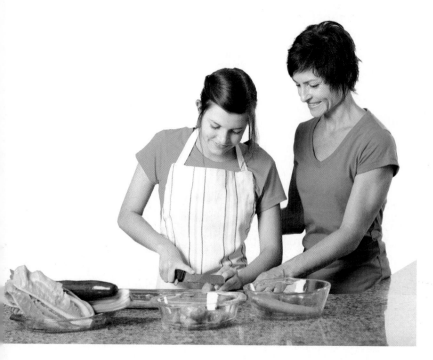

These quick-fix weight-loss strategies can lead to short-term weight loss that is not permanent. Most importantly, dietary and herbal supplements do not require approval by the Food and Drug Administration, as most other drugs do. Side effects, including blurred vision, dizziness, sleeplessness, and irritability, can be so serious that medical treatment or hospitalization is required.

Healthy Strategies for Gaining Weight

Some people are naturally thin, probably due to their genetic make-up and high rate of metabolism. It is possible to be very thin, but also healthy.

If a person is so thin that his health is in danger, however, he needs to develop strategies for achieving a healthy weight. Healthy weight-gain strategies should focus on nutrient-dense foods to provide not only additional calories, but also nutrients to help the body heal, build muscle, and strengthen bones (Figure 4.11). Foods that supply empty calories from added sugars and solid fats may add pounds, but do not benefit your health.

After achieving a weight-gain goal, people often must work to maintain the weight. Many of the lifestyle changes recommended for those trying to lose weight can be effective for people trying to gain weight. For example, people who are underweight need to monitor their eating to make sure they are eating frequent meals and adding calories whenever possible. They can also benefit from the social support of others in making these changes.

You can gain weight by eating nutrient-dense foods such as whole milk, nuts, and dried fruit.

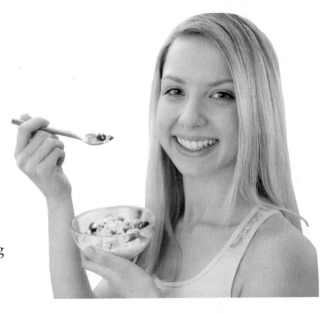

Lesson 4.3 Review

Know and Understand
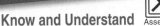
Assess

1. List six strategies for healthy weight loss.
2. Why are fad diets an unhealthy weight-loss strategy?
3. List a strategy for healthy weight gain.
4. Why is limiting screen time important for weight management?

Analyze and Apply

5. Compare and contrast a healthy weight-loss plan with a fad diet. Critique the fad diet.

6. Create your own healthy strategy for either weight gain or weight loss.

Real World Health

Using the Internet, locate a nutritionist or other healthcare professional in your area and ask to interview him or her on the topics of dieting and weight management. Create a list of questions that you want to ask. During the interview, take notes and ask the person to show you the body-fat tests they perform on patients.

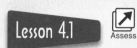

Lesson 4.1 Assess

What Is a Healthy Weight?

Key Terms

body composition
body mass index (BMI)
obesity

overweight
skinfold test
underweight

Key Points

- A variety of factors determine healthy body weight. Body weight is assessed differently for children and teens because they are still growing and developing.
- Measures of body composition and body fat distribution combined with BMI provide the most accurate indication of body weight status.
- There are health risks associated with both underweight and overweight.

Check Your Understanding

1. The ratio of fat, bone, and muscle that makes up your body is called _____.
   A. body fat distribution
   B. body composition
   C. body mass index (BMI)
   D. healthy weight

2. *True or false?* Muscle weighs more than fat.

3. Which of the following statements is true about body composition?
   A. Body composition measures the location of fat deposits on the body.
   B. A person's body composition cannot be changed.
   C. Body composition is determined by measuring waist circumference.
   D. Gender affects body composition.

4. *True or false?* Body mass index (BMI) is interpreted the same way for children, teen, and adults.

5. An adult male weighs 182 pounds and is 5 feet 10 inches tall. Perform the calculation to determine which of the following represents his body mass index (BMI).
   A. 28.1
   B. 21.6
   C. 26.1
   D. None of the above.

6. The skinfold test is a reliable measure of _____ when performed correctly.

7. Adults with a BMI between 25 and 29.9 are considered _____.
   A. underweight
   B. normal weight
   C. overweight
   D. obese

8. Waist circumference is used to assess _____.

9. Underweight is caused by which of the following?
   A. chronic insufficient nutrient intake
   B. underlying medical condition
   C. psychological, social, and emotional problems
   D. All of the above.

10. Which of the following statements are true?
    A. Type 2 diabetes is a health problem commonly associated with obesity.
    B. In type 2 diabetes, the body is unable to process glucose properly.
    C. Both A and B are true.
    D. Neither statement is true.

11. Men and women who store extra fat _____ are at greater risk of developing diabetes, hypertension, and cardiovascular disease.
    A. around their waists
    B. around their hips
    C. during the winter
    D. during the summer

12. **Critical Thinking.** Evaluate whether body mass index (BMI) or waist circumference is a better method to assess an individual's health.

Lesson 4.2 Assess

Factors that Influence Weight

Key Terms

culture
ghrelin
leptin

physiological need
portion size
psychological desire

Key Points

- Although genetic factors can be a significant predictor of BMI, other factors also influence a person's weight and body composition.

- Psychological and social factors sometimes trigger eating even though a physical need to eat does not exist.
- Cultural factors can have an effect on a person's weight.
- A number of socioeconomic factors can influence an individual's weight.

Check Your Understanding

13. Twin and adoption studies are performed to examine the influence of which of the following factors?
    A. psychological
    B. genetic
    C. portion size
    D. Both B and C.

14. Which hormone affects weight by acting as an appetite suppressant?
    A. ghrelin
    B. insulin
    C. leptin
    D. adrenaline

15. *True or false?* Genes are the sole factor affecting body weight.

16. *True or false?* Hunger is a social or psychological factor that triggers eating.

17. According to studies, people eat more when food is served on _____ serving dishes.
    A. larger
    B. smaller
    C. unique
    D. plain

18. A baby's fondness for flavors she was exposed to in the womb is an example of a _____ factor affecting taste preference.

19. *True or false?* Lack of access to safe parks for play and exercise is an example of the effect of socioeconomic status on a child's weight.

20. **Critical Thinking.** Based on what you have learned in this lesson, formulate an opinion on the complexity of weight management.

Lesson 4.3 Assess

Treatment and Prevention of Weight Problems

Key Terms

all-or-nothing mindset
diuretic
fad diets
fasting
food diary

Key Points

- Healthy weight management requires a commitment to permanent, lifelong healthy eating habits.
- Unhealthy weight-loss strategies usually yield temporary results and possible health complications.
- Similar to weight loss, people trying to gain weight must make permanent, healthy changes to gain and maintain weight.

Check Your Understanding

21. *True or false?* A healthy weight-loss strategy is to reward achieving a weight-loss goal with a food item.

22. Which of the following is a successful strategy for losing weight?
    A. Distract yourself by watching television.
    B. Do not share your weight-loss goals with others.
    C. Avoid eating chocolate for the rest of your life.
    D. Keep a daily record of what you eat.

23. *True or false?* An all-or-nothing mindset is an effective strategy for losing weight.

24. Healthy weight-gain strategies should focus on _____ foods.

25. *True or false?* Dietary and herbal supplements must be approved by the Food and Drug Administration (FDA).

26. Give an example of a negative thought about eating or weight management. Rewrite the thought to make it positive.

27. Which of the following is an unhealthy weight loss strategy?
    A. use of diuretics
    B. fasting
    C. juice cleanse diet
    D. All of the above.

28. **Critical Thinking.** Evaluate the effectiveness of using drugs, such as appetite suppressants and diuretics, for healthy weight management.

Skill Development

Health and Wellness Skills

29. **Advocate for Health.** Living a sedentary lifestyle can increase your body weight and your risk for developing diseases. For one week, try to be a true health advocate for your family and friends. Get your family and friends up and moving. Try going for a walk after dinner, playing outside instead of playing video games, or even leading your family in some exercises during commercials while you watch television. Compare your advocacy results with your classmates' results.

30. **Set Goals.** Knowing the different behaviors that lead to weight gain and unhealthy body composition enables you to live a healthy life. Create a daily checklist of things you can do to follow a healthy lifestyle. Try to check off all the items on your list each day.

31. **Practice Healthy Behaviors and Reduce Health Risks.** Go to a nutritionist, dietician, or other health professional, and ask him or her to perform health tests and identify your level of health. Once you have the results, talk to the professional about the changes you can make in your diet and lifestyle to improve your overall health.

32. **Analyze Influences.** Every time you watch television, the media is providing you with both direct and indirect messages. A direct message specifically states what is being sold and might describe the cost, size, or quality of an item. An indirect message draws attention to a product without specifically describing it and might depict people having fun or emphasize the perks that come with an item. For this activity, identify the direct and indirect messages in commercials and printed ads that you see. Then, create a PowerPoint or poster and present your findings to the rest of the class.

33. **Advocate for Health.** Speak with your family members about the genetic health issues present in your family. Develop a list of these health issues and research how you can prevent or delay the onset of these diseases.

Hands-On Activity:

Healthy Food Choices

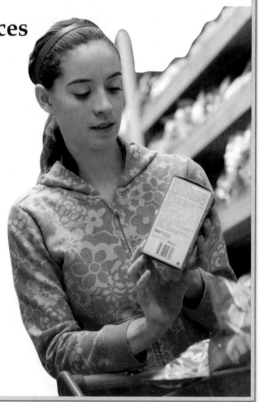

As you learned in this chapter, the choices you make when it comes to food are important for maintaining a healthy weight. To make better food choices, you can remove all unhealthy foods from your home. Take the steps listed below to fill your home pantry with more nutritious food choices that will keep you and your family healthy.

Steps for this Activity

1. Go through the foods at your house—in your pantry, refrigerator, and freezer—and identify and list all of the foods that are unhealthy. If you are uncertain, use the Internet to assess a food's health value.

2. Once you have a list of all the unhealthy foods in your house, create a new list that you will take to the store with the person who does the grocery shopping in your house.

3. Explain that your family is not practicing healthy behaviors and ask if you can replace some unhealthy foods with healthier and more nutritious options.

4. After you have purchased the new, healthy foods, clean out all of the unhealthy foods and donate them to a local food bank.

Core Skills

Math Practice

Changes in Portion Sizes and Effect on Caloric Content		
Food or Beverage	1980s (calories)	Today (calories)
turkey sandwich	320 calories	820 calories
French fries	210 calories	610 calories
bagel	140 calories	350 calories
slice of pizza	500 calories	850 calories
soda	85 calories	250 calories

34. What was the percentage change in calories for a soda from the 1980s to today?
    A. 194%
    B. -194%
    C. 19.4%
    D. 34%

35. Suppose you decide to have a turkey sandwich, French fries, and a soda for lunch. If your daily food plan allows for 2,200 total calories each day, what percentage of your total day's calories does this meal represent?
    A. 13%
    B. 130%
    C. 0.76%
    D. 76%

36. Suppose that two men—one living in 1980 and one living today—each eat one bagel every morning for breakfast. Assuming that their diet and physical activity are the same otherwise, how many more pounds would the man living today gain in a year's time than the man living in 1980? (Hint: There are 3,500 calories in a pound.)
    A. 37 pounds
    B. 17 pounds
    C. 22 pounds
    D. 15 pounds

37. What was the percentage change in calories for a slice of pizza from the 1980s to today?
    A. 41%
    B. 143%
    C. 70%
    D. None of the above.

Reading and Writing Practice

Read the passage below and then answer the questions.

Your body composition is the ratio of the various components—fat, bone, and muscle—that make up your body. The size and shape of two people who weigh the same, but differ in body composition, can look very different.

To better understand the concept of body composition, try to envision what one pound of metal looks like in comparison to one pound of Styrofoam™. The Styrofoam will take up much more space than the metal. In the same way, a person who weighs 160 pounds, with a body composition that includes a higher ratio of fat to bone and muscle, will be larger than a 160-pound individual with a lower ratio of fat to bone and muscle.

Your body composition is an important factor in your weight. Muscle and bone weigh more than fat. A person may weigh more than someone else because she is more muscular, not because she is overweight. Athletes often train for long hours, which builds muscle and increases bone density. It should not be a surprise, therefore, that athletes often have considerably lower body fat averages than nonathletes.

38. Which of the following concepts is the author trying to communicate in this passage?
    A. Individuals with the same body composition will weigh the same amount.
    B. Muscle and bone are denser than fat and, therefore, more compact.
    C. Nonathletes have lower body fat percentages than athletes.
    D. Muscle and bone are denser than metal.

39. Which of the following best explains why athletes often have lower body fat averages?
    A. Their training builds muscle and bone density.
    B. The majority of athletes are male and have more muscle mass.
    C. Athletes weigh less than nonathletes.
    D. All of the above.

40. Analyze how the author introduces and develops key points in this passage. Write an essay describing your analysis and citing specific examples.

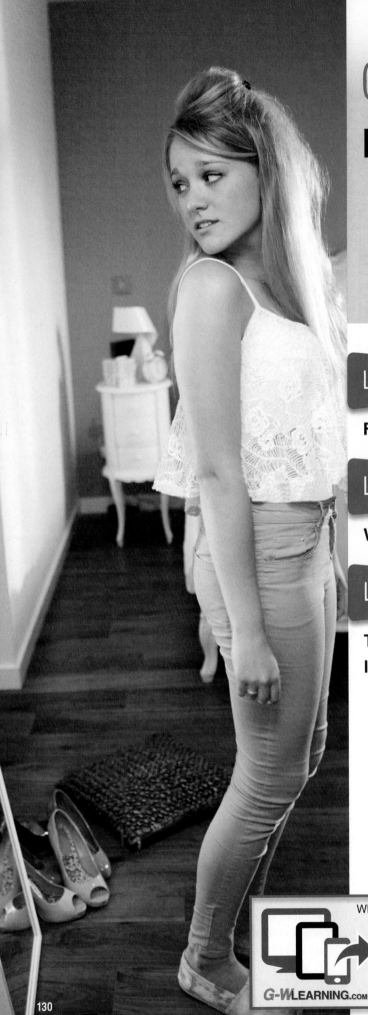

Chapter 5
Body Image

Lesson 5.1

Factors that Influence Body Image

Lesson 5.2

What Are Eating Disorders?

Lesson 5.3

Treating and Preventing Body Image Issues

While studying this chapter, look for the activity icon to:

- **review** vocabulary with e-flash cards and games;
- **assess** learning with quizzes and online exercises;
- **expand** knowledge with animations and activities; and
- **listen** to pronunciation of key terms in the audio glossary.

G-WLEARNING.com

www.g-wlearning.com/health/

Take this quiz to see what you *do* and *do not know* about body image, eating disorders, and their impact on health. If you cannot answer a question, pay extra attention to that topic as you study this chapter.

1. Identify each statement as True, False, *or* It Depends. *Choose* It Depends *if a statement is true in some cases, but false in others.*

2. *Revise each* False *statement to make it true.*

3. *Explain the circumstances in which each* It Depends *statement is true and when it is false.*

Health and Wellness IQ 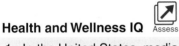 Assess

	True	False	It Depends
1. In the United States, media images of the ideal female body have become thinner over time.	True	False	It Depends
2. A thin body is viewed as the ideal in feminine beauty in all cultures.	True	False	It Depends
3. In the United States, media images of the ideal male body have become more muscular over time.	True	False	It Depends
4. Men and women are equally likely to develop anorexia nervosa.	True	False	It Depends
5. People who have bulimia nervosa feel in control of their weight.	True	False	It Depends
6. Eating disorders can lead to long-term health problems and death.	True	False	It Depends
7. Images of very thin women in the media do not impact women's feelings about their bodies.	True	False	It Depends
8. Individual therapy is more effective than family therapy in the treatment of eating disorders.	True	False	It Depends
9. Sorne countries have banned the use of very thin models in advertisements.	True	False	It Depends
10. Businesses have not done anything to help prevent body image issues.	True	False	It Depends

Setting the Scene

How do you feel about your body? Do you marvel at its strength and agility, which allow you to do things like play basketball, hold a small child safely, and do heavy lifting at your part-time job? Do you appreciate the organs in your body that accomplish amazing feats? For example, your heart pumps about 2,000 gallons of your blood each day, and your reproductive system enables you to create a new life.

Many teenagers don't think about these things when asked how they feel about their bodies. Instead, they think about how much weight they need to gain or lose, or they worry about a particular body part they wish they could change. These types of feelings are common among teenagers whose bodies are changing rapidly in many ways. The thoughts and feelings people have about their bodies, however, can affect their physical and emotional health in powerful ways. Some people develop a distorted view of how they look, or attempt to achieve an unattainable or unrealistic ideal.

In this chapter you'll learn about factors that influence how people view their bodies and some resulting problems, such as eating disorders. You'll also learn strategies that can help you avoid developing these problems.

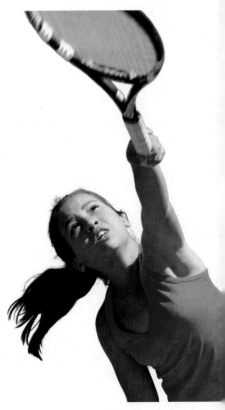

Factors that Influence Body Image

Key Terms ⬀ E-Flash Cards

In this lesson, you will learn the meanings of the following key terms.

anabolic steroids
body image
creatine
dietary supplement
muscle dysmorphia

Before You Read

Self-Assessment

Before you read and as you are reading this lesson, choose four of the following outcome sentences and complete each one on a separate sheet of paper.
I feel…
I learned…
I'm beginning to wonder…
I rediscovered…
I'm still not sure of…
I was surprised that…

Lesson Objectives

After studying this lesson, you will be able to

- identify several factors that can influence a person's body image;

- compare and contrast the factors that lead people of different genders and cultures to be dissatisfied with their bodies; and

- analyze how the media can impact the body image of teenagers.

Warm-Up Activity

Magazine Models
Magazines contain countless advertisements that show models selling some type of product. Obtain a few different magazines that contain these kinds of ads. List all of the physical traits that the female models have in common. Then list all of the physical traits that the male models share. What do your findings tell you about the physical ideals being presented in the media?

Female Models, Common Traits	Male Models, Common Traits

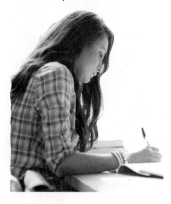

Your thoughts and feelings about how you look make up your **body image**. Your body image doesn't describe what your body *actually* looks like—but how you *think* it looks. How your body actually looks and how you feel about it are not necessarily related. For example, someone who is fit and considered attractive by many people may dislike aspects of his or her body. If so, this person has a poor body image. On the other hand, someone whose body type is not considered ideal or attractive by many people may still feel good about his or her body. This person has a positive body image.

People who have a positive body image have an accurate perception of the shape and size of their bodies. They see the parts of their bodies as they truly are. They appreciate and value their bodies. They recognize that a person's physical appearance has no impact on his or her character, values, and worth.

Although men and boys can have poor body images, girls and women are more likely to have negative thoughts about their bodies. One reason for this is that girls and women are defined by their physical appearance more often than men and boys. For example, women in leadership positions are often criticized or complimented on their outfits, hairstyles, and other physical attributes (Figure 5.1). Articles or news reports profiling men rarely include such information. This is just one example of how society is more inclined to judge girls and women by their physical appearance.

In this lesson you will learn about factors that influence body image, including family and peers, images in the media, ethnicity, and sports.

body image
term that describes a person's thoughts and feelings about how he or she looks

Family and Peers

Parents can influence their child's body image by emphasizing the importance of body weight and shape. Girls who believe their parents value being thin are more likely to be concerned about their weight. One study

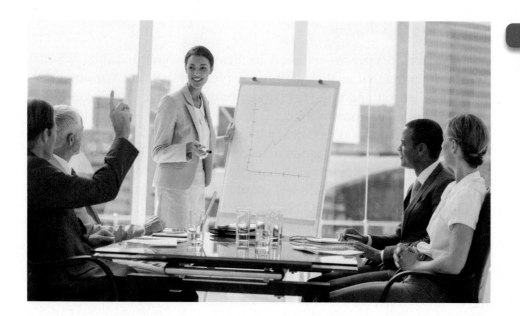

Figure 5.1

Unfortunately, in some workplaces the physical appearance of female employees may receive more attention than their work performance.

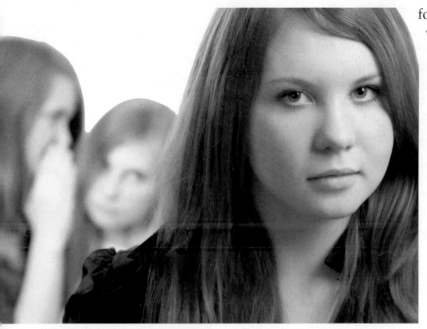

Figure 5.2

Teenagers sometimes feel insecure about their body shapes and sizes, especially when they feel pressured by their peers to look a certain way. *What can teens do to counter the peer pressure they experience?*

found that 40% of 9- and 10-year-old girls who were trying to lose weight by dieting were urged to do so by their mothers. These family pressures can lead to serious eating disorders.

A teenager's body image is also influenced by his or her friends. To fit in with a peer group, teenagers may feel pressured to have a certain body shape or size (Figure 5.2). Teenagers who hang out with friends who have a similar body type—very thin or very muscular, for example—can feel pressured to conform to that body type. Extra pressure may be added when teenagers worry that their bodies won't be attractive to potential dating partners.

Unfortunately, teenagers sometimes make unhealthy choices when attempting to change their body shape or size. Teenage boys may feel pressured to use steroids or other types of drugs to become more muscular, even though these drugs can have very serious side effects. Eating disorders are triggered, at least in part, by the pressure to be thin.

Some teenagers may even choose cosmetic surgery to change some aspect of their appearance, such as the shape of their noses or eyes. More than 200,000 people between 13 and 19 years of age have plastic surgery each year. The most common procedure is *rhinoplasty*, or reshaping of the nose. A report by the American Society of Plastic Surgeons revealed that many teenagers view plastic surgery as a way to fit in with their peers.

All teenagers feel self-conscious about their bodies at some time, and wish they could change some aspects of their appearance. This feeling usually goes away with time, and with age.

In the Media

Every day, people are exposed to messages communicating what is considered attractive in their culture. Advertisements for various products—such as shampoo, lipstick, and clothing—convey messages about what is regarded as attractive. People are also regularly exposed to images of celebrities, actors, and models, which set the standard for attractiveness. For example, the average woman in the United States wears a size 12 to 14, but the average model featured in a magazine wears a size 0 to 4. These images can influence how people feel about their bodies. If their bodies don't look like the idealized images, people can feel that they don't measure up.

Besides associating particular physical traits, such as thinness, with physical attractiveness and desirability, the media also associates these physical traits with wealth, health, success, and happiness. Advertising tries to convey the message, "If you look this way, you will be rich, healthy, successful, and happy."

Critics of the advertising industry say consumers are led to believe that happiness can be achieved if they look a certain way and use certain products. Many studies have shown that the best predictors of happiness do not include how people look. People who describe themselves as "happy" tend to have close relationships with others, and have opportunities to engage in work they find meaningful and satisfying.

Female Body Image

Think quickly—who is the most attractive female television or film star? Whoever came to mind is almost certainly thin. Virtually all images of women in American media, including women in movies, on television, in music videos, and on the covers of magazines, show very thin women.

Interestingly, the preference for thin girls and young women in media is relatively new. Movie and magazine depictions of women have become consistently thinner over the years. Marilyn Monroe, the most famous sex symbol of the 1950s, would be considered overweight (at least as a model) by current standards.

Research in Action

Does the Preference for Thinness Begin in Preschool?

A study was performed to determine whether the preference for the thin ideal is seen in very young children. The assumption was that these children would have had less exposure to media images of thin models and celebrities. The researchers asked preschool girls from 3 to 5 years of age to play a board game—either *Candy Land* or *Chutes and Ladders*.

To play the game, each girl had to select a game piece to represent the character she would be in the game. Each girl chose from three game pieces representing three characters. The characters were exactly the same except for their body sizes—one character was thin, one was average, and one was overweight.

If the girls had no preference for a particular body type, then about 33% of the girls should have chosen each of the three figures. Instead, researchers found that 69% of the girls chose the thin figure, 20% chose the average figure, and only 11% chose the overweight figure. The girls showed a strong preference for the character who was thin.

When asked to explain why they chose a particular figure, many of the girls expressed negative attitudes about the overweight figure. One girl said, "I hate her because she has a fat stomach."

Another girl said, "I don't want to be her, she's fat and ugly." Sadly, this research suggests that the preference for thinness emerges very early in life.

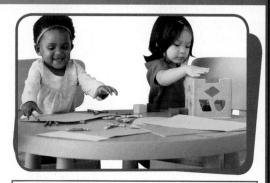

Thinking Critically

1. Given that these girls were very young, why do you think they showed such a strong preference for the thin figure? Was this preference a result of influence from the media, culture, or family?

2. This study only examined girls' body image preferences. What would you expect if the same study examined boys? Would researchers find the same preference for the thin ideal? Why or why not?

3. Many people find the idealization of thinness disturbing, especially in such young girls. Do you think the preference for thinness can or should be changed? Why or why not?

Figure 5.3

Teenage girls spend an average of 15 minutes a day reading teen magazines, many of which set unrealistic expectations for women. *How have pictures in magazines and on television shaped your expectations for your body?*

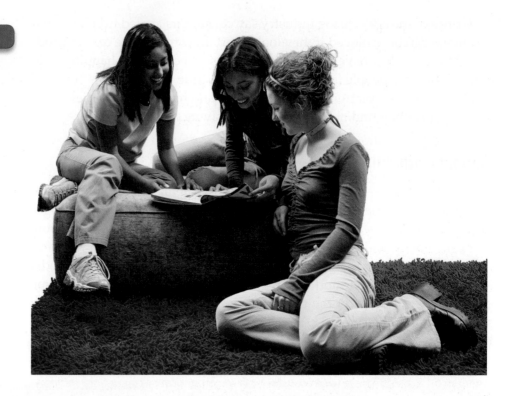

Popular media employs images of women who are consistently young and thin, promoting a standard of attractiveness against which women are measured (Figure 5.3). One study found that teenage girls who were surveyed said their ideal body size was five feet seven inches tall and 100 pounds. These dimensions are both taller than the average woman (by more than 3 inches) and substantially lighter (by over 50 pounds). A person with these body dimensions would have a BMI of less than 16. People with this BMI meet the criteria for having a serious illness, as you'll learn about later in this chapter.

Researchers in another study showed women and men silhouettes of female figures of various sizes, from thin to heavy. Participants were asked to identify the figure they considered the ideal, or the most attractive. In addition to their own preference, the women were asked to guess which silhouettes would be chosen as the ideal by other women and by men.

In the majority of cases, the figure the women chose as other women's ideal body was thinner than the figure they chose as their own ideal. The figure that women chose as men's ideal was also thinner than the figure the men in the study chose as their ideal. The women believed that men preferred a thinner female body than the men actually preferred.

Male Body Image

Like females, males are feeling increased pressure to conform to an unrealistic body image. As images of women in the media have become increasingly thin over time, images of men have become increasingly muscular. Many images in the media show men with "six-pack" abdominals, muscular chests, and large biceps. Most male bodies do not look like this, but the bodies of male models, celebrities, and sports stars portrayed in the media do.

Partly as a result of exposure to the muscular ideal, some men develop *muscle dysmorphia*. This disorder is characterized by an extreme concern with becoming more muscular. Boys and men with muscle dysmorphia see themselves as smaller than they really are, and are highly focused on bulking up to make their bodies more muscular (Figure 5.4).

The drive to achieve an unrealistically muscular figure has led some boys and men to take extreme measures, such as using *dietary supplements* and steroids to change their body shape and size. Dietary supplements, such as *creatine*—a naturally occurring amino acid that helps the body build protein—are taken in an attempt to build muscle mass.

To bulk up, some boys and men endanger their health by taking anabolic steroids or other illegal drugs. *Anabolic steroids* are artificial hormones that are used to treat certain types of muscular disorders. People also use them illegally to strengthen and increase the size of their muscles. An estimated 1 in 10 male high school athletes has tried creatine or another dietary supplement, and nearly 1.6% of high school seniors have taken steroids.

Using performance-enhancing or muscle-building drugs and supplements is not recommended by medical experts because these substances can cause both short- and long-term physical and psychological problems. These problems can include severe mood swings, hallucinations, difficulty sleeping, nausea and vomiting, high blood pressure, and an increased risk of developing heart disease, stroke, and cancer.

In addition, some of these drugs are illegal, and getting caught using them can have serious consequences. Teams with players who have used steroids may have their wins taken away. High school athletes can be thrown off their team, and may be made to feel embarrassed and ashamed of their use of illegal substances.

Ethnicity and Body Image

Although people from all backgrounds are exposed to particular body builds and types in the media, these ideals are not embraced to the same extent by everyone. Different groups in society may have different values and preferences when it comes to ideal weight and appearance. People are taught specific beliefs and norms about body image that are preferred by their own distinct group, culture, or community.

For example, some research suggests that, compared with Caucasians, African-Americans are less likely to view a very thin female body as the ideal. African-American girls and women tend to prefer a heavier weight than do Caucasians. Compared with Caucasians, African-American girls and women are also less preoccupied with their weight and dieting, and are more satisfied with their weight. The thin ideal of the female body represented in the media reflects the values of Caucasians.

muscle dysmorphia
a disorder characterized by an extreme concern with becoming more muscular

dietary supplement
a product that can be ingested to give a person's body more of a specific nutrient; can be harmful when used in excess

creatine
an amino acid that helps the body build protein; can be taken as a dietary supplement to help a person build muscle mass

anabolic steroids
artificial hormones used to treat muscular disorders; are sometimes illegally used to help people build muscle mass

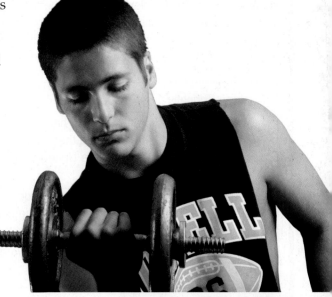

Figure 5.4

Males can sometimes be insecure about the size and tone of their muscles and may lift weights to build muscle mass. *When do you think weight lifting is healthy? At what point might it become unhealthy?*

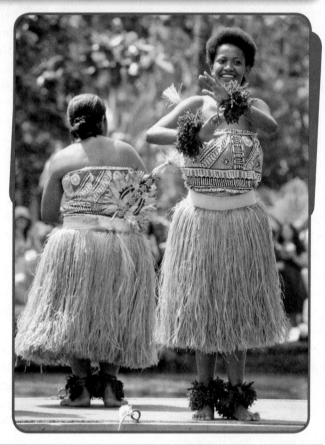

In the United States, the belief that thin women are the most attractive is clearly prevalent. This preference for thinness, however, is not seen in all cultures. Researchers in one study asked more than 7,000 people in different countries to rate their own bodies and to state what they viewed as the ideal female body. The percentage of participants who preferred a very thin female body was

- 40% in the United States and other countries where food is generally plentiful;
- 17% in countries where there is sometimes not enough food for all people; and
- 0% in countries where there is often not enough food for all people.

People in countries with limited food supplies—where there is not enough food to satisfy the nutritional needs of all the people—had a stronger preference for women who are heavier than people in countries where food is plentiful. Researchers believe that in societies with limited food supplies, women who are heavier are viewed as healthier, more fertile, and possibly wealthier than women who are thinner.

Thinking Critically

1. You read that the preference for thin women is stronger in affluent countries than it is in poorer countries. If that is true, should there also be a difference in the preference for thin versus heavy women in different parts of the United States? What do you think these preferences would be? Explain your answer.

2. Predict how the preference for the thin ideal in women might change over time. What are some factors that might cause this preference to strengthen? What factors might cause this preference to weaken?

3. This study only examined the ideal body image for women. What would you predict similar research would show if men in different countries were asked to rate their current and ideal male body shape? Explain your answer.

Compared with their white counterparts, African-American men also tend to view a larger female figure as more attractive. One study examined the body size preferences of men who were registered on an online dating website. White males were more likely than nonwhite men to seek thin and toned women to date. Both African-American and Latino men were more likely than white men to look for dating partners with larger bodies.

Sports and Body Image

Another factor that can influence a person's body image is involvement in particular sports and activities. Teenagers who are involved in sports that place importance on being thin are at greater risk of developing a poor body image. Dancers, gymnasts, and ice skaters often face pressure to be thin because certain moves are easier to perform at lighter weights.

Athletes' appearance can also influence how their performance is evaluated by judges. Athletes who participate in these activities may feel particular pressure from coaches and even parents to maintain a thin body (Figure 5.5). People who participate in these activities are also more likely to compare themselves to others who are very thin. Staying small and light becomes especially difficult, if not impossible, when these athletes reach puberty and their body shape and weight changes as their bodies mature.

In contrast, teenagers who participate in sports that do *not* emphasize thinness—such as softball, basketball, and soccer—feel less pressure to be thin. These teenagers are able to develop a more positive body image. Participation in sports such as these allows teenagers to learn new skills, experience the health and fitness benefits of regular exercise, and develop close friendships with teammates. People who participate in these sports also feel good about what their bodies are capable of doing—hitting a home run, scoring a goal, or making a basket.

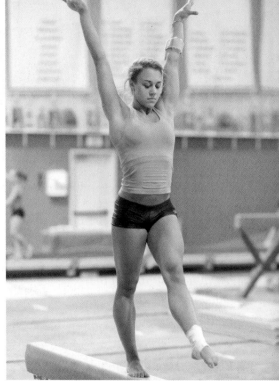

Figure 5.5

Athletes may feel pressure from coaches or family members to maintain a thin body. *Do you ever feel pressured to maintain a certain kind of body? Explain.*

Lesson 5.1 Review

Know and Understand

1. Define *body image.*
2. List four factors that influence a person's body image.
3. Explain why many girls who are a normal weight try to lose weight.
4. Describe the role that a person's ethnicity can play in the development of his or her body image.
5. Identify how parents can influence the body image of their children.

Analyze and Apply

6. Compare and contrast the various factors that are associated with body dissatisfaction in males versus females. Compare and contrast the factors that are associated with body dissatisfaction in Caucasians versus African-Americans.
7. Analyze the power of the media to affect people's body satisfaction. Use examples from the text to support your analysis.

8. Evaluate the impact of popular sports on the body image of the teenagers who participate in them. Why do some sports tend to have a positive impact on a teenager's body image, while other sports can have a negative effect?

Real World Health

List your five favorite people and write a sentence or two for each, describing why that person is so special to you. Then read what you have written to determine whether or not any of the following factors—the size and shape of their bodies, the type of clothes they wear, and their attractiveness—play a role in making those people special to you. Write a paragraph describing how important these factors are to you. Write a second paragraph discussing whether you believe your appearance is important to people who are close to you. Which of your traits and characteristics do you believe these people value?

What Are Eating Disorders?

Key Terms E-Flash Cards

In this lesson, you will learn the meanings of the following key terms.

acid reflux disorder
anorexia nervosa
binge-eating disorder
bulimia nervosa
constipation
eating disorder
hypoglycemia
infertility
lanugo
laxative

Lesson Objectives

After studying this lesson, you will be able to

- list the different types of eating disorders;
- describe the symptoms of each eating disorder;
- summarize the medical complications of eating disorders; and
- analyze the complex causes of eating disorders.

Warm-Up Activity

Eating Disorders
For this group activity, your teacher will assign each group an eating disorder. You and your group will draw the outline of a body on a poster, as shown below. Use the drawing to illustrate all the medical complications, personality traits, and behaviors associated with your assigned eating disorder. Be sure to use at least 20 facts. Type all of the facts from the poster onto a worksheet to distribute to your classmates. Be creative and make your poster colorful.

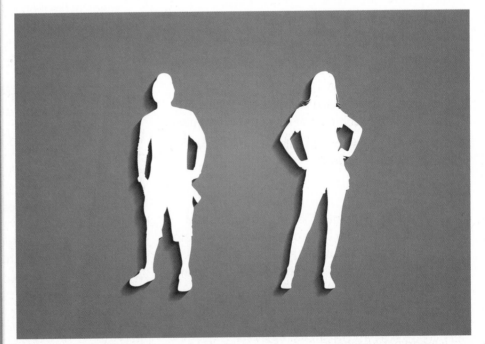

Before You Read

Eating Disorder Mindmap
*Place the key term **eating disorders** in the middle of a mindmap similar to the one shown here. As you read the lesson, brainstorm and create a mindmap around your key term.*

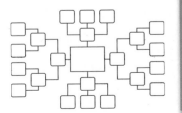

An ***eating disorder*** is a serious illness that causes major disturbances in a person's daily diet. These disturbances can include eating only extremely small amounts of food, or eating huge quantities of food in a small amount of time. People with eating disorders often focus so much on their food and weight that they have difficulty concentrating on other things.

Although eating disorders may develop during childhood or later in life, they most commonly begin during the teenage years.

Relatively few people are actually diagnosed as having eating disorders. Many people, however, engage in some type of disordered eating behavior or use unhealthy strategies to lose weight. This is especially true of girls and women.

Types of Eating Disorders

All types of eating disorders involve disturbances in eating behavior. These disorders, however, vary considerably in their symptoms. There are three main types of eating disorders: anorexia nervosa, bulimia nervosa, and binge-eating disorder.

Anorexia Nervosa

An estimated 0.9% of females and 0.3% of males in the United States develop ***anorexia nervosa***, a disorder in which people have an intense fear of gaining weight and lose far more weight than is healthy for their height. On average, this disorder begins at age 19. Anorexia tends to be more prevalent in Caucasians from upper- and upper-middle-class backgrounds, than in people from other ethnic groups and socioeconomic backgrounds.

People who have anorexia nervosa demonstrate symptoms such as

- extreme thinness (emaciation);
- a relentless pursuit of thinness;
- intense fear of gaining weight;
- distorted body image, self-esteem that is heavily influenced by perceptions of body weight and shape, or a denial of the seriousness of low body weight; and
- lack of menstruation among girls and women.

The most obvious signs of anorexia nervosa are an extremely thin body and very restricted eating. To maintain a very thin body, a person with this disorder eats only small amounts of food each day—for example, a few cornflakes for breakfast, a piece

eating disorder
a psychological illness characterized by a serious disturbance in a person's eating behavior

anorexia nervosa
an eating disorder in which a person has an intense fear of gaining weight, eats too little, and loses far more weight than is healthy for his or her height

Figure 5.6

To lose weight, people with anorexia nervosa go to extremes—perhaps eating a lettuce leaf for a meal, for example. Obviously, a single lettuce leaf does not provide the nutrients a person's body needs.

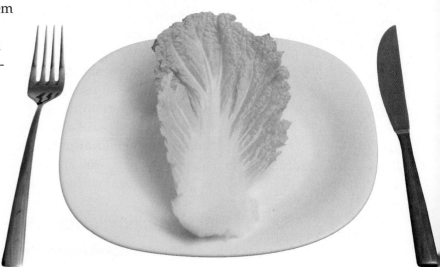

bulimia nervosa
an eating disorder in which a person has recurrent episodes of binge eating followed by purging

binge-eating disorder
an eating disorder in which a person repeatedly consumes a huge amount of food in a short period of time

of an apple for lunch, and a lettuce leaf for supper (Figure 5.6 on the previous page). An anorexic person may also engage in distinct eating rituals as a way to avoid eating. For example, he or she may cut food into very small portions or eat very slowly.

People with anorexia nervosa tend to have particular personality types. They often hold themselves to very high standards in regard to their appearance and their work or school habits. They may show high levels of orderliness and cleanliness. Ironically, these types of behaviors often lead others to see people with anorexia as well-organized and "perfect." In reality, these people are unhealthy and possibly in danger due to their extreme behavior.

Girls and women who participate in weight-focused activities—such as ballet, gymnastics, cheerleading, and modeling—are especially vulnerable to developing this disorder. Some estimates suggest that 6–7% of women who attend professional schools for modeling and dance meet the criteria for having anorexia.

Bulimia Nervosa

Bulimia nervosa is an eating disorder in which a person has recurrent episodes of binge eating followed by purging. During binge eating, enormous quantities of food are consumed at one time. People typically feel out of control while binge eating. Purging refers to efforts people make to get rid of the large number of calories consumed during a binge episode. These efforts typically include vomiting or excessive exercise. The symptoms of bulimia nervosa include a continuing pattern over time of these two types of behavior. This disorder has a prevalence rate of approximately 1.5% in American women and 0.5% in American men.

On average, this disorder begins at age 20. Bulimia is easier to hide than anorexia, in part because people with bulimia are typically a normal weight. Bulimics have often struggled with weight issues for some time and may have histories of binge eating, weight fluctuation, and frequent exercise or dieting.

People with bulimia nervosa often experience negative emotions, which both lead to and result from this unhealthy behavior pattern. Binge-purge episodes are often triggered by some type of negative emotion, such as anxiety, tension, or fatigue. Many people with bulimia nervosa are depressed and anxious, and may engage in binge eating as a way of comforting themselves. They also report feeling out of control while they are binge eating, which leads to feelings of guilt and self-hatred afterward. Sadly, an estimated 20–30% of bulimics have made at least one serious suicide attempt.

Bulimia nervosa is also often associated with other types of problems. People with bulimia are more likely than their peers to engage in destructive behavior such as drug and alcohol abuse. According to estimates, as many as 35% of women with bulimia have experienced some type of sexual abuse.

Binge-Eating Disorder

Although anorexia nervosa and bulimia nervosa are the most widely known eating disorders, the most common eating disorder is *binge-eating disorder*.

Sarah is a 15-year-old sophomore in high school. Several months ago, she was selected to be on the cheerleading squad. Although Sarah has always been thin, she has become increasingly concerned about her weight since she joined the squad. She compares herself to the other girls on the squad, which leads her to feel that she should lose weight.

Sarah went on a strict diet and weighs herself several times a day. During meals with other people, she cuts her food into very small pieces, which is time-consuming and forces her to eat slowly. Although Sarah knows she is losing weight because her clothes feel looser, she still feels overweight and worries that she needs to lose even more weight.

Thinking Critically

1. What do you think are the primary factors that led Sarah to develop a negative body image?

2. What are some strategies that could help Sarah feel better about how she looks?

3. What advice would you give other teenagers in Sarah's situation so they don't develop negative feelings about their bodies?

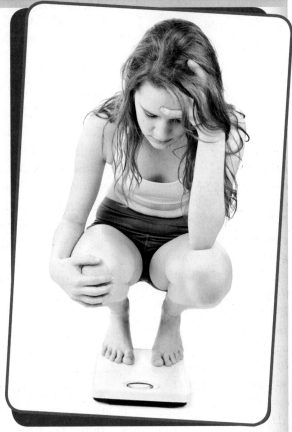

Binge-eating disorder is characterized by compulsive overeating in which people consume huge amounts of food, typically over a period of about two hours. During such a binge, people feel completely out of control and unable to stop eating. An estimated 3.5% of females and 2.0% of males report having experienced binge-eating disorder at some point in their lives. The average age at which this disorder develops is 25.

The key features of binge-eating disorder are frequent episodes of uncontrollable binge eating and feelings of extreme distress during or after bingeing. Unlike people with bulimia nervosa, people who have binge-eating disorder do not regularly attempt to "make up" for the binges by vomiting, fasting, or exercising excessively.

Because they eat as fast as they can, people with binge-eating disorder don't register what they are eating or how it tastes. They eat even when they're not hungry and continue eating long after they're full. Not surprisingly, binge-eating disorder often leads to obesity and is prevalent in up to 30% of people who seek weight-loss treatment. People with this disorder often experience feelings of guilt, disgust, and depression. They worry about what their destructive eating behavior is doing to their bodies, and feel terrible that they do not have the self-control to stop it.

Problems Caused by Eating Disorders

Eating disorders can lead to very serious and, in some cases, life-threatening medical complications. The nature of these problems varies depending on the behaviors associated with each of these disorders.

Anorexia Nervosa

Many of the problems caused by anorexia nervosa result from starvation and include decreased bone density (Figure 5.7), brittle hair and nails, dry and yellowish skin, and growth of fine hair all over the body (*lanugo*). More serious problems can include mild anemia (an insufficient number of red blood cells); muscle wasting and weakness; severe *constipation* (infrequent or delayed hard, dry bowel movements); low blood pressure; and feeling tired and cold. In addition, anorexia can cause heart and brain damage, organ failure, and *infertility* (inability to reproduce).

Some of these health problems disappear once the person gains enough weight. For example, feeling tired all the time, feeling cold, and anemia are problems caused by severe thinness, and cease to be problems once the person is no longer very thin.

Unfortunately, anorexia nervosa causes other problems that continue even after the person has gained weight again. For example, adolescence is an extremely important time for bone density growth. Low calcium intake during this life stage can't be made up later in life. People who had anorexia during their teenage years have a greater risk for osteoporosis and bone fractures for the rest of their lives.

Bulimia Nervosa and Binge-Eating Disorder

Problems caused by bulimia nervosa include a chronically inflamed and sore throat, swollen salivary glands in the neck and jaw area, a worn tooth enamel, and increasingly sensitive and decaying teeth. Other problems

lanugo
the growth of fine hair all over the body; often a result of anorexia nervosa

constipation
a condition characterized by infrequent or delayed hard, dry bowel movements

infertility
a condition in which a man or woman is physically unable to reproduce

---

Figure 5.7

Osteoporosis, which can result from an eating disorder, is a disease characterized by brittle bones. Compared with the healthy bone tissue on the left, the bone tissue of the person with osteoporosis is weak and brittle, and more likely to fracture. *Why do you think people with anorexia starve themselves despite the harm it does to their bodies?*

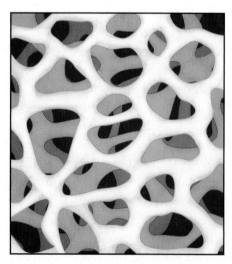

Normal

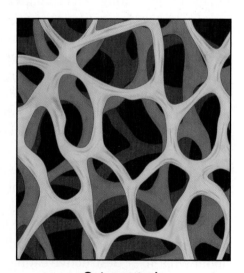

Osteoporosis

include intestinal problems such as *acid reflux disorder* (movement of acid-containing chyme from the stomach into the lower esophagus); intestinal distress and irritation from *laxative* (medication used to encourage bowel movement) abuse; severe dehydration from purging of fluids; and electrolyte imbalance (too low or too high levels of sodium, calcium, potassium and other minerals), which can lead to a heart attack.

Many of the problems associated with bulimia nervosa are caused by the repeated purging following binges. For example, frequent vomiting may cause tearing and bleeding in the esophagus, burning of the throat and mouth by stomach acids, and damage to tooth enamel. Frequent purging can lead to deficiencies in various nutrients, as well as anemia, which can cause both weakness and tiredness. Fortunately, many of these problems go away after the purging behavior stops.

Other problems observed in people with bulimia nervosa and binge-eating disorder are caused by the binges. Consuming extremely large amounts of food in a very short period of time can damage the stomach and intestines. Binges can also lead to *hypoglycemia*, which is a deficiency of sugar in the blood. Following a binge of sweets, the pancreas releases excessive amounts of insulin, which drives down blood sugar levels and can lead to feelings of dizziness, fatigue, and depression.

acid reflux disorder
a gastrointestinal problem in which acid-containing chyme moves from the lower stomach into the esophagus

laxative
a medication that is used to encourage and aid bowel movements

hypoglycemia
a deficiency of sugar in the blood; often a result of excessive amounts of insulin being released to lower blood sugar levels

Mortality

Most importantly, people with eating disorders experience high rates of mortality. An estimated 4–6% of people with eating disorders die as a result of the disorders. People with anorexia nervosa are 18 times more likely to die early compared with people of similar age in the general population. Most of these deaths are a result of heart failure, organ failure, or suicide (Figure 5.8).

Factors Contributing to Eating Disorders

Although virtually everyone in our culture is exposed to images of thin women in the media, relatively few people develop eating disorders. This suggests that while media images may contribute to the development of a negative body image, other factors play a larger role in disordered eating. While experts don't know what specifically causes these disorders to develop, they believe that both biological, or genetic, factors and family dynamics may play a role.

Biological and Genetic Factors

Experts believe biological and genetic factors may trigger the development of eating disorders. Women who have a close relative, such as a mother or sister, with an eating disorder are more likely to develop an eating disorder themselves. Anorexia is eight times more common in people who have relatives with the disorder than in people who do not. Eating disorders are also much more likely to afflict both individuals in pairs of identical twins than those in pairs of fraternal twins.

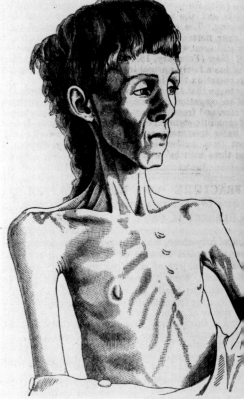

Figure 5.8

This sketch of a young woman with anorexia nervosa was published in a medical journal in1888.

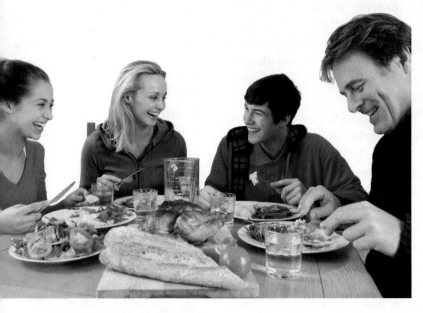

Family Dynamics

In some cases, children learn or develop unhealthy eating patterns from watching their parents. For example, teenage girls who use extreme weight-loss methods—such as fasting, crash dieting, and skipping meals—are more likely to have mothers who also use such methods. Even if the mothers do not directly encourage their daughters to engage in such behaviors, the mothers model their attitudes and behaviors.

Negative interaction patterns within a family may also trigger disordered eating. Children who develop anorexia nervosa sometimes have parents who are very controlling and overly involved in their lives. Patients diagnosed with anorexia nervosa typically describe their parents as people who set extremely high standards of achievement. These parents are frequently disapproving.

Similarly, the families of people with bulimia nervosa share particular characteristics. These characteristics include high levels of conflict and hostility and low levels of nurturance and support. People who lack supportive relationships with family members may binge and purge to cope with feelings of isolation and stress. Parents of people with bulimia nervosa are also more likely to have had problems such as alcoholism, substance abuse, and obesity.

Certain characteristics are also associated with the families of children with low rates of disordered eating. For example, studies show that these families tend to have meals together on a regular basis (Figure 5.9). So families that eat together regularly are less likely to have a teenager with an eating disorder.

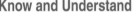

Figure 5.9

Teenagers who have meals with their families are less likely to develop anorexia. *Why do you think eating as a family can reduce a person's risk of developing an eating disorder?*

Lesson 5.2 Review

Know and Understand 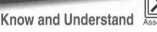 Assess

1. List three eating disorders discussed in this chapter.

2. Describe health problems that can be caused by anorexia nervosa.

3. Describe health problems that can be caused by bulimia nervosa.

4. Discuss health problems that can be caused by binge-eating disorder.

Analyze and Apply

5. Compare and contrast the behaviors that are characteristic of anorexia nervosa, bulimia nervosa, and binge-eating disorder.

6. Analyze the effect family dynamics may have on the risk for developing an eating disorder.

Real World Health

As a high school student, you have great influence over younger students. Create a presentation appropriate for an elementary or middle school class that gives information about the three eating disorders. Be sure to include the signs, symptoms, and medical complications. Don't forget to add some interesting facts found in this chapter. Lastly, give your audience at least 10 tips for how they can improve their body image.

Treating and Preventing Body Image Issues

Lesson Objectives

After studying this lesson, you will be able to

- compare different approaches for treating eating disorders;

- evaluate how images of celebrities and models are altered to enhance certain features or make them appear thinner;

- analyze the impact of enhanced photos on the body image of a young person who views them; and

- describe how the media's use of size diversity when selecting models might impact teens' body image and the incidence of eating disorders.

Key Terms E-Flash Cards

In this lesson, you will learn the meanings of the following key terms.

airbrush

cognitive-behavioral therapy

family-based therapy

idealized image

therapist

Before You Read

KWL Chart: Eating Disorders
Create a chart similar to the one shown below and list information under the headings "Know," "Want," and "Learned." Under the "Know" heading, brainstorm what you already know about the prevention and treatment of eating disorders. Under "Want," brainstorm what you would like to learn about this topic. After you have read this chapter, list what you learned about eating disorder prevention and treatment under "Learned."

K What you <u>K</u>now	W What you <u>W</u>ant to know	L What you have <u>L</u>earned

Warm-Up Activity

"Rules" for Being Thin
People with eating disorders often live by extreme rules. Listed below are several rules that people with an eating disorder might create and consider important. In groups, develop "The 5 Healthy Rules" by modifying each of the statements listed below to reflect more healthful behavior.

The Thin Rules

1. You are only attractive if you are thin.
2. You must feel guilty about what you eat.
3. You must punish yourself for eating fatty foods.
4. You must keep track of your calorie intake.
5. If you're losing weight, you're good. If you're gaining weight, you're bad.

The Healthy Rules

1. _____
2. _____
3. _____
4. _____
5. _____

Although people who have eating disorders can suffer serious health consequences, they are often reluctant to seek treatment. Getting treatment, however, is vital to recovery from disordered eating. In this lesson, you'll read about treatments that have been effective. You'll also learn about strategies that can help prevent eating disorders and body image issues.

Treating Eating Disorders

Many people with eating disorders are embarrassed to admit their behavior and may believe that their disorders will go away without treatment. Some of these people are afraid that treating their disorder will cause them to gain weight.

Eating disorders rarely go away without proper treatment, so it is important for people struggling with these disorders to get help. By getting help, they can feel better about themselves and avoid serious, long-term health consequences. Eating disorders are mental disorders and should be treated by mental health professionals.

Individual Therapy

Many people find that talking with a therapist is very helpful in managing a mental or emotional illness, including eating disorders. A **therapist** is a professional trained to diagnose and treat people with mental illnesses and disorders. Therapists include psychologists, psychiatrists, social workers, and counselors. Individual therapy consists of meeting one-on-one with a therapist. Therapists help their patients better understand problems that may contribute to their eating disorders. For example, people with anorexia nervosa are often perfectionists. Therapists can help these people learn to manage their drive for perfectionism in healthier ways. In addition, therapists can help people with bulimia improve their negative self-image (Figure 5.10).

Another type of individual therapy often used to treat eating disorders is **cognitive-behavioral therapy**. This type of therapy focuses on clarifying patients' distorted thoughts and behaviors regarding food, weight, and body shape.

Cognitive-behavioral therapy often employs techniques to

- help patients create more normal eating patterns by encouraging them to eat slowly and to eat regular meals;
- expand the types of foods patients are comfortable eating;
- change patients' faulty beliefs about food, such as "If I gain one pound, I'll gain a hundred," and "Any sweet is instantly converted into fat;"
- help patients develop more realistic body ideals, partially by teaching them that media images are often illusions created by digitally altering and airbrushing to correct imperfections; and
- change patients' thoughts and attitudes about eating, food, and their bodies by teaching them to avoid linking their self-esteem with their weight.

In cases of bulimia nervosa and binge-eating disorder, therapists may also help patients understand the thoughts, feelings, and circumstances that lead to their episodes of binge eating and purging. Then patients are taught other ways to cope with those feelings.

therapist
a professional who is trained to diagnose and treat people with mental illnesses and disorders

cognitive-behavioral therapy
a type of therapy that focuses on clarifying patients' distorted thoughts and behaviors

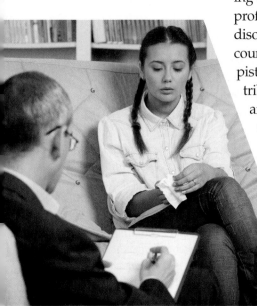

Figure 5.10

Therapy can be a powerful tool for battling an eating disorder. *Have you ever been to a therapist? What therapy centers are in your area?*

Improving Body Image

If you find that you are experiencing body image issues, try some of the following strategies.

- Ask yourself if images you view in the media reflect reality. Are these images digitally manipulated or airbrushed to present a more idealized image?

- Remember that advertisements are carefully crafted for the purpose of convincing you to buy something. By making you feel you need to fix or improve some aspect of your appearance, advertisers entice you to spend money buying their products.

- Make a list of things you like about your body—your hands, your hair, or your eyes, for example. Try to focus on these positive features instead of dwelling on the parts of your body you don't like.

- Focus on what your body can *do*, not just your appearance. Can you kick a soccer ball, dance in a school performance, hike up a mountain, or swim a lap of freestyle? Reminding yourself of these skills will help you view your body in a more positive light.

- Avoid unrealistic images of people in magazines, on television, and online whenever possible. Remember these images are often manufactured and very few people have these idealized body types. If it's difficult to look at the images without making comparisons to yourself, avoid them completely. Doing something small, such as refusing to buy fashion or body-building magazines, is a strategy that will help you feel better about yourself, save money, and send a message of protest.

- Focus on all the features you like about yourself—your intelligence, your sense of humor, your kindness to others—and not just your physical appearance.

Family Therapy

As you know, the patterns of interaction in a patient's family are thought to influence the development of disordered eating. As a result, many therapists recommend some combination of individual and family therapy when treating eating disorders. *Family-based therapy* involves parents or guardians, as well as siblings of the patient, in treatment. Therapists help parents and guardians to separate their child from the disorder, and to address how this disorder affects their child's development (Figure 5.11).

In one study of adolescents with bulimia nervosa, participants received 20 therapy sessions over the course of six months. Some adolescents received family therapy, while other participants received individual therapy. At the end of treatment, 39% of those in family therapy had stopped their disordered eating behaviors, compared with only 18% of the teenagers who received individual therapy. Family therapy has been similarly helpful to teenagers with anorexia nervosa.

family-based therapy
a type of therapy that involves parents or guardians, and siblings of patients in treatment

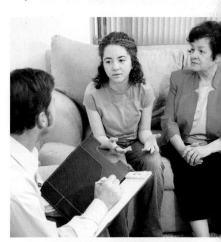

Figure 5.11

Research has shown that family dynamics can play a significant role in the development of eating disorders, so it is not surprising that family therapy sessions can help end the disorders.

Challenges of Treatment

Although people with eating disorders do get better, they have a relatively high rate of relapse. Among those with anorexia nervosa or bulimia nervosa, about 60% have a full recovery, about 20% have a partial recovery, and about 20% have no real improvement. Many people with anorexia continue to be underweight and require repeated hospitalizations. Their bodies may be unable to repair the damage caused by years of disordered eating. For example, they are at high risk of developing the bone disease osteoporosis.

Among people with bulimia nervosa, about one-third of those who fully recover experience a relapse within two years. These depressing statistics suggest that recovery from eating disorders is best viewed as a process. Patients and their families should not expect instant results.

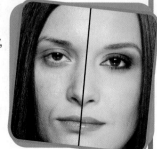

Health in the Media

Airbrushing Media Images

In 2011, the British Advertising Standards Authority, which regulates advertising in that country, banned the publication of two makeup advertisements. The ads were said to violate advertising standards by presenting misleading images of women.

Both advertisements promoted the use of skin foundation to cover imperfections and enhance beauty. One ad featured a photograph of actress Julia Roberts, and the other featured model Christy Turlington. The images of both women were airbrushed to improve their appearance. This made it difficult for the public to determine whether the flawless skin they saw in the ads resulted from the products advertised or from the altering of the photographs.

Thinking Critically

1. Generate a list of actions you could take to try to decrease the use of misleading images in the media.

2. Given the product being advertised, how would you evaluate the action taken by the British Advertising Standards Authority?

idealized image
an image or standard of beauty that does not exist in real life

airbrush
to alter an image using specialized software to conceal imperfections

Preventing Body Image Issues

Many people—especially girls and women—have body image issues and show symptoms of disordered eating. Doctors and therapists have developed a number of strategies and programs to prevent such issues.

As you learned earlier in this chapter, one factor contributing to negative body image is the unrealistically thin images of women presented in the media. In one program's approach, participants are taught to recognize how images of people are manipulated to create an *idealized image*, or an image that does not exist in real life. For example, these images are almost always *airbrushed* or digitally altered to eliminate blemishes, cellulite, or wrinkles; to add tans; and to reduce bulges. Images of men are also altered to present a more idealized image.

In another program's approach, high school girls participating in a workshop discussed the nature and origins of the thin ideal. They were then asked to write a letter to a hypothetical younger girl discussing the harmful effects of believing in this ideal. The girls were taught to focus on positive thoughts about their own bodies and to develop strategies for coping with and countering the thin ideal. This program led to improvements in the body satisfaction of participants, reduced concerns about weight, and decreased symptoms of disordered eating.

What Businesses Are Doing

Another strategy for improving body image is the presentation of more realistic images of people in the media. This is intended to help improve body satisfaction in normal-weight girls and women, and to decrease the pressure they feel to conform to an extremely thin ideal.

Dove Advertising Campaign. Some companies are opposing industry practices by using more realistic images of women in their advertising campaigns. For example, the Unilever company developed a highly successful advertising campaign for Dove soap called the *Campaign for Real Beauty.* The ads featured the slogan "real women have curves." In contrast to the images of unrealistically thin and unhealthy females that populate most advertisements, this campaign featured six women of various shapes and sizes, rather than models. Real, natural beauty was promoted in this campaign. These women, who ranged from size 6 to size 14, appeared throughout the national campaign.

Banning Overly Thin Models. Given the negative impact of the thin ideal, some health advocates have proposed a ban on the use of underweight models in advertising. In 2012, *Vogue,* one of the best-selling fashion magazines in the world, began to ban the use of very thin models. According to this policy, the magazine would not use models that appear to have eating disorders. This decision could reduce the number of images of very thin women in magazines, especially if other magazines follow suit.

What Governments Are Doing

US lawmakers have introduced legislation to educate the public and promote the use of healthier images in the media. Unfortunately, several efforts to create such legislation have failed.

Other countries have taken stronger action. For example, Spain and Italy now require that models have a BMI of at least 18.5 before they can participate in prestigious fashion-week shows. There are no such regulations about models' BMI in the United States (Figure 5.12).

In March of 2012, Israel became the first country to pass legislation banning the use of extremely thin models in local ads and publications. According to the law, a model must produce a recent medical report to prove that her BMI is higher than 18.5. According to the World Health Organization, a BMI lower than 18.5 is an indication of malnourishment. The Israeli law also requires publications to tell readers when an image has been edited to make a model appear thinner.

The editing of photos to make models look thinner has recently become controversial. When a cover photo of actress Kate Winslet was edited to make her appear taller and slimmer than she is in real life, she complained publically, saying: "… I don't want to look like that. They made my legs look quite a bit thinner. They also made me look about six feet tall, which I'm not, I'm 5′ 6″… Me and my sisters and my mum are quite proud of our [muscular], strong legs and hips—and all the rest of it."

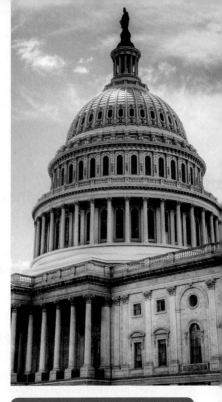

Figure 5.12

Some countries have been much more aggressive than others in trying to curb body image problems through legislation. *Do you think the US government should pass legislation banning certain types of advertising related to body image? Why or why not?*

Lesson 5.3 Review

Know and Understand

1. List two ways therapists help individuals with eating disorders manage their condition.
2. Evaluate the effectiveness of therapy for a person with an eating disorder when family members participate versus when they do not participate.
3. Describe how government regulations concerning airbrushed magazine photos and model BMIs could help improve body image and decrease eating disorders.
4. Explain what Dove's *Campaign for Real Beauty* tried to accomplish.

Analyze and Apply

5. Analyze the impact that airbrushed photos of male models, celebrities, and athletes can have on males.
6. Search online to find original and digitally altered versions of photos of a celebrity. Write a brief comparison of the images.

7. Some professional athletes speak out against their images being airbrushed when they appear in magazines and other media. Analyze the impact that taking this stance against digitally altered images can have on the body image of these athletes' fans.

Real World Health

One of the most powerful contributors to body dissatisfaction is exposure to harmful images in the media. A person who is dissatisfied with his or her body may diet, which can lead to the development of an eating disorder. Write a letter to the editor of your favorite magazine and express your desire to see models of different shapes and sizes in the magazine. Support your argument with at least 10 facts about body image and eating disorders that you read in this chapter.

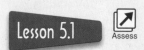

Lesson 5.1

Factors that Influence Body Image

Key Terms

anabolic steroids
body image
creatine
dietary supplement
muscle dysmorphia

Key Points

- An individual's body image is influenced by family and friends, the media, his or her ethnicity, and any sport in which he or she participates.
- Because people of different ethnic backgrounds have different ideals of beauty, eating disorders are more common in some cultures than in others.
- Just as media images of women have become thinner over time, media images of men have become more muscular.
- Teens compare their bodies to the unrealistic bodies they see in the media.

Check Your Understanding

1. *True or false?* Males do not experience body dissatisfaction.

2. *True or false?* Body image is defined as what a person's body looks like.

3. Advertisements for beauty products are an example of which of the following factors that influences body image?
   A. family and peers
   B. the media
   C. ethnicity
   D. sports

4. Which of the following statements is true about the female body image?
   A. There has always been a preference for thin girls and women in the media.
   B. Many women believe men prefer a thinner female body.
   C. The preference for thin girls and women in the media is relatively new.
   D. Both B and C are true.

5. A type of disorder that is characterized by an extreme concern with being more muscular is known as _____.

6. Which of the following statements about anabolic steroids is true?
   A. Anabolic steroids are naturally occurring amino acids.
   B. Anabolic steroids can cause both short- and long-term physical and psychological problems.
   C. Anabolic steroids are artificial hormones.
   D. Both B and C are true.

7. Discuss why African-Americans are less likely to see a very thin female body as ideal.

8. Which of the following statements is true?
   A. Certain sports increase an athlete's positive body image.
   B. Certain sports decrease an athlete's positive body image.
   C. Neither statement is true.
   D. Both A and B are true.

9. **Critical Thinking.** Analyze factors that have led to the increase in male body dissatisfaction over the last few decades.

Lesson 5.2

What Are Eating Disorders?

Key Terms

acid reflux disorder
anorexia nervosa
binge-eating disorder
bulimia nervosa
constipation
eating disorder
hypoglycemia
infertility
lanugo
laxative

Key Points

- All types of eating disorders are severe disturbances in daily eating patterns, but symptoms of each disorder vary.
- People who have anorexia nervosa are characterized by extremely thin bodies and severe, self-imposed restrictions on eating.
- People with bulimia nervosa exhibit a pattern of consuming huge amounts of food and then attempting to purge, or expel, this food from their bodies to prevent weight gain.
- Binge-eating disorder, the most common eating disorder, is characterized by the consumption of large amounts of food without any purging behaviors.
- Eating disorders are dangerous illnesses that can lead to serious health problems and even death.
- In addition to the media, biological and genetic factors are believed to play a role in the development of eating disorders.

Check Your Understanding

10. List the three most common eating disorders.

11. Which eating disorder is the most common?

12. *True or false?* An estimated 20–30% of people who have bulimia attempt suicide at least once.

13. What is the average age for the onset of binge-eating disorder?
    A. 15 years old
    B. 20 years old
    C. 25 years old
    D. 30 years old

14. List the major differences between anorexia nervosa and bulimia nervosa.

15. Why is it easier for people with bulimia nervosa to hide their condition than it is for people with other eating disorders?

16. The growth of fine hair all over the body is a side effect of anorexia nervosa called _____.

17. Compared with their peers, people who have anorexia nervosa are _____ more likely to die early.
    A. 3 times
    B. 8 times
    C. 15 times
    D. 18 times

18. Frequent purging associated with bulimia nervosa can contribute to which of the following?
    A. tearing and bleeding in the esophagus
    B. damage to tooth enamel
    C. deficiencies in various nutrients
    D. All of the above.

19. *True or false?* Biological, or *genetic*, factors and family dynamics are believed to play a greater role in the development of an eating disorder than media images.

20. **Critical Thinking.** Hypothesize why anorexia has the highest mortality rate of all the eating disorders.

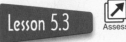

Lesson 5.3

Assess

Treating and Preventing Body Image Issues

Key Terms

airbrush
cognitive-behavioral therapy
family-based therapy
idealized image
therapist

Key Points

- Eating disorders are mental disorders and must be treated by mental health professionals.
- Counseling, especially when it includes the family, is important to the recovery of someone with an eating disorder.
- The ability to recognize when images have been digitally altered helps individuals feel better about their own bodies.
- By emphasizing only one standard of beauty, which is unrealistic, the media play a large role in making people feel dissatisfied with their bodies.
- In other countries, legislation has been introduced that requires models to have healthy BMIs.

Check Your Understanding

21. *True or false?* Eating disorders often resolve themselves.

22. _____ focuses on clarifying patients' distorted thoughts and behaviors regarding food, weight, and body shape.
    A. Family-based therapy
    B. Cognitive-behavioral therapy
    C. Dysmorphia
    D. None of the above.

23. List three strategies described in the text to prevent poor body image.

24. *True or false?* Airbrushing is a technique used by the media to create idealized images.

25. Spain and Italy are being proactive by banning models who are too thin from being used in advertisements. What is the minimum BMI required to model in these two countries?
    A. 15
    B. 15.5
    C. 18.5
    D. 28.5

26. **Critical Thinking.** Develop a hypothesis about how the media might create a healthier body image for Americans by using models of all shapes and sizes.

Health and Wellness Skills

27. **Advocate for Health.** *Just Try it, Don't Diet*: Use your advocacy skills to produce a poster that will be used by your school to promote healthy eating instead of dieting. The poster will be part of an anti-dieting campaign aimed at teenagers. Another goal of the campaign is to boost the self esteem of teenagers by helping them view their bodies more positively. The poster should be visually stimulating and include a catchy slogan, as well as five facts about why dieting is unhealthy.

28. **Analyze Influences.** Write a paragraph about the factors that influence an individual's concept of what is attractive and unattractive. Post your paragraph on a class blog and exchange feedback with a classmate. Then update your blog post using your classmate's feedback.

29. **Self Management.** Make a "Top 10" list of behaviors or attitudes that can help enhance the body image and overall health of teenagers. For example: Always wear clothes that fit properly. This helps a person feel comfortable in his or her clothes and helps foster body satisfaction.

30. **Analyze Influences.** Listen to the song "Video" by India.Arie and answer the following questions:

   A. What message is the artist trying to convey to people in this song?

   B. What is your view or opinion about this media message?

   C. Pick out your favorite line (a complete thought or sentence) from the song. Write it down and explain why you chose that line.

Hands-On Activity
Mirror, Mirror

As you learned in this chapter, your body image describes how you feel about your appearance, but it does not describe how you actually look. If you have a negative self-image, you can alter your thinking to view yourself more positively. Take the following steps to consider your inner beauty and improve your self-image.

Steps for this Activity

1. On a separate sheet of paper, write seven statements to describe your inner beauty. The list should include your strengths, talents, and other characteristics you take pride in. Do *not* list physical traits.

2. On the back of the sheet, write a few paragraphs to answer the following questions:

   • Was it difficult to come up with seven statements about your inner beauty? If so, why do you think it was difficult?

   • Can you think of a time in your life when you exhibited or used each strength, talent, and characteristic? Briefly describe these experiences.

   • Analyze why it is healthier for people to focus on their inner beauty than their outer beauty.

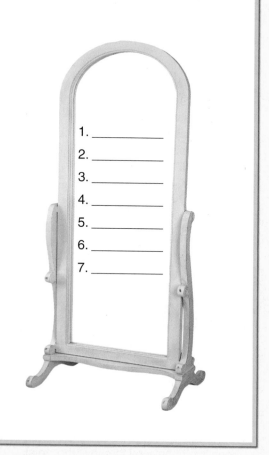

1. _____
2. _____
3. _____
4. _____
5. _____
6. _____
7. _____

Core Skills

Math Practice

Eating Disorder Statistics		
	Period 1	**Period 2**
Total Hospitalizations due to Eating Disorders	23,807	28,155
male	2,265	?
female	21,524	?
Type of Eating Disorder		
anorexia nervosa	8,932	10, 413
bulimia nervosa	7,286	6,770
other	7,589	10,972
Average Hospital Cost per Patient	$7,046	$9,628

31. What was the percentage change in total hospitalizations due to eating disorders from period 1 to period 2?
    A. 15%
    B. 18%
    C. -15%
    D. -18%

32. In period 2, 89% of the total hospitalizations were female patients. How many females were hospitalized?
    A. 2,508
    B. 19,156
    C. 21,188
    D. 25,058

33. Using the average hospital cost per patient, determine the total hospital cost in period 1 for patients with anorexia nervosa.
    A. $167,744,122
    B. $85,997,296
    C. $62,934,872
    D. $62,934

34. What was the percentage change in average hospital cost per patient from period 1 to period 2?
    A. 36.6%
    B. 0.36%
    C. 26.8%
    D. 0.26%

Reading and Writing Practice

Read the passage below and then answer the questions.

Another factor that can influence a person's body image is involvement in particular sports and activities. Teenagers who are involved in sports that place importance on being thin are at greater risk of developing a poor body image. Dancers, gymnasts, and ice skaters often face pressure to be thin because certain moves are easier to perform at lighter weights. Athletes' appearance can also influence how their performance is evaluated by judges. Athletes who participate in these activities may feel particular pressure from coaches and even parents to maintain a thin body. People who participate in these activities are also more likely to compare themselves to others who are very thin.

In contrast, teenagers who participate in sports that do not emphasize thinness—such as softball, basketball, and soccer—feel less pressure to be thin. These teenagers are able to develop a more positive body image. Participation in sports such as these allows teenagers to learn new skills, experience the health and fitness benefits of regular exercise, and develop close friendships with teammates. People who participate in these sports also feel good about what their bodies are capable of doing—hitting a home run, scoring a goal, or making a basket.

35. Why does body weight matter in sports such as gymnastics, dancing, and skating?
    A. Because the media has set the standard for the weight of those athletes.
    B. Because these sports set weight limits.
    C. Because some of the moves are harder to perform at a heavier weight.
    D. Because of the costumes used for these sports.

36. In sports that seem to emphasize weight, who is pressuring athletes to be thin?
    A. coaches
    B. parents
    C. judges
    D. Both A and B.

37. Write a paragraph describing the effect you believe sports should have on a teen's body image.

Unit 3 Fitness and Personal Health

Big Ideas

- Being physically active and getting regular exercise benefits your health in many ways.

- Most teenagers are regularly sleep deprived and suffer consequences to their health and wellness.

- By performing simple acts of personal hygiene and basic healthcare, you promote your health and wellness.

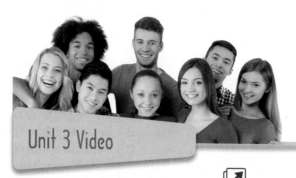

Unit 3 Video

Exercise! The Infomercial Videos

Which product can make you healthy and strong, increase your energy level, boost your positive emotions, extend your life, and help you look good? And it's free! The benefits of physical activity and exercise are promoted in this spoof of an infomercial.

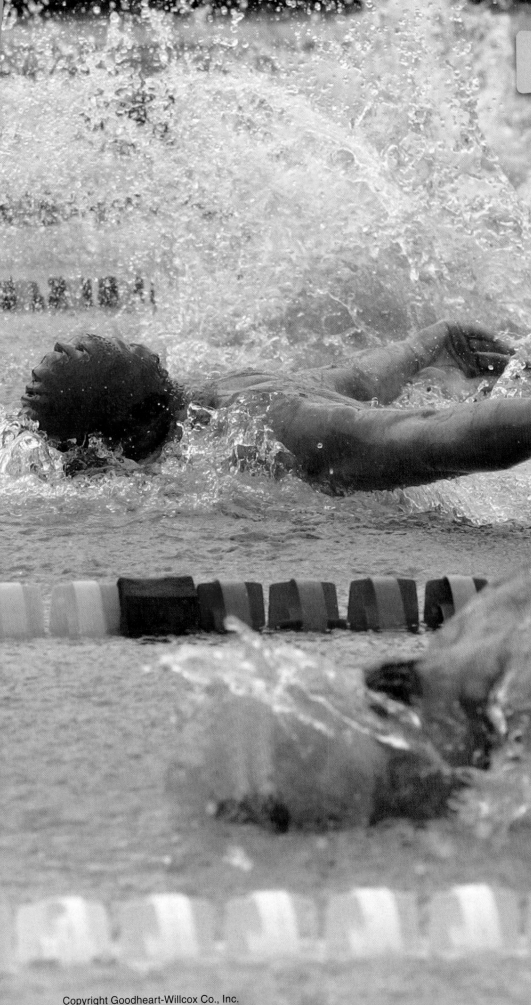

Assess the Usefulness of Each Source

You've gathered information about your topic from authoritative sources. Now, carefully read the information and answer the following questions for each source:

- Who is the author(s) and what are his or her credentials and affiliation (a professor of public health at X College, for example). Don't use the information if this is unclear.
- In the case of a study, who paid for the study? Avoid information paid for by groups with vested interests—a study about the health effects of chocolate funded by a candy company, for example.
- When was the information published or posted, or the study conducted?
- What does the author cite as his or her sources of information? Are these authoritative sources (see Unit 2)? If not, don't use the information.
- Which main points is the author(s) trying to convey? Does the information help you answer your research question?

Compare and contrast the different sources of information and identify which are the most credible and most relevant to your research question. Identify and note any facts you can use from these sources. Create a tentative bibliography of the sources you intend to use.

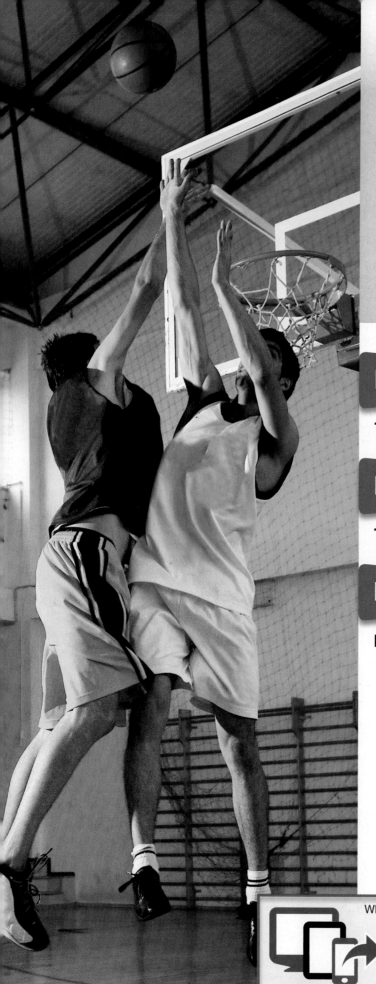

Chapter 6
Physical Fitness

Lesson 6.1

The Benefits of Improved Physical Fitness

Lesson 6.2

The Components of Physical Fitness

Lesson 6.3

Fitness Safety

While studying this chapter, look for the activity icon  to:

- **review** vocabulary with e-flash cards and games;
- **assess** learning with quizzes and online exercises;
- **expand** knowledge with animations and activities; and
- **listen** to pronunciation of key terms in the audio glossary.

G-WLEARNING.com

www.g-wlearning.com/health/

Take this quiz to see what you do *and* do not *know about physical fitness. If you cannot answer a question, pay extra attention to that topic as you study this chapter.*

1. *Identify each statement as* True, False, *or* It Depends. *Choose* It Depends *if a statement is true in some cases, but false in others.*
2. *Revise each* False *statement to make it true.*
3. *Explain the circumstances in which each* It Depends *statement is true and when it is false.*

Health and Wellness IQ Assess

	True	False	It Depends
1. People who engage in regular physical activity are less likely to develop cardiovascular disease.	True	False	It Depends
2. People who engage in regular physical activity live longer.	True	False	It Depends
3. Coordination is closely related to balance.	True	False	It Depends
4. Regular physical activity has no effect on muscle strength.	True	False	It Depends
5. You should stretch before engaging in any type of physical activity.	True	False	It Depends
6. All high school students participate in physical education classes.	True	False	It Depends
7. If you are just starting an exercise program, you should begin by exercising for long periods of time to give yourself confidence to continue.	True	False	It Depends
8. Engaging in physical activity leads to better academic performance.	True	False	It Depends
9. Drinking high-calorie juices, sodas, or sports drinks is the best way to hydrate your body while working out.	True	False	It Depends
10. The acronym FITT stands for frequency, intensity, time, and type.	True	False	It Depends

Setting the Scene

What types of physical activity have you engaged in during the last month? Did you go for a walk, run, or bike ride? Did you participate in a team or individual sport? Did you dance with friends at a party? Did you vacuum, sweep, or rake leaves?

These are all examples of physical activity. Physical activity is any type of action that requires movement, during which your body expends energy. This chapter examines the benefits of physical activity, different types of physical fitness, and strategies for safely increasing fitness and avoiding injury.

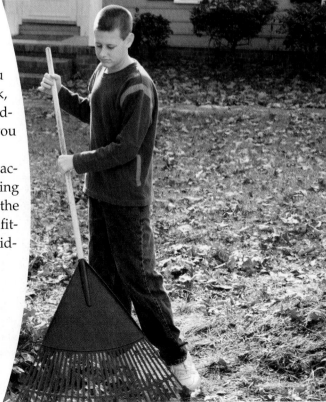

The Benefits of Improved Physical Fitness

Key Terms 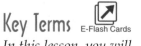 E-Flash Cards

In this lesson, you will learn the meanings of the following key terms.

endorphins

exercise

fitness

physical activity

Physical Activity Guidelines for Americans

sedentary behavior

Before You Read

Stress and Physical Activity

Draw a line down the middle of a sheet of paper to create two columns. In the column on the left, list the top ten stressors that you are experiencing right now. In the column on the right, identify how regular physical activity could help manage each stressor. Share and discuss your lists with your classmates.

My top ten stressors	How physical activity can help

Lesson Objectives

After studying this lesson, you will be able to

- summarize how physical activity can lower risks for diseases such as cancer;
- describe the benefits of physical activity related to bone and muscle strength;
- identify ways in which physical activity helps control weight and improve sleep;
- recognize how physical activity can improve academic performance;
- differentiate between exercise and physical activity; and
- summarize strategies for improving your fitness.

Warm-Up Activity

Do I Get Enough Physical Activity?

On a separate sheet of paper, list all of the regular physical activity and all of the structured exercise that you have participated in over the last seven days. Label each item as a sport, chore, physical education class activity, or the regular physical activity of your daily routine. Write a reflection explaining whether you feel you get enough exercise. What changes could you make to include more physical activity and exercise in your daily life?

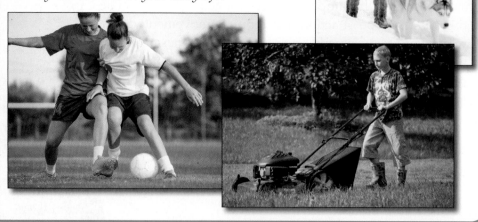

P eople who are physically fit have enough energy to perform their regular daily life activities. They also have enough energy, strength, and flexibility to meet unexpected physical demands (Figure 6.1). This means that people who are physically fit can easily climb a flight of stairs, carry a heavy package, or walk through a shopping mall. In short, *fitness* is the body's ability to respond to the physical demands placed upon it. People who are fit can meet the day's physical challenges with energy to spare.

In this lesson, you will learn how engaging in physical activity benefits your health. You will also learn strategies for improving your physical fitness.

What Are the Benefits of Physical Activity?

Engaging in regular physical activity is one of the most important actions you can take to help your physical and psychological health. One of the most significant benefits of physical activity is a lowered risk for certain diseases.

Lower Risk of Cardiovascular Disease

Even moderate amounts of exercise can lead to major benefits for your cardiovascular system. These benefits include reduced risk of cardiovascular disease, reduced risk of stroke, lower blood pressure, and lower blood cholesterol levels.

How does regular exercise reduce your risk of developing cardiovascular problems? The job of the cardiovascular system is to carry oxygen in the blood throughout the body. When you engage in physical activity, your heart beats faster and your breathing increases to provide your muscles with sufficient oxygen. If you exercise regularly, your heart will strengthen as it gets its own workout whenever you exercise. Exercise also strengthens the lungs, which must work harder to get plenty of oxygen to the muscles during your workout.

Physical activity is also associated with living longer. Heart disease and stroke are two leading causes of death in the United States. People who get at least 150 minutes (2 hours and 30 minutes) of moderate-intensity activity each week are less likely to develop these diseases than people who don't exercise. Engaging in regular physical activity can add years to your life (Figure 6.2).

Lower Risk of Cancer

Engaging in regular physical activity also reduces your risk of developing some types of cancer. Research on the link between physical activity and cancer demonstrates that physically active people have a lower risk of colon cancer and may have a lower risk of lung cancer than people who do not exercise. Research also shows that physically active women may have a lower risk for breast cancer and endometrial cancer (cancer of the uterus) than women who do not exercise.

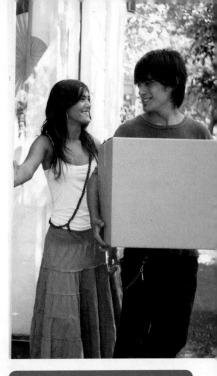

Are you physically fit? Are you able to perform routine tasks without feeling exhausted or strained?

fitness
the body's ability to meet daily physical demands

Some Health Benefits of Physical Activity

↑ Strength of immune system to better ward off illness

↑ Sleep quality

↓ Risk of cancers (colon, lungs, and for females, uterus and breast)

↓ Risk of diabetes

↓ Risk of overweight and obesity

↑ Mental health (mood, ability to cope with stress)

↑ Intellectual health (learning, thinking, concentration, judgment)

↓ Risk of cardiovascular diseases (heart attack, stroke)

↑ Strength of lungs

↑ Strength of muscles

↑ Strength of bones

↓ Pain due to arthritis

Key
↑ Improves
↓ Lowers

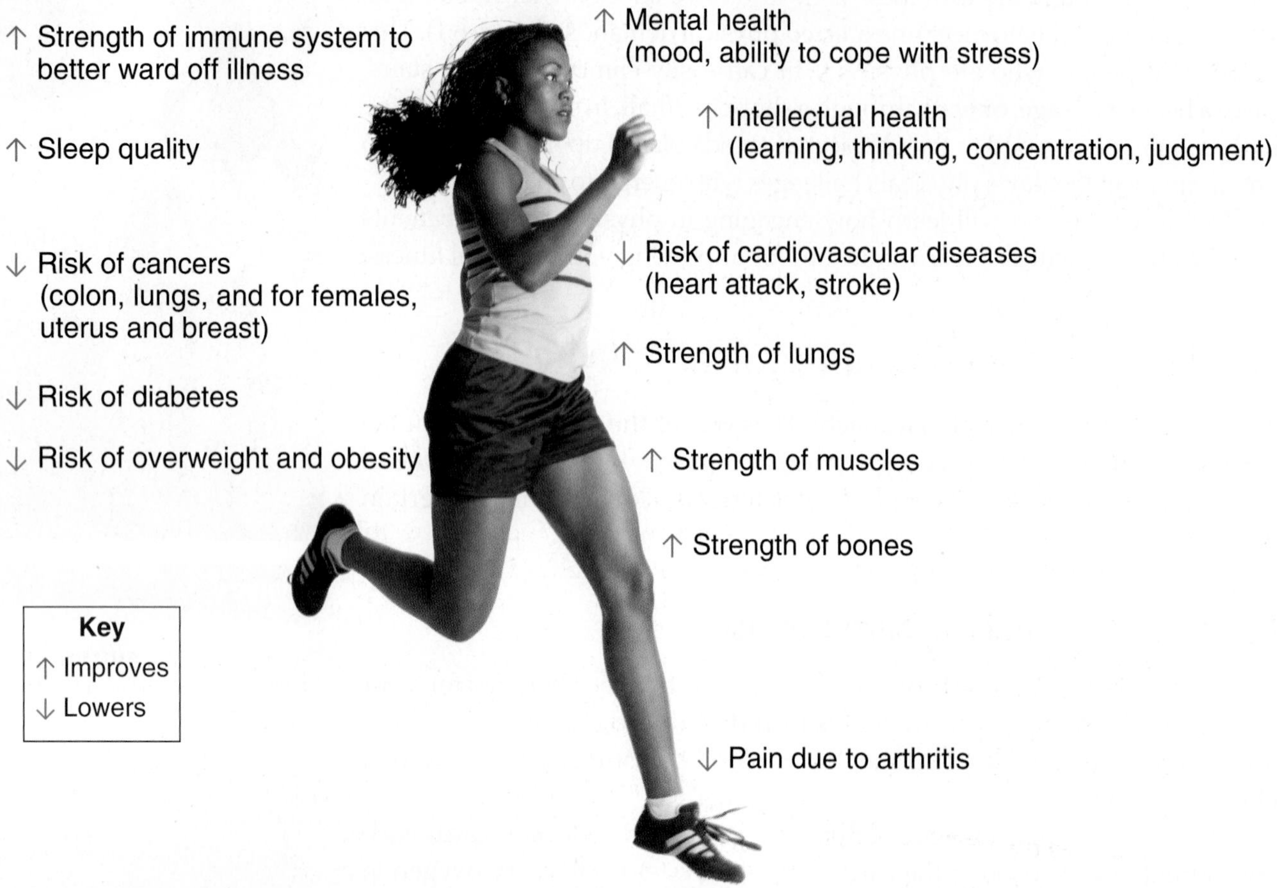

Figure 6.2

Shown above are just some of the ways that physical activity can benefit your physical, emotional, and intellectual health. *In what ways can physical activity benefit your social health?*

Researchers don't know exactly how physical activity reduces the risk of developing particular types of cancer. Physical activity does, however, influence how your body functions, including its production of particular hormones, the rate of metabolism, and the work done by your immune system to fight off disease and infection. The effects of physical activity on these functions may explain how physical activity reduces the risk of developing these types of cancer.

Stronger Bones and Muscles

Engaging in regular physical activity helps your bones and muscles in several ways. Engaging in physical activity increases the amount of fluid in your joints, which helps strengthen the cartilage that covers the ends of your bones. In addition, regular physical activity increases the strength of your bones and ligaments, which means you are less likely to become injured or develop osteoporosis. Regular physical activity also improves the strength of your muscles and increases the blood flow to and from your muscles.

The benefits of regular exercise on bone and muscle strength also include the following:

- slowing the natural loss of bone density that comes with age
- helping to increase or maintain muscle mass and strength
- reducing the likelihood of a fall

- reducing the pain caused by arthritis and other conditions that affect the joints
- increasing the ability to perform normal tasks of daily life

Better Weight Control

Regular physical activity is especially important for people who are trying to lose weight or maintain a healthy weight. More physical activity means your body burns more calories for energy than it would normally. When you burn more calories and reduce the number of calories you eat, you experience a calorie deficit (calories burned is greater than calories taken in). A calorie deficit leads to weight loss. Physical activity combined with a more nutritious diet that contains fewer calories can help you control your weight.

Engaging in regular physical activity can also improve weight control by changing a person's body composition. People who engage in strength training, which includes push-ups, sit-ups, or lifting weights, can increase

Research in Action

Feeling Depressed? Try Some Exercise!

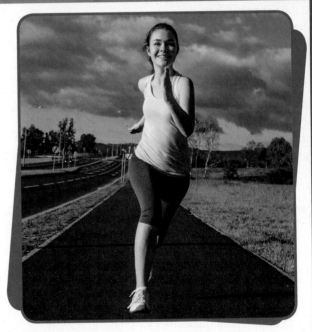

In a recent study, researchers attempted to determine whether exercise could help improve the moods of people who are depressed.

To test this hypothesis, researchers assigned 156 adults with *clinical depression* (a severe level of depression that disrupts daily life) to one of three groups. People in Group One engaged in aerobic exercise (three 45-minute sessions a week). Group One did not receive any drugs to combat depression. People in Group Two received drugs to relieve the symptoms of depression, but did not engage in aerobic exercise. People in Group Three engaged in aerobic exercise and received drugs. Each group continued their exercise or use of medication for 16 weeks.

After 16 weeks, the researchers examined people in all three groups over time to see if their levels of depression changed. Researchers found that people who engaged in aerobic exercise, even when they received no drugs to help with their symptoms of depression, showed improvements in their mood for as long as six months. In fact, people in all three groups improved at the same rate. This study provides important evidence that exercise can be as effective as drug treatment in treating depression.

Thinking Critically

1. After you have finished reading this lesson, evaluate which of the three treatments you would recommend for people experiencing depression. Why?

2. Analyze the reasons why exercise helps treat depression.

their muscle mass. Muscles are active tissues that consume calories to use for energy. In contrast, fat stored in the body uses very little energy. This means that a person whose body consists of more muscle and less fat burns calories at a higher rate (Figure 6.3). This higher rate of metabolism helps people lose weight and maintain that weight loss over time.

Improved Sleep

People who engage in regular physical activity experience a better quality of sleep than those who do not exercise. Compared with people who do not exercise, physically active people fall asleep more quickly, enjoy deeper and more restful sleep, awake less often during the night, and stay asleep longer. In fact, research shows that strength training is as effective at improving sleep quality as sleep medications.

Improved Mental Health

People who engage in regular physical activity also experience improvements in their mental health, including lower levels of depression and anxiety. Have you ever been in a bad mood, but then exercised and felt better? This happens because engaging in physical activity can

- cause the brain to release chemicals called *endorphins*, which make you feel good;
- distract you from problems you may be facing;
- increase social interaction with other people who are exercising; and
- lead to increased blood flow to the brain, which contributes to an improved mood.

Engaging in physical activity also makes people feel better about themselves. As a result, they have higher levels of self-confidence and self-esteem.

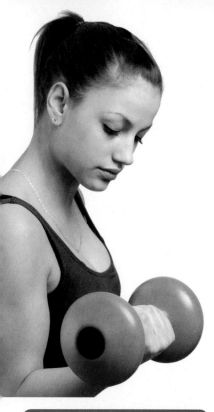

Figure 6.3

Many people mistakenly think that they need to run long distances to burn calories and lose weight. *How will this girl's weight lifting help her control her weight?*

endorphins
chemicals found mainly in the brain that affect emotions and relieve pain

Health across the Life Span

Rates of Aerobic Activity by Age

According to a nationwide survey of nearly half a million American adults, only 21% of adults met both the cardiovascular and muscle-strengthening guidelines for physical activity. Whether people meet the recommended physical activity guidelines varies widely among age groups. The survey found that

- 29.6% of people 18 to 24 years of age meet the recommended guidelines;
- 24.3% of people 25 to 44 years of age meet the recommended guidelines;
- 19.2% of people 45 to 54 years of age meet the recommended guidelines;

- 15.9% of people 55 to 64 years of age meet the recommended guidelines;
- 13.6% of people 65 to 74 years of age meet the recommended guidelines; and
- 6.4% of people 75 years of age and older meet the recommended guidelines.

Analyzing Data

1. What conclusions can you draw from this data?

2. Select one of the age groups mentioned here, then formulate and evaluate a plan to increase the physical activity levels of people within that group.

Improved Academic Performance

Engaging in regular physical activity helps improve thinking, learning, and judgment skills. Not surprisingly, improvements in these skills can lead to better performance in school. Students who participate in regular physical activity demonstrate

- increased academic achievement, including higher grades;
- improved academic behavior, such as spending more time focused on a task; and
- improved concentration and focus in class.

Improving Your Physical Fitness

Although the health benefits of engaging in regular physical activity are clear, most people don't get enough physical activity. Many people spend much of their day engaging in *sedentary behavior* instead, meaning activities that consist of sitting or lying down and using very little energy. Sedentary behaviors include driving, engaging in screen time (TV, movies, Internet, video games), and reading. Statistics show that

- only 49% of adults meet the *Physical Activity Guidelines for Americans* for aerobic physical activity;
- only 21% of adults meet the Physical Activity Guidelines for Americans for both aerobic and muscle-strengthening activities; and
- 24% of American adults don't engage in any physical activity.

The United States Department of Health and Human Services (HHS) recommends that people between 6 and 17 years of age participate in at least one hour of physical activity every day. Do you get at least this much physical activity? What types of exercise do you do on a regular basis? Do you jog, swim, or skate? Do you lift weights, or do push-ups or sit-ups? Do you stretch or do yoga or Pilates? Do you mow lawns, rake leaves, or carry boxes? These are all examples of physical activity, and each of these activities leads to a different type of physical fitness.

We often think of the terms *physical activity* and *exercise* as meaning the same thing. A difference does exist, however, between these two terms. *Exercise*—meaning a type of physical activity that is planned, structured, and purposeful—is actually just one type of physical activity. *Exercise* could describe the cycle of exercises you do in PE class, a varsity sports team's daily practice, or running every day to prepare for a half-marathon.

The term *physical activity* is broader because it includes structured exercise as well as other activities that use energy. Biking to school, playing Frisbee with friends, and dancing to music alone in your bedroom are not what we would typically call *exercise*, but they are all definitely *physical activity* (Figure 6.4 on the next page).

sedentary behavior
activities such as sitting or lying down that use very little energy

Physical Activity Guidelines for Americans
a set of recommendations developed by the government, health professionals, and policymakers to help Americans improve their health through appropriate physical activity

exercise
term that describes a type of physical activity that is planned, structured, and purposeful

physical activity
broad term that describes structured exercise as well as other activities that use energy

Figure 6.4

Physical activity includes exercise and other activities—such as dancing—that use energy. *List five physical activities that most people can add to their daily routines.*

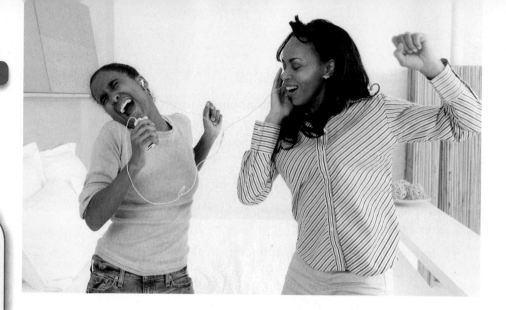

Personal Profile

How Physically Fit Are You?

These questions will help you assess whether you are currently physically fit.

I engage in 60 minutes or more of physical activity each day. **yes no**

I do vigorous-intensity aerobic physical activity such as running, playing sports, or taking a dance class at least three days a week. **yes no**

I do muscle-strengthening activities such as push-ups or sit-ups at least three days a week **yes no**

I do bone-strengthening activities such as jumping rope or running at least three days a week. **yes no**

I regularly do yoga, Pilates, or some type of stretching. **yes no**

I make physical activity a regular part of my day by biking to school, walking up stairs instead of taking an elevator, and doing sit-ups or push-ups while watching television. **yes no**

I have enough energy to perform various daily life activities such as carrying groceries or books, walking up stairs, and walking around a shopping center. **yes no**

I make sure to stretch my muscles to cool down after exercising. **yes no**

Add up the number of yes answers to assess your physical fitness. The more yes answers you have, the more physically fit you are.

Deciding to exercise is a good lifestyle choice if you want to be physically fit. You do not need to engage in structured exercise, however, to improve your fitness level. Your health and fitness can benefit from many different types of physical activity.

Many easy strategies exist for you to begin and maintain a fitness program. By setting SMART goals—goals that are specific, measurable, action oriented, realistic, and timely—you can start taking steps toward improving your physical fitness.

Integrate Physical Activity into Your Daily Life

Ideally, you should have a fitness program that matches up well with your daily life. To achieve this, try to find ways of being physically active that don't require too much time or money. For example, it is easier—and cheaper—to jog around your neighborhood or follow a yoga video than it is to join an expensive health club or gym.

Most people feel that they are too busy to find time to exercise. They feel that they have too many other tasks to accomplish each day. Even the busiest people should be able to find a few hours each week to exercise.

When you make physical activity a part of your daily or weekly routine, you will find the time to do it more easily. The first and most important step is to set aside time each week—even as little as 10 minutes at a time—to engage in some type of physical activity. Soon the exercise will become part of your daily life and it may even feel strange to not exercise.

Choose Physical Activities You Enjoy

It is much easier to maintain an exercise program if you find types of physical activity that you enjoy. Some people find engaging in team sports, such as basketball, soccer, or field hockey, particularly fun. Other people prefer to exercise alone, and might find swimming, jogging, or climbing stairs more enjoyable than team sports. Consider whether you like to exercise outside or inside, and whether you like to exercise alone or with other people. Also consider which physical activities are appropriate for your levels of fitness and development.

Exercise with a Friend

You are more likely to have success maintaining your fitness program if you have the support of your friends and family members. Try to find someone who is interested in engaging in physical activity with you. Do you know someone who might be interested in going for a brisk walk after school, taking a bike ride on the weekends, or joining a yoga class? Most people find it more difficult to make excuses and skip their exercise session if they know that someone is expecting them to be there.

You could also develop new friendships by joining a group with other people interested in a particular type of physical activity. You might meet new people at an aerobics class at a local gym, a pick-up baseball game at a local playground, or a hiking club.

Take Advantage of School and Community Programs

Most children and teenagers attend schools that offer physical education classes. Participating in physical activity during school is a great way to increase fitness. Both the National Association for Sport and Physical Education (NASPE) and the American Heart Association (AHA) recommend that all students engage in regular physical education classes in school. These recommendations include the following:

- Elementary school students should participate in more than 150 minutes of physical education per week.

- Middle and high school students should participate in more than 225 minutes of physical education per week.

Schools can increase the amount of physical activity in a student's day by ensuring that physical education classes are taught by qualified teachers and are provided to all students in all grades. Unfortunately, too few high school students participate in physical education classes on a regular basis.

Many schools and communities provide free or low-cost opportunities to engage in physical activity. You could join an intramural club or interscholastic sports team offered through your school. Community centers often provide opportunities for noncompetitive physical activity, such as lessons in different types of sports, dance and yoga, and weight training.

Health in the Media

Want to Increase Your Fitness? Turn Off the Television!

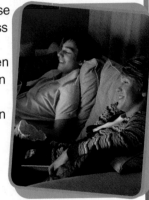

One of the best ways to increase your physical activity and your fitness level is to decrease the hours you spend watching television. Children and teenagers who watch television for at least six hours a week are typically less physically active than those who watch fewer hours of television. In fact, time spent watching television appears to have a greater negative effect on physical activity levels than other types of screen time, including time spent on the computer and playing video games.

Watching television is also associated with lower levels of physical activity in adults. In one study, people reported watching an average of 3.6 hours of television per day. Researchers found that for each hour of television a person watched, he or she was 16% less likely to engage in recommended physical activity.

Thinking Critically

1. Generate a hypothesis to explain the finding that television viewing has a greater impact on inactivity than other forms of screen time.

2. The impact of television viewing on inactivity in adults seems out of balance with the other results of the study. Evaluate possible reasons why adults are more affected by television viewing than children or teens.

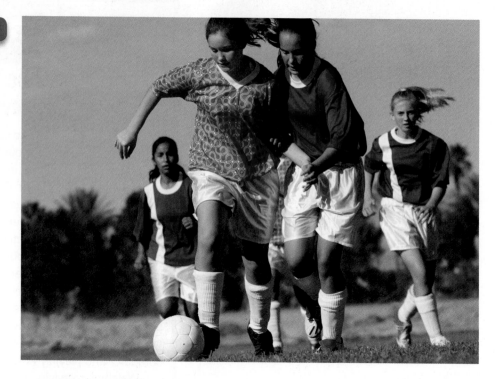

Figure 6.5

Free or low-cost exercise programs, especially those involving team sports, are available through schools and community centers. These programs can improve your fitness and lead to new friendships.

Many communities offer facilities you can use for free or at a reduced cost such as the following:

- parks and green spaces for playing Frisbee, throwing a baseball, or playing soccer (Figure 6.5)
- outdoor sports facilities such as baseball or softball fields, and tennis and basketball courts
- indoor sports facilities such as weight rooms, fitness centers, and racquetball courts
- walking and biking trails, and skate parks
- public pools

Lesson 6.1 Review

Know and Understand Assess

1. Explain how physical activity reduces the risk for developing cardiovascular problems.
2. List three ways physical activity reduces the risk for some cancers.
3. List two ways physical activity helps control weight.
4. Describe how physical activity affects sleep quality.
5. List five developmentally appropriate activities you would enjoy.

Analyze and Apply

6. Based on this lesson, make a case for mandatory physical education classes in high schools.

7. Why might many people spend much of the day engaging in sedentary behavior?
8. Research and analyze the roles of games and sports in the physical activity of people in different cultures.

Real World Health

Physical activity and exercise have many benefits that go beyond your physical health. Identify at least 10 benefits of exercise as identified in this lesson of the chapter. Label each benefit according to whether it affects your physical health, emotional health, or social health. Then, for each type of health, identify a problem you are experiencing in your life that physical activity and exercise might help solve.

The Components of Physical Fitness

Lesson Objectives

After studying this lesson, you will be able to

- summarize the various components of fitness;
- recognize how cardiorespiratory fitness is achieved;
- determine and monitor desired target heart rates;
- list guidelines for developing a strength-training plan;
- explain how endurance is measured;
- apply safe stretching techniques; and
- develop a personal fitness plan.

Warm-Up Activity

Agree or Disagree

Recreate the chart shown below on a separate piece of paper. Before reading the lesson, record whether you agree or disagree with each of the statements. When you have finished reading the lesson, consider the statements again based on any new information you may have read. In the final column, record whether you agree or disagree now, and check to see whether your opinion has changed based on new evidence.

Before Reading	Statements	Page	After Reading
1. Agree/Disagree	The intensity of a workout can be measured by how hard you feel your body is working.		Agree/Disagree
2. Agree/Disagree	Walking to school or work each morning can help you get more physical activity.		Agree/Disagree
3. Agree/Disagree	A marathon runner requires more oxygen than a sprinter.		Agree/Disagree
4. Agree/Disagree	Fitness plans are personal to you and your fitness-related needs.		Agree/Disagree
5. Agree/Disagree	About 31% of adults worldwide don't get enough physical activity.		Agree/Disagree
6. Agree/Disagree	There is no standard maximum heart rate for everyone.		Agree/Disagree

Key Terms E-Flash Cards

In this lesson, you will learn the meanings of the following key terms.

aerobic
agility
anaerobic
cardiorespiratory fitness
components of fitness
cross training
flexibility
health-related fitness
intensity
overload principle
progression principle
range of motion
skill-related fitness
specificity principle
target heart rate

Before You Read

The Parts of Fitness

Look at a bicycle and identify its individual parts. Now think about the different aspects of fitness. What types of movements, skills, and actions make up personal fitness? Write a paragraph that compares the parts of a bike and the parts of fitness, and explain how each part contributes to overall physical health.

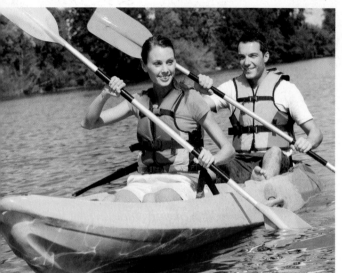

Obviously, people engage in very different activities in their daily routines. This means that people have different fitness requirements. For example, a varsity college athlete will face different fitness challenges than a casual jogger. A soldier, firefighter, or police officer will confront different fitness challenges than a teacher, bookkeeper, or lawyer (Figure 6.6).

As people engage in different physical activities, they develop some parts of their fitness more than others. In this lesson you will learn about many different types of fitness. How fast, and how long, can you run? How many sit-ups and push-ups can you do? Are you able to touch your toes? These activities represent different types, or *components of fitness*. Many physical fitness experts divide the components of fitness into two broad categories: *health-related fitness* and *skill-related fitness*.

As you will see, people can rate higher or lower in the different components of fitness. After learning more about the components of fitness, you will probably want to determine your level of fitness for each one. You can then develop a plan to improve your weaker fitness components.

Figure 6.6

Do you participate in any recreational physical activities such as canoeing? If you don't have access to a canoe or body of water, what types of activities could you do in your area and get the same kind of workout?

components of fitness
different types of fitness, such as strength and flexibility

health-related fitness
type of fitness used to easily perform daily activities

aerobic
activity involving the use of oxygen to fuel processes in the body

anaerobic
activity occurring in the absence of oxygen

cardiorespiratory fitness
term that describes how efficiently the cardiovascular and respiratory systems deliver oxygen to the muscles during prolonged physical activity

Health-Related Fitness

Health-related fitness is the type of fitness you need to perform daily activities with ease and energy. Fitness experts talk about the different aspects of health-related fitness in different ways. This lesson will discuss cardiorespiratory fitness, endurance, muscular strength, and flexibility. Another component of health-related fitness is body composition, which you read about in chapter 4.

When people think about exercise and fitness, they often think of aerobic exercise, which is a cardiorespiratory type of fitness. *Aerobic* means *in the presence of oxygen*. During aerobic exercise, oxygen is delivered to the muscles, which gives them the energy they need to continue exercising.

Not all types of exercise, however, require oxygen to provide energy. In *anaerobic* exercise, such as weight lifting, glycogen provides the energy your body needs. Anaerobic activity occurs in short bursts, while aerobic activities occur over a longer stretch of time. Consider the difference between a sprinter (anaerobic) and a marathon runner (aerobic) to remember the difference between these two terms, which you will encounter often as you learn more about fitness (Figure 6.7).

Cardiorespiratory Fitness

Cardiorespiratory fitness refers to how well the heart and lungs work together to deliver oxygen and nutrients to the muscles and cells. This type of fitness is aerobic because the body relies on oxygen to provide the energy needed to continue exercising. Many different types of activities (running, gardening, dancing, shoveling snow) provide cardiovascular fitness.

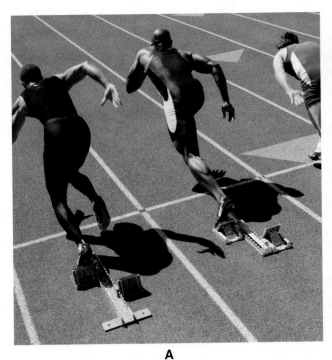
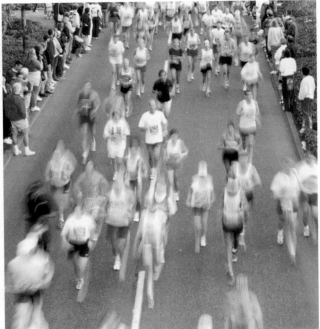

A   B

People who engage in regular cardiorespiratory exercise maintain the health of their heart and lungs in several ways. They strengthen the heart, improve blood flow throughout the body, and improve the body's ability to quickly transport oxygen and nutrients to all of its muscles and cells. This increased strength and ability leads to greater endurance. The stronger your heart and lungs become, the longer they can endure increased levels of physical activity.

Increasing cardiorespiratory fitness requires that you engage in physical activity for a certain amount of time, or *duration*, each week and at a certain level of intensity. The frequency at which you engage in the activities and the types of activities you engage in also impact your fitness. Some people use the acronym *FITT* (frequency, intensity, time, and type) to help them focus on these key factors. Manipulating these factors will allow you to gradually and safely improve your fitness.

Time, Types, and Frequency. People who want to achieve cardiorespiratory fitness need to engage in various types of physical activity for at least 150 minutes, or 2½ hours, each week. Many people prefer to divide this time into smaller, more frequent sessions, such as 30 minutes of physical activity five days a week, or 50 minutes three days a week.

You can also engage in physical activity several times a day for relatively brief periods of time. For example, you achieve the same cardiovascular benefits whether you go for a 30-minute walk, or three 10-minute walks. The time and frequency of your workouts are related to intensity.

Intensity. People must perform physical activity at a certain level of intensity to achieve cardiorespiratory fitness. **Intensity** is measured by the amount of energy your body uses per minute while engaging in an activity (Figure 6.8 on the next page). You can judge the intensity of a given physical activity based on how it affects your heart rate and breathing.

Figure 6.7

A) Sprinting, which occurs in short bursts, is an example of anaerobic activity. B) Running a marathon is an example of an aerobic activity. *Why is running a marathon considered an aerobic activity? Give another example of an anaerobic and an aerobic activity.*

intensity
a quality that is measured by how much energy the body uses per minute during physical activity

Figure 6.8 Approximate Calories Burned for Different Physical Activities

Moderate Physical Activity	Calories Burned in 30 Minutes of Activity				
	100-lb. person	120-lb. person	135-lb. person	150-lb. person	200-lb. person
hiking climbing stairs	136	164	184	205	273
gardening softball	114	136	153	170	227
calisthenics mopping scrubbing floors	102	123	138	153	205
bicycling (< 10 mph) brisk walking (> 3 mph)	91	109	123	136	182
weight lifting (light workout)	68	82	92	102	136

Vigorous Physical Activity	Calories Burned in 30 Minutes of Activity				
	100-lb. person	120-lb. person	135-lb. person	150-lb. person	200-lb. person
rock climbing (ascending)	250	300	338	375	500
running (10 min. mile) bicycling (>10 mph)	227	273	300	341	455
football tennis (singles) calisthenics (push-ups, sit-ups) jumping rope	182	218	245	273	364
soccer rollerblading	159	191	215	239	318
swimming basketball (half court) shoveling snow	136	164	184	205	273
dancing (vigorous)	125	150	169	187	250

During an activity of moderate intensity, your heart rate and breathing are faster than normal, but you can still carry on a conversation. During an activity of vigorous intensity, your heart rate and breathing are considerably faster than normal, and you are unable to carry on a conversation.

Target Heart Rate. How intense should your workout be? Your goal is to increase your heart rate, but not by too much. For moderate-intensity activity, a person's *target heart rate* should be 50–70% of her maximum heart rate. For vigorous-intensity activity, a person's target heart rate should be 70–85% of her maximum heart rate.

What is the maximum heart rate? A single, standard maximum does not exist. A person's maximum heart rate depends on his or her age. You can calculate your maximum heart rate by subtracting your age from 220. For example, if you are 16 years of age, your maximum heart rate is 204 beats per minute (or *bpm*).

220 – age in years = Maximum heart rate in beats per minute (bpm)

220 – 16 = 204 bpm

target heart rate
the heart rate to aim for while performing aerobic exercise that leads to optimal cardiorespiratory fitness; varies by age

Once you have determined your maximum heart rate, you can calculate your target heart rate for different levels of physical activity. Suppose that you are a 16-year-old with a maximum heart rate of 204 bpm. Using that information, you would perform the following calculations to find your target heart rates for moderate-intensity physical activity (50–70%) and vigorous-intensity physical activity (70–85%):

$204 \times 50\% = 102$ bpm

$204 \times 70\% = 142.8$ bpm

$204 \times 85\% = 173.4$ bpm

As you can see from these calculations, a 16-year-old should try to engage in physical activities that cause a heart rate between 102 and 173 bpm. If the goal is moderate-intensity physical activity, this person should maintain a heart rate between 102 and 143 bpm. If the goal is vigorous-intensity physical activity, this person's heart rate should be between 143 and 173 bpm (Figure 6.9).

Taking Your Pulse. An easy way to monitor the intensity of physical activity is to check your *pulse* (your heart rate) to see if it is within the target range during the activity. You can check your pulse at the neck, wrist, or chest, although the wrist is often the easiest place to find a pulse. Taking your pulse at the wrist is very easy if you follow these steps:

- Find your pulse on the artery of the wrist in line with your thumb.
- Place the tips of your index and middle fingers over the artery and press lightly (Figure 6.10).
- Start counting on a beat, which is zero (not one).
- Count the number of heartbeats for a full 60 seconds. You can also count for six seconds and multiply by 10.

Heart Rate Monitors. Heart rate monitors can also measure your pulse. Traditionally, such monitors had to be worn snugly around the chest so that they could measure how fast the heart was beating. Newer heart rate monitors are worn around the wrist. These monitors measure your pulse by shining a light into the blood vessels in your wrist and measuring changes in blood volume each time your heart beats and blood is pushed through your body. Less light reflected back into the sensor on your wrist means more blood volume and a faster pulse.

RPE Tests. Another way to monitor the intensity of physical activity during a workout is to rate how hard you feel your body is working. The Borg Rating of Perceived Exertion (RPE) test is based on the physical sensations—heart rate, sweating, breathing, and muscle tiredness—that a person experiences during physical activity. This is a subjective measuring method, which means it is only based on a feeling; there are no facts to back up that feeling. Nevertheless, research has shown that these types of assessment are fairly good measures of actual intensity.

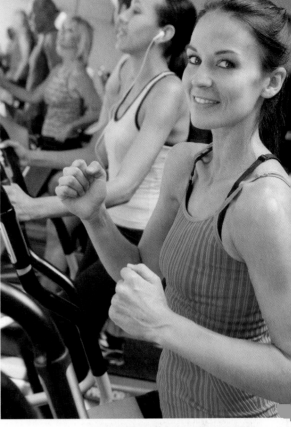

Figure 6.9

It is a good idea to get into the habit of monitoring your heart rate as you work out. *Who might be monitoring her heart rate in this photo? Explain.*

Figure 6.10

When taking your pulse at your wrist, place the tips of your index and middle fingers on the artery that lines up with your thumb.

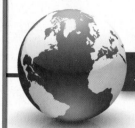

Local and Global Health

Rates of Physical Activity around the World

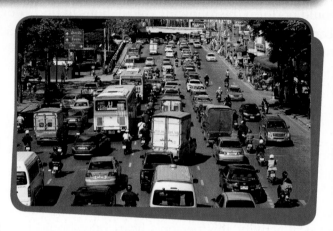

Although about 25% of American adults report not engaging in any type of physical activity in the past month, there are substantial differences in the level of physical activity among people who live in different states. In Oregon, Minnesota, Colorado, and Vermont, less than 19% of adults report not engaging in any physical activity in the last month. In contrast, more than 30% of adults in Kentucky, Mississippi, Oklahoma, and West Virginia report not engaging in any physical activity in the last month.

Big differences in levels of physical activity also exist among people who live in different countries. In some parts of the world, almost 50% of women and 40% of men don't participate in enough physical activity. These areas include

- North America (the United States, Canada, and Mexico);
- South America (Argentina, Peru, Chile, Ecuador, and Bolivia); and
- the Eastern Mediterranean (Afghanistan, Egypt, Iraq, Pakistan, Saudi Arabia, Somalia, and Sudan).

Many factors contribute to this overall lack of physical activity. These factors include

- a lack of recreational physical activity;
- an increase in sedentary behavior, such as watching television and using the computer;
- an increase in driving and public transportation use, and a decrease in biking and walking; and
- environmental factors such as violence, air pollution, and lack of access to safe parks and recreation facilities.

Thinking Critically

1. What do you think causes these differences of physical activity levels among different states and countries? How could you test your idea?

2. How do you think the worldwide rates of physical activity will change over time? What are some factors that might lead rates of physical activity to increase? decrease?

3. What strategies could governments take to increase the rate of physical activity in their countries? Which strategies do you think would be most effective? Explain your answer.

Ratings on the RPE test are made using a scale of 6 to 20. A score of 6 means "no exertion at all" and 20 means "maximal exertion." While you are exercising, you should rate how hard you feel your body is working using this range of numbers. You can then adjust the intensity of your workout by speeding up or slowing down to reach the desired level of workout intensity. Exertion rates between 12 and 14 are considered a moderate level of intensity.

Endurance

Another important component of health-related fitness is a person's endurance. There are two types of endurance—aerobic and muscular. Some experts consider aerobic endurance to be equal to the cardiorespiratory fitness that you read about earlier in this lesson. *Aerobic endurance* describes a person's ability to engage in cardiorespiratory activity over a period of time (Figure 6.11). The level of aerobic endurance a person can achieve depends on the rate at which the heart can continue to pump blood and the rate at which the body can break down carbohydrates and fat to produce the energy the body needs.

Muscular endurance refers to the length of time for which a particular group of muscles can continue to exert force. Muscular endurance is different from muscular strength. Muscular endurance has to do with the duration of performance, whereas strength has to do with the amount of force used to move or lift an object.

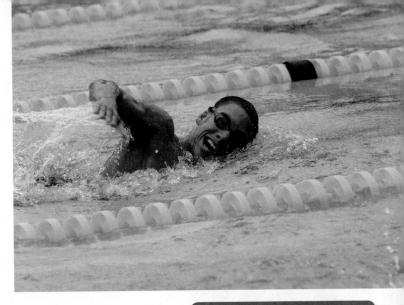

Swimming moderate to long distances is an excellent activity for building your cardiorespiratory endurance. *How long can you swim without resting?*

Some types of physical activity require high levels of both aerobic and muscular endurance. For example, marathon runners must have great muscular endurance for their leg muscles to continue working over long distances for hours at a time. These runners must also have great aerobic endurance for their heart to continue pumping at higher than normal intensity levels for such an extended period of time. Marathon runners often consume snacks that are high in carbohydrates, such as bananas, dried fruits, and energy drinks, while running to provide the body with the energy it needs to maintain a high level of endurance for two, three, or four hours of running.

Muscular Strength

Muscular strength is the ability of a muscle to exert force against resistance. Imagine that you are arm wrestling a friend. Assume that you have stronger arm muscles than your friend. As you push against your friend's weaker arm muscles, your force will overcome his resistance, and you will win the match.

Muscle strength can be measured in many ways. For example, you can measure how much weight (resistance) you can lift, how much weight you can push, and how much weight you can pull.

Types of Strength Training. The goal of strength training is to increase the strength of your muscle and bone. The resistance needed for strength training can be provided by a variety of sources. The following are examples of ways to provide resistance during strength training:

- Your body weight serves as resistance when performing push-ups, sit-ups, or leg squats.

- Resistance bands or tubes are lightweight and provide constant tension to build muscle strength. The thicker the band, the more resistance it provides.

- Free weights, such as barbells and dumbbells, can be used to provide maximum resistance.

- Weight machines guide your motion to ensure the target muscle is being exercised.

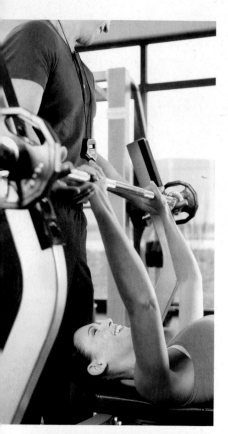

Figure 6.12

Always work with a spotter when lifting free weights that challenge your lifting capabilities.

Guidelines for Strength Training. Strength training should be performed for 20 to 30 minutes, two or three times a week, to build muscle mass and bone density.

You should target all the major muscle groups during your training. These include the chest (or *pectorals*), back, arms and shoulders, abdominals, and legs and buttocks. Different types of exercises are designed to target different muscle groups.

Do not perform any type of strength training unless you know the proper form for each exercise. Proper form includes finding a consistent tempo and paying attention to your breathing. Using improper form can lead to injuries and less-than-desirable increases in strength and endurance. The following are some guidelines for strength training:

- Start with a 5- to 10-minute warm-up, which includes a low- or moderate-intensity cardiorespiratory activity to get blood flowing to your muscles. You will learn more about proper warm-ups and cooldowns in the next lesson.

- Select a weight (resistance) level that tires your muscles after 12 to 15 repetitions. This weight will be different for different exercises.

- Do two or three *sets* (groups of repetitions followed by rest) of an exercise. For example, you could choose to do three sets of squats, with each set consisting of 10 repetitions.

- As you become stronger, you won't feel tired doing the same number of repetitions as you did when you first started. When this happens, you will probably want to increase the weight you are using. You may choose to do fewer sets with increased weight to build strength, or you could build muscular endurance by doing more sets.

- Work out with a partner if you lift heavy weights. This person, called a *spotter*, can help you avoid dropping the weight on yourself if it becomes too difficult for you to manage (Figure 6.12).

- Rest the muscles in a particular group for at least one full day after strength training to give the muscles time to recover. Strength training works in part by causing tiny tears in the muscle tissue, which then allows the muscles to grow stronger as the tears are repaired.

- Stop immediately if you feel sharp pain or experience swollen joints, which is a sign that you've done too much. Some muscle soreness is a normal part of strength training, but intense pain indicates a problem.

flexibility
the ability to bend without injury or breakage

range of motion
a measure of flexibility that tells how far a joint or body part can be moved

Flexibility

You probably know what it means to be flexible. People who are flexible are able to fully and easily move their muscles and joints. Your **flexibility** is determined by the elasticity of your muscles and connective tissues, such as your ligaments and tendons. One measure of flexibility is **range of motion**, which tells how far a joint can move in a particular direction.

Some people are very flexible, meaning that they are easily able to move their muscles and joints into difficult positions. Ballet dancers and gymnasts, for example, have great flexibility and are able to perform moves such as backbends and the splits. Other people are not so flexible, and might have a hard time bending over to tie their shoes (Figure 6.13).

Increasing Flexibility. To increase your flexibility, you simply need to regularly (and safely) stretch your muscles. Fitness guidelines suggest that everyone should engage in some type of stretching activity at least two or three days each week. Guidelines for increasing your flexibility include the following:

- Before stretching, engage in 5 to 10 minutes of low- or moderate-intensity cardiorespiratory activity, such as jumping jacks, skipping rope, or light jogging, to increase the heart rate and blood flow to the muscles.
- After your muscles are warmed up, stretch your muscle so that you can feel tightness, but not pain.
- Hold this stretch for 10 to 30 seconds, but do not bounce (this can lead to overstretching or even small tears in the muscle).
- While holding the stretch, you should breathe naturally to provide oxygen to your muscles.
- Repeat each stretch 2 to 4 times. Repetition will help you really work the muscle and increase flexibility (Figure 6.14).

Advantages and Disadvantages of Flexibility. Some people benefit from having flexibility in certain parts of their bodies. For example, baseball pitchers need great flexibility in their shoulders, and ballet dancers need flexibility in their hamstrings and inner thighs. Everyone benefits from having some flexibility because it helps improve performance in many types of physical activity and lowers the risk of experiencing an injury.

People who are not very flexible, meaning they have a limited range of motion, often have tight or stiff muscles. They may have difficulty performing normal daily life activities, such as tying their shoes.

More flexibility is usually a good thing, but you can be too flexible. In fact, people who are extremely flexible have an increased risk of injuring their joints.

Skill-Related Fitness

Skill-related fitness refers to the kind of fitness a person needs to perform successfully in a particular sport or leisure activity. The different aspects of skill-related fitness include speed, agility, balance, power, coordination, and reaction time.

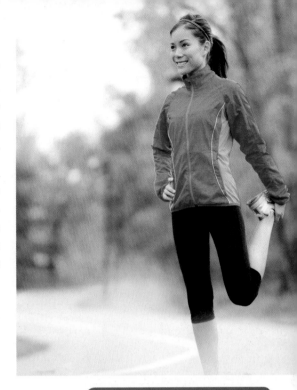

Figure 6.13

How would you rate your flexibility?

Figure 6.14

Stretching improperly can cause injuries. For example, when doing this groin stretch, you should pull your upper body down gently over your legs, bending from the hips. Do not bounce up and down.

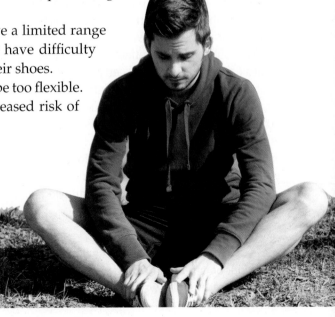

skill-related fitness
type of fitness that improves a person's performance in a particular sport

agility
the ability to quickly change the body's momentum and direction

Speed

If you have participated in or watched sporting events, you know what speed is. Some people are simply faster than others, which makes speed an important aspect of many different sports. Runners and swimmers must be fast, especially if they are racing short distances. Sprinting requires more speed than long-distance running or swimming.

Agility

Another type of skill-related fitness is *agility*, which is the ability to rapidly change the body's momentum and direction. This skill involves accelerating in a particular direction from a position of standing still, or rapidly changing from movement in one direction to movement in another direction. Agility also describes a person's ability to navigate obstacles they may encounter and need to go under, over, or around. A running back on a football team, for example, must have agility to maneuver around and away from players on the other team to avoid getting tackled.

CASE STUDY — How to Make Time for Physical Activity in a Full Schedule

Elise is a high school senior involved in many activities at her school. She is a good student and hopes to receive a scholarship for college. For this reason, Elise studies several hours each night. She also sings in the high school chorus, which involves rehearsals in the evenings, and has a part-time job waitressing. Elise's doctor told her that she needs to exercise for her health, but she can't find the time in her busy schedule.

Elise soon begins to recognize signs of poor fitness. She sometimes experiences shortness of breath when waitressing during busy times at the restaurant. She also worries that her lack of fitness could negatively affect her singing and other activities she enjoys. Elise read in her health book that improving her physical fitness could help her academic performance. As a result, she decides to work with the school nurse to plan a strategy for engaging in physical activity a few times a week. She is excited about the plan they develop, which includes

- taking a 20-minute walk with friends after school and before she starts studying;

- biking to school and her waitressing job when the weather is nice; and

- buying a set of hand weights she can use to work on strength training while she is watching television on the weekends.

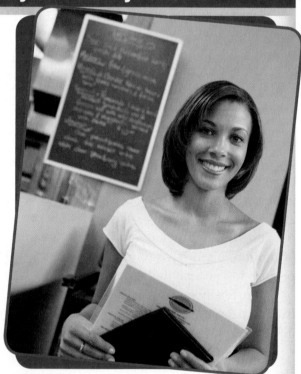

Thinking Critically

1. Evaluate Elise's fitness plan to determine the likelihood that she will succeed at her fitness goal.

2. Do you think Elise's problem is common for teens? What are some other factors you believe contribute to teens' lack of physical activity?

Balance

Balance means holding a particular body posture and position on a stable or unstable surface. Balance is obviously an important part of some sports, such as diving and gymnastics, as well as many leisure activities. Can you do a handstand or ride a unicycle? These are examples of fitness skills that require considerable balance. Balance varies from person to person, and most people find that this skill declines as they get older. Many people fail to appreciate their balancing skills until they lose them.

Power

Power is a combination of strength and speed. Some athletes are strong but not fast; others are fast but not strong. The athlete who combines strength and speed can be powerful. Power is an important skill in many sports, such as football and baseball. An outstanding volleyball striker is usually one of the more powerful players on the team (Figure 6.15).

Coordination

Do you think of yourself as being coordinated? Can you perform various movements easily and gracefully? Soccer players, hockey players, and other athletes who must have agility also have high levels of coordination. Coordination is also closely related to balance.

Some people are naturally more coordinated than others. Many athletes who perform complex movements do so smoothly, however, as a result of practice. Natural ability and practice lead to better coordination.

Figure 6.15

What skill-related components of fitness are most needed by these athletes if they are to be successful?

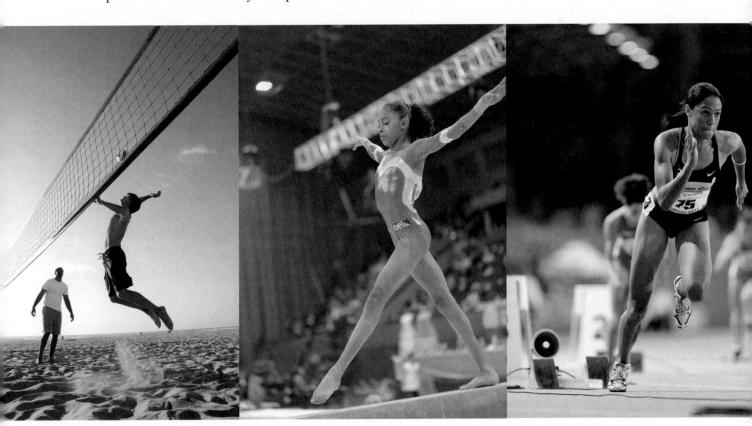

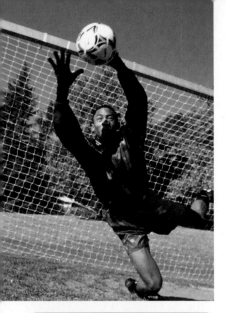

Figure 6.16

Many athletes need to exhibit good reaction time. *What position players in what sports come to mind when you think of reaction time?*

overload principle
standard which states that gradual increase of a physical demand on the body will improve fitness

specificity principle
standard which states that exercising a particular component leads to improvements in the fitness of only that component

progression principle
standard which states that FITT factors should be increased over time to improve fitness

Reaction Time

Reaction time refers to the quickness of a response. How fast do you react to someone else's movement? If you are faster than most at responding, you might have the qualities to be an outstanding tennis player, a good hitter in baseball, or a soccer goalie (Figure 6.16).

Designing a Personal Fitness Plan

Now that you know the components of fitness, you are better able to create a personal fitness plan. Most people, even those who are already physically fit, can improve some aspects of their fitness. That is why fitness plans are "personal," so that you can work on the parts of your fitness most in need of improvement. The components of fitness that you need to focus on might be very different from those that your best friends need to prioritize.

Training Principles

When developing your fitness plan, you will want to keep in mind a few basic principles: overload, specificity, and progression. Combined with the four ways of varying your workout—frequency, intensity, time, and type (*FITT*)—these principles will guide you as you monitor and adjust your fitness plan to maximize its benefits.

The **overload principle** states that you must put a greater demand on your body to improve it. You won't be able to run for a longer distance unless you try to run a longer distance. You won't be able to lift more weight unless you try lifting heavier weights. You need to "overload" your cardiorespiratory system and your muscles to strengthen them.

The **specificity principle** states that certain activities will lead to improvements in certain components of fitness. Stretching exercises for your legs improve the flexibility of your leg muscles, but not your arm muscles. If you lift a weight, the muscles used to lift the weight will be strengthened, but that particular exercise will have no effect on your other muscles. This means that you need to choose activities that focus on the components of fitness that you want to improve.

The **progression principle** says that you must increase your FITT factors over time to improve your fitness. If you want to maintain your current levels of fitness, you can develop a plan and stick to that plan forever. If you want to improve your fitness beyond its current level, however, you will need to increase one or more of the FITT factors periodically to increase flexibility, strength, or endurance.

First Steps

The first step in designing your fitness plan is to determine your current level of fitness within the different components. These baseline measurements will give you a sense of where you are now and help you understand what you want to improve. These measurements will also help you chart your progress as you proceed with your program.

You could begin by measuring the following areas of fitness:

- pulse rate after you walk a mile
- the time it takes you to walk a mile
- how many push-ups you can do at one time
- how far you can reach forward, toward your toes, while sitting with your legs straight in front of you
- your waist circumference
- your weight or BMI

Next, you need to develop a specific fitness plan that will help you achieve your goals. The fitness plan you create will be based on the goals you want to achieve, such as increasing flexibility, building strength, or increasing cardiorespiratory endurance.

It is a good idea to create a balanced fitness plan, even if you are targeting a particular fitness component. This means that your plan should include at least 150 minutes of moderate-intensity aerobic exercise each week (or 75 minutes of vigorous aerobic activity) plus at least two days of strength training.

Staying on Track

Staying on track with your fitness plan can be difficult, but it can be done. It is helpful to select activities you can do, given the available space and equipment (Figure 6.17). Does your school have a gym you can use?

Figure 6.17 Physical Activities You Can Do to Increase Fitness

Moderate-Intensity Activities	Vigorous-Intensity Activities	Muscle-Strengthening Activities	Bone-Strengthening Activities
• walking briskly • raking leaves • biking (slower than 10 miles per hour) • skateboarding • mowing the lawn • basketball • volleyball • hiking • rollerblading • canoeing • shoveling snow • doubles tennis	• soccer • jumping rope • martial arts, such as karate • singles tennis • field or ice hockey • aerobics • cheerleading • gymnastics • jogging or running • swimming laps • rollerblading or skating at a brisk pace • cross-country skiing • football • basketball • soccer • aerobic dancing • biking (10 miles per hour or faster) • hiking uphill or with a heavy backpack	• push-ups • sit-ups • rock climbing • using weight machines • lifting handheld weights • using resistance bands	• jumping rope • running • gymnastics • volleyball • tennis • basketball

Do you have a bike? Do you have access to a swimming pool? Remember, many fitness activities—such as jumping rope and doing push-ups—require only a small amount of space, and very minimal equipment.

Find times in your day and in your week that you know you can free up for exercise. If you are unrealistic in setting your schedule, you will probably fail to stick with your fitness plan. You should also look for ways to use your time efficiently. For example, you might be able to watch your favorite television show while riding a stationary bike or walking on a treadmill in front of the TV. It is important to think about ways you can build exercise into your daily schedule.

Cross Training. You may want to engage in *cross training*. This type of training means you participate in one activity to help you improve in another. A tennis player, for example, might include regular upper body weight lifting in a fitness program to strengthen his or her serve. A basketball player might take a dance class to improve his or her agility. Even if you don't purposefully engage in cross training, you should try to include different activities in your weekly plan so that you don't get bored doing the same activity multiple times a week. Choosing different activities also reduces your chance of injuring a single body part. It also lets you work on different types of fitness that rely on different parts of your body (Figure 6.18).

Keeping Records. Documenting your fitness plan can also help you stay on track. This includes writing your plan and then noting specific times and numbers for each exercise in each workout. Be specific when documenting your plan. This will help you assess your progress to determine whether you need to modify your goals. Self-assessment can easily be done by monitoring and documenting your progress. You can also take advantage of prepared assessment programs, which your physical education instructor can recommend.

cross training
training in different activities to improve performance in a sport and reduce the risk of injury

SKILLS FOR HEALTH AND WELLNESS

Increasing Fitness

The following strategies can help you start, and maintain, a fitness program.

- Create a written weekly schedule of physical activities. Choose times and days that work best for you.

- Select physical activities that you enjoy doing. For instance, some people like competitive team sports, such as basketball or volleyball. For others, group activities, such as a yoga class or a running club, are most rewarding. Some people prefer individual activities, such as lifting weights or swimming.

- Find family members or friends who want to exercise with you. It is often more fun to exercise with a partner.

- Find ways to incorporate physical activity into your daily life. Do sit-ups or push-ups while you watch television, walk upstairs instead of taking an elevator, or go for a walk after dinner instead of watching television.

- Start slowly if you are new to exercise. You don't want to overdo it and become injured. Set smaller goals at first and work toward bigger goals.

- Exercise safely to avoid injury that could cause you to stop being physically active. Use the right equipment for your activity; take time to warm up and cool down; and drink water before, during, and after engaging in physical activity.

Be Safe and Effective. Above all, you should choose exercises and fitness activities that are safe and effective. This will ensure that you stay on track and meet your fitness goals.

Some fitness products are advertised as being highly effective at helping people burn calories, increase strength, or change their body's shape in some way. These advertisements may not be entirely truthful. Before you buy a new fitness product, such as special shoes, carefully evaluate the evidence showing this product's effectiveness and safety.

If a new fitness product sounds too good to be true, it probably is. Find out more about the product from an objective source, such as a newspaper article or an adult you trust, before spending money or time on something that may not really help improve your fitness.

Learning More. As you monitor and continue to improve your fitness, you may want to learn more about how your body works. If you chose to study kinetics or biomechanics, for example, you would learn how to use to your benefit the internal and external forces that act on your body. Understanding principles such as force, pressure, torque, compression, and tension can help you avoid injuries. Studying these topics on your own or in college classes later in life can be interesting and help you reach your maximum fitness levels.

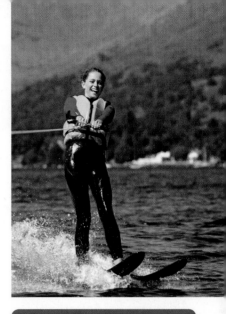

Figure 6.18

Most people who water ski do so for fun. Suppose, however, that this girl is water skiing as part of a cross training program. *In what other sports might she improve her skills as a result of her water skiing?*

Lesson 6.2 Review

Know and Understand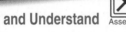

1. Name the health-related and skill-related components of fitness.

2. How much physical activity per week is recommended for cardiorespiratory fitness?

3. What fitness factors are represented by the acronym *FITT*?

4. Where can you check your pulse?

5. Calculate the target heart rate range for moderate-intensity physical activity for a 22-year-old (round up to the nearest whole number).

6. List four types of resistance used in strength training.

7. Explain the three training principles discussed in this lesson.

Analyze and Apply

8. Compare and contrast the health-related benefits of activities such as weight lifting and running marathons.

9. Select a sport or physical activity and evaluate the three most important components of fitness it requires to be successful.

10. Explain the effect of cardiorespiratory activity on your body during and after exercise.

11. Select an advertisement for a fitness product or program and evaluate it for effectiveness and safety.

12. Design a personal fitness plan that uses training principles to maximize your health benefits.

Real World (Health

In this lesson you learned about ways to increase your physical fitness levels. You read that you need to exercise for a minimum of 10 minutes to start a fitness plan. Create an advocacy contest to get your entire school to "Take Time for Ten." Create a poster or brochure that explains your contest and what people must do to win. Include people of diverse backgrounds and abilities and be sure to include a prize!

Fitness Safety

Key Terms E-Flash Cards

In this lesson, you will learn the meanings of the following key terms.

amenorrhea
female athlete triad

Lesson Objectives

After studying this lesson, you will be able to

- apply safe and proper weight lifting techniques;
- recognize types of back pain and injuries;
- implement strategies for preventing back pain;
- apply guidelines to prevent injuries from physical activity; and
- summarize common fitness concerns for women.

Before You Read

Staying Hydrated

Sports drinks and energy drinks are advertised as good ways to stay hydrated while engaging in physical activity. Use the Internet and what you may already know to analyze the difference between energy drinks and sports drinks. Do you think there are any differences between these two products? Do you think energy drinks are a health concern for today's teens? Explain your answers.

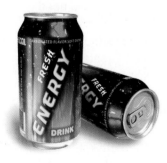

Warm-Up Activity

Staying Safe

This lesson is about preventing fitness-related injuries. Before reading the lesson, make five predictions of safety strategies that you think might be included in the lesson. For each prediction, explain why you think this is an important guideline for avoiding injuries. Use your previous personal experience as well as information you may have learned elsewhere.

My Predictions

1. _____
2. _____
3. _____
4. _____
5. _____

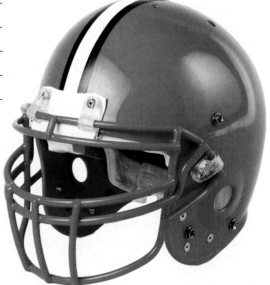

A s you know, engaging in regular physical activity is an important part of staying healthy. You probably also know that you can't engage in regular physical activity if you are injured. This means that taking the necessary precautions and following accepted guidelines when exercising are critical to your health. This lesson will examine actions you can take to avoid common injuries and maximize your physical activity experiences.

Start Slowly and Don't Overdo It

If you are just starting a fitness program, you should take care to start slowly (Figure 6.19). It can be tempting to exercise too much or too strenuously when you are first getting started. You should resist this temptation because overexercising can be harmful. If you overdo any type of physical activity during the first couple of days, you increase your chances of an injury.

Once you feel more comfortable with physical activity, you can increase the time, frequency, and intensity of your exercise. For example, you could eventually walk, roller skate, or bike for 30 minutes instead of just 10 to 20 minutes. You could jog instead of walk, or increase the amount of weight you lift during strength training. Gradually increase the demands on your body over a period of time and be patient rather than trying to do too much too soon.

Warm Up and Cool Down

No matter what type of physical activity you are doing—aerobic, strength training, or flexibility—it is important to warm up your muscles before you begin. A simple 5- to 10-minute warm-up helps get much-needed blood to your muscles, which helps to prevent injuries.

The warm-up should include two distinct components:

- a low- to moderate-intensity cardiorespiratory activity, such as light jogging, jumping jacks, or brisk walking

- at least 5 minutes of muscle stretching, starting at the top of your body and moving to your lower body

Some experts recommend doing a light version of the activity you are about to do as your warm-up. For example, just before a basketball game, you might shoot some baskets and retrieve missed shots. Before a tennis match, you might casually hit some balls back and forth with a partner.

You should also cool down after engaging in physical activity. The cooldown helps your heart rate return to a normal, lower level. A cooldown should include some gentle stretching, which helps prevent your muscles from feeling stiff and sore the next day. Any light activity can serve as your cooldown. Many people simply slow down to low levels of their current activity for a cooldown.

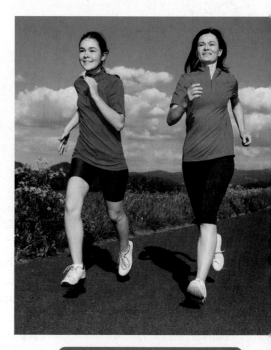

Figure 6.19

If you have been inactive and decide to start a fitness program, start slowly — don't overdo it. And even if you have been exercising regularly for some time, you need to gradually warm up at the beginning of each workout. *Why is it important to warm up?*

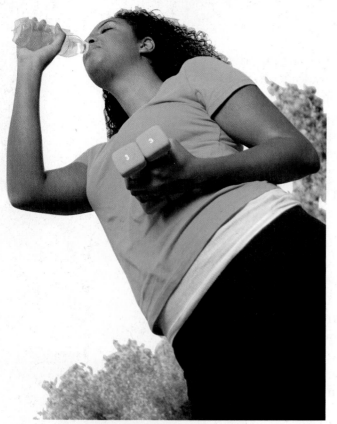

Drinking water before, during, and after engaging in physical activity will prevent fluid loss that can lead to heat-related illnesses. *What are some heat-related illnesses?*

Stay Hydrated

Your body sweats during physical activity, which decreases the amount of fluids in your body. This fluid loss causes blood volume to decrease and, as a result, the heart must work harder to circulate blood throughout your body. A loss of fluid can also lead to muscle cramps, dizziness, and fatigue.

It is, therefore, essential to drink lots of water before, during, and even after engaging in physical activity (Figure 6.20). Make sure to bring water when you exercise, and remember to drink frequently.

Sports and Energy Drinks

Some people think that it is a good idea to use a sports drink or an energy drink to help the body recover after working out. Be aware, however, that sports drinks and energy drinks are very different.

Sports drinks are flavored beverages designed to help restore water and electrolytes that are lost through sweating. These drinks have specific amounts of carbohydrates, minerals, electrolytes (sodium, potassium, calcium, magnesium), and other vitamins and nutrients.

In contrast, energy drinks are designed to help improve energy, concentration, stamina, and athletic performance. These drinks may contain caffeine, vitamins, carbohydrates (sugar), and other supplements. Using a drink that contains caffeine (as all energy drinks do) after exercising is not a good idea. Caffeine does not help replenish the water your body has lost during exercise. It can also have side effects that hinder performance, such as headaches, abnormally fast heartbeat, nausea, and jitteriness.

Chocolate Milk

Are sports drinks that contain carbohydrates and electrolytes better than water for staying hydrated? It depends on how long you plan to exercise. For most types of physical activity, plain water is exactly what your body needs. If, however, you will be exercising for more than an hour, getting some extra calories from a sports drink or fruit juice (diluted with some water) is a good idea. Chocolate milk is an even better idea.

Sports beverage companies rely on consumers believing that sport drinks are the best way to replenish the body after a workout. These companies don't broadcast the fact that chocolate milk provides more needed nutrients than sports drinks do. Chocolate milk contains three grams of carbohydrates for every one gram of protein, which helps muscles recover. It also contains whey protein, which helps build and repair muscles, and the protein *casein*, which helps reduce muscle breakdown. Chocolate milk also costs less than sports drinks.

Use Proper Equipment

When you exercise or play sports, you should be sure to use the necessary safety equipment. You should also make sure that your equipment fits well. Don't use hand-me-downs or used equipment that is overly worn or the wrong size for you. Common safety equipment for popular activities includes the following:

- Helmets should be worn for organized sports such as baseball, softball, and football. You should also wear a helmet when participating in many recreational activities, including biking, skiing, and rollerblading (Figure 6.21).

- Mouth guards protect your teeth and tongue and are needed in sports such as lacrosse, ice hockey, and football.

- Eye protection, such as goggles or a face mask, is recommended for participants in many sports, such as ice hockey goalies, swimmers, and baseball catchers.

- Padding for wrists, knees, hips, shoulders, and elbows prevents injuries common in sports such as ice hockey, football, soccer, and lacrosse, as well as ice-skating, rollerblading, and snowboarding.

- Reflective gear makes you more visible when you are riding your bike or running along the side of a road.

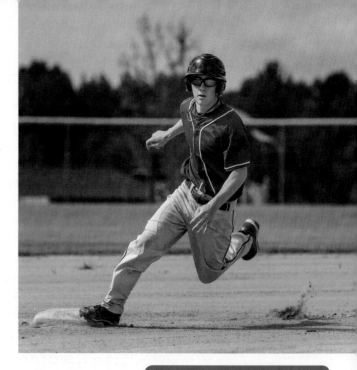

Figure 6.21

Helmets are one of the most valuable pieces of safety equipment. They should be worn during physical activities such as bicycling, and for sports such as baseball and football.

Follow the Rules

Many types of physical activity, especially sports, have certain rules that must be followed. These rules are created, at least in part, to help people stay safe. It is important to know and follow the rules of your chosen activity to keep you and the people you are playing with safe and free from injury.

Rules can vary considerably based on the activity. For example, a rule stating that all activity on the field must stop when the referee blows the whistle is important in sports such as football, soccer, lacrosse, or ice hockey. A rule that traffic laws must be obeyed is important for activities such as biking, running, or rollerblading. Because rules can vary depending on the location or organization in which an activity occurs, you should always make sure to know the particular rules under which you are playing.

It is also important to follow rules for taking care of sporting equipment and facilities. Sports equipment is expensive, so you should keep your equipment in good condition and store it in a safe place. Follow rules at your sports facilities, which may include not bringing in food or drink, wiping off equipment when you are finished with your workout, and wearing proper clothing and shoes.

Practice Good Sportsmanship

Another important aspect of playing sports is practicing good sportsmanship, which means you play fair and treat people with respect. You should use good sportsmanship with people on your team, people on the opposing team, spectators, coaches, and officials. Good sportsmanship includes shaking hands with members of the opposing team at the end of the game, accepting the officials' calls (even if you don't believe they were right), and acknowledging good performance by members of both teams.

Sometimes it can be hard to congratulate the other team when your team has just lost a close game. It is important to remember, however, that sports should be about learning new skills and having fun, not just winning. Treating members of the other team how you'd like to be treated shows respect for yourself, your teammates, coaches on both sides, officials, and the game.

Use Caution in Extreme Conditions

Exercising or playing sports outside in extreme conditions such as high heat and humidity, temperatures below 0°F, rain or snow, high altitudes, and low visibility requires extra precautions.

Heat and Humidity

Try to avoid exercising outside when it is hot and humid. Doing so can lead to serious problems, including the following:

- dehydration (a lack of body fluids)
- heat exhaustion (which can include nausea, dizziness, weakness, headache, weak pulse, disorientation, and fainting)
- heat stroke (which can lead to shock, coma, and even death)

If you are engaging in physical activity outside in high temperatures, steps you can take to stay safe include the following:

- Drink at least 8 ounces of fluid—preferably water—every 20 minutes while you are exercising.
- Drink more water once you are finished exercising to help your body replenish the fluid it lost.
- Wear light-colored and lightweight clothing.
- Use misting sprays to keep cool.
- Be aware of the signs and symptoms of heat-related health problems, including confusion, dizziness, fainting, headache, nausea, and weakness. If you are experiencing any of these symptoms, immediately tell your coach or someone who is with you.

Cold Weather

Exercising in very cold weather can also be dangerous. If you are engaging in physical activity outside in very cold temperatures, you need to stay safe. Steps you should take to ensure your safety include the following:

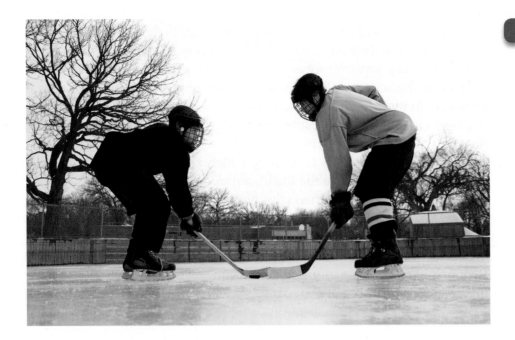

Figure 6.22

Participating in outdoor sports during very cold weather can be dangerous. *What steps do these hockey players need to take to protect themselves?*

- Check the temperature—including the wind chill factor—carefully before you go outside.
- Dress warmly with several layers of clothing.
- Make sure to protect your head, hands, feet, and ears, which are especially vulnerable to frostbite (Figure 6.22).
- Drink plenty of fluids, just like you would when exercising in hot weather.
- Know the signs and symptoms of frostbite and hypothermia, including numbness, loss of feeling or a stinging sensation, intense shivering, slurred speech, and a loss of coordination.

High Altitudes

Another extreme condition that some people may face is exercising at high altitudes, meaning areas in which you are high above the level of the ocean. Areas of high altitude have lower levels of oxygen in the air, which means you have to breathe faster and more deeply to take in enough oxygen. This can make engaging in physical activity even more difficult than usual.

If you exercise or engage in any physical activity in a mountainous area, you should take precautions to do so safely. Ideally, you should try not to exercise when you first arrive in an area of high altitude. This will give your body a chance to *acclimate*, or get used to, the change in oxygen level. When you do exercise, make sure to reduce the time and intensity of your workout.

Take Care of Your Back

After colds and the flu, back pain is the third most common reason that people see their healthcare providers. Although pain can occur in any part of the back, the most common location for injury is the lower back, which supports most of the body's weight. Many types of physical activity, especially if they are done improperly, can lead to back injuries (Figure 6.23).

One of the best ways to reduce your risk of experiencing back pain is to engage in regular exercise. Exercise reduces the likelihood of back pain by improving your posture, strengthening your back, and improving your flexibility.

Doing exercises, such as sit-ups, which strengthen your abdominal muscles also helps reduce the likelihood of developing back pain. Strong abdominal muscles strengthen your body's core and give your back more support.

Most back pain goes away on its own over time. In some cases, however, it is important to seek medical treatment. If you experience severe back pain that does not improve, or which was the result of a fall or other injury, talk to a school nurse or a doctor.

Fitness Concerns for Women

Some girls who play sports or exercise intensely are at risk for a health problem called *female athlete triad*, which is a combination of three conditions:

- Disordered eating, which can include avoiding certain foods, eating too few calories, or eliminating consumed calories in an unhealthy way (such as by vomiting or exercising excessively). Engaging in some types of disordered eating can develop into eating disorders, such as anorexia nervosa and bulimia nervosa.

- *Amenorrhea* (meaning abnormal absence of menstrual period), which is a sign that the body doesn't have sufficient fat tissue to function normally. Amenorrhea can be caused by eating too little or by exercising too much.

- Osteoporosis (meaning weak bones), which can lead to stress fractures. This condition is caused by getting too little calcium and

female athlete triad
a health problem characterized by three conditions—amenorrhea, disordered eating, and osteoporosis

amenorrhea
a condition in which a female's menstrual cycle is abnormally absent

---

Figure 6.23 Strategies for Safe Lifting

- If an object is too heavy or awkward to lift or carry alone, get help.
- Spread your feet apart to shoulder width when lifting to give you a wide base of support.
- Stand as close as possible to the object you are lifting, and lift it close to your body.
- Bend at your knees, not at your waist.
- Tighten your stomach muscles as you lift and lower the object.
- Use your leg muscles to lift, not your back muscles.
- Keep your back as straight as possible; do not bend forward or twist while holding the object.

---

vitamin D, which can have a permanent effect on bone strength for the rest of your life.

A female athlete can have one, two, or all three conditions in the triad. If you or someone you know is experiencing any of these conditions, it is very important to talk to an adult you trust (Figure 6.24). Each of these conditions can lead to serious, and even life-threatening, health problems, so seeking help is very important.

Seek Medical Advice

If you have an ongoing health condition, such as arthritis, diabetes, or high blood pressure, it is a good idea to talk with your doctor before you start on a particular exercise program. A healthcare provider can help you determine the activities and the levels of intensity that are safe for you.

Medical help may become necessary while you are actively engaging in a physical activity. Inform your parents or guardian if you

- experience severe pain;
- see swelling around a particular part of your body; or
- experience pain that makes it difficult for you to engage in normal daily activities, such as walking and sleeping.

If you do experience an injury, be sure to follow your doctor's instructions. These instructions could include taking appropriate medications, performing recommended exercises and stretches, or receiving physical therapy. Be sure to follow the doctor's recommendations regarding amount of time to refrain from certain physical activities. Returning to the activity that led to your injury too soon after the injury increases your risk of re-injury.

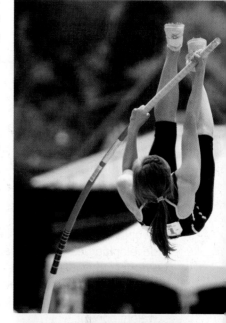

Figure 6.24

What three health problems make up the female athlete triad?

Lesson 6.3 Review

Know and Understand Assess

1. Why is it important to start slowly with any new fitness program?
2. What is the purpose of a warm-up when working out? a cooldown?
3. Explain why chocolate milk is preferable to a sports drink for hydration.
4. List at least four examples of physical activity safety equipment.

Analyze and Apply

5. Analyze the effect of hydration on your heart.
6. Evaluate the need for rules in sports and other physical activities.

7. Evaluate the safety concerns described in this lesson as they relate to you and to your community.

Real World Health

Staying hydrated is important whether or not you are engaging in physical activity. According to some experts, a good guideline for minimum water intake per day is determined by dividing a person's weight in pounds by two. For example, someone who weighs 150 lbs should drink a minimum of 75 ounces of water per day. Make a chart and record how many ounces of water you drink daily. Write a few sentences each day reflecting on how and why you were successful or not successful in staying hydrated.

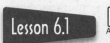

The Benefits of Improved Physical Fitness

Key Terms

endorphins
exercise
fitness
physical activity

Physical Activity
Guidelines for
Americans
sedentary behavior

Key Points

- People who exercise regularly lower their risk of developing heart disease and some cancers.
- Physical activity increases bone and muscle strength and improves sleep quality.
- Regular physical activity is important for long-term weight control.
- Physical activity does not have to be structured to improve your fitness level.
- Using certain strategies can increase the likelihood that your fitness program will succeed.

Check Your Understanding

1. What amount of physical activity is associated with reduced risk for heart disease?
   A. 150 minutes of vigorous-intensity activity per week
   B. 30 minutes of vigorous-intensity activity a day
   C. 150 minutes of moderate-intensity activity per week
   D. 30 minutes of moderate-intensity activity a day

2. Physical activity increases the amount of _____ in your joints.

3. Which of the following is a benefit of strong bone and muscle?
   A. increased loss of bone density
   B. reduced pain from arthritis and other conditions affecting the joints
   C. decreased levels of circulating endorphins
   D. Both B and C

4. True or false? Regular physical activity can help with weight control by changing a person's body composition.

5. A body that consists of _____ muscle and _____ fat burns calories at a higher rate.

6. True or false? Strength training is less effective at improving sleep quality than sleep medications.

7. Which of the following describes how physical activity improves mental health? (see top of next column)

A. causes the brain to release chemicals that make you feel good
B. increases your focus on problems you are having
C. decreases anxiety by eliminating opportunities for social interaction
D. None of the above

8. True or false? Regular physical activity generally improves academic achievement.

9. Surfing the Internet is an example of _____.
   A. anaerobic activity
   B. range of motion
   C. sedentary behavior
   D Both A and C

10. True or false? The United States Department of Health and Human Services recommends at least 30 minutes of physical activity every day for people between 6 and 17 years of age.

11. True or false? You must engage in structured exercise to improve your fitness level.

12. **Critical Thinking.** Evaluate how physical activity may lower risk for certain cancers.

13. **Critical Thinking.** Analyze strategies for implementing a successful fitness program.

The Components of Physical Fitness

Key Terms

aerobic
agility
anaerobic
cardiorespiratory fitness
components of fitness
cross training
flexibility
health-related fitness

intensity
overload principle
progression principle
range of motion
skill-related fitness
specificity principle
target heart rate

Key Points

- Health-related fitness consists of several components: cardiorespiratory fitness, endurance, muscular strength, flexibility, and body composition.
- Cardiorespiratory fitness is improved by engaging in physical activity for a certain amount of time each week at a certain level of intensity.
- Muscular endurance is the ability of a set of muscles to continue to exert force over time.

- The ability to fully and easily move muscles and joints is determined by your muscles and connective tissues.
- Skill-related fitness consists of several components: speed, agility, balance, power, coordination, and reaction time.
- A personal fitness plan focuses on the component of fitness most in need of improvement.

Check Your Understanding

14. To increase cardiorespiratory fitness, you must engage in _____ activity at a certain level of intensity for a certain amount of time each week.
    - A. anaerobic
    - B. aerobic
    - C. stretching
    - D. strengthening

15. Which of the following best describes moderate-intensity activity?
    - A. Your heart rate and breathing are considerably faster than normal, and you are unable to carry on a conversation.
    - B. Your heart rate and breathing are normal, and you are able to carry on a conversation.
    - C. Your heart rate and breathing are faster than normal, but you can still carry on a conversation.
    - D. None of the above

16. What is the maximum heart rate for a 24-year-old?
    - A. 196 bpm
    - B. 220 bpm
    - C. 204 bpm
    - D. 244 bpm

17. Using the formula in this chapter, calculate your target heart rate and list five exercises you could use to increase your heart rate during a workout.

18. When performing a push-up, your body weight serves as _____ against which your muscles must exert force.

19. *True or false?* You should rest the muscles in a particular group for at least one full day after strength training to give the muscles time to recover.

20. The ability to rapidly change the body's momentum and direction with accuracy describes which skill-related fitness component?
    - A. balance
    - B. speed
    - C. strength
    - D. agility

21. _____ is measured by the range of motion in a body's muscles and joints.

22. **Critical Thinking.** Explain why 5 to 10 minutes of low- or moderate-intensity cardiorespiratory activity is recommended before you begin stretching.

23. **Critical Thinking.** Compare and contrast aerobic versus anaerobic activities.

24. **Critical Thinking.** Explain how a skill from one physical activity can be used in another physical activity.

Lesson 6.3
Assess

Fitness Safety

Key Terms
amenorrhea female athlete triad

Key Points
- A weight-lifting routine should include safe and correct lifting techniques.
- Back pain is a common reason people see healthcare providers.
- Following a few guidelines for safe physical activity can prevent injuries.
- Individuals with existing health conditions should talk to their doctor before starting an exercise program.
- Female athletes are at risk for a unique set of health concerns.

Check Your Understanding

25. A warm-up should consist of at least _____ of muscle stretching
    - A. 1 minute
    - B. 30 minutes
    - C. 5 minutes
    - D. 1 hour

26. *True or false?* You should begin a fitness program by exercising strenuously right away.

27. Which of the following is best for staying hydrated during physical activity?
    - A. energy drinks
    - B. fruit juice
    - C. soda
    - D. chocolate milk

28. Strong _____ muscles strengthen your body's core and give your back more support.

29. *True or false?* The warm-up helps your heart rate return to a normal, lower level.

30. Which of the following is a condition included in the female athlete triad?
    - A. herniated disc
    - B. endorphins
    - C. amenorrhea
    - D. obesity

31. Choose one athlete you admire and assess his or her sportsmanship.

32. **Critical Thinking.** Why is hydration important during physical activity?

Health and Wellness Skills

33. **Practice Healthy Behaviors.** Exercise, along with a healthy diet, is one of the key factors in obesity prevention. For each day of the week, list one or two things you can do to get active. This can include going to sports practice, walking your dog, jogging with your friends, walking to class, or playing Frisbee. After each day, make a note of whether you engaged in physical activity at all. What can you do to become more physically active in your daily life?

34. **Communicate with Others.** Choose one of the skill-related components of fitness mentioned in this chapter—speed, agility, balance, power, coordination, or reaction time. Research five exercises that someone could do to improve the component of fitness that you chose. Then create a booklet that contains that information. For each exercise, include an explanation of how it is done, a picture that illustrates the exercise, at least three steps for performing the exercise safely and correctly, and an explanation of how the exercise

improves your chosen component of fitness. Share your finished booklets with the class.

35. **Advocate for Health.** Imagine that you have been challenged to create a fully developed fitness app for an app developer. This is an app that teenagers and adults will use to stay on track with their fitness programs. When presenting your app to the class, include its name, how it works, a drawing of the icon used for the app, how much the app would cost, and how it would be effective in helping people track their fitness progress.

36. **Research Community Resources.** In small groups, research the resources that promote fitness and wellness in your community. Choose three resources and create a poster summarizing their mission statements, histories, benefits, and details about participation. Present your poster to the class, and as a class, brainstorm one additional resource your community could offer.

Hands-On Activity
Creating a Fitness Plan

In this chapter, you learned that fitness plans are personal and specific to you. The components of fitness that you need to focus on might be very different from those that your best friends need to prioritize. This activity will help you create a fitness program that is unique to you and that will benefit your health.

Steps for This Activity

1. Determine the following information about yourself:
    - pulse rate after you walk a mile
    - the time it takes you to walk a mile
    - how many push-ups you can do at one time
    - how far you can reach forward, toward your toes, while sitting with your legs straight in front of you
    - your waist circumference
    - your weight or BMI

2. Evaluate the different types of exercise and physical activity. Choose the ones that you are most interested in, or would most like to do.

3. In your plan, include 10 advantages you have that will help you be successful. For example, your family may own a lot of sporting equipment, or you may already have a gym membership.

4. In your plan, include 10 obstacles that you will need to plan around such as a heavy academic load or family responsibilities. For each obstacle, list one strategy you will use to overcome that obstacle.

5. Create a SMART goal for each of the five health-related components of fitness.

6. Create a poster or chart that displays 30 days and explains all of the exercises that you hope to use. Also include the duration of those exercises and which health-related component of fitness each exercise addresses. Don't forget to vary the FITT factors in your fitness plan.

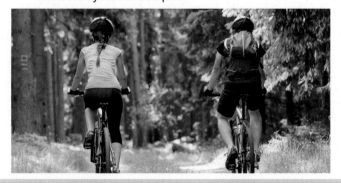

Core Skills

Math Practice

The following bar graph shows the percentage of youth who were physically active in 2012 according to the number of days they were active. Study the graph and then answer the following questions.

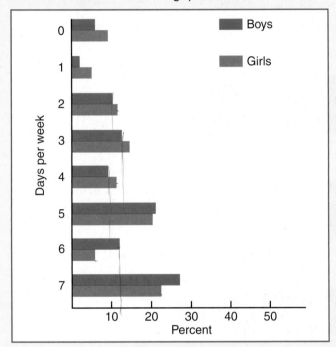

37. Approximately what percentage of boys were physically active three days per week?
    A. 13%
    B. 19%
    C. 8%
    D. 27%

38. The percentage of boys who were physically active seven days per week is _____ the percentage of girls who were physically active seven days per week.
    A. less than
    B. equal to
    C. greater than
    D. greater than or equal to

39. Approximately what percentage of girls were physically active five or more days per week?
    A. 30%
    B. 60%
    C. 38%
    D. 48%

Reading and Writing Practice

Read the passage below and then answer the questions.

Most children and teenagers attend schools that offer physical education classes. Participating in physical activity during school is a great way to increase fitness. Both the National Association for Sport and Physical Education (NASPE) and the American Heart Association (AHA) recommend that all students engage in regular physical education classes in school. These recommendations include the following:

- *Elementary school students should participate in more than 150 minutes of physical education per week.*
- *Middle and high school students should participate in more than 225 minutes of physical education per week.*

Schools can increase the amount of physical activity in a student's day by ensuring that physical education classes are taught by qualified teachers and are provided to all students in all grades. Unfortunately, too few high school students participate in physical education classes on a regular basis.

40. What is the main idea of this passage?
    A. Most physical education classes are taught by unqualified teachers.
    B. Schools can play an important role in improving students' fitness levels.
    C. Most students participate in physical activity outside of school.
    D. Middle and high school students should participate in more physical activity per week than elementary school students.

41. Based on this passage, what do you think the author's point of view is regarding physical education in schools?
    A. The amount of time dedicated to physical education is sufficient.
    B. More quality time should be dedicated to physical education.
    C. There is too much time dedicated to physical education.
    D. None of the above

42. Based on the passage you just read, write two or three paragraphs about your experience with physical education in schools.

Chapter 7
Sleep

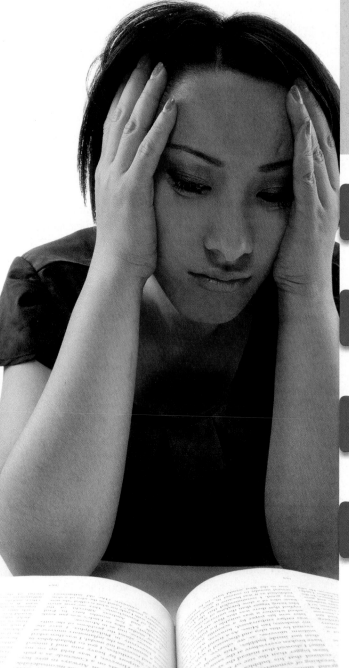

Lesson 7.1

Getting Enough Sleep

Lesson 7.2

The Science behind Sleep

Lesson 7.3

Common Sleeping Problems

Lesson 7.4

Strategies for Getting the Sleep You Need

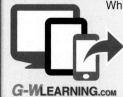

While studying this chapter, look for the activity icon to:

- **review** vocabulary with e-flash cards and games;
- **assess** learning with quizzes and online exercises;
- **expand** knowledge with animations and activities; and
- **listen** to pronunciation of key terms in the audio glossary.

G-W LEARNING.com

www.g-wlearning.com/health/

Take this quiz to see what you do and do not *know* about sleep and its impact on health. If you cannot answer a question, pay extra attention to that topic as you study this chapter.

1. *Identify each statement as* True, False, *or* It Depends. *Choose* It Depends *if a statement is true in some cases, but false in others.*

2. *Revise each* False *statement to make it true.*

3. *Explain the circumstances in which each* It Depends *statement is true and when it is false.*

Health and Wellness IQ Assess

1. Some people can get by on less sleep than others.	True	False	It Depends
2. It is possible to train yourself to need less sleep.	True	False	It Depends
3. Most people dream every night.	True	False	It Depends
4. People who don't get enough sleep are at a higher risk of becoming obese.	True	False	It Depends
5. Driving while drowsy is not especially dangerous.	True	False	It Depends
6. Taking a nap is a good way to catch up on your sleep.	True	False	It Depends
7. Heavy snoring is a sign of a sleep disorder.	True	False	It Depends
8. People who sleepwalk typically remember sleepwalking when they wake up.	True	False	It Depends
9. Teenagers need more sleep than adults.	True	False	It Depends
10. Teenagers have difficulty going to sleep at the same time as adults.	True	False	It Depends

Setting the Scene

How did you feel when you woke up this morning? Did you spring out of bed to face the new day, feeling completely refreshed and rested? Or did you hit the snooze button a few times before crawling out of bed, dragging yourself to school, and nearly nodding off in class?

If you don't get enough sleep, you're not alone. Surveys have found that many teenagers are sleep deprived. In this chapter you'll learn about the consequences of getting too little sleep, the science of sleep, and common sleep disorders. Perhaps most importantly, you'll learn effective strategies to make sure that you get the sleep you need.

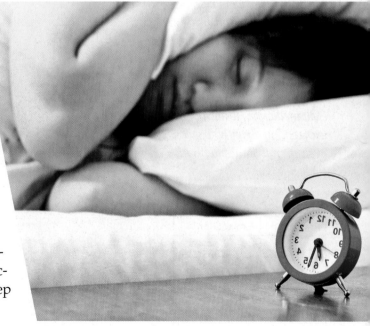

Getting Enough Sleep

Key Terms E-Flash Cards

In this lesson, you will learn the meanings of the following key terms.

hypothalamus
short sleepers
sleep deficit

Lesson Objectives

After studying this lesson, you will be able to

- compare amounts of sleep needed at various lifespan stages;
- recognize reasons why teens don't get adequate sleep; and
- summarize the effects of insufficient sleep.

Before You Read

A Lack of Sleep

Before reading this lesson, try to answer the question, "how do you think lack of sleep affects your overall health?" In a chart like the one shown below, list at least five predictions of sleep-related health problems based on your own experiences. Along with each prediction, write a brief explanation about how lack of sleep contributes to health problems.

Prediction	Explanation

Warm-Up Activity

Your Sleeping Habits

Consider your own sleeping habits and then answer the following questions on a separate piece of paper.

- *Do you get enough sleep?*
- *How do you think the amount of sleep you get affects your academic performance?*
- *What are three factors that affect how much sleep you get each night?*

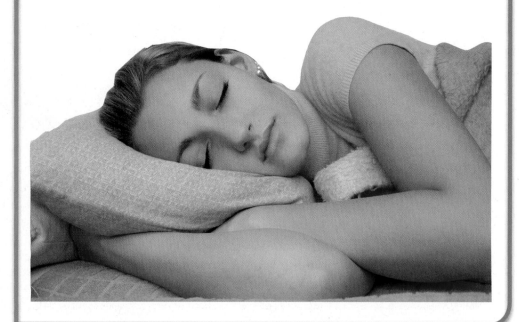

T eenagers need about nine hours of sleep per night. If you're like many teenagers, you do not get this ideal amount of time to rest. Lack of sleep can have major consequences on your psychological and physical health. In this lesson, you'll learn why many teenagers don't get enough sleep, and the health consequences of sleep deprivation.

Varying Sleep Needs

The amount of sleep that people need varies at different ages. Infants and children need considerably more sleep than adults. Surprisingly, teens also require more sleep than adults, but often do not get enough sleep to meet their needs.

Why do so many teenagers experience *sleep deficit*? One reason is that many teenagers have busy lives and stay up later to accomplish everything. If a typical teenager's school day starts before 8 a.m., however, teenagers must go to sleep by 9 p.m. or 10 p.m. to receive the recommended nine hours of sleep.

There is also a biological reason why teenagers may not get as much sleep as they need. This difference explains why teenagers can have difficulty falling asleep as early as adults or younger children do.

Many adults are sleep deprived as well. Even within the same age group, however, there can be variation in how much sleep people need. Some people are known as *short sleepers*, meaning they can function well on less sleep than other people. Short sleepers have a genetic mutation that regulates their sleep-wake cycle. These people often feel fully awake after sleeping for only four to six hours. Other people may need more than nine hours of sleep to feel fully rested.

sleep deficit
a shortage of sleep that leads to tiredness and to other health problems

short sleepers
people who can function well on less sleep than others

Health across the Life Span

Hours of Sleep Required by Age

Although everyone needs sleep to stay healthy, the amount of sleep your body needs changes with age. The recommended amount of sleep per 24-hour period for different age ranges can be seen in the table at the right.

Analyzing Data

1. What is the average number of hours of sleep recommended for a four-year-old?

2. Why do you think babies and young children need more sleep than adults? Explain your answer.

Age	Recommended Hours of Sleep
Birth to 2 months	12 to 18
2 to 11 months	14 to 15
1 to 3 years	12 to 15
3 to 5 years	11 to 13
5 to 12 years	9 to 11
12 to 18 years	8.5 to 9.5
18 years and older	7 to 9

Insufficient sleep leads to more than grogginess or grumpiness; it is linked to a number of dangerous conditions and diseases. *Do you feel well-rested most mornings?*

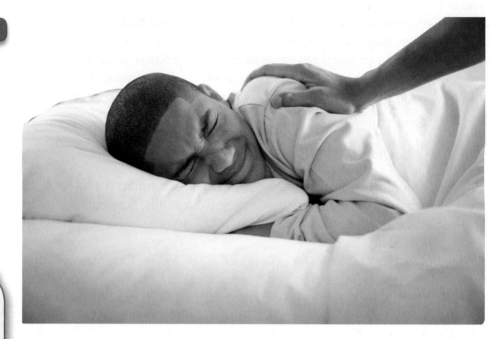

The Impact of Insufficient Sleep

Adequate sleep is essential for a person's development and for the maintenance of good physical and mental health. Unfortunately, there is no way to train your body to get by on less sleep. Moreover, getting insufficient sleep for even a short period of time can lead to problems with judgment, reaction time, and other functions. Inadequate amounts of sleep can have a serious impact on health, accidents, and performance in both school and athletics.

Disease

Getting enough sleep is just as important to good health as eating well or exercising (Figure 7.1). Scientific studies have repeatedly shown that people who routinely fail to get enough sleep are more likely to develop a number of serious health conditions, including

- diabetes;
- cardiovascular disease;
- hypertension;
- stroke;
- coronary heart disease; and
- irregular heartbeats, or *cardiac arrhythmias.*

Obesity

People who get insufficient sleep are also more likely to be obese, which is associated with numerous health problems. Children are especially at risk of experiencing weight problems if they don't get enough sleep.

It is unclear why getting insufficient amounts of sleep leads to obesity. One possibility is that sleeping for short amounts of time changes a person's *metabolism*, or the rate at which he or she burns off calories. Another possibility is that insufficient sleep, especially in children, influences the function of the **hypothalamus**, the part of the brain that regulates appetite and the consumption of energy.

hypothalamus
a part of the brain that regulates appetite and energy consumption

Accidents

People who are sleep deprived show serious impairments in their ability to pay attention, concentrate, and react quickly. A sleep deficit of just one hour a day for three days in a row can lead to impairments that cause serious injuries and even death.

Car Accidents. Driving while feeling tired is very dangerous. A drowsy driver could miss a stop sign or a red light and cause an accident. In some cases, sleepy drivers fall asleep at the wheel and drive off the road (Figure 7.2). People who drive while drowsy are just as likely to have an accident as those who drive while intoxicated.

Although people sometimes drink coffee or caffeinated sodas to try to stay awake, stimulant use fails to compensate for severe sleep deprivation. Several symptoms indicate that people are too tired to drive safely. These include having trouble staying focused on the road, being unable to stop yawning, and being unable to remember driving the last few miles.

Workplace Accidents. Inadequate sleep is also linked to many workplace accidents, some of which have caused major environmental problems, serious injuries, and even deaths. One study found that reducing the shift length a doctor can work could reduce the number of medical errors made by 36%.

The problems associated with sleep deprivation have led to a number of laws and regulations designed to help people get appropriate amounts of sleep. These laws include those that mandate

- rest periods for medical residents between work shifts;

- minimum rest periods for airline pilots between flights; and

- the maximum number of hours a truck driver can drive during a workweek.

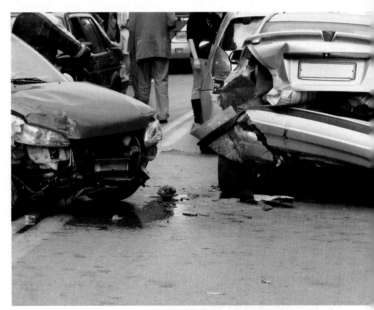

Figure 7.2

Lack of sleep can slow your reaction time on the road, putting yourself and others at risk for an accident. *What kinds of mistakes do you make when you're tired?*

School Performance

Students who arrive at school having slept too little often have problems concentrating, paying attention, solving problems, and retaining information. Students who are especially tired may even fall asleep during class. Not surprisingly, insufficient sleep leads to lower grades and poor academic performance.

Tabitha, a junior in high school, is busy with many activities. She is taking several honors classes, plays goalie on the school soccer team, and works part-time at a clothing store. In the weeks before midterm exams, Tabitha drinks several cups of coffee after dinner so she can stay up late studying. When she tries to study, however, she has difficulty concentrating.

While taking the exams, Tabitha is tired and has trouble focusing on the questions. Tabitha is also tired during her soccer games that week. The other team scores several goals that she normally would have blocked. Tabitha realizes that she needs a new strategy for studying.

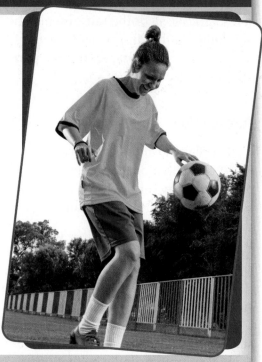

Thinking Critically

1. How do you think lack of sleep affected Tabitha's school and game performance?

2. What are some strategies that could help Tabitha do better on her next set of exams?

To help students come to school more rested, some school districts have postponed the high school start time. For example, students at some high schools begin their days at 8:30 a.m. instead of 7:30 a.m. Even this relatively small change can lead to improvements.

Schools that made this change report a variety of positive benefits including improvements in student grades, attendance, behavior, alertness, motivation, and health. The schools also report benefits such as reductions in discipline problems, tardiness, and visits to the school nurse. In some communities, the switch to later school start times has been followed by a drop in the number of car accidents.

Lesson 7.1 Review

Know and Understand 📲 Assess

1. List your family members' ages and identify the recommended amount of sleep for each.

2. Explain why teens are more likely than others to experience sleep deficit.

3. Describe the possible impact of insufficient sleep on your health.

Analyze and Apply

4. Based on what you've learned in this lesson, compose a public service announcement to persuade your peers to get adequate sleep.

5. Analyze your school's daily schedule as it relates to what you learned about sleep in this lesson. Could the schedule be altered so as to make students more productive due to the typical teenager's sleep patterns? If so, develop a new schedule for your school.

Real World Health

People who drive while drowsy are just as likely to have an accident as people who drive intoxicated. Create a poster with a creative slogan that informs students about the dangers of driving while tired. Include at least three facts or statistics about drowsy driving, and make the poster colorful and appealing. If you can, hang the poster somewhere in your school.

Lesson 7.2

The Science behind Sleep

Lesson Objectives

After studying this lesson, you will be able to

- explain the system that directs the body to sleep and wake;
- compare and contrast the five stages of sleep;
- describe the roles that dreams may play in health; and
- summarize the effect of sleep on the body's systems.

Warm-Up Activity

Your Sleep Schedule

Teenagers have a different biological clock than adults. Teenagers tend to fall asleep later in the evening and awake later in the morning. In a chart like the one shown below, outline your sleep schedule, including the time you fall asleep, the time you wake up, and any naps you take during the day.

Then, interview an adult about his or her sleep schedule and record the information. Finally, compare the two sleep schedules. How do the schedules differ? How do you think your biological clock affects your academic performance?

My Sleep Schedule	An Adult's Sleep Schedule
Weekdays	Weekdays
Weekends	Weekends

Key Terms E-Flash Cards

In this lesson, you will learn the meanings of the following key terms.

circadian rhythm

jet lag

melatonin

neuron

suprachiasmatic nucleus (SCN)

Before You Read

KWL Chart: Sleep and Dreams

Create a KWL chart to map what you know, what you want to know, and what you have learned about sleep and dreams. In the first column, brainstorm what you already know about this subject. In the second column, list several topics related to sleep and dreams that you'd like to know more about. Finally, in the third column, write what you learned after reading this lesson.

K What you Know	W What you Want to know	L What you have Learned

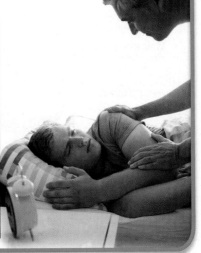

T he body and brain are quite active during sleep, and these activities are essential to staying healthy. Activities associated with learning, memory, and body growth and repair occur during sleep.

The Body's Biological Clock

Regular changes occur in your body on a daily basis. For example, your body temperature, blood pressure, and levels of different hormones rise and fall regularly.

Circadian rhythms are naturally occurring physical, behavioral, and mental changes in the body that typically follow the 24-hour cycle of the sun (Figure 7.3). For example, the body temperature drops during the night and rises during the day.

Most circadian rhythms are controlled by the body's master biological "clock." This clock, called the **suprachiasmatic nucleus (SCN)**, is a group of nerve cells in a part of the brain called the *hypothalamus*. The SCN controls many physiological responses in the body, including the sleep-wake cycle, body temperature, hormone levels, and brain wave activity.

Sleep and Circadian Rhythm

Your body's biological clock determines when you feel tired and when you feel awake. There are generally two periods of the day during which the body feels like sleeping—at night and in the early part of the afternoon, between 1 p.m. and 3 p.m. In many cultures, the early part of the afternoon is a dedicated rest time, or *siesta*.

The SCN works in two ways to regulate sleep. First, it monitors the amount of light in the environment. It leads the body to be more active when there is more light and less active when there is less light. The SCN also causes the pineal gland to release the hormone *melatonin* during the late evening, which increases feelings of relaxation and sleepiness, and signals that it is time to go to sleep (Figure 7.4). Compared with adults,

circadian rhythm
physical, behavioral, and mental changes in the body that occur naturally and typically follow the 24-hour cycle of the sun

suprachiasmatic nucleus (SCN)
a cluster of nerve cells in the hypothalamus that controls sleep, body temperature, hormone levels, and brain activity

melatonin
a hormone released by the pineal gland that increases feelings of relaxation and tiredness

Figure 7.3

The body's biological clock follows the cycle of the sun, from sunrise to sunset. *Follow this diagram around the "clock" beginning at 6:00 a.m., sunrise, on the left side of the clock. What time is 18:00? What do you think your body would do if you turned off all of your alarms and removed all the clocks from your house?*

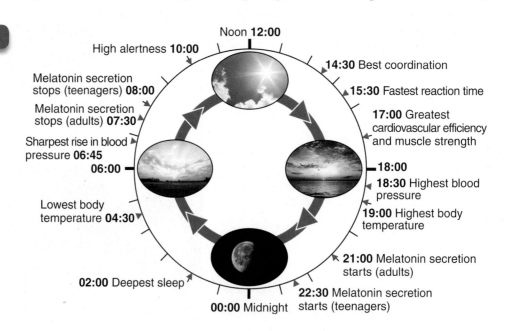

Noon **12:00**
High alertness **10:00**
14:30 Best coordination
Melatonin secretion stops (teenagers) **08:00**
15:30 Fastest reaction time
Melatonin secretion stops (adults) **07:30**
17:00 Greatest cardiovascular efficiency and muscle strength
Sharpest rise in blood pressure **06:45**
06:00
18:00
18:30 Highest blood pressure
Lowest body temperature **04:30**
19:00 Highest body temperature
21:00 Melatonin secretion starts (adults)
02:00 Deepest sleep
22:30 Melatonin secretion starts (teenagers)
00:00 Midnight

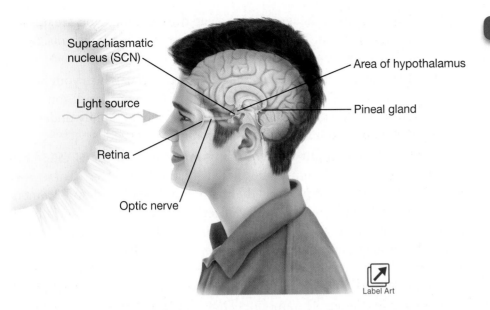

Suprachiasmatic nucleus (SCN)

Light source

Retina

Optic nerve

Area of hypothalamus

Pineal gland

Label Art

Figure 7.4

The retina and the optic nerve transmit visual information—including the level of light in the environment—to the brain. The SCN in the brain's hypothalamus monitors the amount of light. When light fades, as it does in the evening, the SCN signals the pineal gland to release melatonin, a hormone that makes you drowsy. When light in the environment becomes brighter, the release of melatonin by the pineal gland is suppressed, and you become more alert.

teenagers' melatonin is typically released later in the evening and remains at high levels in the blood until later in the morning. This biological difference contributes to the difficulty teenagers have falling asleep earlier in the evening and waking up early the next morning.

Disruptions to Circadian Rhythm

When the natural circadian rhythm is disrupted, the body's biological clock takes a while to readjust. This explains *jet lag*, which is a fatigue that people feel after changing time zones when they travel. When people travel by plane from California to New York, their bodies feel like they "lost" three hours. When their alarms ring the next morning at 7 a.m., they are tired because it is only 4 a.m. according to their biological clocks.

People who work at night or work long shifts may routinely have trouble getting adequate amounts of sleep. They may try to sleep during the day to compensate for the sleep they miss at night. This is hard to do, however, since the body is programmed to be more active during periods of sunlight. People who must sleep during the day may have trouble falling asleep and may feel drowsy during work.

jet lag
the fatigue that people experience after changing time zones during travel

Stages of Sleep

Each night, you usually pass through five distinct stages of sleep.

- **Stage 1**. This is a stage of light sleep, during which you may experience vivid sensations, or *hallucinations*. Many people experience a sensation of falling, which may jolt their bodies awake. During this stage, you drift in and out of sleep, and can be awakened easily.

- **Stage 2**. In this stage, your body temperature starts to drop, and your heart rate slows down. You may have bursts of great brain activity, called *sleep spindles*.

- **Stage 3**. This is a transitional stage between light sleep and deep sleep. Your brain waves become even slower.

- **Stage 4**. This is a stage of deep sleep during which you are difficult to awaken. The movement of your eyes and your muscle activity stop completely.
- **REM sleep**. This is an active stage of sleep during which your breathing changes, becoming irregular, shallow, and more rapid. Your heart rate and blood pressure rise. Your eyes dart about rapidly under your eyelids, and your muscles are temporarily paralyzed.

REM sleep is thought to have many important functions. The brain regions used for learning are stimulated during REM sleep. There is an increased production of proteins that help your body build and maintain tissues and fight off infections. REM sleep is thought to be especially important for normal brain development during infancy. This helps explain why infants spend more time in REM sleep than adults.

A complete sleep cycle—from Stage 1 through REM sleep—lasts about 90 to 110 minutes. Over the course of a night, you go through this sleep cycle three, four, or five times. The amount of time you spend in each stage of sleep, however, changes considerably as the night progresses (Figure 7.5). The first period of REM sleep usually occurs about 70 to 90 minutes after you fall asleep. The first sleep cycles of your night's rest period contain relatively short REM periods and long periods of deep sleep (Stage 4). The REM sleep periods get longer while the deep sleep periods get shorter in each successive sleep cycle.

Dreaming

Although you may typically forget your dreams, you do dream every night. On most nights, you spend more than two hours dreaming, with most dreams lasting between 5 and 20 minutes. The content of your dreams varies considerably from night to night. They are sometimes closely related to what is going on in your daily life. At other times, dreams may appear bizarre and fantastical.

Although most dreams occur during REM sleep, they can also occur during other sleep stages. Dreams that occur during REM sleep—when the brain is particularly active—are remarkably vivid and rich in action,

Figure 7.5

The blue line traces a person's sleep through a typical night. The graph shows five cycles of sleep, each of which includes the four stages of non-REM and then REM. *Does the graph show shorter or longer periods of REM as the night goes on? Why is REM sleep important for you as a high school student?*

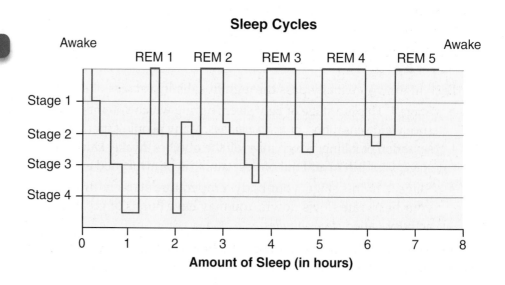

Sleep Cycles

Researchers wanted to examine whether the amount of sleep people get influences how likely they are to get sick. In one study, researchers asked a group of people to report how many hours they slept each night. Then, with the permission of study subjects, researchers injected them with a cold virus.

The researchers then studied all of the people who had been exposed to this cold virus. People who slept less than seven hours a night were nearly three times more likely to develop a cold than those who slept eight hours or more. This study provides evidence that getting an adequate amount of sleep helps your body defend itself against infections, including cold viruses.

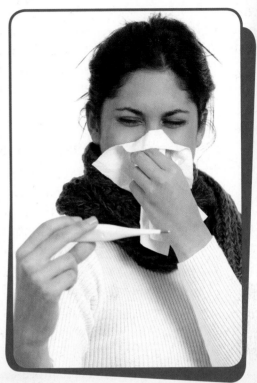

Thinking Critically

1. This study examined the impact of sleep on preventing the common cold. Do you think sleep could impact other types of health problems, such as the flu? Explain your reasoning.

2. One explanation for these findings is that more sleep leads to a better immune system. Are there other possible explanations for these findings? Consider whether people who get more sleep differ in some way from those who don't.

complexity, and emotion. People who wake up at the end of a REM sleep period are more likely to remember their dreams.

It isn't clear how dreams influence psychological and physical well-being because it is difficult to study dreams. This difficulty is because people often don't remember their dreams upon waking. Some sleep researchers believe that dreams play a valuable role in daily life. They believe dreams help people remember information, resolve conflicts, and regulate their moods. Dreams may provide important information about a person's deepest feelings, thoughts, and motives.

The Impact of Sleep on Body Systems

Your brain works in many important ways during sleep to help your body function and stay healthy. The following section examines the impact of sleep on different body systems.

Nervous System

People who get inadequate sleep feel drowsy and have difficulty concentrating and remembering things. Their physical performance, including coordination, is also impaired. This helps explain why sleep-deprived people are more likely to have motor vehicle accidents. Sleep deprivation also increases impulsive decision making. These impulsive decisions are symptomatic of a nervous system that is not working properly.

Researchers believe there are several ways that sleep benefits the nervous system. During sleep, *neurons*—the cells that make up nerve tissue—have a chance to shut down, rest, and repair. During sleep, the brain also creates important connections between neurons that can improve memory and learning. Research shows that people who get adequate sleep are better able to learn new information. Information may be processed and stored during sleep, which helps people learn and remember more information.

neuron
a type of cell that makes up the body's nerve tissues

Immune System

Getting an adequate amount of sleep is an important part of keeping the immune system functioning well. The immune system protects the body from illnesses. People who get adequate amounts of sleep produce enough immune cells to fight infection. In contrast, people who are sleep deprived show fewer immune cells in their bodies, meaning their bodies may be unable to defend against infections.

Endocrine System

Sleep also helps the endocrine system function well. The endocrine system regulates hormone levels in the body. These hormones influence many basic processes in your body. For example, during periods of deep sleep, the body releases growth hormones in both children and young adults.

During sleep, the endocrine system also speeds up the production of proteins. Proteins are essential for cell growth. They are also needed to help repair cells that are damaged by stress. This is why getting adequate sleep may improve your appearance.

Lesson 7.2 Review

Know and Understand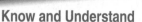

1. What controls the body's physiological responses such as the sleep-wake cycle and brain wave activity?

2. During which stage of the sleep cycle does body temperature begin to drop and heart rate slow?

3. List three important functions believed to occur during REM sleep.

4. Describe a typical dream that occurs during REM sleep.

5. Identify ways in which sleep benefits the nervous system.

Analyze and Apply

6. Compare and contrast the various stages of the sleep cycle.

7. Analyze the impact of dreaming on an individual's well-being. Use examples from the text to support your analysis.

Real World Health

Write a letter to your school board advocating for a later high school start time. Provide concrete information on teen sleep cycles and outline any other information that would help your argument.

Lesson 7.3

Common Sleeping Problems

Lesson Objectives

After studying this lesson, you will be able to

- recognize symptoms of common sleep disorders;
- explain factors that may contribute to sleep disorders; and
- identify treatments for common sleep disorders.

Warm-Up Activity

Getting Quality Sleep

Getting quality sleep can make you feel refreshed and energized for the next day, but sometimes quality sleep is hard to get. Describe a time when you tried but could not fall asleep or stay asleep. What were the circumstances surrounding your difficulty sleeping? What factors may have caused your sleep to not be restful or complete?

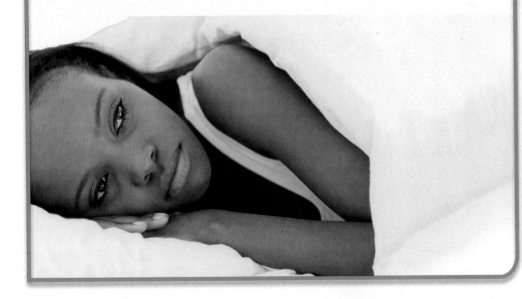

Key Terms E-Flash Cards

In this lesson, you will learn the meanings of the following key terms.

bruxism
continuous positive airway pressure (CPAP) therapy
insomnia
narcolepsy
parasomnia
restless legs syndrome (RLS)
sleep apnea

Before You Read

Sleep Disorders

In a table like the one shown below, list all the sleep disorders you know about and include a list of symptoms for each disorder. If multiple disorders have some symptoms in common, highlight each repeated symptom in a different color.

Sleep Disorders	Symptoms

Chronic, long-term sleep disorders can cause problems at work and at school. They interfere with a person's family life and social activities. Most importantly, sleep disorders can sabotage a person's health. Fortunately, most sleep disorders can be treated once the person recognizes the problem and seeks help.

Insomnia

insomnia
a condition in which the body is unable to fall asleep or stay asleep

At some point in their lives, almost everyone experiences *insomnia*, which is an inability to fall asleep or to stay asleep. Some people with insomnia wake up several hours early and are unable to go back to sleep. People who have insomnia don't get adequate amounts of sleep and this often affects their ability to function the next day at work or school (Figure 7.6).

Insomnia can be caused by many different factors, including stress; jet lag; diet; and health conditions such as cancer, cardiovascular disease, and lung disease. Acute, or *short-term*, insomnia is common and can be caused by problems that occur in daily life.

On the other hand, chronic, or *long-term*, insomnia lasts a month or longer. Chronic insomnia is a symptom or side effect of another problem, such as a medical condition, substance use, or a sleep disorder.

Insomnia may be treated in many ways. Treatment can initially include sleeping pills. Long-term use of sleeping pills is discouraged, however, because using them can interfere with good sleeping habits.

Figure 7.6

Insomnia is an inability to fall asleep and can be either short-term or long-term. *Do you have problems with insomnia? If so, have you identified any solutions?*

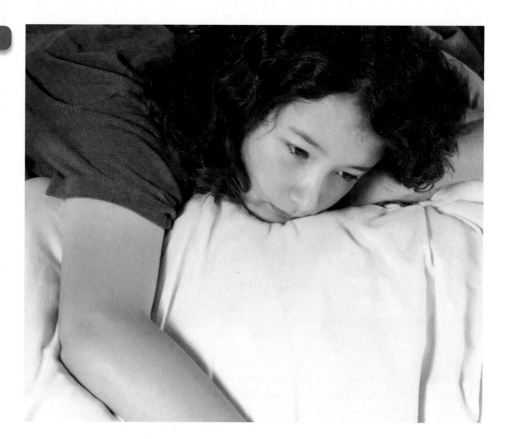

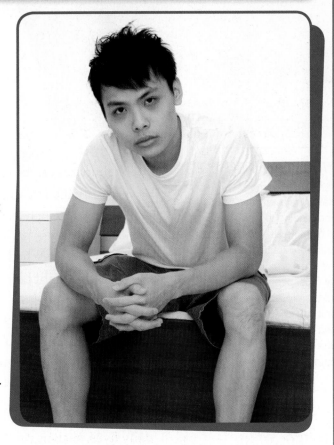

People all over the world struggle with getting adequate sleep. People in some countries, however, fare better than others. In a study of people around the world, researchers found that the French sleep more hours per night than people in the other countries studied. The French sleep an average of 530 minutes a night, or almost nine hours. People in the United States sleep an average of 518 minutes a night, or about eight and a half hours.

In which country do people get the least amount of sleep? People in Korea sleep an average of 469 minutes a night, or a little less than eight hours.

People in different countries also have varying impacts of work stress on their sleep. Americans are more likely to lose sleep because of work-related stress than people in other countries. Thirty percent of the Americans in this study reported that work stress caused them to have difficulty sleeping. In comparison, 27% of the Germans, 24% of the British, and 20% of the Japanese reported that work stress impacted their sleep. Only 12% of the people surveyed in the Netherlands reported that stress from work led to sleep problems.

Thinking Critically

1. Why do you think Americans are more likely to suffer from work-related sleep problems than people in other countries? Do you think the percentage of Americans who have difficulty sleeping due to work stress has increased over the last 50 years? Do you think this percentage will get higher or lower in the future? Explain your answer.

2. You read that the average number of hours people sleep varies among countries. What factors do you think would cause this data to vary? For example, do you believe that living in a big city would impact the average amount of sleep people receive, as compared with living in a small town? Why or why not?

3. Given the health consequences of sleep deprivation, what strategies might be effective in ensuring that people get enough sleep?

Parasomnia

Parasomnia is a classification of sleep disorders that occur when people are partially, but not completely, aroused from sleep. These disorders can occur when people are first falling asleep, when they are between sleep stages, or when they are aroused from sleep. The most common types of parasomnia include nightmares, sleepwalking, restless legs syndrome, and teeth grinding.

parasomnia
a class of sleep disorders in which a person is partially, but not completely, aroused from sleep

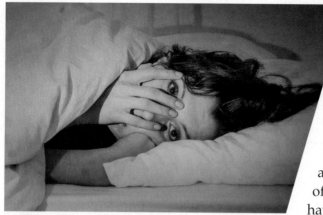

Have you ever been worried about going to sleep because of nightmares you have had on previous nights? Nightmares are not a serious problem for most people, but if you frequently fail to get to sleep, or if you frequently wake up and can't get back to sleep due to nightmares, talk to your parents about seeking help.

Nightmares

Have you ever woke up terrified after being chased by someone who wanted to do you harm? Perhaps you've dreamt that your teeth fell out or that you forgot to prepare an oral report for a class. These are some common nightmare scenarios.

Nightmares are highly disturbing dreams associated with negative feelings, such as anxiety, fear, and sadness. These dreams, which are quite common, often seem real, and may lead people to wake up and have difficulty falling back asleep. Nightmares usually occur during the last hours of sleep in a given night.

Nightmares can be caused by many factors, including

- daily life stresses or major changes;
- trauma, such as an accident or injury;
- exposure to books, television programs, and movies, especially right before bed;
- eating right before bed, which can cause an increase in energy and brain activity;
- illness, especially if accompanied by a fever; and
- alcohol, illegal drugs, and some types of medications.

Young children often have nightmares about monsters or scary scenarios. The scary images or scenarios are sometimes based on something they saw on television or read about immediately before going to bed. Older children typically have nightmares that focus on fears connected to their daily lives, such as problems at school or at home.

Having nightmares or being afraid of having nightmares can cause some people to develop a fear of going to sleep (Figure 7.7). People who have this problem should talk to a doctor.

Sleepwalking

Sleepwalking is a sleep disorder that leads people to get out of bed and walk around while they are in a state of deep sleep. Sleepwalking can take a number of different forms. A person who is sleepwalking may walk slowly around a bedroom. Another person may run fast around the house. When sleepwalking, people may also speak incoherently.

Although the eyes of a sleepwalking person are typically open, he or she will not respond to questions. The affected person will also not remember sleepwalking.

Sleepwalking may be caused by different factors, including

- genetic makeup;
- environmental factors such as stress and lack of sleep;
- alcohol and drug use; and
- various medical conditions, including arrhythmias (abnormal heart rhythms), fever, and some types of psychiatric disorders.

Restless Legs Syndrome (RLS)

Restless legs syndrome (RLS) is a disorder that causes people to experience crawling, prickling, or tingling in their lower legs and feet. People with RLS may have feelings of aches and pains in their legs, and an urge to constantly move their legs to relieve these sensations. This disorder is one of the most common sleep disorders, especially among older people. Not surprisingly, people with RLS have difficulty falling sleep.

Teeth Grinding

Most people occasionally grind and clench their teeth. This behavior is known as *bruxism*. Teeth grinding can be caused by stress or anxiety, having an abnormal bite, or missing or crooked teeth. Many people who grind their teeth are unaware they do it because it often occurs during sleep. They may learn they grind their teeth from other people. Although this behavior is usually harmless, persistent teeth grinding can lead to tooth damage, a sore jaw, headaches, and even hearing loss (Figure 7.8).

Fortunately, there are some highly effective strategies for reducing bruxism. A dentist can determine whether you are grinding your teeth and may suggest wearing a mouth guard during sleep to protect your teeth. A dentist may also recommend the following:

- Avoid chewing on pencils, pens, or gum, which accustoms your jaw muscles to more clenching.
- Focus on relaxing your teeth and jaw while you are awake.
- Place the tip of your tongue between your teeth, which helps prevent teeth clenching.
- Relax your jaw muscles before you go to sleep by holding a warm washcloth on the side of your face, or by massaging and stretching your jaw to help it relax.

Since stress can lead to bruxism, other strategies focus on reducing overall stress. For example, starting an exercise program can be helpful in managing stress. People who experience bruxism should also reduce their consumption of caffeinated foods and drinks, which tend to increase teeth grinding. Drinking more water can be helpful since dehydration may increase teeth grinding. In severe cases of bruxism, doctors may recommend a prescription drug to help relieve symptoms.

Sleep Apnea

Sleep apnea is a potentially serious disorder in which a person actually stops breathing for short periods of time during sleep. This disorder is usually associated with loud snoring, but not everyone who snores has this disorder. Many people with this disorder don't have the problem diagnosed. Sleep apnea is most common among older people, and is more common in men than in women.

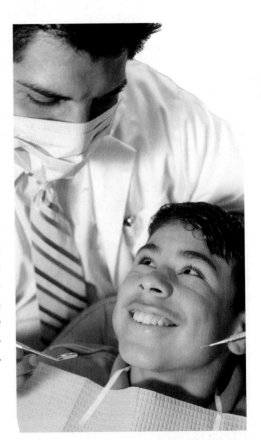

Figure 7.8

Bruxism, or teeth grinding, may lead to dental problems. If you grind your teeth, it is important to talk with your dentist about it.

restless legs syndrome (RLS)
a disorder in which people experience prickling, tingling, or other irresistible urges to move their legs

bruxism
a condition in which a person grinds or clenches his or her teeth while sleeping

sleep apnea
a serious disorder in which a person stops breathing during sleep

Types of Sleep Apnea

There are two types of sleep apnea—obstructive and central. *Obstructive sleep apnea* is caused in part by fat buildup, or the loss of muscle tone, that occurs with aging. These physical changes cause the windpipe to collapse when the muscles relax during sleep. Teenagers can also develop obstructive sleep apnea, but in those cases it is often caused by swollen tonsils that make it more difficult to breathe.

Obstructive sleep apnea follows a particular cycle, which may be repeated hundreds of times a night. The sleeping person's effort to inhale air creates suction that collapses the windpipe. This blocks the airflow for 10 seconds to a minute while the sleeping person struggles to breathe. When the person's blood oxygen level falls, the brain responds by awakening the person enough to tighten the upper airway muscles and open the windpipe. The person may snort or gasp, and then resume snoring.

Central sleep apnea occurs when the brain fails to send the right signals to the muscles that control breathing. This type of sleep apnea may be caused by other medical conditions, such as heart failure and stroke, or by sleeping at a high altitude. Central sleep apnea is less common than obstructive sleep apnea.

Symptoms of Sleep Apnea

People with sleep apnea can suffer numerous side effects due to inadequate sleep and a lack of oxygen in their blood. These include

- excessive daytime sleepiness;
- irritability or depression;
- morning headaches;
- a decline in mental functioning;
- cardiovascular problems, including high blood pressure, irregular heartbeats, and an increased risk of heart attacks and stroke; and
- accidents, including automobile accidents.

Treatment of Sleep Apnea

Once obstructive sleep apnea is diagnosed, there are a number of possible treatments available. People may be advised to lose weight or to try sleeping on their sides instead of their backs. Some dentists specialize in creating dental appliances that pull the jaw forward and keep the airway open. In some cases, surgery is required to remove tissue from the throat, clear nasal obstructions, or to correct other medical problems. Surgery may also be needed to treat contributing conditions such as congestive heart failure.

People may also use a special machine while sleeping that increases air pressure in the throat, and keeps the airway open to assist breathing. This type of machine, which is called **continuous positive airway pressure (CPAP) therapy**, consists of either a mask that covers the nose and mouth

continuous positive airway pressure (CPAP) therapy
a type of therapy in which a machine is used to open the airways during sleep; a treatment for sleep apnea

or nasal prongs (Figure 7.9). This nonsurgical option can be very effective for treating sleep apnea.

Narcolepsy

Narcolepsy is a disorder that causes people to have difficulty regulating their sleep. For most people, sleep regulation occurs naturally and without effort. People with narcolepsy have frequent *sleep attacks* at various times of the day, even if they have had a normal amount of nighttime sleep.

During a sleep attack, people fall asleep suddenly for a period lasting several seconds or even more than 30 minutes. These sleep attacks can be embarrassing and dangerous. They may occur when people are walking, driving, and performing other forms of physical activity. Symptoms typically appear first during adolescence.

Episodes of narcolepsy may be triggered by strong emotions or surprise. The causes of narcolepsy are, however, still unclear. This disorder tends to run in families, so a person's genes are known to play a role in its development. People whose parents have narcolepsy are more likely to develop it themselves than are people who have no family history of the disorder. Narcolepsy may also be caused by brain damage resulting from a head injury or neurological disease.

Narcolepsy can be treated with drugs, such as stimulants or antidepressants that help control the symptoms. People who have narcolepsy may also take frequent naps during the day, which reduces excessive sleepiness.

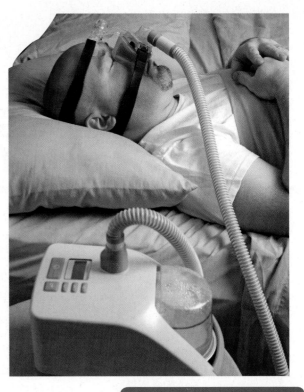

Figure 7.9

A CPAP machine opens a person's airways, which helps maintain regular breathing.

narcolepsy
a disorder characterized by "sleep attacks" in which a person suddenly falls asleep at various times during the day

Lesson 7.3 Review

Know and Understand Assess

1. Compare factors that contribute to acute insomnia versus chronic insomnia.

2. List four types of parasomnias.

3. Identify possible treatments for sleep apnea.

4. What two factors contribute to the side effects of sleep apnea?

5. Identify two triggers for narcolepsy.

Analyze and Apply

6. Older people are more likely to experience insomnia than younger people. Why do you think this is?

7. Distinguish between obstructive sleep apnea and central sleep apnea.

Real World Health

Imagine that you have been named the director of your local sleep clinic. It is your responsibility to educate your community about sleep disturbances and disorders. Using this chapter as a guide, create a brochure to educate local teens about the signs and symptoms of all the different sleep disturbances and disorders.

Strategies for Getting the Sleep You Need

Key Terms 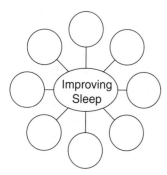 E-Flash Cards

In this lesson, you will learn the meanings of the following key terms.

stimulant

tryptophan

Lesson Objectives

After studying this lesson, you will be able to

- understand the importance of following a sleep schedule;
- explain guidelines for napping;
- recall how to use exercise as a sleep strategy;
- recognize substances that interfere with sleep;
- identify relaxation techniques that help you prepare for sleep;
- recall ways to create an environment that is conducive to sleep; and
- summarize strategies for using light to regulate your sleep cycle.

Before You Read

Sleep Mindmap

Write the phrase Improving Sleep in the middle of a mindmap like the one shown below. As you read this lesson, brainstorm and write what you learn about improving your sleep in the surrounding circles.

Improving Sleep

Warm-Up Activity

Sleep Environment

Your sleeping environment is extremely important to your getting a good night's rest. Describe, in detail, the conditions of the room where you sleep. Don't forget to include details such as temperature, the size and comfort of your bed, noise levels, and siblings who share your room.

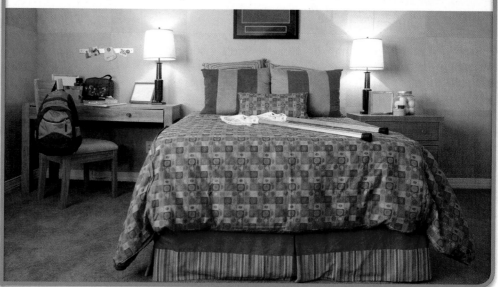

Getting enough sleep is an essential part of staying healthy, yet many teenagers get insufficient sleep. If you're one of these teenagers, keep in mind that different sleep strategies work best for different people. The strategies that work best for you may be different from the strategies that work best for your parents, siblings, or friends.

Set (and Follow) a Schedule

One of the best ways to make sure you get enough sleep is to set and follow a sleep-wake schedule. This means you go to bed at approximately the same time each night and get up at approximately the same time each morning. A good sleep schedule should be in sync with your body's natural circadian rhythm. The predictable pattern makes it easier for the body to fall asleep and wake up (Figure 7.10).

Use the same schedule throughout the week—not just Monday through Friday. Many people get too little sleep during the week and then try to "catch up" on the weekends. When you sleep in for two or three extra hours on the weekends, your body clock is disrupted, which just makes it more difficult to get up on Monday morning.

There are times when you may want to change your sleep schedule. For example, during the summer, you may be able to sleep later when school is not in session. You can help your body adjust to a new sleep schedule by making small, gradual changes in the time you go to bed and wake up. Going to bed and waking up just 15 or 20 minutes later each day helps reset your biological clock to the new time, and will help you get better sleep.

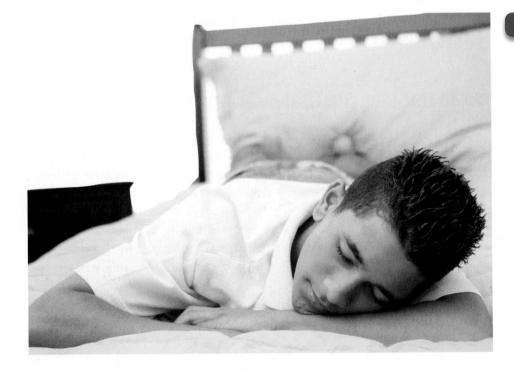

Figure 7.10

Following a consistent sleep schedule will make it easier for you to fall asleep and wake up. *What is your sleep schedule? How closely do you follow it?*

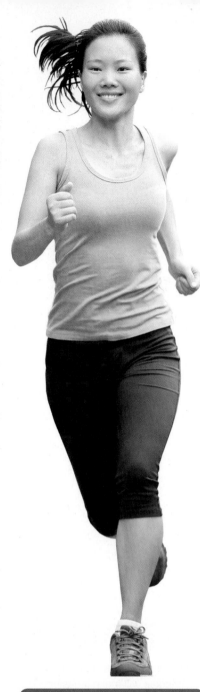

Nap Strategically

Napping is a better way of catching up on sleep than sleeping in late on the weekends. Napping during the day can help you get some extra sleep without disrupting your regular sleep schedule.

Napping has other benefits as well. People who take even a short nap—for 20 to 60 minutes—feel more alert, and find it easier to learn new skills and use their memory. They are also more creative.

If you choose to take naps during the day, remember the following strategies:

- Set an alarm so you don't get too much sleep during the day.
- Nap in the early afternoon when your body's biological clock tells your body it is time to rest. Stop taking daytime naps if you start having trouble falling asleep at night.
- Do not nap after dinner; this can disrupt your regular sleep schedule. If you are drowsy after dinner, do something active to avoid falling asleep.

Exercise Regularly

Exercising for as little as 20 to 30 minutes a day can help people get to sleep—and stay asleep. Find ways to add at least this much exercise to your day in whichever way feels best for you. Remember that you don't need to do the 20 to 30 minutes of exercise all at once. Sometimes it can be easier to find smaller periods of time for exercise. Fortunately, exercising for five to ten minutes several times during the day will still help you get to sleep at night.

You should try to exercise at least five or six hours before you plan to go to sleep. Stimulation in the evening can make it difficult to fall asleep. It is best to exercise in the morning or afternoon if you can (Figure 7.11).

Figure 7.11

Exercising for at least 20 minutes a day can help you fall asleep. Try to engage in that exercise five to six hours before your bedtime.

stimulant
a substance that increases the body's activity and makes it more difficult to sleep

Avoid Substances That Interfere with Sleep

Substances called ***stimulants*** produce a temporary increase in activity in the body and make it difficult to sleep. Caffeine is one of these substances. You should avoid any drink or food that contains caffeine, including coffee, chocolate, energy drinks, soft drinks, nonherbal teas, and diet drugs.

Another substance that can interfere with sleep is nicotine, which is a stimulant found in tobacco. People who are addicted to nicotine often wake up early in the morning. They are experiencing nicotine withdrawal after not having a cigarette all night.

Your eating habits also influence how well you sleep. It is particularly important to avoid eating large meals or snacks in the hours leading up to your bedtime.

Getting Sufficient Sleep

If you have trouble getting enough sleep, try some of these strategies and see which ones work for you.

- Go to bed at the same time each night and get up at the same time each morning.
- Exercise each day, ideally before the evening.
- Avoid large meals or snacks late in the evening.
- Avoid caffeine—including coffee, sodas, and chocolate—in the late afternoon and evenings.
- Use your bed for sleep only, and not for studying or watching television.
- Nap in the afternoon, not in the evening.
- Sleep in a quiet, dark room that is kept at a moderately cold temperature.
- Make sure your mattress and pillows are comfortable.
- Relax your body and mind before you get into bed and try to sleep.
- Try some light stretching or deep breathing to clear your mind.
- See a doctor if your trouble persists.

A light snack before bed can promote sleep for some people. Eating foods that contain tryptophan may help calm the brain and allow you to sleep better. *Tryptophan* is an amino acid that aids the body in making chemicals that help you sleep. Experiment with foods to determine your optimum evening meals and snacks. If you need a bedtime snack, try half a turkey sandwich or a banana.

tryptophan
an amino acid that aids the body in producing chemicals that cause sleep

Relax before Bedtime

When people try to fall asleep, they sometimes focus on stressful experiences or worry about upcoming events. Not surprisingly, people who go to bed feeling stressed, worried, and angry have trouble falling asleep.

If you are worrying about something you need to remember the next day, write a quick note to yourself. This will help you feel confident that you will remember, and you will no longer need to keep that item in your mind.

A peaceful bedtime routine sends a powerful signal to your brain that it's time to relax and let go of the day's stresses. Practicing relaxation techniques before bed is a great way to wind down, calm the mind, and prepare for sleep. Here are some simple relaxation techniques to try.

- Take slow, deep breaths.
- Relax all of the muscles in your body, starting at your toes and working up to your head.
- Think about being in a peaceful, calm place, such as a warm beach or a lush forest.
- Read a book or magazine, or listen to an audiobook.
- Take a warm bath or shower.
- Listen to quiet music.
- Perform yoga, meditation, or gentle stretching to relax your body and your mind.

How Screen Time Interferes with Sleep Time

If you are often tired, your screen-viewing habits may be causing the problem. Researchers studied teenagers who spend more time viewing television and computer screens than their peers. They found that the teenagers who logged more screen time got to sleep later and slept fewer hours a night than their peers. These teens also reported feeling more tired overall. These sleep problems were even worse for teenagers who had televisions in their bedrooms.

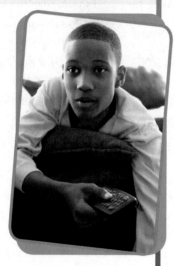

Why does watching television in the evenings interfere with sleep? One reason is that many shows are suspenseful, violent, and dramatic. Viewing exciting or violent content in the media leads to physiological changes in the body, such as higher levels of hormones. These hormones increase feelings of arousal, which may make it more difficult to relax and go to sleep.

Additionally, the light from television and computer screens suppresses melatonin, a hormone that tells the brain it is time to sleep. So, using a screen late at night can make falling asleep more difficult.

Extensive television viewing during adolescence may even lead to the development of sleep problems during young adulthood. Researchers in one study found that 14-year-olds who watched more television than their peers had more sleep problems years later at 16 and 22 years of age.

Thinking Critically

1. This feature described two different explanations for the link between watching television and difficulty getting to sleep. Can you think of other factors that could explain why or how screen time interferes with sleep? Explain your reasoning.

2. What do you think explains the finding that more television watching during the teenage years leads to sleep problems later on? What evidence would you need to test your theory?

If you can't sleep, or if you wake up in the middle of the night and can't get back to sleep, get out of bed and do something relaxing. Feeling anxious about not sleeping makes it even harder to get to sleep. Read a book or listen to soft music until you feel tired. Avoid watching television or checking your phone or computer, since these activities will stimulate you.

Create a Comfortable Sleep Environment

It is easier to get to sleep in an environment you find comfortable. Even if you share a bedroom with a sibling, you can take certain actions to improve the sleep environment.

- Reduce the room's temperature. Most people sleep best in a slightly cool room with a temperature around 65°F.

- Keep the bedroom dark. If light comes through a window, install an inexpensive room-darkening shade. If you share a bedroom with a sibling, consider wearing an eye mask to create a feeling of darkness or negotiate a lights-out time.

- Maintain quiet. If you can't eliminate noise completely, consider wearing earplugs, or sleeping with a fan or a white noise machine to mask sounds.

- Make your bed as comfortable as possible. You should have enough room in your bed to stretch and turn comfortably. If your mattress is uncomfortable, you might need a new one. Speak with your parent or caregiver about it. Adding a less expensive foam mattress cover may solve the problem. An inexpensive new pillow can also help.

Control Exposure to Light

Melatonin is a naturally occurring hormone that helps regulate the sleep-wake cycle. Light affects the body's production of melatonin. When it is dark, your body produces more melatonin, which makes you feel sleepy. When it is light, less melatonin is produced, which leads you to feel more awake and alert. Exposure to sunlight in the morning and throughout the day regulates your body's biological clock and helps you feel more active.

Many aspects of modern life can disrupt your body's natural production of melatonin and your sleep-wake cycle. For example, spending time in a school or office that doesn't let in natural light can make you feel sleepier. On the other hand, if you spend the evening exposed to bright lights from a television or computer screen, your body may produce less melatonin, which makes it harder to feel sleepy.

Try natural methods of regulating your sleep schedule. The following are strategies you can use:

- Spend time outside during the day whenever possible (Figure 7.12). Eat lunch outside or go for a walk in the late afternoon.

- Keep curtains and blinds open during the day to increase the amount of natural light in your room or office. Move your desk or chair near a window.

- Minimize the time you spend in front of a television or computer screen at the end of the day.

- Avoid reading from an electronic device that emits extra light just before you go to bed. Reading a physical book with a bedside lamp exposes your body to less light, which makes it easier to fall asleep.

- Use a night-light in the bathroom to avoid turning on a bright light in the middle of the night.

- When you wake up, open the blinds or curtains and turn on bright lights to jump-start your body's clock and help you feel more awake and alert.

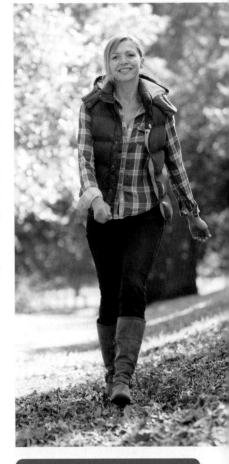

Figure 7.12

It might surprise people to know that spending time outdoors during the day can help them sleep at night. *How would you explain why this is so to someone who doubted it?*

Lesson 7.4 Review

Know and Understand Assess

1. Why might sleeping an extra two or three hours on the weekend make waking up on Monday morning more difficult?

2. What is usually the best time of day to nap?

3. List three eating habits that will help you sleep more soundly.

4. Why is it important to relax before bedtime?

5. What are two ways to combat noise issues when trying to sleep?

6. How is exposure to light related to sleep?

Analyze and Apply

7. Create a list of strategies to use when you wake in the middle of the night and cannot get back to sleep.

Real World Health

Reread the section in this lesson about creating a comfortable bedroom environment. Then, compare and contrast your sleeping environment with the recommendations listed here. What changes need to be made to your environment? What other improvements could be made that were not on the list?

Chapter 7   Review and Assessment

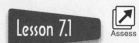

Lesson 7.1
Assess

Getting Enough Sleep

Key Terms

hypothalamus   sleep deficit
short sleepers

Key Points

- Teens require more sleep than adults, but most do not get enough sleep to meet their needs.
- Insufficient sleep has a negative effect on health, weight, accident avoidance, and performance in school and athletics.

Check Your Understanding

1. How much sleep is recommended for 12- to 18-year-olds?
   A. 12–15 hours per day
   B. 9–11 hours per day
   C. 8.5–9.5 hours per day
   D. 7–9 hours per day

2. *True or false?* There is a biological reason that may contribute to teens getting insufficient sleep.

3. _____ function better on less sleep than other people.
   A. Short sleepers
   B. Toddlers
   C. Athletes
   D. Women

4. Scientific studies have shown that people who routinely fail to get enough sleep are more likely to develop which of the following health conditions?
   A. osteoporosis
   B. diabetes
   C. cardiovascular disease
   D. Both B and C.

5. Insufficient sleep influences the function of the _____, the part of the brain that regulates appetite and the expenditure of energy.

6. *True or false?* Some school districts have implemented nap breaks during the high school day to improve academic performance.

7. **Critical Thinking.** Identify jobs other than those listed in this chapter that you believe should have sleep requirements mandated. Cite your reasoning.

Lesson 7.2
Assess

The Science behind Sleep

Key Terms

circadian rhythm   neuron
jet lag   suprachiasmatic nucleus
melatonin   (SCN)

Key Points

- Changes that occur in your body following a 24-hour cycle affect when you sleep and wake.
- Sleep transitions through five stages, which then repeat over the course of the night.
- Dreams may play a valuable role in helping people remember information, resolve conflicts, and regulate moods.
- Sleep is important for proper functioning of the nervous, immune, and endocrine systems.

Check Your Understanding

8. _____ are naturally occurring physical, behavioral, and mental changes in the body that typically follow the 24-hour cycle of the sun.

9. *True or false?* Neurons aren't released in teenagers' brains until later in the evening, making it difficult to fall asleep earlier and wake up earlier.

10. *True or false?* Jet lag is the result of the natural circadian rhythm being disrupted.

11. During which stage of sleep are regions of the brain used in learning stimulated?
    A. Stage 2
    B. Stage 3
    C. Stage 4
    D. REM sleep

12. Describe the nature of dreams that occur during REM sleep.

13. Which body system is important for memory and learning?
    A. nervous system
    B. biological clock
    C. suprachiasmatic nucleus (SCN)
    D. immune system

14. **Critical Thinking.** Hypothesize why the circadian rhythm follows the 24-hour cycle of the sun.

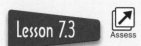

Common Sleeping Problems

Key Terms

bruxism

continuous positive airway
   pressure (CPAP)
   therapy

insomnia

narcolepsy

parasomnia

restless legs syndrome
   (RLS)

sleep apnea

Key Points

- Insomnia can be caused by a number of different factors. Many people experience short-term insomnia.
- Parasomnias are sleep disorders that occur when people are partially aroused from sleep.
- Sleep apnea is a potentially serious disorder that often goes undiagnosed.
- Narcolepsy has little to do with the amount of sleep a person has had.

Check Your Understanding

15. _____ is the inability to fall asleep or stay asleep.

16. List four factors that can cause insomnia.

17. Restless legs syndrome (RLS), nightmares, sleepwalking, and teeth grinding are examples of _____.
    A. parasomnias
    B. bruxism
    C. sleep apnea
    D. narcolepsy

18. *True or false?* People with bruxism can suffer numerous side effects due to inadequate sleep and a lack of oxygen in their blood.

19. Which of the following statements is true about sleep apnea?
    A. Everyone who snores has sleep apnea.
    B. Teens can develop sleep apnea.
    C. The only treatment for sleep apnea is surgery.
    D. None of the above.

20. What happens during a sleep attack?

21. **Critical Thinking.** Based on what you've learned about sleep apnea, can you think of any corrective measures other than those mentioned in the lesson?

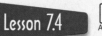

Strategies for Getting the Sleep You Need

Key Terms

stimulant

tryptophan

Key Points

- Following a consistent sleep schedule makes it easier to fall asleep and wake up.
- Napping should not disrupt your normal sleep cycle.
- Regular exercise helps you fall asleep and stay asleep.
- Consuming some types of substances before bed can interfere with sleep.
- Relaxing before bedtime can improve your chances of falling asleep.
- The bedroom environment can affect your ability to fall asleep.
- Exposure to light has an impact on your sleep-wake cycle.

Check Your Understanding

22. What is the best schedule to follow to help your body fall asleep and wake up most easily?

23. *True or false?* The best time to take a nap is early afternoon.

24. For the best sleep, it is best to exercise _____.
    A. as little as possible
    B. for a minimum of one hour
    C. 20 to 30 minutes per week
    D. five or six hours before going to bed

25. List three substances that can interfere with sleep.

26. Exposure to light affects the body's production of _____, which helps regulate the sleep-wake cycle.
    A. narcolepsy
    B. tryptophan
    C. melatonin
    D. neurons

27. **Critical Thinking.** Using the information in this lesson, create a daily plan that will help you get the sleep you need.

Health and Wellness Skills

28. **Practice Healthy Behaviors and Reduce Health Risks.** Teenagers are busier than ever and usually don't get enough sleep, but time management skills can help with setting and sticking to a bedtime each night. Map out a detailed schedule for a five-day school week. Your schedule should be an hour-by-hour chart that includes travel time, grooming, family time, study time, and extracurricular activities. In your schedule, set a bedtime that will allow you a good amount of sleep based on what you learned in this chapter. Once you have finished your schedule, list five obstacles you may face in sticking to your chosen bedtime. Lastly, list five strategies you could use to overcome these obstacles.

29. **Communicate with Others.** Think about a person, place, or object that could embody sleep. Then, create a poster that uses this person, place, or object to illustrate the five stages of sleep. Describe or depict the five stages and what occurs in each stage. Use your imagination to convey all the important information in an accessible and appealing way. Present your poster to the class.

30. **Comprehend Concepts.** Now that you understand circadian rhythms, consider your own biological clock. Imagine that all of your body systems are transmitting information to a reporter who works for the W-SLEEP network. Write this reporter's article as he or she analyzes your circadian rhythms and the effects they have on your day. Include information such as when you are most cheerful, most cranky, most alert, or most drowsy.

31. **Access Information.** Choose one of the common sleep problems you read about in this chapter. Then, use the Internet or your library to research how a healthy diet, proper stress management, and exercise may help battle this sleep disturbance. Write a short paragraph about your findings.

Hands-On Activity

Drowsy Driving

Chris was really busy this week. His teachers all seemed to be giving him more homework than he could possibly do. He had basketball practice every night, SAT prep class two evenings, and extra chores because his grandparents were visiting. Finally, it's Friday and Chris has some free time. He has a date that he is extremely excited about. However, when Chris leaves the house, he starts nodding off at the wheel and hits the rumble strips on the road twice. Chris has learned in health class about the dangers of drowsy driving, but he does not want to cancel his date. How should Chris handle this situation?

Steps for this Activity

1. In groups of two or three, cut a piece of paper into eight squares and write one possible decision Chris could make on each square. Divide the pieces of paper evenly among your group.

2. For each of the possible decisions you have, list the possible consequences on a separate sheet of paper.

3. Write a short paragraph comparing this set of decisions to your own values. Then pass the set of decisions to your right.

4. Continue passing the squares of paper to your right until everyone has seen, considered, and written about all of the possible decisions that Chris could make.

5. Finally, announce the decision you would make based on all the possibilities offered. Discuss in your group why each person chose as he or she did. As a group, consider which decision you would collectively choose. Are there any alternatives you didn't include?

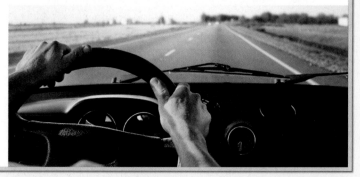

Core Skills

Math Practice

Global Sleep Time Average (Minutes Per Day)

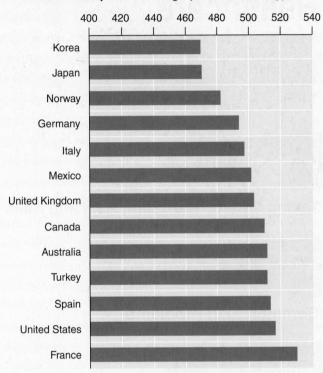

32. What is the sleep time, in hours, on an average day in France?
    A. 7.8 hours
    B. 5.3 hours
    C. 8.8 hours
    D. 6.3 hours

33. Which country's population receives the least amount of sleep on an average day?
    A. United States
    B. Italy
    C. Japan
    D. Korea

34. What percent of the day do people in Australia sleep?
    A. 35%
    B. 28.5%
    C. 50.5%
    D. 8%

Reading and Writing Practice

Read the passage below and then answer the questions.

Your body's biological clock, or the suprachiasmatic nucleus (SCN), *determines when you feel tired and when you feel awake. There are generally two periods of the day during which the body feels like sleeping— at night and in the early part of the afternoon, between 1 p.m. and 3 p.m. In many cultures, the early part of the afternoon is a dedicated rest time, or siesta.*

The SCN works in two ways to regulate sleep. First, it monitors the amount of light in the environment. It leads the body to be more active when there is more light and less active when there is less light. It also releases the hormone melatonin during the late evening, which increases feelings of relaxation and sleepiness, and signals that it is time to go to sleep. Compared with adults, teenagers' melatonin is typically released later in the evening and remains at high levels in the blood until later in the morning. This biological difference contributes to the difficulty teenagers have falling asleep earlier in the evening and waking up early the next morning.

35. What is the author's main idea in this passage?
    A. Teenagers' bodies don't produce enough melatonin, so it is difficult for them to fall asleep.
    B. Melatonin regulates the suprachiasmatic nucleus (SCN).
    C. Many cultures incorporate a period of rest into the afternoon schedule.
    D. The body's biological clock regulates sleep in two ways.

36. What is melatonin's role in sleep?
    A. It senses the level of light in the environment.
    B. It increases feelings of relaxation and sleepiness.
    C. It leads the body to be more active.
    D. All of the above

37. Based on the information in this passage, write a persuasive argument for introducing the *siesta* concept into the high school schedule.

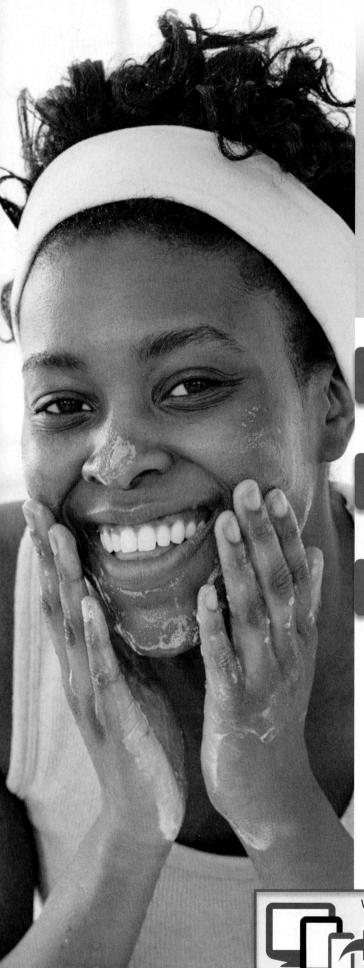

Chapter 8

Personal Hygiene and Basic Healthcare

Lesson 8.1

Taking Care of Your Skin, Hair, and Nails

Lesson 8.2

Common Skin Problems

Lesson 8.3

Keeping Your Mouth, Eyes, and Ears Healthy

While studying this chapter, look for the activity icon to:
- **review** vocabulary with e-flash cards and games;
- **assess** learning with quizzes and online exercises;
- **expand** knowledge with animations and activities; and
- **listen** to pronunciation of key terms in the audio glossary.

G-WLEARNING.com

www.g-wlearning.com/health/

What's Your Health and Wellness IQ?

Take this quiz to see what you do *and* do not *know about personal hygiene and its role in protecting your health. If you cannot answer a question, pay extra attention to that topic as you study this chapter.*

1. *Identify each statement as* True, False, *or* It Depends. *Choose* It Depends *if a statement is true in some cases, but false in others.*

2. *Revise each* False *statement to make it true.*

3. *Explain the circumstances in which each* It Depends *statement is true and when it is false.*

Health and Wellness IQ Assess

1. The skin consists of three different layers.	True	False	It Depends
2. You can't get a sunburn on a cloudy day.	True	False	It Depends
3. Getting a tattoo removed from the skin is painful and expensive.	True	False	It Depends
4. To keep your teeth clean, you should never eat sticky foods.	True	False	It Depends
5. Untreated gum disease can seriously damage your gums and jawbone.	True	False	It Depends
6. Squeezing a pimple will help it heal faster.	True	False	It Depends
7. Shampooing hair too often can cause dandruff.	True	False	It Depends
8. Wearing sunglasses can protect eyes from harmful UV rays.	True	False	It Depends
9. Listening to music at a high volume can damage your hearing.	True	False	It Depends
10. Hearing loss can occur so gradually that a person may not notice it happening.	True	False	It Depends

Setting the Scene

Do you brush and floss your teeth every day? Do you regularly wash your face, body, and hair? Do you use sunscreen every time you go out in the sun?

These are steps you can take to keep your skin, teeth, eyes, and ears healthy. You may not consider these activities to promote your health. Even simple acts of personal hygiene, however, help your body stay healthy. For example, regularly brushing and flossing your teeth prevents cavities. Regular brushing and flossing also helps you avoid serious damage to your gums, jawbone, and the nerves of your mouth.

This chapter will describe the importance of personal hygiene and basic healthcare, including how to take care of your skin, hair, eyes, and ears.

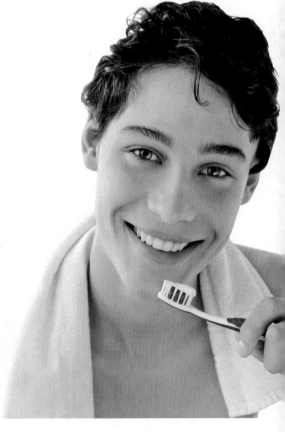

Taking Care of Your Skin, Hair, and Nails

Key Terms 📷 E-Flash Cards

In this lesson, you will learn the meanings of the following key terms.

antiperspirant
dandruff
deodorant
dermis
epidermis
hypodermis
lice

Before You Read

Roundabout Reflections

Your teacher will divide you into groups and assign each group some main headings and subheadings from this lesson. Write your group's assigned headings on a piece of paper and then brainstorm related words and ideas. After 30–45 seconds, pass your papers clockwise so the next group can add their ideas. Repeat this process until each group has added their ideas under every heading. After reading the lesson, add what you learned to each paper.

Lesson Objectives

After studying this lesson, you will be able to

- describe the three distinct layers of skin;
- explain ways to control body odor;
- demonstrate techniques for hair care; and
- practice effective nail care.

Warm-Up Activity

Personal Grooming Chart
Each day, we all groom ourselves in ways we hardly think about. Consider your morning, daily, and evening routines that involve taking care of your skin, hair, and nails. In a chart like the one shown below, document these grooming routines or activities.

Skin Care	Hair Care	Nail Care

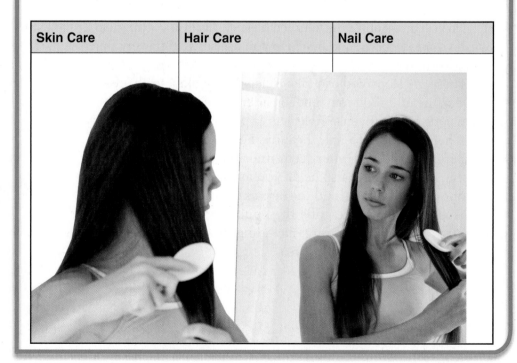

W hen you were a child, problems such as smelly arm pits and oily hair were probably not issues. After you reached adolescence, however, personal hygiene became more important—and it became your responsibility. This lesson describes some basic steps you can take to ensure that your body is healthy and clean and that you present your best self to the world.

Your Skin

The skin plays a very important role in keeping you healthy. First, the skin protects everything inside the body, including the muscles, bones, ligaments, and internal organs. The skin serves as a barrier for keeping bacteria and viruses from entering your body. Your skin also plays an important role in regulating your body temperature.

Anatomy of the Skin

The skin, which is the largest organ in the body, is the outer covering of the entire body. The skin consists of several different components, including water, protein, lipids (fats and oils), and minerals. Although you may think of the skin as just one type of body tissue, it actually consists of three distinct layers (Figure 8.1).

The outer layer of the skin is called the *epidermis*. The epidermis, which is made up of four layers of its own, is the thinnest layer of the skin. This layer protects the body from infection by stopping foreign substances from entering the skin. The epidermis also contains cells that produce the skin's pigment, or *melanin*. People who have a darker complexion have more melanin in their skin than people with fairer skin.

The middle layer of the skin is called the *dermis*. This layer contains small tubes called *hair follicles* that hold the hair roots. These follicles determine what your hair looks like—whether it is curly, straight, thick, or thin. As hair grows, it pushes out of the follicle and through the skin. Once it passes through the skin, however, the cells of the hair are no longer alive. Every follicle is attached to a gland that produces oil, or *sebum*. When these glands produce too much oil, a person's skin or hair may look greasy.

In addition, the dermis contains sweat glands, blood vessels, and nerve endings. This layer also includes two proteins that provide support and elasticity to the skin—collagen and elastin. With age, the body creates less of these proteins, which leads to the appearance of wrinkles and sagging skin. The dermis also contains the nerve endings that allow you to feel pain, pressure, and temperature.

The inner layer of the skin is called the *hypodermis*. This layer consists of fat, blood vessels, and nerve endings. It also connects the skin to the bone and muscle underneath.

epidermis
the outermost layer of skin, which protects the body from foreign substances and contains pigment-producing cells

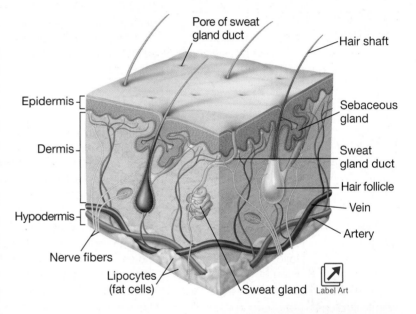

Epidermis
Dermis
Hypodermis
Nerve fibers
Lipocytes (fat cells)
Pore of sweat gland duct
Hair shaft
Sebaceous gland
Sweat gland duct
Hair follicle
Vein
Artery
Sweat gland
Label Art

Figure 8.1

The epidermis, dermis, and hypodermis make up the *skin*, the largest organ in the body.

dermis
the middle layer of skin, which contains hair follicles

hypodermis
the innermost layer of skin, which contains fat, blood vessels, and nerve endings; attaches to underlying bone and muscle

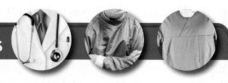

Health and Hygiene

Explore these rewarding careers related to hygiene and basic healthcare.

Career	Typical Education and Training	Typical Job Duties and Demands	Career Resources
Dermatologist	four-year college degree followed by four years of medical school, plus one year of internship and three years of specialized residency training	Dermatologists are medical doctors who specialize in skin care. They are able to evaluate and provide care for patients with disorders of the skin, hair, and nails, including skin cancers, moles, hair loss, scars, and inflammatory skin disorders.	American Academy of Dermatology, American Board of Dermatology
Skincare Specialist	cosmetology or esthetician program, followed by passing a state exam for licensing	Skincare specialists work in salons or spas to cleanse a person's face and body to enhance their appearance.	American Association of Cosmetology Schools, Associated Skin Care Professionals, National-Interstate Council of State Boards of Cosmetology, Professional Beauty Association (PBA)
Dentist	four-year college degree followed by dental school, must pass written and practical exams to qualify for a license	Dentists diagnose and treat problems related to patients' teeth, gums, and other parts of the mouth. They provide advice and instruction on caring for teeth and gums to maintain good oral health.	American Dental Association, American Dental Education Association
Dental Hygienist	associate's degree in dental hygiene, followed by a state license	Dental hygienists clean teeth, examine patients for oral diseases, and provide preventative dental care. They also educate patients on ways to improve and maintain oral health.	American Dental Hygienists Association, Commission on Dental Accreditation, American Dental Association
Ophthalmologist	four-year college degree, followed by four years of medical school, plus one year of internship and three years of specialized residency training	Ophthalmologists are medical doctors who specialize in eye and vision care. They are able to provide all types of eye care from prescribing glasses and contact lenses to performing eye surgery. They may also conduct research into the causes and cures for eye diseases and vision problems.	American Board of Ophthalmology
Optometrist	four-year college degree, followed by a four-year Doctor of Optometry Degree	Optometrists perform eye exams to check for vision problems and diseases. They prescribe eyeglasses or contact lenses as needed.	Association of Schools and Colleges of Optometry, American Optometric Association

Exploring Careers

1. Think about your interests, strengths, and weaknesses. With these in mind, which career appeals most to you? Which career does not interest you?

2. Do you know someone in one of these careers? If so, ask this person why he or she chose this career and what she or he likes most and least about the work.

Body Odor

Your body goes through a number of changes during puberty. One of these changes is greater activity in your sweat glands. Following puberty, your sweat glands produce greater amounts of perspiration, or *sweat*. These glands also begin to produce different chemicals, which cause sweat to have a strong odor. Many people notice this stronger odor under their arms. Other parts of your body might also have stronger smells.

To prevent body odor, take a bath or shower every day using a mild soap and warm water. This will help wash away any bacteria that contribute to the odor. Wear clean clothes each day. You should also use a **deodorant**, which covers up the odor of sweat, or an **antiperspirant**, which actually stops or dries up perspiration.

Hair

Although you have more than 100,000 hairs on your head, you lose about 50 to 100 hairs every day through normal activities such as washing, brushing, or combing your hair. These hairs are replaced by new hairs, which grow from the same follicle.

Common Hair Problems

A common problem for teenagers is having oily hair. Every follicle is attached to a gland that produces sebum. When these glands produce too much oil, such as during puberty, a person's hair may look greasy.

Some teenagers notice white flakes of dead skin in their hair and on their shoulders. This is **dandruff**, which is caused by flaking of the skin on the scalp. Dandruff is usually worse in the fall and winter, when indoor heating can dry out skin. Dandruff can also be caused by infrequent shampooing, which allows oils and skin cells from the scalp to build up. Shampooing too often or using too many hair care products, however, may irritate the scalp and also lead to dandruff.

Some teenagers become infected with **lice**, which are tiny insects that attach to the hair and feed on human blood. Lice are easily transmitted from one person to another through direct head-to-head contact or by sharing combs, brushes, or hats. Although lice do not cause any major health problems, they are very itchy and can therefore be uncomfortable.

Preventing and Treating Hair Problems

Here are some strategies you can use to keep your hair healthy and looking good:

- Wash your hair regularly to keep it clean.

- Eat a healthful diet. Some hair problems are partly caused by a lack of certain vitamins and fats.

- If you have dandruff, try using a medicated shampoo. If the dandruff continues, see your doctor or dermatologist.

deodorant
a product designed to cover up body odor

antiperspirant
a product designed to stop or dry up sweat

dandruff
dead skin that flakes off the scalp due to dryness, infrequent shampooing, or irritation

lice
small insects that attach to hair and feed on human blood

Personal Profile

Are You Taking Care of Your Personal Hygiene?

I take a bath or shower every day. **yes no**

I use sunscreen whenever I'm going to be outside. **yes no**

I brush my teeth at least twice a day. **yes no**

I floss my teeth every day. **yes no**

I wash my face twice a day. **yes no**

I wear safety goggles when doing activities that could damage my eyes. **yes no**

I get my eyes examined regularly. **yes no**

I avoid exposure to loud noises. **yes no**

Add up the number of yes answers. The more yes answers you have, the better you are at taking care of your body's hygienic needs. After completing this course, take this test again to see if your skills have improved.

- Avoid sharing items that have touched your hair with other people.

- If you become infected with lice, use a medicated shampoo to kill the lice and their eggs (or *nits*). You also need to wash all bedding, towels, and other items that have touched your hair in hot water.

Nails

Fingernails and toenails are made up of layers of a hard protein called *keratin*. This hard surface protects the sensitive tissues on the tips of your toes and fingers. Nails grow out from the area at the base of the nail. As new cells continuously grow, older cells are pushed out.

Healthy fingernails and toenails are smooth, free of spots or discoloration, and consistent in color. Some irregularities in the nails, such as white spots or vertical ridges, are normal. Other problems, however, such as nail discoloration, curled nails, or redness and swelling around the nail, can sometimes indicate health problems.

Fortunately, it is relatively easy to keep your nails strong and healthy. First, you should always keep your nails dry and clean. This prevents bacteria and other organisms from growing under your fingernails. If you must soak your hands, such as while washing dishes, or if you must use harsh chemicals, wear gloves. You should also trim your fingernails regularly using clippers, manicure scissors, or a nail file (Figure 8.2).

In addition, you should moisturize your hands regularly, including your fingernails and cuticles. Do not bite your fingernails, pick at your cuticles, or pull off your hangnails. Doing so can cause infections.

Before using the services of a salon for nail care, make sure the salon and the nail technician are licensed. All tools should be properly sterilized between customers to avoid spreading infections.

Figure 8.2

Trimming your nails is an important part of keeping them clean and healthy. *How often do you need to trim your nails? What factors do you think contribute to nail trimming frequency?*

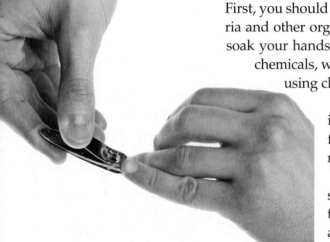

Lesson 8.1 Review

Know and Understand

1. List two functions of the skin.
2. Describe three ways to help prevent body odor.
3. How are lice transmitted from one person to another?
4. What attributes of fingernails might indicate health problems?

Analyze and Apply

5. What steps would you take to investigate a salon before booking a nail care treatment?

Real World Health

Personal Hygiene Products Visit your local drugstore or grocery store and tour the sections of the store that contain skincare, hair care, and nail care products. List three products from each category that best fit your needs. Write a brief summary about why you chose these products and how they fit your specific needs. Discuss your assessments of the different products with your classmates' opinions of the products they chose. After the discussion, would you change any of your choices?

Lesson 8.2

Common Skin Problems

Lesson Objectives

After studying this lesson, you will be able to

- describe common skin problems;
- discuss ways to prevent and treat acne;
- discuss ways to protect skin from ultraviolet light damage; and
- evaluate the effect of body art on health.

Warm-Up Activity

If You Were Your Own Skin
You spend every day of your life surrounded by and protected by your skin. But if you are like most people, you probably don't think much about your skin. You probably take it for granted. So think about your skin for a few minutes and then write your thoughts on a piece of paper. Think about your skin's strengths and weaknesses, what your skin has to endure and "put up with" during a typical day, what would have to happen for your skin to consider it a really good day, or a really bad day. Share your thoughts with the class.

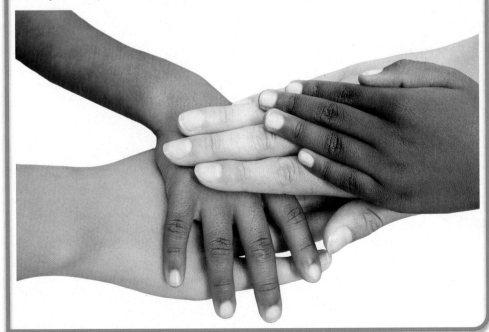

Key Terms E-Flash Cards

In this lesson, you will learn the meanings of the following key terms.

acne

body art

cystic acne

eczema

pores

sunscreen

ultraviolet (UV) light

Before You Read

Skin Problems Chart
Draw a chart like the one shown below. Before reading this lesson, list what you know and what you want to know about common skin problems. While you're reading, take note of topics that catch your interest. Finally, after reading the lesson, write what you have learned.

K What you Know	W What you Want to know	L What you have Learned

S kin problems — including rashes and sunburns — are common occurrences. In this lesson, you will learn more about these and other common skin problems, and how they can be prevented and treated.

Acne

acne
a skin condition in which inflamed, clogged hair follicles cause pimples

pores
hair follicles underneath your skin that contain oil-producing glands

At some point, most teenagers suffer from **acne**, a skin disease that causes pimples. Acne is partly caused by the increased level of hormones that occur during puberty. These hormones lead to higher levels of oil production in the body, which makes it more likely for pimples to form.

Pimples are created when **pores**, or hair follicles that are under your skin, become clogged with oil. All pores contain *sebaceous glands*, which produce sebum. This substance provides oil that helps keep your skin and hair from drying out. As the outer layer of skin is sloughed off, however, these dead skin cells can become stuck together inside a pore by the sebum. This creates a blockage, meaning the sebum that is produced by the pore cannot come to the surface of the skin as it normally does.

Over time, oil and bacteria leak into the skin surrounding this pore, which causes infection and inflammation, including redness, swelling, and pus (Figure 8.3). A pimple called a *whitehead* gets its name from the whitish pus inside a clogged pore that has only a tiny opening to the skin's surface. In contrast, a *blackhead* is a yellow or blackish bump inside a clogged pore that is more open to the air. When air gets inside the follicle, it causes the oil inside the follicle to become darker.

Figure 8.3

Pimples occur when hair follicles are blocked by sebum. *What steps do you take to wash your face and prevent pimples each day?*

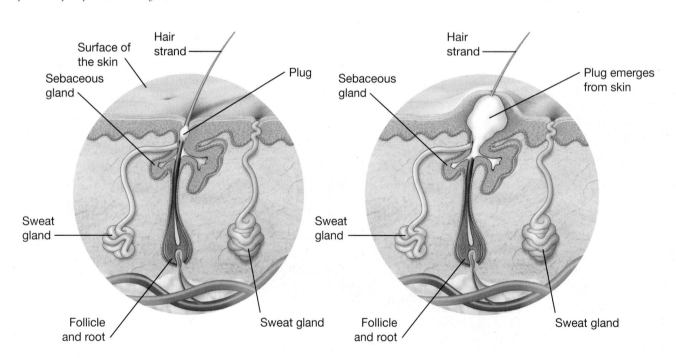

A. A plug forms in a hair follicle.

B. The plug becomes infected by bacteria and a whitehead or blackhead forms.

Animation

Fortunately, there are steps you can take to prevent acne breakouts and help them clear up quickly when they do occur. The following strategies can help:

- Wash your face gently twice a day. After washing your face, rinse well so that the soap does not stay on your skin.

- Do not squeeze pimples. This can lead to permanent acne scars.

- Avoid touching your face with your fingers, which can spread bacteria and cause inflammation and irritation to other parts of your face or body.

- Make sure that anything that touches your face is clean, including glasses, headbands, and hats. Keep your hair clean and pulled away from your face.

- If you wear makeup, buy brands that are oil-free and *noncomedogenic* or *nonacnegenic*. Throw away old makeup, which can contain bacteria. Be sure to wash all makeup off your skin before you go to sleep.

- Make sure to use sunscreen, since a sunburn can make acne appear even worse.

- Be careful when shaving your face. Try to shave lightly, and not too frequently, to avoid accidentally cutting a skin blemish (Figure 8.4).

If you have a serious problem with acne, you should consult a dermatologist. A dermatologist can give you useful information about caring for your skin type. People who have **cystic acne** have a particularly severe type of acne that does not clear up without medication.

It is especially important to seek help for severe acne. People who feel self-conscious about this skin problem can experience emotional distress about their skin's appearance. Over time, this can lead to low self-esteem and a negative body image.

Eczema

Eczema, or *dermatitis*, is a condition that affects the skin in one or more parts of the body. Although this condition is not dangerous, it causes swollen, red, dry, and itchy patches of skin, which can be irritating. When these patches are scratched, they can become infected.

Eczema is a chronic disease, which means it typically reoccurs over time. Some people are more prone to developing this condition than others. Eczema is not contagious, meaning you cannot catch it from someone else.

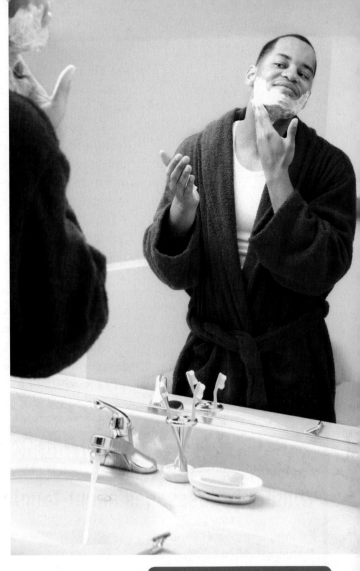

Figure 8.4

When shaving, do so lightly and not too frequently. *How often do you have to shave to look neat?*

cystic acne
a severe type of acne that requires medical treatment

eczema
a chronic skin condition characterized by patches of red, itchy, dry, or swollen skin

Eczema flare-ups can be triggered by colds or other minor illnesses, as well as irritating substances. Stress is also associated with eczema flare-ups.

Do not scratch the affected area of skin or you may cause an infection. To relieve dryness and itching, you can apply a lotion or cream when the skin is damp, such as after you bathe or wash your hands. This locks in moisture and can help reduce itching. Symptoms of eczema can be treated using over-the-counter products.

Skin Cancer and Sunburn

ultraviolet (UV) light
an invisible type of radiation that emanates from the sun, tanning beds, and sunlamps

sunscreen
a product that protects the skin by absorbing and scattering UV rays

Skin cancer is the most common form of cancer in the United States. Most cases are caused by exposure to *ultraviolet (UV) light*, an invisible kind of radiation that comes from the sun, tanning beds, and sunlamps.

Anyone can get skin cancer, but some people are at greater risk of developing skin cancer than others. People who have skin that reacts quickly to the sun by turning red or beginning to freckle have a higher risk of developing skin cancer. A family history of skin cancer also increases risk of developing the disease.

Although the link between having a sunburn and developing skin cancer is clear, many people fail to adequately protect themselves from becoming burned. It is very important to protect your skin *whenever* you are outside.

The simplest way to protect yourself is to stay out of the sun whenever possible. If you need to be outside, especially during the midday hours when the sun's rays are the strongest, there are several simple ways to protect your skin.

When spending time outside, find a shady spot. Wear clothing that protects any exposed skin. Certain fabrics even have built-in SPF protection. Wear a hat with a large brim to protect your face, head, ears, and neck (Figure 8.5 on the next page). You should also wear sunglasses to protect your eyes from UV rays.

Using a *sunscreen* is also very important if you must spend time outside. Sunscreens protect the skin by absorbing, reflecting, or scattering UV light. A sunscreen's effectiveness in blocking UV rays is indicated by its sun protection factor (*SPF*). The higher the SPF of a sunscreen, the greater the protection it provides from UV rays. It is important to use sunscreen, including a lip balm, with a sun protection factor of at least 15.

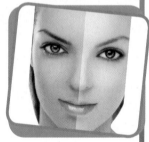

Health *in the Media*

Unhealthy Messages about Tanning

You've probably seen ads featuring tanned models. Some health experts are concerned that these advertisements perpetuate the dangerous idea that tanning is good—even healthy—and that tanned people are more attractive. Unfortunately, tanned skin is not necessarily healthy skin.

Researchers in one study took photos of women and altered them so the women appeared tanned. Then researchers submitted both the regular and tanned photos to a website that allows people to rate the attractiveness of the people in photos posted to the site. The researchers found that the exact same women were rated as more attractive when they were tanned than when they were not. The tanned-skin version of the model was twice as likely to be rated as more attractive than the non-tanned version.

Thinking Critically

1. Why do you think many people find tanned skin more attractive than pale skin?

2. Can people achieve a tanned appearance without damaging their skin? Explain your response.

Did you know that your skin can be damaged by the sun's UV rays after just 15 minutes of exposure? Here are some useful strategies to remember when using sunscreen:

- Make sure to use sunscreen *whenever* you are outside—not just in the summer and on sunny days. Clouds do not block UV rays, so rays from the sun can damage your skin even on cloudy days.

- In case you are outside longer than you expected to be, keep sun protection handy in your car, purse, or backpack.

- For the best protection, apply a thick layer of sunscreen 30 minutes before going outdoors. Cover all parts of your body that will be exposed to the sun.

- Remember to reapply sunscreen often—every two hours, or more often if you perspire or swim.

Finally, it is very important to avoid tanning beds, tanning booths, and sunlamps. The UV rays produced by these machines are just as dangerous as those from the sun. The UV rays produced by these machines are also just as likely to cause skin cancer.

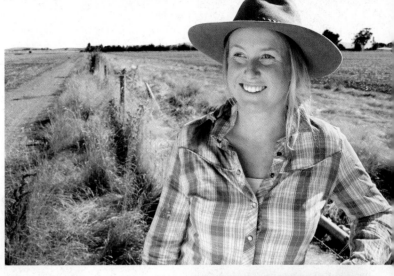

Figure 8.5

Dressing in clothes that will shield against sunlight is a good way of protecting yourself from UV rays.

Body Art

Since ancient times, people have chosen to decorate their bodies in permanent ways. Two of the most common types of decoration, or **body art**, are tattoos and piercings. These types of body decorations may potentially impact health.

body art
permanent decorations that are applied to the body; examples include tattoos and piercings

Tattoos and Piercings

Tattoos are designs on the skin made by inserting colored ink under the skin, which is done with a needle. A survey of American adults found that about 24% of them—almost one in four—reported having a tattoo. Of those who were tattooed, 16% had their first tattoo before they turned 18.

Body piercing involves making a hole in the skin in which jewelry can be inserted. The most common body part to be pierced is the earlobe. Other body parts that are often pierced include ear cartilage, the belly button, the nose, and the tongue.

Health Problems Caused by Tattoos and Piercings

Although getting a tattoo or a body piercing may seem harmless, health problems can occur whenever needles are inserted into the body.

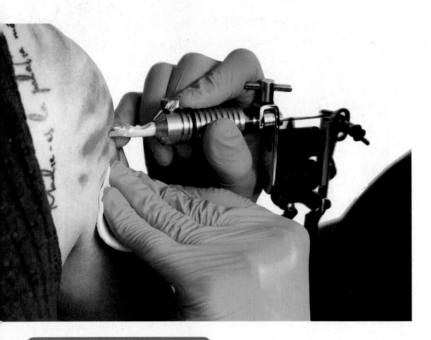

If they are not sterilized, the needles used for piercings and tattoos can spread infections that are carried in the blood, such as hepatitis or HIV. Some people with body art can also experience an allergic reaction, typically to the jewelry that is worn in the pierced area, or to the tattoo ink. Once you have gotten a piercing or tattoo, it is important to follow instructions to care for it and decrease the possibility of infection.

To decrease the risk of these complications, people should have tattoos and piercings done at clean, safe, well-regarded facilities (Figure 8.6). Some states require a particular license to perform piercings or tattoos.

People should always deliberate carefully before getting a tattoo or a piercing. Several issues, in addition to potential health problems, need to be considered. For example, do you really want to keep a tattoo forever? It is possible to have a tattoo removed. However, this is a painful, expensive, and time-intensive process that often leaves scarring.

You should also consider whether a piercing or a tattoo in a particular part of your body may have long-term consequences for jobs or relationships. For example, people with tongue piercings often have a noticeable clicking sound when they talk, which can alienate potential employers.

Figure 8.6

Anyone who decides, after long and careful thought, to get a tattoo, should do so at a clean and well-regarded tattoo parlor. *How could you find out whether a tattoo parlor is safe and clean?*

Lesson 8.2 Review

Know and Understand

1. Explain how pimples form.
2. Explain how eczema is treated.
3. List two characteristics of people who have a higher risk of developing skin cancer.
4. What does a sunscreen's SPF indicate?
5. Name two health problems that can be caused by tattoos and piercings.

Analyze and Apply

6. Compare and contrast eczema and acne.
7. Weigh the benefits and risks of using a tanning booth. Why might someone choose to tan?

Real World Health

Skin Self-Exam Look over the list of risk factors for skin cancer listed in this lesson and consider whether you have a low risk, medium risk, or high risk for skin cancer. How many strategies to prevent skin cancer do you practice consistently? While your doctor probably checks your skin during your annual exams, you may also want to perform a *skin self-exam*.

To self-examine your skin, check your body—even in hard-to-reach areas—and document any moles, freckles, or other blemishes. Are there any marks that you have never noticed before? Have any marks recently changed? Are there any spots that you want to discuss with your doctor? Write a summary of your findings, as well as possible questions you might have for your next medical exam.

Keeping Your Mouth, Eyes, and Ears Healthy

Lesson Objectives

After studying this lesson, you will be able to

- identify parts of the mouth;
- summarize ways to prevent and treat problems with the mouth and teeth;
- identify parts of the eye and their functions;
- describe common vision problems;
- identify parts of the ear and their functions; and
- describe common hearing problems.

Key Terms E-Flash Cards

In this lesson, you will learn the meanings of the following key terms.

cavities
cochlea
cornea
decibels
eardrum
gingivitis
halitosis
iris
lens
optic nerve
oral cavity
periodontitis
plaque
pupil
retina
saliva

Warm-Up Activity

Healthy Mouth
Imagine that one of your friends doesn't practice oral hygiene and consistently has dirty teeth and bad breath. How would you explain the importance of brushing and flossing without hurting your friend's feelings? Work with a partner to write a short script or story outlining how you would deal with this scenario. Compare scripts and stories in class. Were some more "diplomatic" than others?

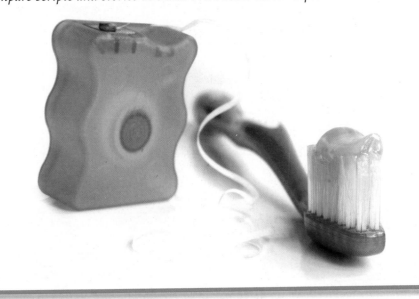

Before You Read

Brainstorming
In a mindmap write all the health and wellness resources you know. These could include healthcare facilities, methods of healthy living, or educational resources. After reading the lesson, go back and fill in further information you learned.

You may be wondering how having clean teeth matters in terms of your health. Having good oral hygiene affects much more than your smile. For example, your teeth impact your ability to speak clearly, and to chew and swallow different types of foods.

Through everyday activities, you may be putting strain on your eyes and ears. These are important sensory organs that help you live life to the fullest, so it is important to take good care of them. This lesson will discuss some common health problems associated with your eyes and ears, and ways to keep them in good working condition.

Oral Cavity

oral cavity

the area of your mouth that includes the lips, teeth, and tongue

The very first area of your mouth is called the **oral cavity**, or *mouth cavity*. The mouth includes the lips, teeth, and tongue.

One of the primary functions of the mouth is to take in food and break it down so that it can be digested. Through chewing, teeth help break down larger pieces of food into smaller ones. The mouth also produces *saliva*, which contains an enzyme that helps break down food into smaller particles. These two processes allow food to be swallowed, meaning that it travels through the esophagus and into the stomach.

saliva

a substance produced in the mouth, which contains enzymes that break down food

Understanding Teeth

Teeth consist of three distinct parts (Figure 8.7). The *crown* is the visible portion of the tooth. It is protected by a hard, white substance made of

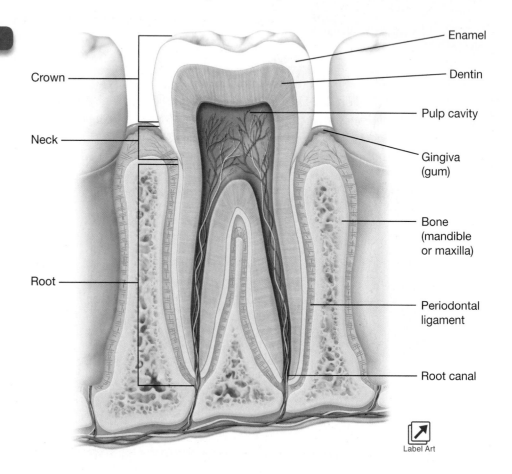

Figure 8.7

A tooth is composed of a crown protected by enamel, a neck, and a root. There's a good chance that you take your teeth for granted — they probably do their job and cause you few if any problems. *Talk to your parents and grandparents about their teeth. Have they had any serious problems with their teeth? Did they take good care of their teeth when they were younger?*

Crown

Neck

Root

Enamel

Dentin

Pulp cavity

Gingiva (gum)

Bone (mandible or maxilla)

Periodontal ligament

Root canal

Label Art

calcium called *enamel*. The *neck* connects the crown to the root of the tooth at the gum line. The *root* contains blood vessels and nerve endings that connect the tooth to the jaw.

A normal adult mouth contains 32 teeth (Figure 8.8). Different types of teeth have different shapes, locations in the jaw, and functions. These types include

- *incisors* (8 total)—the four teeth at the very front of the mouth on the upper and lower jaws;

- *canines* (4 total)—the pointy teeth right beside the incisors;

- *premolars* (8 total)—teeth between the canines and the molars;

- *molars* (8 total)—flat teeth in the rear of the mouth; and

- *wisdom teeth* (4 total)—the teeth at the very back of the mouth, which are the last permanent teeth to come in, usually between 17 and 21 years of age.

plaque
a sticky, colorless substance formed by bacteria in the mouth; coats the teeth and slowly dissolves enamel

cavities
holes in the teeth caused by plaque eating away at tooth enamel

Common Mouth Problems

Many people experience problems with their mouths at some point. These problems can interfere with important daily life functions such as chewing, swallowing, and even talking.

Tooth Decay

When you eat or drink something, an enzyme in your saliva breaks down the food particles and sugars so they can be digested. This process turns everything you eat or drink into a type of acid. This acid then combines with the bacteria in your mouth, as well as saliva and small food particles, to form plaque. **Plaque** is a sticky, colorless film that coats the teeth and dissolves their protective enamel surface. If plaque is not removed, it mixes with minerals to become *tartar*, a harder substance. Tartar requires professional cleaning to be removed.

If you do not brush and floss your teeth daily, food particles remain in your mouth and promote bacterial growth. This results in tooth decay. Over time, tooth decay causes **cavities**, or holes in the teeth that occur when plaque eats into a tooth's enamel. Cavities are also known as *dental caries*. When the decay continues, the hole gets deeper and eventually reaches the nerve layer under the enamel known as the *dentin*. This causes painful nerve damage. The *death of the tooth* occurs when the decay reaches the deepest layer of the tooth (the *pulp cavity*).

Central incisor
Lateral incisor
Canine
First molar
Second molar

Deciduous teeth

Central incisor
Lateral incisor
Canine
First premolar (bicuspid)
Second premolar (bicuspid)
First molar
Second molar
Third molar (wisdom tooth)

Permanent teeth

Label Art

Figure 8.8

Your mouth contains five different types of teeth. *What do you think are the specific functions of each type of tooth?*

Jamal has always enjoyed sticky candy, especially gummy candies. Although Jamal brushes his teeth in the morning, he never brushes his teeth later in the day. If he's tired, he sometimes forgets to brush his teeth before bed.

During a dentist appointment, Jamal learns he has three cavities. The dentist explains that sticky candies attach to the teeth and are very difficult to remove unless brushing happens right away. Bacteria feed off the sugar and produce acid, which then eats away at the teeth. The longer the sugar remains on the teeth, the more time bacteria will have to feed.

Jamal's father makes an appointment for him to come back and get the cavities filled. The procedure will cost about $500.

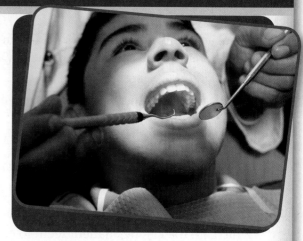

Thinking Critically

1. What are the repercussions of Jamal's hygiene habits?

2. What steps can Jamal take in the future to prevent cavities?

Gum Disease

Your teeth are surrounded by a pinkish tissue called the *gums*. The gums lie on top of the bones of the jaw, and cover the entire root of each tooth. The gums help keep your teeth in place.

Gum disease occurs when plaque and tartar build up on the teeth. The bacteria in plaque cause toxins to form in the mouth, which irritates the gums. Over time, this irritation can lead to **gingivitis**, an inflammation of the gums, and **periodontitis**. Periodontitis, or *periodontal disease*, is an infection caused by bacteria getting under the gum tissue and destroying the gums and bone. Early signs of gum disease include swelling and bleeding of the gums. If gum disease goes untreated, it can damage the gums and jawbone.

gingivitis
an inflammation of the gums

periodontitis
an infection in which bacteria gets beneath the gums and destroys gum and bone

Cold Sores

Cold sores, or *fever blisters*, are small blisters that appear on the lips and inside the mouth. These blisters are red, swollen, and painful, especially when touched. Cold sores typically last several days, but can last as long as two weeks. Cold sores are caused by a virus spread from person-to-person through passing saliva in some way, such as sharing a utensil.

Teeth Misalignment

A misalignment between the upper and lower teeth may result in an *overbite*, a condition in which the upper teeth protrude significantly over the lower teeth. An *underbite* is a condition in which the lower teeth protrude significantly past the upper teeth.

Wisdom teeth may become stuck under the gum tissue, or may only be able to partially come through the gums. This can be caused by lack of room in the jaw. When this occurs, the condition is called *impacted wisdom teeth*. In this case, the teeth may need to be removed because they can become infected or displace other teeth.

Other Common Mouth Problems

Bad breath, or **halitosis**, can be caused by poor dental hygiene. Bad breath is also caused by gum disease and eating certain foods. Bad breath can be a sign of various health problems, such as respiratory tract infections.

Teeth grinding, or *bruxism*, occurs when a person repeatedly clenches and grinds their teeth. This problem may be caused by stress, anxiety, or sleep disorders. Many people who have bruxism are unaware of it because the grinding occurs while they are asleep. If bruxism is not treated, it can cause damage to the teeth and jaw over time.

halitosis
the condition of having bad-smelling breath

Treating and Preventing Teeth and Mouth Problems

Sometimes teeth and mouth problems can be treated at home. For example, a person with bruxism can wear a mouth guard while sleeping to minimize teeth grinding. For other mouth problems, people need to see a dentist for treatment. For example, tooth sensitivity may indicate a cavity in the tooth, which requires professional treatment. Similarly, many teenagers wear devices such as braces, which need to be applied by an orthodontist.

Many common problems with the teeth and mouth are caused largely by choices people make. You have some control over whether you develop these problems, and they tend to be easier to fix. The following are strategies you can use to prevent some of the most common teeth and mouth problems:

- Brush your teeth, including your tongue, at least twice a day. Use a soft-bristle brush and toothpaste that contains fluoride.

- Get a new toothbrush when the bristles wear out, which is usually about every three months.

- Floss your teeth every day to help remove food particles that are stuck between your teeth and cannot be reached by brushing (Figure 8.9).

- Avoid using any type of tobacco, including cigarettes and chewing tobacco.

- Eat healthful foods, including fruits and fiber-rich vegetables. Avoid eating sticky foods that are high in sugar and starch, such as candy, cakes, and soda. If you do eat these types of foods, brush your teeth as soon as possible afterward.

- If you have bad breath and you brush and floss regularly, use an antiseptic mouth-rinse, which reduces the bacteria that causes bad breath.

Figure 8.9

Flossing helps remove food that is stuck between teeth. *How often should you floss? Why?*

- See your dentist twice a year. Your dentist will catch mouth problems early on, when they can be more easily treated.

- Wear a mouth guard during activities that can result in broken teeth, such as football or ice hockey.

- If cold sores are painful, you can treat them using a skin cream or ointment that will speed up the healing and help ease the pain.

Eyes

Most people rely on their sense of vision more than any of their other senses. You need good vision for many activities in your daily life, from kicking a soccer ball and taking a photograph to driving a car. Keeping your eyes healthy is important. How do your eyes let you see the world? What are some good strategies for keeping them healthy?

Understanding Vision

Many different parts of your eyes must work together to show you the world (Figure 8.10). Light first passes through the *cornea*, a clear tissue that covers the front of the eye.

Next, light reaches the *iris*, which is the colored part of the eye. Light passes into the inner eye through a small opening in the middle of the iris—the *pupil*. The pupil changes size, which influences the amount of light that can enter the inner eye. In bright light, the pupil is small and lets in relatively little light. In dim light, the pupil is large and considerable light enters the eye.

cornea
the clear tissue covering the front of the eye

iris
the colored part of the eye that constricts and dilates the pupil

pupil
the black opening in the middle of the iris through which light passes

Figure 8.10

The eye is a complex structure that receives and focuses light for your brain to interpret.

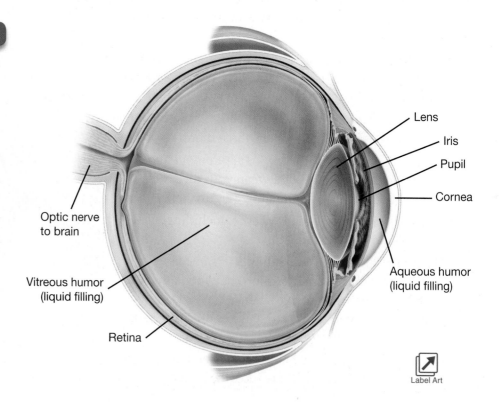

Lens
Iris
Pupil
Cornea
Aqueous humor (liquid filling)
Optic nerve to brain
Vitreous humor (liquid filling)
Retina

Label Art

After the light moves through the pupil, it reaches the *lens*, a clear part of the eye. The lens focuses the light onto the *retina*.

The retina is a light-sensitive tissue that contains millions of photoreceptor cells, called *rods* and *cones*. These cells convert light into nerve impulses or electrical signals. These nerve impulses travel from the retina to the brain through the *optic nerve*. The brain interprets these impulses into the images you see.

Common Vision Problems

For many people, especially young people, their vision works well. Other people, however, experience vision problems. For example, in some people, the eyeball is shaped in such a way that it does not focus where it need to focus—on the retina (Figure 8.11 on the next page).

Vision problems are more common in older people because aging can cause changes in parts of the eye. People whose parents have vision problems are also more likely to have vision problems themselves.

The following are the most common vision problems:

- **Nearsightedness** (or *myopia*) is a condition in which objects close to the eye appear clear, while objects farther away appear blurry. In the eye of someone who is nearsighted, light focuses in front of the retina instead of on the retina.

- **Farsightedness** (or *hyperopia*) is a condition in which distant objects are seen more clearly than nearby objects. In the eye of someone who is farsighted, light focuses behind the retina instead of on the retina.

- **Astigmatism** is a condition in which the eye does not focus light evenly onto the retina. As a result, objects appear blurry and stretched out.

- **Presbyopia** is a condition that affects adults beginning in middle age. In this condition, the lens of the eye loses its elasticity, and it becomes harder to see close objects clearly.

lens
a clear part of the eye that focuses light on the retina

retina
the innermost, light-sensitive area of the eye, composed of photoreceptors that convert light into nerve impulses and electrical signals

optic nerve
the tissue by which nerve impulses travel from the retina to the brain

Health across the Life Span

Hearing Changes

In the United States, 8.6% of the population has some type of hearing problem. The following data shows the percentage of people in each age group who have hearing problems:

- 3 to 17 years of age: 1.8%
- 18 to 34 years of age: 3.4%
- 35 to 44 years of age: 6.3%
- 45 to 54 years of age: 10.3%
- 55 to 64 years of age: 15.4%
- 65 years of age and older: 29.1%

Analyzing Data

1. In what age group are hearing problems most common?

2. If less than 2% of teens have hearing problems, what is the value of having hearing tests before 18 years of age?

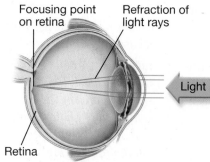

Focusing point on retina | Refraction of light rays

Light

Retina

A. Normal vision: light rays focus on the retina

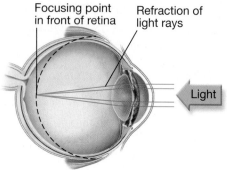

Focusing point in front of retina | Refraction of light rays

Light

B. Myopia (nearsightedness): light rays focus in front of the retina

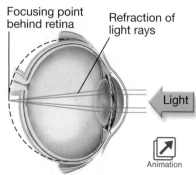

Focusing point behind retina | Refraction of light rays

Light

Animation

C. Hyperopia (farsightedness): light rays focus beyond the retina

Figure 8.11

Nearsightedness, farsightedness, and astigmatism are all problems within the anatomy of the eye.

eardrum
the part of the middle ear that vibrates in response to sound

cochlea
a spiral tube in the inner ear that senses sound vibrations and transmits them to the auditory nerve

Fortunately, these problems can usually be corrected with glasses or contact lenses. Surgery may also be able to correct, or at least improve, some vision problems. LASIK (or *laser in-situ keratomileusis*) is a surgery that works by reshaping the cornea, which allows light to reach the retina, and helps improve vision.

Protecting Your Eyes

There are several simple strategies to help you keep your eyes as healthy as possible throughout your lifetime. You should always wear protective eyewear when playing contact sports. You should also use protective gear during activities that can create flying debris that could hit the eyes, such as mowing the lawn, sawing wood, or sanding.

When spending long periods of time outdoors, you should wear sunglasses to block harmful UV rays. Look for sunglasses that claim to block at least 99% of UVB and UVA rays, or provide UV 400 protection. If you wear contact lenses, make sure to care for your lenses properly to avoid infection. Perhaps the simplest step you can take to protect your eyes is to get regular eye exams.

Ears

What do the following activities have in common: target shooting, woodworking, playing in a band, attending rock concerts, and using a leaf blower? All of these activities can contribute to hearing loss. Many teenagers regularly expose themselves to loud noises, often through headphones. The sense of hearing allows you to listen to music you enjoy, talk with friends, and be alerted to approaching cars and other dangers. Did you know your ears also play a role in helping you keep your balance? In this section you will learn about parts of the ear and how they function, common hearing problems, and strategies for maintaining your hearing.

Parts of the Ear

The ear has three main parts, and each serves a different but important role. The outer ear, which is called the *pinna*, is the large part of the ear that people can see. The main job of the pinna is to help bring sounds into the ear, where they enter the ear canal, the part of the ear that extends inward. The ear canal is where earwax is produced. This part of the ear also amplifies sounds so that they can be clearly heard and interpreted.

After sound is gathered by the outer ear and sent through the ear canal, it reaches the middle ear. The middle ear includes the **eardrum**, which vibrates when sounds reach it. This part of the ear also includes three small bones—the hammer, the anvil, and the stirrup.

The inner ear converts sound vibrations produced in the middle ear into neural impulses that the brain recognizes as sound. This part of the ear includes the **cochlea**, which is a spiral tube. The cochlea is covered with

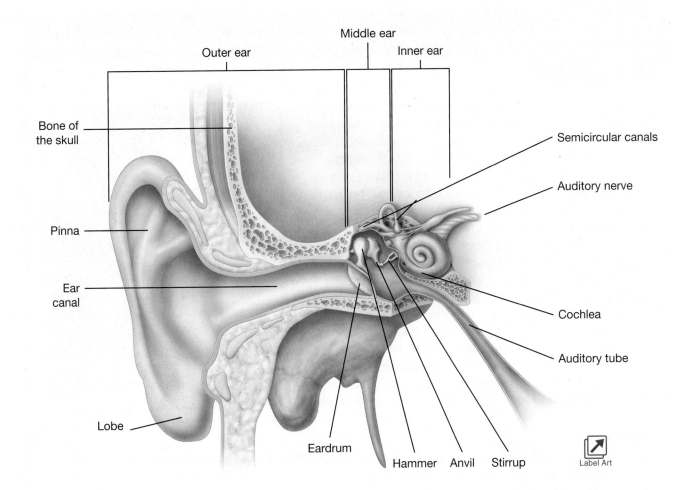

Middle ear
Outer ear
Inner ear

Bone of the skull

Semicircular canals

Auditory nerve

Pinna

Ear canal

Cochlea

Auditory tube

Lobe

Eardrum

Hammer   Anvil   Stirrup

Label Art

nerve cells, or ear hairs, which pick up different vibrations. These vibrations are then sent to the brain through the auditory nerve (Figure 8.12). The inner ear also includes the *semicircular canals*, which are attached to the cochlea. These canals are filled with fluid and move when you move, which helps you keep your balance.

Common Hearing Problems

The most serious health problem associated with the ears is permanent loss of hearing. Hearing loss is typically caused by damage to the inner ear. This damage is often the result of repeated exposure to excessively loud sounds, which can cause damage to the nerve cells in the cochlea. This may mean exposure to loud music through headphones. One recent study found that 12.5% of children and teenagers (6 to 19 years of age) experience hearing loss caused by using headphones or earbuds at too high a volume.

Sound intensity, or loudness, is measured in units called **decibels**. You can experience hearing loss by listening to sounds at or above 85 decibels over an extended period of time. The louder the sound, the less time it takes for hearing damage to occur.

Hearing loss can also be caused more suddenly by a ruptured eardrum. This can be caused by loud blasts of noise, sudden changes in pressure, insertion of an object into the ear, or an infection. In fact, just one exposure to a very loud sound, blast, or impulse (at or above 120 decibels) can cause hearing loss.

Figure 8.12

The ear receives sound as a series of vibrations, which are then interpreted by the brain.

decibels
the units by which sound intensity, or loudness, is measured

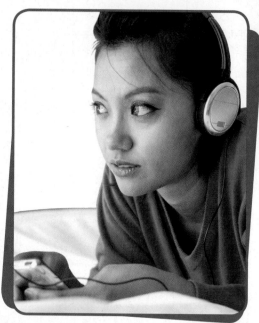

Did you know that listening to loud music—especially on headphones—can lead to permanent hearing damage? Researchers in one study examined the music listening habits of 289 teenagers (13 to 17 years of age). These teenagers were asked how long they spent listening to music using headphones each day, and at how loud a volume. Next, researchers tested the teenagers' hearing in both quiet and noisy environments. Can you predict what they found?

First, 80% of teenagers regularly listen to music on headphones, with 21% of teenagers listening from 1–4 hours each day, and 8% listening for more than 4 hours a day. The hearing test revealed that 25% of teenagers are already at severe risk for hearing loss based on the duration and volume of the music they listen to on headphones. Because hearing loss caused by continuous exposure to loud music occurs gradually, this type of damage is often initially hard to recognize. Unfortunately, that means a considerable amount of permanent hearing damage may already be done before the harm is noticed.

Thinking Critically

1. Given the results of this study, what do your own music listening habits tell you about the hearing damage that you may experience?

2. Do you think the type of music being listened to should be taken into consideration with this data? Do you think listening to classical music loudly on headphones would cause as much damage as listening to rock music?

Unfortunately, many people do not notice that they are losing their hearing because damage from noise exposure is usually gradual. By the time they notice, they have substantial symptoms of permanent hearing loss. Early signs of hearing damage include

- difficulty hearing relatively soft sounds, such as doorbells;

- difficulty understanding speech during telephone conversations or in noisy environments; and

- pain or ringing in the ears, or *tinnitus*, after exposure to excessively loud sounds.

Protecting Your Hearing

Once hearing is lost, it cannot be completely brought back. It is important, therefore, to protect your ears. There are several simple ways to do so. Avoid exposure to very high levels of noise, such as at rock concerts, dances, or construction sites, whenever possible. You should also avoid listening to music at high volume levels (above 85 decibels), especially even when using headphones.

Maintaining Good Personal Hygiene

Using the following strategies can help you keep your skin, hair, nails, and teeth healthy.

- Don't pick at or squeeze pimples—this pushes the infection deeper into your skin and can lead to permanent acne scars.

- Take a bath or shower every day using a mild soap and warm water to prevent body odor. Wash your face gently twice a day with warm water and a mild soap, and rinse well.

- Apply a deodorant, which covers up odor, or an antiperspirant, which dries up perspiration, daily.

- If you must be out in the sun, cover up and use sunscreen—at least SPF 15—on all parts of your body that will be exposed to the sun. Be sure to apply the sunscreen 30 minutes before going outdoors.

- Brush your teeth, including your tongue, at least twice a day with a toothpaste that contains fluoride.

- Floss your teeth every day to help remove food particles that are stuck between your teeth and can't be reached by brushing.

- Wear a mouth guard during an activity that may cause you to break a tooth, including sports such as football, lacrosse, or ice hockey.

- Wash your hair regularly, using a gentle shampoo.

- Trim your fingernails regularly using clippers or a nail file. Avoid using your fingernails to pick, poke, or pry things open.

- Wear protective eyewear when playing contact sports, such as basketball, lacrosse, or hockey. Use eyewear during activities that could lead to eye damage, such as mowing the lawn, sawing wood, or sanding.

- Avoid places that have high levels of noise, such as construction sites.

- Avoid listening to music at high volume levels, especially when using earphones.

Lesson 8.3 Review

Know and Understand

1. List the five types of adult teeth.
2. What causes cold sores?
3. Why are wisdom teeth removed?
4. List three health or hygiene problems for which halitosis can be a symptom.
5. Describe five ways to prevent teeth and mouth problems.
6. Explain two of the most common vision problems.
7. List three strategies to help keep eyes healthy.
8. List the three main parts of the ear.
9. What might cause the eardrum to rupture?

Analyze and Apply

10. What can happen if plaque is not removed from the teeth?

11. Why do you think being stressed can cause bruxism?
12. Explain in your own words the process that allows the eye to see images.
13. Why is it important to start protecting your hearing when you are young?

Real World Health

Decibel Diagram Decibels (dBs), the units that measure sound intensity, can be a factor in hearing loss. Using the Internet, research how many decibels are associated with some of the sound-related activities you engage in daily. Then create a diagram ranking your activities by decibels from low to high. Include a description, picture, and the dBs measured in each activity on your diagram.

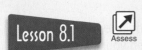

Taking Care of Your Skin, Hair, and Nails

Key Terms

antiperspirant
dandruff
deodorant
dermis

epidermis
hypodermis
lice

Key Points

- Skin plays important roles in health.
- The skin consists of three layers—the dermis, the epidermis, and the hypodermis.
- Body odor can become an issue during puberty.
- Most common hair problems can be easily prevented and treated.
- Nail care includes cleaning, trimming, and moisturizing.

Check Your Understanding

1. *True or false?* The skin is the largest organ in the body.

2. Which layer of the skin is the outer layer?
   A. epidermis
   B. dermis
   C. hypodermis
   D. exidermis

3. Which layer of the skin contains hair follicles?
   A. epidermis
   B. dermis
   C. hypodermis
   D. exidermis

4. Which layer of skin connects to the bone and muscle underneath?

5. Describe the difference between deodorant and antiperspirant.

6. _____ is white flakes of dead skin in the hair caused by flaking of skin on the scalp.

7. Which of the following is not a strategy for preventing hair problems?
   A. Wash your hair regularly to keep it clean.
   B. Eat a healthful diet.
   C. Share hair-related items such as hats, brushes, and combs.
   D. Use a medicated shampoo if you have dandruff.

8. Fingernails and toenails are made up of a hard protein called _____.

9. *True or false?* Nail discoloration and curled nails can sometimes indicate health problems.

10. **Critical Thinking.** Why does body odor increase during puberty?

Common Skin Problems

Key Terms

acne
body art
cystic acne
eczema

pores
sunscreen
ultraviolet (UV) light

Key Points

- Common skin problems include acne and eczema.
- Protection from UV radiation can help prevent skin cancer.
- Body art such as tattoos and piercings may include health risks.

Check Your Understanding

11. A skin disease that causes pimples is called
    _____.
    A. acne
    B. eczema
    C. skin cancer
    D. pores

12. Describe the difference between a whitehead and a blackhead.

13. Pimples are created when _____, or hair follicles that are under your skin, become clogged with oil.
    A. acne
    B. dermatitis
    C. sebaceous glands
    D. pores

14. *True or false?* Roughly scrubbing your face every morning will help prevent acne breakouts.

15. A skin condition that causes swollen, red, dry, and itchy patches of skin is called _____.
    A. acne
    B. eczema
    C. skin cancer
    D. pores

16. *True or false?* Eczema is contagious.

17. Most cases of skin cancer are caused by exposure to _____.

18. *True or false?* People who have skin that reacts quickly to the sun by turning red or beginning to freckle have a higher risk of developing skin cancer.

19. *True or false?* Clouds block UV rays, so you do not need to wear sunscreen when it is cloudy outside.

20. Tattoos and piercings are two of the most common types of _____.

21. **Critical Thinking.** What factors would you consider before getting a tattoo or body piercing?

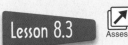

Lesson 8.3

Assess

Keeping Your Mouth, Eyes, and Ears Healthy

Key Terms

cavities
cochlea
cornea
decibels
eardrum
gingivitis
halitosis
iris

lens
optic nerve
oral cavity
periodontitis
plaque
pupil
retina
saliva

Key Points

- The oral cavity includes lips, teeth, and tongue.
- Tooth decay and gum disease can be prevented through good dental hygiene.
- Many different parts of the eye work together to make sight possible.
- The three main parts of the ear play different but important roles.
- Hearing loss is usually caused by damage to the inner ear.

Check Your Understanding

22. _____ contains an enzyme that helps break down food in the mouth.

23. Which part of the tooth contains blood vessels and nerve endings that connect the tooth to the jaw?
    A. the crown
    B. the neck
    C. the root
    D. enamel

24. _____ is a sticky, colorless film that coats the teeth and dissolves their protective enamel surface.

25. Inflammation of the gums is called _____.
    A. gingivitis
    B. periodontitis
    C. halitosis
    D. bruxism

26. *True or false?* Periodontitis is an infection that occurs when bacteria gets under the gum tissue and begins to destroy the gums and bone.

27. The _____ is the colored part of the eye.
    A. iris
    B. pupil
    C. lens
    D. retina

28. *True or false? Myopia* is another term for astigmatism.

29. Briefly describe the three main parts of the ear— the outer ear, middle ear, and inner ear. What functions do each part of the ear have?

30. Which of the following is another name for the outer ear?
    A. anvil
    B. cochlea
    C. pinna
    D. ear canal

31. Sound intensity is measured in units called _____.

32. **Critical Thinking.** What choices can you make now to help you enjoy healthy teeth for years to come?

33. **Critical Thinking.** If you had the choice, would you prefer to correct your vision with surgery or to wear eyeglasses or contacts? Explain.

Skill Development

Health and Wellness Skills

34. **Access Information.** Imagine that one or more of your grandparents are suffering from poor vision or hearing loss. Research both of these health problems and find out what kinds of "aids" might be available for their use. Where in your community could you find these types of devices? Is a doctor's visit required for their use or purchase? What type of doctor would your grandparents need to see?

35. **Advocate for Health.** Skin cancer is the most common form of cancer in the United States. Create a poster or brochure to educate members of your community about the causes, risk factors, identification methods, and preventive measures for skin cancer.

36. **Make Decisions.** Conduct some research on health problems associated with tattoos, reasons for tattoo regret, and the process of tattoo removal. Be conscious about gathering your information from credible sources. After gathering your information, write a personal statement as to whether or not you will get a tattoo. Explain your choice.

37. **Analyze Influences.** Watch, listen to, or read some commercials or advertisements for products that might negatively affect one or more of the health behaviors covered in this chapter. Choose one commercial or advertisement and write a short paragraph about how the product advertised might affect consumer health in a negative way.

Hands-On Activity

Tooth Enamel and Eggshells

Eggshells, like enamel, contain calcium. In this activity you will see what different substances can do to the enamel that protects your teeth.

Materials Needed

In groups and with your teacher, decide who will bring the following supplies to class: six or more white-shelled, hardboiled eggs; six clear plastic cups; a glass of each of soda, coffee, juice, a sports drink, water, and vinegar; a permanent marker; toothbrushes and toothpaste; and plastic wrap.

Steps for this Activity

1. Fill each of the six cups with one of the liquids. Then, put an egg in each cup and label each cup according to its contents.

2. Cover the cups with plastic wrap and let the eggs soak overnight. Let the egg in vinegar soak for several days. Discuss what you think will happen to the eggshells.

3. On the second day, check the eggs (except for the egg in vinegar) to see how the eggshells have been affected by the different liquids. Use toothbrushes and toothpaste to try cleaning the eggs. In a group, discuss how the different types of liquids affected the "enamel" on the eggshells and how much brushing it took to get each eggshell clean. Which liquid had the greatest impact on the eggshells? the smallest effect? Which of the liquids would be healthy choices? Which would be unhealthy?

4. Check the egg soaking in vinegar after letting it soak for several days. Vinegar simulates the effects of acid in the mouth. In your group, discuss what happened to the eggshell soaked in vinegar. How might the acid in your mouth affect the enamel on your teeth? Research this question if you are unsure.

5. Write a paragraph explaining the importance of brushing and flossing daily based on what you learned.

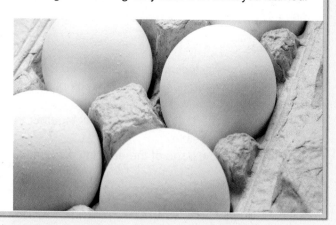

Core Skills

Math Practice

The following study investigated perceptions and knowledge about health risks in relation to tattoos and piercings. Researchers gathered data from students at high schools and universities in the Italian province of Naples. The results are shown below.

Of 9,322 high school students
- 31.3% were pierced;
- 11.3% were tattooed;
- 79.4% knew about infectious risks associated with body art;
- 46% knew about noninfectious risks; and
- 3.5% acknowledged the risk of viral disease transmission.

Of 3,610 university students
- 33% were pierced;
- 24.5% were tattooed;
- 87.2% knew about infectious risks;
- 59.1% knew about noninfectious risks; and
- 15% acknowledged the risk of viral disease transmission.

Seventy-three percent of the high school students and 33.5% of the university students had body art done at unauthorized facilities. Approximately 7% of both samples reported complications from their body art.

38. How many high school students in the study had tattoos?
    - A. 1,053
    - B. 11.3
    - C. 2,918
    - D. 334

39. What percentage of the high school students acknowledged the risk of viral disease transmission?
    - A. 15%
    - B. 3.5%
    - C. 24.7%
    - D. 2%

40. Of the university students, how many knew about infectious risks?
    - A. 3,148
    - B. 872
    - C. 1,805
    - D. 2,514

41. How many of the 9,322 high school students had body art done at unauthorized facilities?
    - A. 3,610
    - B. 3,123
    - C. 652
    - D. 6,805

Reading and Writing Practice

Read the passage below and then answer the questions.

When you eat or drink something, an enzyme in your saliva breaks down the food particles and sugars so they can be digested. This process turns everything you eat or drink into a type of acid. This acid then combines with the bacteria in your mouth, as well as saliva and small food particles, to form plaque. *Plaque is a sticky, colorless film that coats the teeth and dissolves their protective enamel surface. If plaque is not removed, it mixes with minerals to become* tartar, *a harder substance. Tartar requires professional cleaning to be removed.*

It is easy to brush away plaque shortly after eating. If you do not brush and floss your teeth daily, however, food particles remain in your mouth and promote bacterial growth between teeth, around the gums, and on the tongue. This results in tooth decay. Over time, tooth decay causes cavities, *or holes in the teeth that occur when plaque eats into a tooth's enamel. Cavities are also known as* dental caries. *When the decay continues, the hole gets deeper, and eventually reaches the nerve layer under the enamel known as the* dentin. *This causes painful nerve damage. The death of the tooth occurs when the decay reaches the deepest layer of the tooth (the* pulp cavity*).*

42. What is the author's main idea in this passage?
    - A. Brushing teeth helps prevent tooth decay.
    - B. Brushing and flossing daily is a rule.
    - C. Cavities can cause nerve damage.
    - D. Teeth can die.

43. How does plaque relate to tartar?
    - A. Plaque can lead to tartar.
    - B. Tartar can lead to plaque.
    - C. Plaque helps eliminate tartar.
    - D. Tartar helps eliminate plaque.

44. What is another term for *cavities*?
    - A. *pulp cavity*
    - B. *dentin*
    - C. *dental caries*
    - D. *plaque*

45. Write a paragraph about your daily dental hygiene routines. Share your paragraphs in class.

Unit 4 Understanding and Avoiding Hazardous Substances

Chapter 9	Tobacco
Chapter 10	Alcohol
Chapter 11	Medications and Drugs

Big Ideas

- Tobacco products contain an addictive substance that makes it difficult for people to quit using tobacco.

- Teenagers who abuse alcohol raise their risk of serious injury or death from accidents, alcohol poisoning, and violence.

- People who abuse drugs—including some over-the-counter medicines—increase their risk of health problems, addiction, and death.

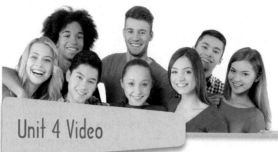

Unit 4 Video

A Day in the Life Videos

As you follow a teenager through her school day, she describes the impact of tobacco, alcohol, and drugs on her peers and on society. She shares what she learns in her classes that reinforces her decision to avoid hazardous substances.

Organize Your Facts and Ideas

Study your notes and reflect on the information you've collected. Put yourself in the shoes of a reader who doesn't know the subject. What would this reader want to know first, second, third, and so forth? Which terms and concepts would this reader want to have defined and explained?

Creating an outline will help you answer these questions in a clear, logical order. The outline will also help you avoid unnecessary work.

Write your research question followed by a list of the main points you plan to discuss in the order you will present them. Each item on the list should be no longer than a few sentences. Then under each main point, list brief sub-points you plan to discuss in the order they will be presented.

Meet with your group and present your outline. Justify the organization and explain how it helps you answer your research question. Incorporate suggestions from your group into the outline.

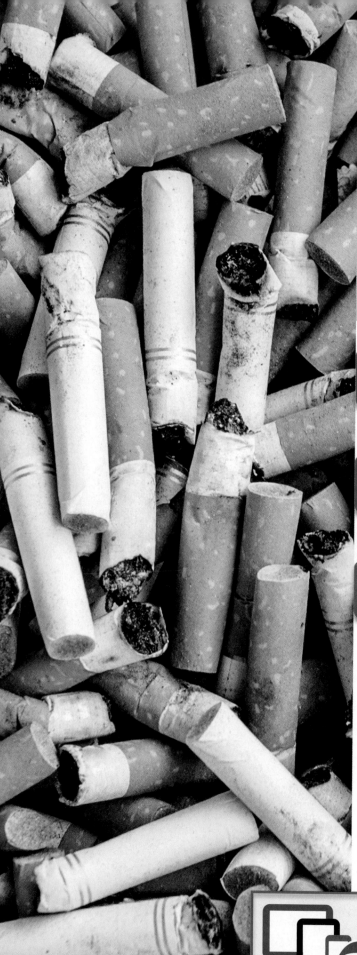

Chapter 9

Tobacco

Lesson 9.1

The Health Effects of Tobacco

Lesson 9.2

Why People Use Tobacco

Lesson 9.3

Treating and Preventing Nicotine Addiction

While studying this chapter, look for the activity icon to:

- **review** vocabulary with e-flash cards and games;
- **assess** learning with quizzes and online exercises;
- **expand** knowledge with animations and activities; and
- **listen** to pronunciation of key terms in the audio glossary.

G-W LEARNING.com

www.g-wlearning.com/health/

What's Your Health and Wellness IQ?

Take this quiz to see what you do *and* do not *know about the negative consequences of using tobacco products. If you cannot answer a question, pay extra attention to that topic as you study this chapter.*

1. *Identify each statement as* True, False, *or* It Depends. *Choose* It Depends *if a statement is true in some cases, but false in others.*

2. *Revise each* False *statement to make it true.*

3. *Explain the circumstances in which each* It Depends *statement is true and when it is false.*

Health and Wellness IQ Assess

	True	False	It Depends
1. People who smoke are addicted to the carbon monoxide present in tobacco smoke.	True	False	It Depends
2. Smoking is a relatively easy habit to break.	True	False	It Depends
3. Smoking leads to stained teeth and bad breath.	True	False	It Depends
4. People who are regularly exposed to secondhand smoke are at increased risk of developing cancer.	True	False	It Depends
5. On average, long-term smokers die 13 to 15 years earlier than nonsmokers.	True	False	It Depends
6. Smoking is extremely harmful to the lungs, but does not typically affect heart health.	True	False	It Depends
7. Tobacco smoke contains carcinogens.	True	False	It Depends
8. Nicotine addiction is only physical.	True	False	It Depends
9. Spending time with people who smoke increases the chances that you will smoke.	True	False	It Depends
10. Increasing the cost of cigarettes has little impact on reducing smoking among teenagers.	True	False	It Depends

Setting the Scene

Companies that sell tobacco products need you and other teenagers to become their future customers. They want you to believe that buying their products will make you more attractive and popular. They want you to believe that their customers drive expensive cars and lead exciting, active lives—while using tobacco.

Every day in the United States, nearly 4,000 people younger than 18 smoke their first cigarette. This is unfortunate because starting to smoke during adolescence can lead to a lifetime of health issues. Friends and family members of smokers also develop health problems from inhaling secondhand smoke. In this chapter you will learn about the health effects of tobacco products and why some people choose to use these products. You will also learn specific strategies for kicking a tobacco habit and preventing tobacco use.

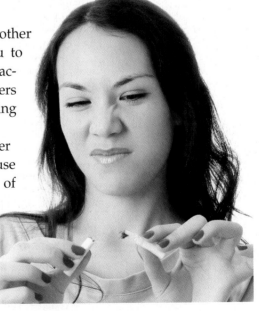

The Health Effects of Tobacco

Key Terms 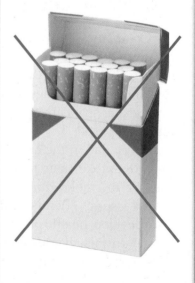 E-Flash Cards

In this lesson, you will learn the meanings of the following key terms.

asthma

carbon monoxide

carcinogens

chronic bronchitis

chronic obstructive
pulmonary disease
(COPD)

emphysema

leukoplakia

nicotine

secondhand smoke

smokeless tobacco

tar

tobacco

Before You Read

It Says, I Say, So

Create a visual chart like the one shown below to connect information in the text with the knowledge you already have. Add as much information as you can, and make your columns as long as you need them to be.

IT SAYS	I SAY	SO
What the text says	What I think the text means	How do I interpret this?

Lesson Objectives

After studying this lesson, you will be able to

- identify various forms of tobacco and the addictive substance in tobacco products;
- assess the hazardous effects nicotine has on the cardiovascular and respiratory systems;
- describe harmful substances in tobacco products and smoke that result in serious illnesses and diseases; and
- analyze the impact of secondhand smoke on individuals.

Warm-Up Activity

Cigarette Smoking and Death

The table below presents the top 10 leading causes of death in adults in the United States. Before you read this chapter, make a new list predicting how this table might look if everyone chose not to smoke. Explain your reasoning.

Leading Causes of Death in Adults	Number of Deaths
Heart Disease	614,348
Cancer	591,699
Chronic Lower Respiratory Diseases	147,101
Accidents (unintentional injuries)	136,053
Stroke (cerebrovascular diseases)	133,103
Alzheimer's disease	93,541
Diabetes	76,488
Influenza and Pneumonia	55,227
Nephritis, nephritic syndrome, and nephrosis	48,146
Intentional self-harm (suicide)	42,773

S moking is the leading cause of preventable death in the United States. This lesson examines different types of tobacco products, the physical effects of tobacco use on the body, and the health impact of being around others who smoke.

Tobacco Products

Tobacco is a plant used for the production of tobacco-related products, such as cigarettes and chewing tobacco. Tobacco leaves contain the chemical *nicotine*, a toxic substance that gives tobacco products their addictive quality. The most common method of using tobacco is smoking cigarettes. Other methods of tobacco use include cigars, pipes, smokeless tobacco, vaporizers, electronic cigarettes (e-cigarettes), and other electronic nicotine delivery systems (ENDS). Some people believe that these methods of tobacco use are safer, healthier, or less addictive than regular cigarettes. The reality is that all forms of tobacco use are associated with addiction and serious health consequences (Figure 9.1).

tobacco
a plant that is used to produce cigarettes and other products; contains nicotine

nicotine
an addictive, toxic substance present in tobacco products

Health Risks of Using Tobacco over Time

Nervous System
- Stroke
- Exposure to nicotine during adolescence is linked to lasting adverse affects on brain development
- Addiction

Mouth
- Cancers of the mouth
- Gum disease and loss of teeth
- Loss of ability to taste and smell

Cardiovascular System
- Increased heart rate and blood pressure
- Constricted blood vessels and buildup of plaque
- Carbon monoxide interferes with the ability of blood cells to carry oxygen
- Increased risk of heart attack or stroke (nonsmokers who inhale secondhand smoke have a greater risk of stroke)

Immune System
- Weakened immune system, leaving smokers more susceptible to colds, the flu, and other illnesses and diseases

Reproductive System
- Smoking while pregnant is linked to birth defects
- Infertility
- Impotence in men

Eyes
- Vision loss

Lungs
- Lung cancer, chronic bronchitis, and emphysema
- Smoking during adolescence—when the lungs are still growing—may permanently stunt the growth of the lungs so they never perform at full capacity
- More lung infections and asthma attacks

Digestive System
- Cancers of the stomach, liver, pancreas, and esophagus
- Colorectal cancer

Endocrine System
- Insulin resistance and diabetes

Urinary System
- Cancers of the kidney and bladder

Appearance and Hygiene
- Bad breath
- Smelly hair and clothes
- Yellow-brown stained teeth
- Stained fingertips and fingernails
- Premature aging of the skin (more wrinkles)
- Loss of teeth due to gum disease

Figure 9.1

Tobacco use affects the entire body, and its harmful effects are not always reversible.

Figure 9.2 Chemicals Found in Cigarettes

Chemical	Other Locations
acetone	found in nail polish remover
acetic acid	an ingredient in hair dye
ammonia	a common household cleaner
arsenic	used in rat poison
benzene	found in rubber cement
butane	used in lighter fluid
cadmium	active component in battery acid
carbon monoxide	released in car exhaust fumes
formaldehyde	embalming fluid
hexamine	found in barbecue lighter fluid
lead	used in batteries
naphthalene	an ingredient in mothballs
methanol	a main component in rocket fuel
nicotine	used as insecticide
tar	material for paving roads
toluene	used to manufacture paint

Tobacco and Your Body

On average, long-term smokers die 13 to 15 years earlier than nonsmokers. Tobacco use increases a person's risk for developing cancers of the mouth, pharynx, esophagus, lung, and bladder. People who smoke also increase their risk for developing coronary heart disease, stroke, emphysema, bronchitis, and respiratory infections.

The Surgeon General of the United States recently issued a report that showed higher risk factors among smokers for developing diabetes, colorectal and liver cancers, vision loss, tuberculosis, and arthritis. People who smoke also have a higher risk factor for minor health problems.

Tobacco products and smoke contain thousands of chemicals and toxic substances that harm the body. Nicotine, carbon monoxide, tar, and carcinogens are just a few of the harmful substances present in tobacco products (Figure 9.2). Many health problems result from damage to the cardiovascular and respiratory systems caused by the harmful substances in tobacco products. These health problems can interfere with a teenager's quality of life and athletic performance.

The Cardiovascular System

The cardiovascular system includes the heart and blood transportation system in your body. Smokers have a higher risk of developing heart disease and hypertension (high blood pressure) than nonsmokers. Smokers are also twice as likely to die from a heart attack as nonsmokers. This is partly because of the substantial impact that nicotine and carbon monoxide have on the cardiovascular system.

Nicotine. When people use forms of tobacco, nicotine enters their bloodstream. Its presence triggers the release of the hormone *adrenaline*, a *stimulant*. Adrenaline triggers an increase in heart rate, breathing rate, and blood pressure. This increase in speed and pressure of blood flow in the body makes the heart work harder to pump blood faster around the body.

Nicotine also causes the blood vessels to constrict. The heart must work harder to pump blood through increasingly narrow vessels. Gradually, nicotine leads to changes in the walls of the blood vessels, which make it easier for fatty substances such as cholesterol (*plaque*) to build up in the arteries. This can disrupt the flow of blood through the body because the fatty deposits restrict the ease of blood transportation. Over time, this buildup increases the risk of a heart attack or stroke, which occur when an artery becomes completely blocked.

carbon monoxide

a poisonous gas found in cigarette smoke; negatively affects cells' ability to carry oxygen

Carbon Monoxide. Cigarette smoke contains high levels of **carbon monoxide**, a poisonous gas. When inhaled, carbon monoxide interferes with the ability of blood cells to carry oxygen. This reduces the amount of oxygen in the blood and the amount of oxygen that reaches the heart.

The Respiratory System

The respiratory system's primary function is to enable breathing. First, the nose takes in air, which then travels down the respiratory tract. The nose, bronchial tubes, and lungs are all lined with tissue containing fine, hair-like projections called *cilia*. The cilia trap and move foreign particles out of the respiratory tract. Air then travels into tubes (*bronchi*) and into the lungs.

When a person smokes, damage is done to the respiratory system that makes breathing more difficult. The burning of tobacco produces a residue known as *tar*, which consists of small, thick, sticky particles. Over time, as smoke repeatedly passes through the bronchial tubes, tar builds up in the lungs. Tar disrupts the ability of the cilia to effectively clear the lungs of foreign particles.

Smoking-related damage to the lungs also contributes to the development of chronic respiratory diseases and can trigger asthma attacks.

Chronic Obstructive Pulmonary Disease (COPD). *Chronic obstructive pulmonary disease (COPD)* refers to a group of diseases that make it more difficult to breathe (Figure 9.3). Most smokers who develop COPD have a combination of chronic bronchitis and emphysema.

tar
a thick, sticky substance produced by burning tobacco; can disrupt the respiratory systems of smokers

chronic obstructive pulmonary disease (COPD)

term for a group of diseases that cause difficulty breathing; includes chronic bronchitis and emphysema

Figure 9.3

Chronic obstructive pulmonary disease (COPD) clogs the bronchioles and damages the lungs, making it more difficult to breathe.

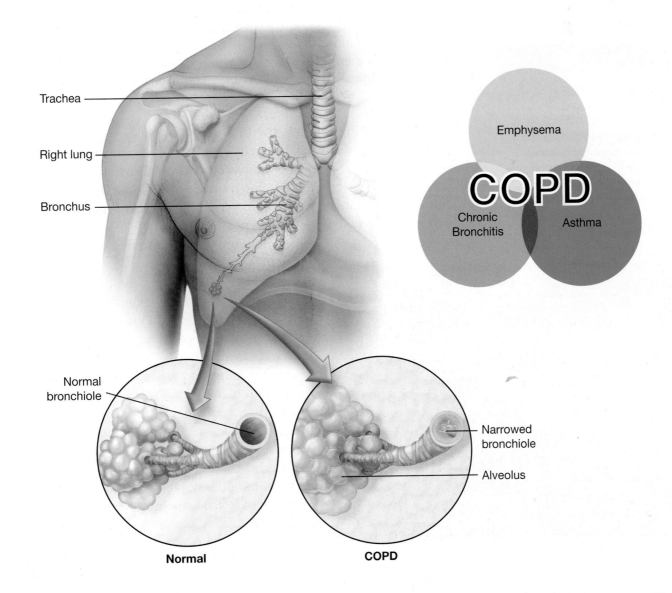

Trachea

Right lung

Bronchus

Emphysema

COPD

Chronic Bronchitis

Asthma

Normal bronchiole

Narrowed bronchiole

Alveolus

Normal

COPD

chronic bronchitis
a condition in which the bronchial tubes swell and become irritated

Chronic bronchitis is an ongoing condition in which the bronchial tubes become swollen and irritated. Smoking causes the mucous membrane in the lungs' bronchial passages to become inflamed, which narrows the pathway to the lungs. This makes it increasingly difficult for the lungs to take in enough oxygen, which is why people with bronchitis often experience coughing spells and have difficulty catching their breath. Smoking and inhaling secondhand smoke are primary causes of chronic bronchitis, but regularly inhaling air pollution and smoke from tobacco products contributes to the condition as well.

emphysema
a disease that permanently enlarges lung airways and destroys lung tissue, making it difficult for a person to breathe

Emphysema is a disease that causes the airways in the lungs to become permanently enlarged. Emphysema destroys the sacs of air that make up lung tissue (*alveoli*), which is where oxygen and carbon dioxide are traded during the breathing process. The destruction of the alveoli makes it more difficult to breathe. As a result, the person has to breathe faster to get enough oxygen into the lungs and into the bloodstream. This extra work places a burden on the heart, leading to more health problems (Figure 9.4).

asthma
a chronic disease characterized by episodes of blocked airflow to the lungs

Asthma and Other Illnesses. *Asthma* is a chronic disease caused by blockages of the airflow to and from the lungs. When a person with asthma inhales tobacco smoke—either by smoking a cigarette or by being around people who are smoking—the lining of the airways becomes irritated. This irritation can then cause an asthma attack. Moreover, because tobacco smoke damages the cilia, they are unable to eliminate unwanted particles in the lungs. This means these particles stay in the airways and continue to trigger asthma attacks.

Similarly, smoking interferes with a person's ability to participate in even casual forms of physical activity. For example, after beginning to smoke, someone who once ran one lap around the track without becoming out of breath may be breathless after running half as far. This is because smoking leads to reduced lung capacity, and the hearts of smokers are already overworked before they begin physical activity.

Smoking also leads to a weakened immune system. Your *immune system* consists of the organs, tissues, and cells in the body that help defend itself from disease-causing agents such as bacteria, parasites, and viruses. Smokers are at greater risk of becoming ill from germs that cause colds and the flu.

Tobacco use can lead to a number of other health problems. Smokers have a higher risk factor than nonsmokers for developing osteoporosis, ulcers, fertility problems, and gum disease. Tobacco use can also interfere with eating by changing the shape of taste buds. When food does not taste as good, some long-term smokers lose their appetite and interest in eating.

Figure 9.4

Below, on the left, is a healthy, normal lung. On the right is a smoker's lung, which has been damaged in many ways. For example, constant irritation from the tar in smoke keeps a smoker's lungs inflamed, resulting in a buildup of scar tissue that reduces the lung's elasticity.

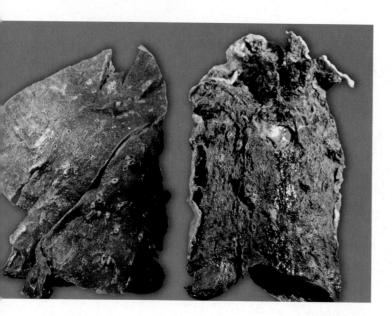

Lung Cancer and Other Cancers. Lung cancer occurs when abnormal cells in one or both lungs grow rapidly and form a mass of cells, which is called a *tumor*. This growth usually happens in the cells that line the air passages. As the tumors grow, they interfere with the lungs' ability to transport oxygen to the bloodstream. Tumors can also spread from the lungs to other parts of the body.

Tobacco smoke contains over 70 **carcinogens**, or cancer-causing agents, that can lead to the abnormal growth of cells in the mouth, throat, and lungs. This is why smokers have higher rates of cancer than nonsmokers.

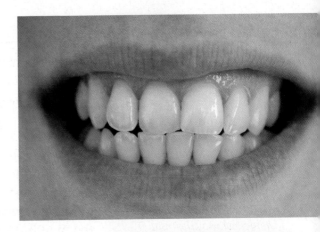

Your Appearance

Tobacco use has numerous negative internal effects, but it also has negative external effects. People who smoke for at least 10 years show more wrinkles in their skin. This is because the nicotine in tobacco causes blood vessels to get smaller, which makes it more difficult for oxygen and nutrients to reach the skin. Tobacco use causes stained teeth, brittle nails, and thin hair. Smokers also tend to have bad breath, and clothes and hair that smell of smoke (Figure 9.5).

Figure 9.5

Tobacco use yellows teeth and can cause bad breath and other oral problems.

carcinogens
substances that cause cancer

The Hazards of Smokeless Tobacco

Forms of **smokeless tobacco** include chewing tobacco, snuff, *snus* (a form of snuff), and dissolvable tobacco. Chewing tobacco involves placing wads, or *plugs*, of tobacco leaves between the cheeks and gums (Figure 9.6). Snuff is a finely cut or powdered tobacco that is inhaled or placed between the cheek and gums. Dissolvable tobacco is taken in the form of flavored mouth drops or strips.

Smokeless tobacco also includes *electronic nicotine delivery systems* (*ENDS*), which produce a tobacco-containing aerosol that users inhale. Types of ENDS include vaporizers, vape pens, hookah pens, e-cigarettes, and e-pipes.

smokeless tobacco
a tobacco-related product that does not require burning; includes chewing tobacco and electronic nicotine delivery systems (ENDS)

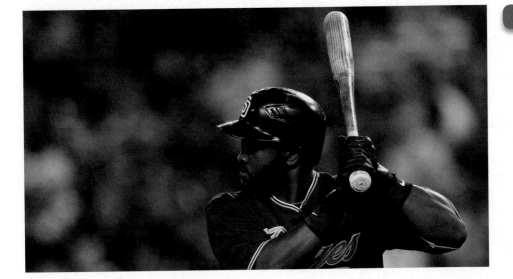

Figure 9.6

When Hall of Fame baseball player Tony Gwynn died of salivary gland cancer at the age of 54, many major league baseball players pledged to quit chewing tobacco. Prior to his death Gwynn had blamed his longtime chewing habit for the development of the cancer. *Do you know high school athletes who chew tobacco? Do you think these athletes are aware of the dangers of smokeless tobacco?*

All forms of smokeless tobacco contain nicotine and carcinogens, so the harmful effects of these substances are the same as if they were smoked. The presence of nicotine also means that smokeless tobacco is just as addictive as cigarettes. In fact, smokeless tobacco is often placed directly into the mouth, so users of these products actually absorb even more nicotine than smokers.

Because using smokeless tobacco does not involve inhaling smoke, people who use it are less likely to develop lung problems than smokers. These people do, however, increase their risk of developing other serious diseases. When using smokeless tobacco, people absorb nicotine through their mouth tissues. The use of these tobacco products can lead to *leukoplakia*, a condition characterized by thickened, white, leathery spots on the inside of the mouth. This condition can develop into oral cancer. Smokeless tobacco use can also lead to an increased risk of cardiovascular disease, respiratory irritation, gum disease, and tooth decay.

The Impact of Secondhand Smoke

Secondhand smoke refers to the tobacco smoke you are exposed to in the environment. People who are regularly exposed to secondhand smoke because they live or socialize with smokers are at greater risk of developing lung cancer or heart disease.

Concerns about the dangerous effects of secondhand smoke on health have led a number of states to pass laws banning smoking in many public areas to protect the health of customers and staff. Secondhand smoke greatly affects certain population groups, including pregnant women, infants, and children.

Pregnant Women and Infants

Exposure to nicotine is particularly hazardous to a developing fetus. When a pregnant woman smokes, the nicotine and carbon monoxide she takes into her body pass through the placenta to the fetus. The immediate impact on the fetus is an increased heart rate and reduction in the amount of oxygen the fetus receives.

Women who smoke while pregnant increase their risk of miscarriage, and of having babies born prematurely or with low birth weight. Babies born to mothers who smoked or breathed secondhand smoke during pregnancy also have a higher risk factor for sudden infant death syndrome (SIDS). SIDS is the unexpected and sudden death of a baby less than one year after birth.

Children

Exposure to secondhand smoke is a major cause of health problems in children. Children exposed to secondhand smoke are more likely to have respiratory problems such as pneumonia, bronchitis, and asthma attacks. Children whose parents smoke also have higher rates of sore throats and ear infections.

leukoplakia

a condition characterized by white, leathery spots inside the mouth; may develop into oral cancer

secondhand smoke

tobacco smoke in the environment that may affect a person even if he or she does not smoke

Personal Profile

Are You at Risk of Tobacco Use?

These questions will help you assess whether your tobacco use or the tobacco use of others is putting your health at risk.

I have smoked a cigarette.
yes no

I have used chewing tobacco or snuff. **yes no**

I spend time with friends who smoke. **yes no**

I spend time with family members who smoke. **yes no**

I sometimes have a craving for a cigarette or chewing tobacco. **yes no**

I smoke a cigarette every day. **yes no**

I smoke more than one cigarette a day. **yes no**

I would find it difficult to go a whole day without smoking. **yes no**

Add up your number of yes answers to assess your own personal risk of developing health problems related to tobacco use.

Behavior-related issues common in children of mothers who smoked during pregnancy include attention deficit disorders, hyperactivity, and aggression. Children of smokers are also more likely to develop smoking habits themselves (Figure 9.7).

If you find yourself sharing the air with smokers, you can take steps to reduce your risk of being exposed to secondhand smoke.

- Avoid spending time in places where smoking may be permitted.

- Do not accept car rides from people who smoke while driving.

- Ask that people smoke only outdoors or in a particular room that is sealed off from the rest of a home or building.

- Increase air circulation in buildings where people are permitted to smoke by opening the windows to let in fresh air.

Perhaps most importantly, you can encourage a friend or family member who smokes to quit smoking, and support his or her efforts toward quitting.

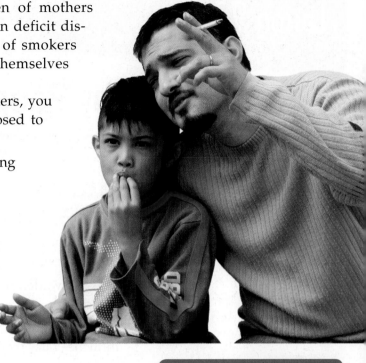

Figure 9.7

Smokers put people around them, including their families, at risk with secondhand smoke. *Where do you usually encounter secondhand smoke? How can you protect yourself from it?*

Lesson 9.1 Review

Know and Understand Assess

1. Define *adrenaline*. How does nicotine affect adrenaline and the body?

2. Explain how nicotine affects the blood vessels. How does this impact on the blood vessels cause smokers to be twice as likely as nonsmokers to die from a heart attack?

3. Describe carbon monoxide and the effect it has on the cardiovascular system.

4. Describe how tar accumulates in the respiratory system and how it affects the lungs.

5. How does smoking or breathing in cigarette smoke impact people with asthma?

6. Most smokers who develop COPD have a combination of what two diseases?

Analyze and Apply

7. Describe why athletes should abstain from tobacco use. How would you explain this to an athlete?

8. Explain how a woman being exposed to secondhand smoke or smoking during pregnancy can impact the developing fetus.

Real World Health

Family Tree Talk to your parents about relatives who were affected by diseases associated with smoking. Make a list of family members, their diseases, and whether or not they are or were smokers. Write a paragraph about the influence that smoking may have had on these family members and their health.

Why People Use Tobacco

Key Terms 📄 E-Flash Cards

In this lesson, you will learn the meanings of the following key terms.

addiction
dependence
peer pressure
substance abuse
tolerance
withdrawal

Before You Read

Give One, Get One
Create a chart like the one shown below. Include as many rows as you need. Before reading the lesson, list facts you already know about people's tobacco use in the Give One column. In the Get One column, list facts you learn as you read the lesson.

Give One (things you already know)	Get One (new information)

Lesson Objectives

After studying this lesson, you will be able to

- analyze the development of addiction according to the stages of substance abuse;
- assess how identity development may relate to the decision to use tobacco;
- explain how attitudes about tobacco use from friends and parents influence rates of tobacco use; and
- evaluate the role of the media in encouraging tobacco use.

Warm-Up Activity

Differences in Smoking Rates
The table below shows differences in smoking rates among adults in the United States based on gender, race, education, and income. Working in groups, after being assigned one of the four topics by your teacher, brainstorm reasons your group thinks these differences exist. Discuss the listed reasons and decide which two or three reasons you think have the most impact. Present your complete list and your two or three most important reasons to the class.

Gender	Race/Ethnicity
17% Adult Men 14% Adult Women	22% Native Americans 20% Non-Hispanic Whites 17% African Americans 17% Hispanics 7% Asian Americans
Level of Education	**Income**
34% GED Degree 4% Graduate Degree	26% Very Low Income 14% Moderate to High Income

U nfortunately, more people start to smoke each day. Most teenagers who begin to smoke do plan to quit, and they believe that quitting will be fairly easy. They soon find that smoking is a very hard habit to break. The majority of teens who smoke become adults who regularly smoke.

Given the expense and the negative effects of tobacco use on health, people's continued use of tobacco is surprising. Most people who use tobacco know that it can cause them to become ill or even die. This lesson examines some of the barriers that lead people to continue to use tobacco.

Addiction

People often talk about addiction in relation to a specific substance. In this case, a *substance* is a drug, such as nicotine, alcohol, or an illegal drug. **Substance abuse** is the use of a drug or intentional misuse of prescription medication that causes harmful, dangerous effects.

Addiction helps explain why many people who start using a substance believe it will be easy to quit, but then have great difficulty quitting. **Addiction** is the physical and psychological need for a given substance or behavior. Addiction to a substance usually develops in four stages (Figure 9.8 on the next page).

substance abuse
the use of a drug (nicotine, alcohol, or illegal drugs) or intentional misuse of medication

addiction
the physical and psychological need for a substance or behavior

Health across the Life Span

Rates of Smoking by Age

A national study conducted by the Centers for Disease Control revealed that the rate of smoking varies considerably across the life span. The rates of smoking by age are represented in the following table.

Why does age make a difference in smoking rates? One major reason is that older adults are more likely to have smoked in the past, but have since quit. About 33% of people 50 to 64 years of age, and about 47% of people 65 years of age and older are former smokers. In contrast, only 12% of people 18 to 29 years of age, and only 23% of those 30 to 49 years of age have quit smoking. People who smoked in the past but have since quit are not counted as smokers for their age range. Smokers in the younger age ranges may end up quitting as they grow older.

Proportion of Age Groups that Smoke	
high school students	9%
adults 18–24	13%
adults 25–44	18%
adults 45–64	17%
adults 65+	8%

Analyzing Data

1. Over time, the health consequences of tobacco use have become more well known. How might this information relate to the numbers of smokers and former smokers in different age groups?

2. Do you think these differences in smoking rates by age will stay the same over time, or will they change? Explain your reasoning.

Figure 9.8 Stages of Substance Abuse

Stage one: experimentation	Experimentation with a substance begins. Substance use may stop at this stage, or may rapidly develop into other stages.
Stage two: regular use	The user develops a habit of regularly using a substance.
Stage three: tolerance	The user's body develops a tolerance to the substance. Gradually, the user feels the need for more and more of a substance to achieve the same effects as before.
Stage four: dependence and addiction	The user becomes reliant on having the substance present in the body to function normally or feel "normal." Substance use also interferes with personal responsibilities and relationships. The user is physically and psychologically addicted to the substance.

Experimentation

Initially, people often choose to use a substance such as cigarettes or chewing tobacco "just to try it." This is the stage of experimentation, when a person is trying a substance and, potentially, using it more regularly. Experimentation with a substance often leads to the regular use of a substance.

Regular Use

After initially trying a substance, people may gradually increase their substance use. Over time, people who smoke a few cigarettes may slowly increase the amount of times they smoke per week. Users are then likely to develop a regular pattern of smoking cigarettes.

Tolerance

People who regularly use a substance develop a tolerance for that substance. A *tolerance* develops when the body needs greater amounts of a substance to experience the effects it felt when a lesser amount was used. The body can quickly develop a tolerance to nicotine and require more cigarettes to achieve the original effect.

Dependency and Addiction

After repeated use, the body adjusts to—or becomes *dependent* on—the feelings that result from the presence of nicotine. **Dependence** occurs when the body relies on the presence of an addictive substance in the system to function "normally" or feel "normal." There are two types of dependence—physical and psychological.

tolerance
a condition in which the body adjusts to given substance, requiring increased amounts of the substance to feel its effect

dependence
a condition in which a person relies on a given substance to function or feel normal

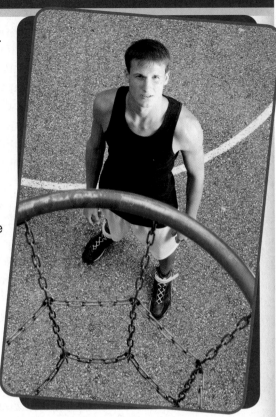

Roberto is 15 years old and a sophomore in high school. As a young child he was bothered by his mother's smoking. Roberto promised himself he would never smoke. During his freshman year, however, he hung out with older students who smoked. One day, he decided that it would be okay to occasionally have a cigarette during the week with friends.

Roberto, who never intended to become a smoker, soon found himself craving cigarettes. Although he only smokes a few cigarettes each week, he has already noticed that he can't run as far as he used to without getting winded. He is also beginning to smoke a couple of extra cigarettes each day. He worries that he may have difficulty making the basketball team again this season.

Critical Thinking

1. Identify the primary factors that led Roberto to begin smoking. What caused him to continue smoking?

2. How does Roberto's situation relate to the stages of substance abuse?

3. How can teenagers who spend time with friends who smoke keep themselves from becoming smokers?

A *physical dependence* occurs when the body relies on having a certain amount of a substance present in the body to function "normally." Without the substance in the body, the dependent person feels uncomfortable, irritable, and even sick.

People who smoke also develop a *psychological dependence*, which causes people to believe that they need the substance to feel "normal." People may also develop patterns for using a substance by associating the substance with certain triggers. Whenever smokers encounter triggers they associate with smoking, they feel a strong psychological need to smoke.

Withdrawal Symptoms

When people are addicted to a substance and they try to stop using it, they experience unpleasant symptoms known as **withdrawal**. For people addicted to nicotine, symptoms can include irritability, difficulty concentrating, fatigue, nausea, and weight gain. They also experience intense cravings for nicotine because their body is now addicted to having this chemical. Withdrawal is one of the reasons why tobacco users have such difficulty quitting. People trying to quit smoking experience withdrawal symptoms for several weeks and even months after they stop. Some ex-smokers continue to have occasional cravings for tobacco for years.

withdrawal
the unpleasant physical or psychological symptoms associated with attempting to stop using a substance

Exploring a New Identity

Some teenagers start to smoke as a way of trying out a new identity. Teens may associate smoking with maturity, sophistication, or glamour. They may believe that, by smoking, they will gain all of these things. Young people may also begin smoking because they want to be viewed as rebellious and tough, perhaps in part because buying cigarettes is illegal for most high school students.

Most teenagers, however, do not view smokers as popular or cool. Surveys have found that teenagers see smokers as unhealthy, foolish, and poor performers in the classroom.

Social Factors

Some people begin using tobacco products because they want to fit in with or imitate community and cultural norms. These social factors have a strong impact on tobacco use (Figure 9.9).

Parents

Parents' attitudes and behaviors about smoking have a strong influence on whether or not teenagers smoke. Teenagers are much less likely to start smoking if their parents set clear expectations, discussing and following through on consequences for smoking. Teens who describe their parents or culture as being strongly against smoking are less likely to smoke than teens who see their parents or culture as open-minded toward smoking.

Figure 9.9

Smoking can lead to social rejection because of other dangerous behaviors that are associated with smoking. *What behaviors do you associate with smoking?*

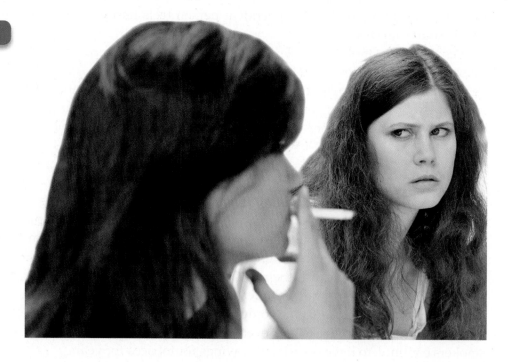

Friends

Another social factor that influences smoking habits is whether or not a teenager's friends smoke. Many teenagers smoke their first cigarette with a friend. Teenagers who have friends who smoke are much more likely to become smokers themselves. The influence of peers who smoke is stronger than the influence of family members who smoke. Not surprisingly, teenagers whose friends smoke are offered cigarettes much more frequently than those whose friends do not smoke.

Teenagers may experience peer pressure to smoke. *Peer pressure* is the influence of peers on an individual. When used to encourage an individual to do something unsafe, unhealthy, or uncomfortable, peer pressure is negative. Teenagers may worry that they will not be liked or accepted by their peer group if they choose not to smoke. Real friends, however, would not want their friends to endanger their health or do something that makes them feel uncomfortable.

peer pressure
the internal feeling that one must conform to the wishes of friends to earn their approval

Media

Celebrities are trendsetters and role models. People often look to celebrities for ideas about fashionable clothing, new hairstyles, and lifestyle choices. One of these lifestyle choices may be smoking, and teenagers are likely to imitate the smoking habits of celebrities they admire.

Lesson 9.2 Review

Know and Understand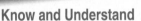

1. Identify the four stages of substance abuse.
2. Define *tolerance*. How does tolerance drive a nicotine addiction?
3. Explain the difference between psychological dependence and physical dependence.
4. Describe how experimentation with identity may lead teenagers to begin smoking.
5. Identify three social factors that may cause a teenager to begin using tobacco.

Analyze and Apply

6. How might withdrawal symptoms cause a person to return to abusing a substance after quitting?
7. How do parents' behavior and attitudes about tobacco influence their children's future decisions about tobacco use?

8. Explain how sports or media figures might influence a teenager to use or not use tobacco.

Real World Health

List every television show or movie you watch over a three-day period, noting those that have characters who smoke. Describe each character and the situation and setting in which smoking occurs. In each instance, describe how the use of a cigarette as a prop conveys information about the character or the story. Could this information have been conveyed in a way that did not use a tobacco product? Write a paragraph about the influence these shows might have on adolescents.

Treating and Preventing Nicotine Addiction

Key Terms 🔲 E-Flash Cards

In this lesson, you will learn the meanings of the following key terms.

laryngectomy
nicotine replacement
response substitution
stimulus control

Lesson Objectives

After studying this lesson, you will be able to

- assess the difficulty of quitting tobacco use;
- summarize strategies used to quit tobacco use;
- outline effective strategies to prevent and discourage tobacco use;
- analyze the government's role in preventing tobacco use and encouraging quitting; and
- utilize refusal, literacy, and critical thinking skills to resist tobacco.

Before You Read

KWL Chart: Treating Addiction

Create a chart like the one shown below. Before you read the lesson, outline what you know and what you want to know about treating and preventing nicotine addiction. After you have read the lesson, outline what you learned.

K What I Know	W What I Want to know	L What I Learned

Warm-Up Activity

Smoking's Impact

Take some time to think about the activities represented by the photos below. Pick two of the four activities and write a paragraph for each activity you chose, describing how smoking would either prevent you from participating in that activity or negatively impact your enjoyment of the activity. Be as specific as possible in describing smoking's impact.

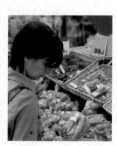
Shopping

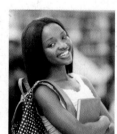
Smiling

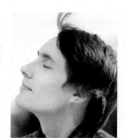
Breathing Clean Air

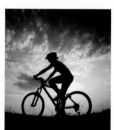
Exercising

G iven the many negative health consequences of smoking, almost half of all smokers try to quit each year. This lesson examines treatment and prevention strategies for nicotine addiction.

Treatment

Unfortunately, smoking is a hard habit to break. Even people who experience life-threatening, smoking-related illnesses have difficulty quitting. For example, about 40% of the people who have had a laryngectomy continue to smoke. A *laryngectomy* is a surgical procedure in which the larynx is removed, requiring the person to breathe through an opening in his or her neck (Figure 9.10). This procedure is typically performed when a person has cancer of the larynx. Similarly, more than half the people who have had a heart attack or surgery resulting from lung cancer continue to smoke.

It's never too late for someone to stop smoking. Smokers who quit successfully experience a number of health benefits. Some of these benefits, such as decreases in blood pressure, heart rate, and coughing, are seen within just a few days of quitting. Other benefits, such as a decreased risk

laryngectomy
the surgical removal of the larynx

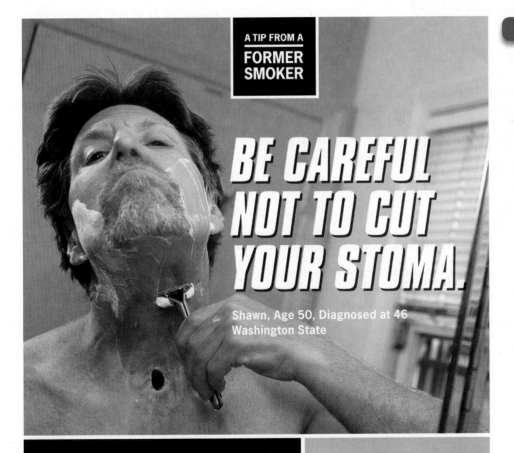

Figure 9.10

Sometimes even the threat of needing a procedure as serious as removing the larynx will not deter a person from smoking. *Do you think this government ad is effective in its attempt to get people to stop smoking? Explain your thinking.*

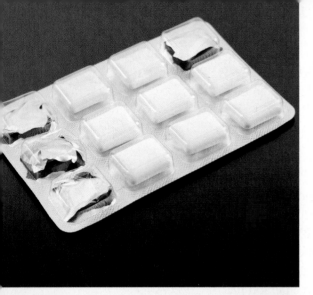

of experiencing a heart attack or developing cancer, are seen within a year after quitting. These benefits increase over time, meaning that the longer an ex-smoker goes without using tobacco, the lower the risk of experiencing these major health problems.

Although quitting tobacco can be difficult, nicotine addiction can be treated. Treatment methods include nicotine replacement, medication, and self-management techniques.

Nicotine Replacement

Some approaches to quitting smoking, or *smoking cessation*, rely on **nicotine replacement**. In this treatment, tobacco users continue to put nicotine into their bodies, which lessens their withdrawal symptoms and cravings, making it easier to quit. In this way, tobacco users can gradually treat their addiction to nicotine by using smaller and smaller amounts. Eventually, people find they are no longer dependent on nicotine. The most commonly used nicotine replacement strategies are nicotine gum and the nicotine patch (Figure 9.11).

Electronic cigarettes, or *e-cigarettes*, and other electronic nicotine delivery systems (ENDS) have also been marketed as a tool for smokers who want to stop using tobacco products (Figure 9.12). E-cigarettes are controversial, however, because the US government has not approved e-cigarettes as a successful and safe form of smoking cessation. E-cigarettes can also lead to nicotine addiction if used by adolescents and other first-time smokers. Because of these risks, the use of e-cigarettes is opposed by the Food and Drug Administration, the American Cancer Society, and the American Heart Association.

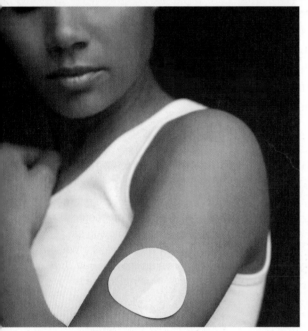

Figure 9.11

Nicotine gum and nicotine patches help tobacco addicts quit smoking. *How helpful do you think these products might be to a person who is quitting smoking?*

nicotine replacement
a method of battling addiction in which tobacco users gradually reduce their nicotine consumption

stimulus control
the technique of avoiding situations that may lead to drug use

Medications Prescribed by a Doctor

Some medications prescribed by a doctor help smokers quit by simulating *dopamine*, a chemical in the brain that leads people to experience the same type of effects caused by nicotine use. People who take these medications may be better able to cope with the withdrawal effects caused by reducing their intake of nicotine.

Self-Management Strategies

Self-management strategies often involve identifying situations that trigger the desire for tobacco use and developing techniques to resist temptation. Once tobacco users understand the situations or feelings that lead them to want to use tobacco, they can respond with two techniques—stimulus control and response substitution. *Stimulus control* involves trying to avoid tempting situations and managing feelings that lead to nicotine use.

With *response substitution*, people learn to respond to difficult feelings and situations with behaviors other than smoking by using stress management, relaxation, and coping skills.

Additional Strategies and Resources

Some people need additional support to quit smoking. The following are additional strategies and resources for treating an addiction to nicotine.

- Attend individual or group counseling.
- Talk to a school guidance counselor, doctor, teacher, or other trusted adult.
- Call a telephone helpline that provides free counseling to those who are trying to quit using tobacco.
- Research online resources for help with quitting.

Figure 9.12

Leading health agencies oppose the use of e-cigarettes as a form of smoking cessation.

response substitution
a technique in which people train themselves to respond to stress with healthy methods of coping and relaxation, rather than smoking

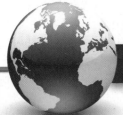

Local and Global Health
Smoking Rates around the World

Rates of smoking vary considerably by country. People who live in wealthier countries are less likely to smoke than those who live in poorer countries. One explanation for this difference is that people who are wealthy tend to have higher levels of education. People with higher levels of education may be more aware of the substantial health hazards of using tobacco.

Rates of smoking also vary by gender. In most countries, men are more likely to smoke than women. Health experts believe these differences in smoking rates may reflect differences in gender roles. For example, women smoking may be viewed as less acceptable than men smoking in some parts of the world. In addition, women may not have access to money or be able to afford cigarettes in some countries.

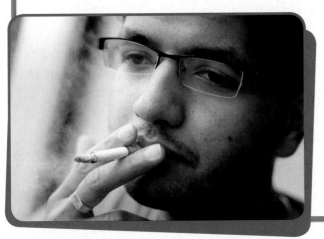

Percentage of Smokers around the World		
	% Men Who Smoke	% Women Who Smoke
East Asia and Pacific	62	5
Europe and Central Asia	53	16
Latin America and Caribbean	39	22
Middle East and North Africa	38	7
South Asia	20	1
Sub-Saharan Africa	28	8

Thinking Critically

1. Hypothesize why smoking rates among men are higher in East Asia, the Pacific, Europe, and Central Asia than in other areas.
2. What steps can governments take to decrease smoking rates in their respective countries? Which strategies would you support? Which would you oppose?

Prevention

Because most adult smokers picked up the habit as teenagers, experts believe the best way to reduce the smoking rate is to prevent smoking. Government-based regulations, awareness of physical and social consequences, and personal skills for refusing tobacco are among the prevention strategies used today.

Government-Based Strategies

Smoking costs society an estimated $289 billion a year in healthcare costs. Given the serious threat to public health associated with the use of tobacco products, governments have often focused on preventing nicotine use and helping tobacco users quit. These strategies may involve state and federal laws that regulate the sale, use, cost, and advertisement of tobacco products.

Banning the Sale of Tobacco Products. The sale of tobacco is prohibited to anyone younger than 18 years of age. As of 2010, the United States also banned the sale of cigarettes in vending machines, except in establishments where people younger than 18 years of age are not allowed. Government programs have also banned the sale of all candy- and fruit-flavored cigarettes.

Banning Smoking in Public Places. Some of the most effective government regulations to prevent smoking are laws that ban smoking in public places (Figure 9.13). These bans help smokers quit in several ways. First, they make it more difficult for people to find places to smoke. The bans reduce the number of places that serve as triggers in a smoker's environment. Smoking bans also help reduce exposure to secondhand smoke, which means fewer heart attacks, less coughing, and improved breathing.

Increasing Taxes on Cigarettes. Cigarettes are expensive. When people continue to smoke, they have a lot less money to buy other things they want and need. Raising federal, state, and municipal taxes on tobacco products can cause people to quit smoking and even discourage them from starting to smoke (Figure 9.14). Higher prices for cigarettes and smokeless tobacco increase the negative consequences of smoking because smokers must cut back on other expenses to continue funding their addiction. Increasing the cost of cigarettes is an especially effective way to decrease smoking in teenagers, who generally do not have much income.

Requiring Warning Labels on Packaging. Another approach to prevent smoking and encourage quitting is to increase people's awareness of the health risk of cigarettes. All cigarette packs and advertisements must have warning labels stating the risks associated with smoking.

Mass Media Antismoking Campaigns

Antismoking campaigns in mass media have also been shown to help prevent smoking. Successful antismoking campaigns emphasize long-term

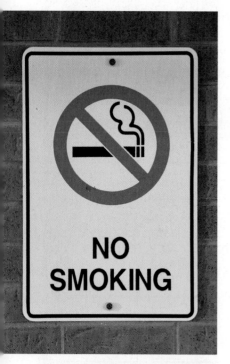

Figure 9.13

Smoking bans encourage people not to smoke and protect people from secondhand smoke. *Are there any places in your community where smoking is still allowed?*

health effects, smelly breath and clothes, strategies for refusing tobacco offers, and the fact that most teenagers do not smoke. Teenagers who regularly see these advertisements and campaigns are less likely to smoke.

Social Costs of Smoking

Awareness of the social cost of smoking is another strategy used to prevent tobacco use. Surveys have found that many nonsmoking teenagers view smoking as "gross." Teenagers who smoke may be viewed as unappealing by their peers, including potential dating partners. Smokers may also have to leave a social situation to have a cigarette, leading them to feel left out.

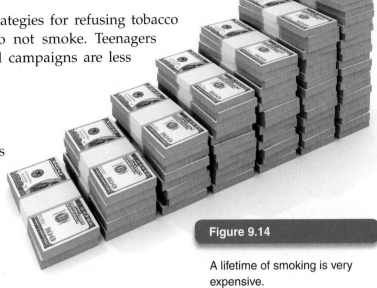

Figure 9.14

A lifetime of smoking is very expensive.

Research in Action

Antismoking Ads Can Work

The tobacco industry spends billions of dollars each year on advertisements that try to convince people to use tobacco products. Advertisements, however, can also be used to convince people not to use those products.

In one study, researchers showed a movie containing scenes of smoking to a group of ninth graders who reported being nonsmokers. Before the movie was shown, half the students watched an antismoking advertisement and the other half did not.

Students who did not see the antismoking advertisement responded more positively when they saw characters smoking than the other group of students. They also reported having more positive attitudes toward smokers and were more likely to smoke in the future.

None of these effects, however, were seen in students who saw the antismoking advertisement before the movie.

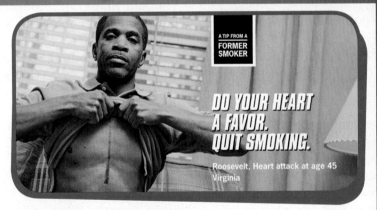

A TIP FROM A
FORMER SMOKER

DO YOUR HEART A FAVOR. QUIT SMOKING.

Roosevelt, Heart attack at age 45
Virginia

These students had more negative attitudes toward the movie characters who smoked and toward smoking in general.

Thinking Critically

1. What do the results of this study indicate about the influence of antismoking campaigns?

2. Based on the results of this study, do you think there should be a law that requires antismoking advertisements to be included in the previews of all movies showing smoking scenes? Why or why not?

Quitting Smoking

If you or someone you know wants to quit smoking, the following strategies can help.

- Set a "quit date" within the next month and circle that date on the calendar. Make a strong commitment to actually stop smoking on that date.

- Tell friends and family members about your quit date and ask them to support your efforts. Ask people who smoke not to smoke around you.

- Get rid of cigarettes and smoking accessories in your environment.

- Develop strategies for coping with nicotine cravings.

- Develop strategies for refusing cigarette offers from other people.

- Remind yourself of the benefits of quitting, including a longer life, more spending money, and increased stamina.

- Reward yourself for quitting. Buy something with the money you saved by not smoking.

- If you slip up and have a cigarette, quickly renew your focus on the goal of quitting. Do not let one lapse lead to a return of the old behavior.

Skills for Resisting Tobacco

Resisting peer pressure to begin smoking can be challenging. Three sets of skills—refusal, literacy, and critical thinking skills—can help you prepare for and respond to situations that may involve tobacco use.

Refusal Skills. If you don't want to smoke or want to quit smoking, spend time with people who do not smoke. Make sure the people around you know you don't want to use tobacco or be around their secondhand smoke. Firmly explain the reasons behind your decision. Stick to your decision and refuse to give in (Figure 9.15).

Figure 9.15

While resisting peer pressure may be difficult, you can improve if you practice your refusal skills. *Imagine that your best friend is offering you a cigarette. How would you turn down the offer?*

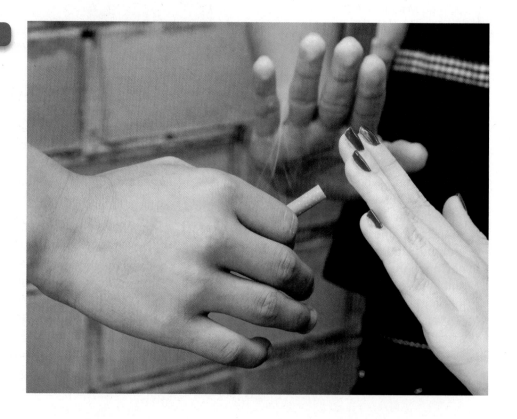

Before you find yourself in situations in which you are offered tobacco, imagine these situations and how you might respond. Play out each situation in your mind and practice responses.

For example, suppose that when you hang out with a certain group of friends, several of them offer you cigarettes. Your response may be, "No thanks, I want to keep my lungs in peak condition for track and field." You may also say, "I don't want my hair, clothes, and breath to smell like cigarettes," or "I like my lungs. I don't want to damage them." Practice your responses. Your true friends will support your decision not to smoke.

Literacy and Critical Thinking Skills. Since they are not allowed to advertise on television, radio, or billboards, tobacco companies use sneaky strategies to convince teenagers to use their products. Because an estimated 480,000 Americans die every year from diseases caused by tobacco, the tobacco industry must somehow convince people to continue buying their products. Media literacy will help you recognize the tobacco industry's sneaky practices, and avoid being tricked by them.

Tobacco companies have changed the types of products they sell to increase their appeal to teenagers. Some tobacco products look like mints, toothpicks, breath strips, and flavored candy. These products also have names that make them appear more like a sugary snack than an addictive tobacco product. To advertise these products, some tobacco companies may try to mimic popular social media trends to appeal to a younger audience.

Use critical thinking skills to analyze tobacco products and messages from tobacco companies. People who understand the manipulative nature of tobacco advertisements are better able to resist them. Analyze advertisements by reminding yourself of the serious physical, social, and financial costs of tobacco use.

Lesson 9.3 Review

Know and Understand Assess

1. What health benefits do smokers experience after just a few days of quitting?
2. List the three main strategies for quitting tobacco use and briefly explain each strategy.
3. Identify four government-based strategies used to discourage tobacco use.
4. Briefly describe the social costs of smoking.
5. Describe three sets of skills you can use to resist tobacco and give an example of each.

Analyze and Apply

6. Many communities run treatment and intervention programs for tobacco use. Research the treatment and intervention resources in your school and community.

7. Explain how the banning of smoking in public areas has affected both smokers and nonsmokers.
8. Compare and contrast the positive and negative effects that the media has on tobacco use.

Real World | Health

A Pack a Day Visit a local grocery or convenience store and determine the average price of a pack of cigarettes. Assuming that someone smokes a pack a day, list the cost of cigarettes for one week, one month, one year, and five years. Write a paragraph on the monetary costs of smoking and what else someone might do with that money over the short- and long-term.

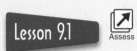

Lesson 9.1

Assess

The Health Effects of Tobacco

Key Terms

asthma
carbon monoxide
carcinogens
chronic bronchitis
chronic obstructive
   pulmonary disease
   (COPD)
emphysema
leukoplakia
nicotine
secondhand smoke
smokeless tobacco
tar
tobacco

Key Points

- Nicotine is the addictive substance that makes tobacco products difficult to quit using.
- Tobacco use impacts the cardiovascular system by increasing the speed and pressure of blood flow, which makes the heart work harder to pump blood and damages the blood vessels.
- Tobacco use and smoke can lead to increased risk factors for respiratory diseases and illnesses.
- Smokeless tobacco is just as addictive as cigarettes.
- Secondhand smoke causes long-term illnesses and diseases and is particularly harmful for pregnant women, infants, and children.

Check Your Understanding

1. The addictive, toxic substance present in all tobacco products is called _____.
   A. nicotine
   B. tar
   C. adrenaline
   D. carbon monoxide

2. A _____ is a cancer-causing agent.
   A. carcinogen
   B. stimulant
   C. blood clot
   D. leukoplakia

3. Which of the following is *not* a form of smokeless tobacco?
   A. chewing tobacco
   B. snuff
   C. hookah
   D. dissolvable tobacco

4. The condition characterized by thickened, white, leathery-looking spots on the inside of the mouth is called _____.
   A. chronic bronchitis
   B. emphysema
   C. gum disease
   D. leukoplakia

5. *True or false?* Exposure to secondhand smoke does not have major health consequences.

6. **Critical Thinking.** If you had a close friend or family member who smoked, how might you advise him or her to quit smoking?

Lesson 9.2

Assess

Why People Use Tobacco

Key Terms

addiction
dependence
peer pressure
substance abuse
tolerance
withdrawal

Key Points

- The four stages of substance abuse are experimentation, regular use, tolerance, and dependence and addiction.
- People who are addicted to a substance have both a physical and psychological dependence on that substance.
- Identity exploration is one factor that leads people to begin using tobacco.
- Attitudes of friends and family toward tobacco use strongly influence an individual's attitudes toward tobacco use.
- Tobacco use in the media may encourage tobacco use among adolescents.

Check Your Understanding

7. Smoking a cigarette "just to try it" is an example of behavior in the first stage of substance abuse, called _____.
   A. dependence
   B. tolerance
   C. regular use
   D. experimentation

8. A _____ occurs when a smoker needs to consume larger amounts of nicotine to experience the same effects that nicotine provided in the past.
    A. dependence
    B. tolerance
    C. withdrawal symptom
    D. stimulant

9. *True or false?* Identity exploration, or trying out a new identity, is one reason why some people begin to smoke.

10. The influence of peers on an individual is called _____ pressure.
    A. peer
    B. media
    C. economical
    D. authoritative

11. **Critical Thinking.** Many of the people who began smoking decades ago were unaware of the addictive power and the negative health consequences of tobacco use. Most people today know about these dangers, yet some still choose to smoke. Why might a person choose to smoke today?

Lesson 9.3

Assess

Treating and Preventing Nicotine Addiction

Key Terms

laryngectomy
nicotine replacement
response substitution
stimulus control

Key Points

- Quitting tobacco use is challenging because of nicotine dependence.
- Treatment options for quitting tobacco include using nicotine replacement, taking medicines prescribed by a doctor, and developing self-management techniques.
- Government-based strategies, mass media antismoking campaigns, awareness of the social costs of smoking, and using skills for resisting tobacco are prevention strategies for tobacco use.

- Refusal skills, literacy skills, and critical thinking skills are necessary skill sets for refusing tobacco offers from peers and the media.

Check Your Understanding

12. *True or false?* A laryngectomy is a surgical procedure in which the larynx is removed, requiring the person to breathe through an opening in his or her neck.

13. Which of the following treatment options involves lessening withdrawal symptoms and cravings by gradually reducing nicotine intake in the body?
    A. nicotine replacement
    B. stimulus control
    C. response substitution
    D. surgery

14. A technique that involves trying to avoid tempting situations and manage feelings that lead to nicotine use is called _____.
    A. nicotine replacement
    B. stimulus control
    C. response substitution
    D. refusal skills

15. Choosing to play basketball with friends instead of smoking a cigarette when experiencing a nicotine craving is an example of _____.
    A. nicotine replacement
    B. stimulus control
    C. response substitution
    D. time management

16. *True or false?* The US government requires all cigarette packs to have warning labels stating the health risks associated with smoking.

17. Having your clothes smell like cigarette smoke is an example of a _____ cost of smoking.
    A. financial
    B. physical
    C. mental
    D. social

18. **Critical Thinking.** Marc is hanging out with a group of friends who begin to smoke cigarettes. They pressure Marc to try one, but he is not interested in smoking. What skills can Marc use to respond to this situation?

Health and Wellness Skills

19. **Access Information.** Tobacco smoke and electronic nicotine delivery systems (ENDS) contain many harmful chemicals. Using the Internet and other resources, identify about a dozen of these chemicals, and research each one. Then list other products that contain each chemical and explain how these chemicals can harm the body.

20. **Communicate with Others.** Peer pressure in schools can create a *social multiplier effect*, which is the concept that the behavior of peers establishes a perceived norm that influences a person's behavior. Because of this effect, it is difficult for people to defy the perceived norm. In small groups, research this effect further and discuss how the effect is present in your school. Using the skills you learned in this chapter, film a video in which you role-play ways to resist peer pressure (including the social multiplier effect) to make wise decisions about substance use.

21. **Advocate for Health.** A public service announcement, or *PSA*, is a message broadcasted to the public through some form of mass media. A PSA attempts to raise awareness about a social or community issue. Research some popular PSAs and then create your own PSA with an anti-tobacco theme.

22. **Analyze Influences.** Write a letter to one of your state-elected officials outlining the influences of tobacco on society, and advocating for anti-tobacco laws.

Hands-On Activity

Smoking and Your Body

While smoking can have a negative effect on your entire body, it can specifically affect your respiratory, cardiovascular, immune, musculoskeletal, and digestive systems. This activity will illustrate how smoking can affect each of these body systems.

Materials Needed

- large crafting paper
- markers
- pens or pencils
- research resources

Steps for this Activity

1. Choose several of your classmates to work with and choose one of the five body systems listed above to research. Your teacher may assign a body system to your group.

2. Research the parts and pathways of your chosen body system, and how smoking affects this body system. Your school librarian can help you find research resources, which might include books, journals, magazines, or the Internet. When completing Internet research, use credible websites that will give medically accurate information. Your school may have access to credible Internet sites specifically designed for this type of research.

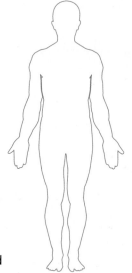

3. Have a group member lie down on a long, wide piece of crafting paper, and then trace the outline of his or her body.

4. Inside the body outline, draw and label the parts and pathways of your group's body system.

5. Outside the body outline, list how cigarettes affect this body system.

6. Hang your group's body poster in the hallway of your school to show other students the dangers of smoking. Obtain permission, if needed.

Core Skills

Math Practice

The graph below shows the trend in smoking rates for adults over a period of almost 50 years. The graph also shows the trend for a 20-year period. Analyze the graph and answer the following questions.

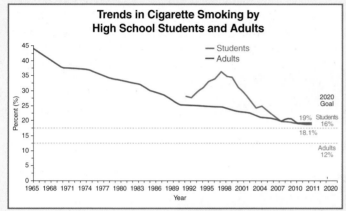

23. What has been the general trend of smoking among adults?
    A. The smoking rate has increased.
    B. The smoking rate has decreased.
    C. There is no trend.
    D. The smoking rate has increased, decreased, and increased again.

24. What has been the general trend of smoking among high school students?
    A. The smoking rate has increased.
    B. The smoking rate has decreased.
    C. There is no trend.
    D. The smoking rate has increased and then decreased.

25. Compare the smoking rate for high school students when data was last collected to the high school student goal (percentage) projected for 2020. What is the difference in percentage between these smoking rates?
    A. 3%
    B. 2%
    C. 1.9%
    D. 1%

Reading and Writing Practice

Read the passage below and then answer the questions.

Addiction to nicotine can happen quickly. Researchers found that 25% of teenage smokers reported feeling addicted within 30 days of having their first cigarette. One in ten of the teenagers reported feeling addicted within only two days of smoking their first cigarette. Nicotine is the chemical in tobacco that causes people to become addicted to tobacco products. Nicotine dependence is one of the most common and powerful types of chemical dependence.

26. What is the author's main idea in this passage?
    A. Studies conducted about nicotine's addictive effects are inconclusive.
    B. Teenagers smoke because they don't think they will become addicted.
    C. One in ten teenagers smoke cigarettes.
    D. Addiction to nicotine can happen quickly.

27. According to the study mentioned, what percentage of teenage smokers reported feeling addicted within 30 days of having their first cigarette?
    A. 30%
    B. 25%
    C. 10%
    D. 1%

28. According to the study, what percentage of teenagers reported feeling addicted within only two days of smoking their first cigarette?
    A. 30%
    B. 25%
    C. 10%
    D. 1%

29. What portion of adults started smoking at age 30?
    A. The study does not say.
    B. The majority of adults.
    C. Almost no adults.
    D. 30% of adults.

30. Write a few sentences in response to the last sentence of the passage. What evidence can you cite from the chapter to support this claim?

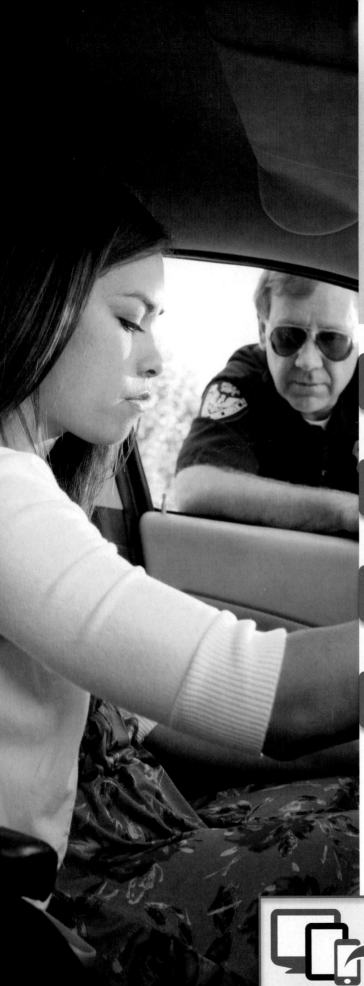

Chapter 10
Alcohol

While studying this chapter, look for the activity icon to:

- **review** vocabulary with e-flash cards and games;
- **assess** learning with quizzes and online exercises;
- **expand** knowledge with animations and activities; and
- **listen** to pronunciation of key terms in the audio glossary.

G-WLEARNING.com

www.g-wlearning.com/health/

Take this quiz to see what you do and do not know about why people use alcohol products, and how alcohol use affects health. If you cannot answer a question, pay extra attention to that topic as you study this chapter.

1. *Identify each statement as* True, False, *or* It Depends. *Choose* It Depends *if a statement is true in some cases, but false in others.*

2. *Revise each* False *statement to make it true.*

3. *Explain the circumstances in which each* It Depends *statement is true and when it is false.*

Health and Wellness IQ Assess

1. Alcohol is a stimulant, meaning it excites or arouses the central nervous system.	True	False	It Depends
2. People who have a blood alcohol concentration (BAC) of .08 or higher are considered "legally impaired."	True	False	It Depends
3. Pregnant women should only consume moderate amounts of alcohol.	True	False	It Depends
4. People who have consumed alcohol often feel very relaxed and happy, and are therefore less likely to show aggression.	True	False	It Depends
5. Each year alcohol use contributes to over 4,300 deaths of people under age 21 in the United States.	True	False	It Depends
6. Alcohol poisoning can cause permanent brain damage.	True	False	It Depends
7. Children of alcoholics are less likely to develop a problem with alcohol when they are adults.	True	False	It Depends
8. High school and college students tend to overestimate their peers' frequency of and comfort with alcohol use.	True	False	It Depends
9. Unintentionally encouraging an addict's unhealthy behaviors is not enabling.	True	False	It Depends
10. Medications can help alcoholics stop drinking.	True	False	It Depends

Setting the Scene

In the United States, you must be 21 years of age to buy alcohol. Some teenagers may not understand why this age limit exists. After all, at 18 years of age you can vote for the president, join the military, and buy cigarettes—you can even buy a gun. The law that sets 21 as the minimum age for purchasing alcohol was adopted in 1984, after concerns were raised about serious problems caused by teenage alcohol consumption. Unfortunately, even with this law, many teenagers have serious problems due to alcohol use. Alcohol use contributes to the deaths of more than 4,300 Americans younger than 21 years of age each year.

This chapter examines how alcohol impacts the body, the short- and long-term consequences of alcohol use, and factors that lead people to use—and abuse—alcohol. You will also learn some strategies for preventing and treating alcohol abuse, and how you can help if someone you know has a problem with alcohol.

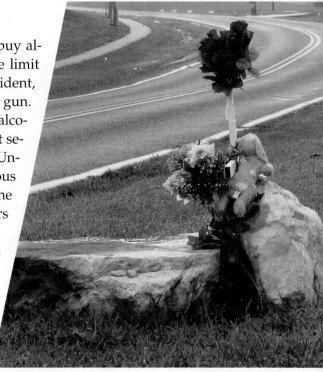

How Does Alcohol Impact Your Body?

Key Terms   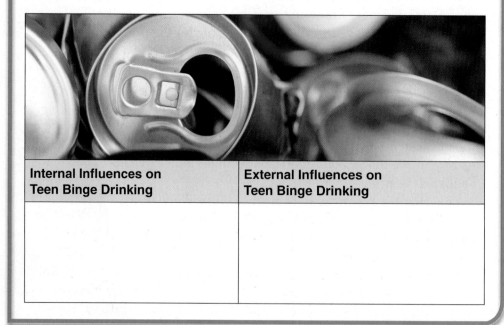 E-Flash Cards

In this lesson, you will learn the meanings of the following key terms.

alcohol

blood alcohol concentration (BAC)

depressant

hangover

inhibition

metabolize

Before You Read

Give One, Get One

Fold a piece of paper in half to make two columns. Label one column "Give One" and the other column "Get One" as shown below. Before reading the lesson, list five words you know that are related to alcohol or alcohol use under "Give One." When you are finished, walk around the room and exchange words with your fellow students to put in the "Get One" column.

Give One	Get One

Lesson Objectives

After studying this lesson, you will be able to

- explain how alcohol is distributed throughout the body;

- analyze the effects of alcohol on the brain;

- assess how blood alcohol concentration (BAC) accumulates in the bloodstream;

- relate the consumption of alcohol to hangover symptoms; and

- identify five factors that influence an individual's BAC level.

Warm-Up Activity

Binge Drinking Influences

In a table like the one shown below, write three internal and three external influences on teen binge drinking. Share your ideas with your classmates and borrow theirs until you have at least 10 influences total in your chart.

Internal Influences on Teen Binge Drinking	External Influences on Teen Binge Drinking

The word **alcohol** is a general term used to describe different chemical compounds with common properties. Ethanol, one of these compounds, is the active ingredient in alcoholic drinks (Figure 10.1). When experts talk about an alcoholic drink they are referring to any drink that contains 0.6 ounces (14.0 grams or 1.2 tablespoons) of pure alcohol. This amount of alcohol can be found in different types of "drinks", including

- 12 ounces of regular beer or a wine cooler;

- 8 ounces of malt liquor;

- 5 ounces of wine; and

- 1.5 ounces of 80-proof (40% alcohol) distilled spirits or liquor, such as gin, rum, vodka, or whiskey. The *proof* stated on a bottle of liquor is twice the percentage of alcohol.

Regardless of how alcohol is consumed, this substance has a powerful effect on all parts of the body.

When someone consumes an alcoholic beverage, the alcohol passes from the stomach into the small intestine, where it is quickly absorbed into the bloodstream and distributed throughout the body. This means that when a person drinks alcohol, every single cell in the body is affected, including the cells in the muscles, the nervous system, and the brain.

alcohol
a general term used to describe a drink that contains a certain amount of ethanol

depressant
a substance that slows the central nervous system and causes chemical changes in the brain

inhibition
the psychological restraint that discourages people from engaging in dangerous behaviors

Effects of Alcohol on the Brain

Alcohol is a **depressant**, which means it is a type of drug that slows down the central nervous system. When alcohol reaches the brain, it changes the level of chemicals called *neurotransmitters*. These chemical changes cause slurred speech, sluggish body movements, and interference with the ability to think clearly.

Alcohol impacts particular parts of the brain in different ways (Figure 10.2 on the next page). In the *cerebral cortex*, which controls thought processing and consciousness, alcohol reduces the brain's ability to process information that is seen or heard. This makes it difficult for a person under the influence of alcohol to think clearly. **Inhibition**, or the psychological restraint that keeps people from taking dangerous risks, is also reduced.

Alcohol also disrupts normal functioning in the *cerebellum*, which controls movement and balance. A person under the influence of alcohol has difficulty walking steadily and coordinating other body movements.

In the *hypothalamus* and *pituitary gland*, which control the release of hormones, alcohol use may increase sexual arousal, but decrease the ability to perform sexually.

The *medulla* controls automatic functions in the body, such as breathing and consciousness. Alcohol use disrupts functioning in the medulla and causes sleepiness, slow breathing, and lower body temperature.

12 ounces of beer   5 ounces of wine   1.5 ounces of liquor

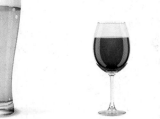

Figure 10.1

Although the total liquid ounces vary considerably in the drinks shown above, the drinks have exactly the same amount of pure alcohol. *If the amount of alcohol is the same, why might a person be less likely to become intoxicated drinking the beer, as opposed to the liquor?*

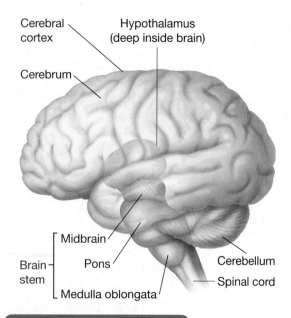

Cerebral cortex

Hypothalamus (deep inside brain)

Cerebrum

Midbrain

Brain stem

Pons

Medulla oblongata

Cerebellum

Spinal cord

Figure 10.2

Alcohol disrupts your inhibition and mental functioning by affecting multiple parts of your brain.

metabolize
term that means to break down ingested substances

blood alcohol concentration (BAC)
the percentage of alcohol that is present in a person's blood

At low levels, drinking alcohol usually leads to relatively small changes in the brain's chemical levels. When people consume small amounts of alcohol, they experience minor effects. People who have had one drink may feel less inhibited, speak more loudly, and use more body movements.

When a person consumes larger amounts of alcohol, however, especially in a short period of time, there is a corresponding large change in chemical levels in the brain. These chemical changes can have substantial effects, including a decrease in reaction time and an increase in accident risk when driving. Overconsumption of alcohol can result in memory loss, which is sometimes referred to as *blacking out*. Large amounts of alcohol can also cause a person's breathing to slow dramatically and body temperature to drop. This can lead to life-threatening health problems and even death.

Blood Alcohol Concentration

Once alcohol is consumed, it stays in the body until the liver can *metabolize* it, or break it down. Generally, the liver can process between .25 and .50 ounces of alcohol every hour.

When someone drinks a lot of alcohol in a short period of time, the body is unable to break down the alcohol fast enough. As a result, the alcohol builds up in the bloodstream. *Blood alcohol concentration (BAC)* is the percentage of alcohol that is in a person's blood. The percentage is based on a comparison of the amount of alcohol in a person's body and the amount of blood. For example, a BAC of 0.08 means there are 8 parts alcohol to 10,000 parts other blood components. People who have a BAC of 0.08 or above are considered legally impaired, also known as *intoxicated* or *drunk*. About two to four alcoholic drinks would result in a BAC of 0.08, depending on a variety of factors. A person who is intoxicated shows substantial physical and mental impairments (Figure 10.3).

Factors Influencing Blood Alcohol Concentration

The main factor that influences how much alcohol affects people is the level of alcohol in their blood. People who consume more alcohol have a higher level of alcohol in their bloodstream, which causes more significant effects. The liver can only metabolize a certain amount of alcohol at a time. People who drink very quickly will, therefore, experience more substantial side effects from drinking. These people will have a greater concentration of alcohol in their blood.

Even if two people drink the exact same amount of alcohol in the same amount of time, their blood alcohol concentration (BAC) level may still be different. This is because the level of alcohol in the blood is also influenced by other factors, such as body weight, gender, food consumption, and ethnicity.

BACs and Impairment

As BAC Increases, So Does Impairment

Same Alcohol Intake (4 drinks) Different BACs

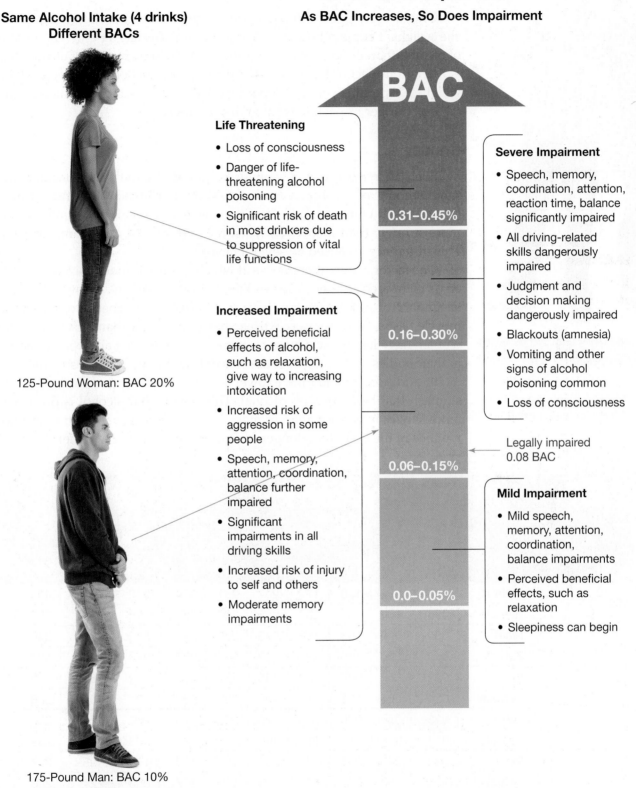

Life Threatening

- Loss of consciousness
- Danger of life-threatening alcohol poisoning
- Significant risk of death in most drinkers due to suppression of vital life functions

Increased Impairment

- Perceived beneficial effects of alcohol, such as relaxation, give way to increasing intoxication
- Increased risk of aggression in some people
- Speech, memory, attention, coordination, balance further impaired
- Significant impairments in all driving skills
- Increased risk of injury to self and others
- Moderate memory impairments

BAC

0.31–0.45%

0.16–0.30%

0.06–0.15%

0.0–0.05%

125-Pound Woman: BAC 20%

175-Pound Man: BAC 10%

Severe Impairment

- Speech, memory, coordination, attention, reaction time, balance significantly impaired
- All driving-related skills dangerously impaired
- Judgment and decision making dangerously impaired
- Blackouts (amnesia)
- Vomiting and other signs of alcohol poisoning common
- Loss of consciousness

Legally impaired 0.08 BAC

Mild Impairment

- Mild speech, memory, attention, coordination, balance impairments
- Perceived beneficial effects, such as relaxation
- Sleepiness can begin

Figure 10.3

The higher a person's BAC, the more impaired he or she becomes. Many factors, including gender and weight, affect BAC.

Body Weight

One of the biggest influences on a person's BAC is how much he or she weighs. People who weigh less are more affected by a given amount of alcohol than people who weigh more. The same amount of alcohol has a different impact if it is distributed throughout the body of someone who weighs 100 pounds versus 200 pounds. This is one reason why alcohol can have a stronger impact on women than on men.

Gender

Even if a man and a woman weigh the same and consume the same amount of alcohol, a woman will have a higher BAC than a man (Figure 10.5). Women usually feel the effects of alcohol more quickly and more strongly than men, even when they are drinking the same amount. This difference is caused by several factors.

One factor is the different rate at which alcohol is metabolized in women as compared to men. Women have a higher amount of fat and a lower amount of muscle in their bodies. Alcohol is absorbed more easily in muscle tissue, because muscle tissue has more water than fat tissue. Since women have less muscle mass than men, alcohol is not absorbed as easily in their bodies and becomes more concentrated in their bloodstream.

In addition, women have lower levels of a particular enzyme in the stomach that helps process alcohol. This means that alcohol is processed more slowly in women than in men, and thus a larger amount of alcohol remains in the body for a longer period of time, causing a higher BAC.

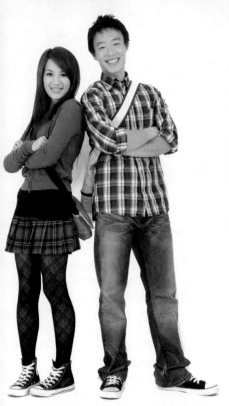

Figure 10.4

If these teens drank the same amount of alcohol, whose BAC would probably be higher? Why?

Figure 10.5 Blood Alcohol Concentration by Gender and Weight											
Number of Drinks		1	2	3	4	5	6	7	8	9	10
Weight (lbs.)											
100	Male	.043	.087	.130	.174	.217	.261	.304	.348	.391	.435
	Female	.050	.101	.152	.203	.253	.304	.355	.406	.456	.507
125	Male	.034	.069	.103	.139	.173	.209	.242	.278	.312	.346
	Female	.040	.080	.120	.162	.202	.244	.282	.324	.364	.404
150	Male	.029	.058	.087	.116	.145	.174	.203	.232	.261	.290
	Female	.034	.068	.101	.135	.169	.203	.237	.271	.304	.338
175	Male	.025	.050	.075	.100	.125	.150	.175	.200	.225	.250
	Female	.029	.058	.087	.117	.146	.175	.204	.233	.262	.292
200	Male	.022	.043	.065	.087	.108	.130	.152	.174	.195	.217
	Female	.026	.050	.076	.101	.126	.152	.177	.203	.227	.253
225	Male	.019	.039	.058	.078	.097	.117	.136	.156	.175	.195
	Female	.022	.045	.068	.091	.113	.136	.159	.182	.204	.227
250	Male	.017	.035	.052	.070	.087	.105	.122	.139	.156	.173
	Female	.020	.041	.061	.082	.101	.122	.142	.162	.182	.202

Food Consumed

When a person consumes alcohol while eating food, or shortly after eating food, the effects of alcohol are felt more slowly. In this case, the stomach must process the alcohol at the same time it is digesting food. As a result, the alcohol is absorbed more slowly into the bloodstream because it cannot be processed as quickly by the stomach (Figure 10.6).

The type of food that is consumed can also impact the length of digestion time and the speed of alcohol absorption. The stomach takes a longer time to process foods that are high in fat. Researchers in one study found that people who drank alcohol after eating a full meal—meaning a meal that included fat, protein, and carbohydrates—took three times as long to absorb the alcohol as people who drank alcohol on an empty stomach.

Ethnicity

Ethnicity may also influence a person's blood alcohol concentration. For example, some research suggests that up to 50% of people who are of Asian heritage have difficulty metabolizing alcohol. This difficulty is caused by a problem with one of the enzymes in the liver that processes alcohol. People with this enzyme problem experience unpleasant side effects after drinking alcohol, including facial flushing, nausea, headache, dizziness, and rapid heartbeat.

The Physiology of a Hangover

The consequences of alcohol consumption continue even after most, or even all, of the alcohol has left a person's body (Figure 10.7 on the next page). Most people who engage in heavy drinking experience a *hangover*, a term that describes the negative symptoms caused by excessive alcohol use. Symptoms may include

- tiredness
- headaches
- muscle aches
- nausea and vomiting
- dizziness and a feeling that the room is spinning
- increased sensitivity to light and sound
- difficulty sleeping
- thirst
- shakiness
- depression, anxiety, and irritability
- difficulty concentrating

When a person drinks alcohol, it enters the bloodstream and circulates throughout the body. When alcohol reaches the brain, it causes the pituitary gland to stop producing a hormone called *vasopressin*. This hormone

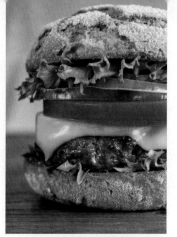
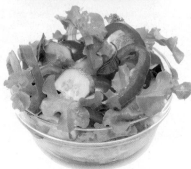

Figure 10.6

How would eating the burger, as compared to the salad affect a person's BAC? Explain.

hangover
term for the uncomfortable physical symptoms caused by excessive alcohol consumption

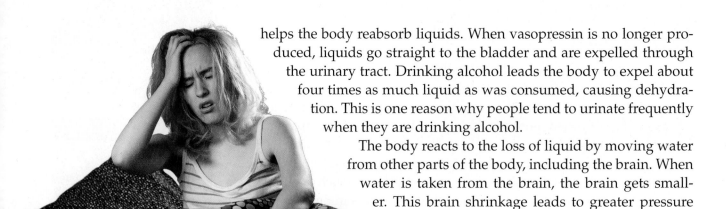

helps the body reabsorb liquids. When vasopressin is no longer produced, liquids go straight to the bladder and are expelled through the urinary tract. Drinking alcohol leads the body to expel about four times as much liquid as was consumed, causing dehydration. This is one reason why people tend to urinate frequently when they are drinking alcohol.

The body reacts to the loss of liquid by moving water from other parts of the body, including the brain. When water is taken from the brain, the brain gets smaller. This brain shrinkage leads to greater pressure on the membranes that connect the brain to the skull. The overall result is a headache, which is another common symptom of a hangover.

The frequent urination associated with drinking alcohol also causes the loss of essential substances from the body, including salt, potassium, and magnesium. Low levels of these nutrients cause problems with nerve and muscle function, which result in a feeling of tiredness, lack of coordination, and overall weakness.

Heavy alcohol use also causes other problems in the body, which contribute to common hangover feelings. Alcohol can irritate the lining of the stomach by increasing the production of stomach acid. This is one reason why people who drink alcohol may experience stomach pain and nausea, and may vomit. Alcohol use also causes increased blood flow, which can lead to headaches. In addition, alcohol use can cause decreases in blood sugar, which lead to feelings of weakness, shakiness, and fatigue.

Figure 10.7

Pretend you are a doctor. Explain to the girl above why her hangover is causing her to feel so miserable.

Lesson 10.1 Review

Know and Understand Assess

1. What is the active chemical compound in alcohol?
2. Describe the effect of a depressant on the central nervous system.
3. Define *blood alcohol concentration (BAC)*.
4. List at least ten possible symptoms of a hangover.
5. Identify four factors that influence the level of blood alcohol concentration in an individual's bloodstream.

Analyze and Apply

6. Why does alcohol consumption reduce a person's inhibition?
7. Why is drinking a lot of alcohol in a relatively short period of time overwhelming for the body?

Real World Health

Imagine that you write an advice column for your school newspaper. It is your job to maturely answer all questions that get submitted to the newspaper. Suppose you receive a letter from a sophomore who wrote the following letter.

"My brother is in college. Ever since he turned 21, he has been drinking heavily every weekend. When I ask him why, he says because it is legal. I am really worried about his health. Can you please tell me how alcohol affects the body, especially the brain?"

Signed, Sophomore Sister

How would you respond to this letter?

The Effects of Alcohol on Health

Lesson Objectives

After studying this lesson, you will be able to

- assess the role alcohol plays in violence and fatal accidents;
- determine the severe consequences of binge drinking and identify signs of alcohol poisoning;
- relate alcohol use to long-term health consequences, including cardiovascular problems, gastrointestinal problems, some forms of cancer, neurological and cognitive functioning problems, and fetal alcohol syndrome;
- explain the risks of underage drinking; and
- identify the health benefits of moderate alcohol use in adults.

Key Terms   E-Flash Cards

In this lesson, you will learn the meanings of the following key terms.

alcohol poisoning
binge drinking
cirrhosis
driving under the influence (DUI)
fetal alcohol syndrome (FAS)

Warm-Up Activity

Decision-Making Process
You and your friends are at a party and your friends decide they want to drive home. You know they have been drinking heavily all night. What should you do? Identify which steps in the decision-making process you would use to address this situation. Write and act out a skit describing the scenario.

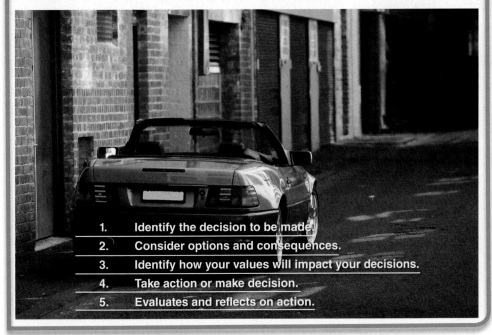

1. Identify the decision to be made.
2. Consider options and consequences.
3. Identify how your values will impact your decisions.
4. Take action or make decision.
5. Evaluates and reflects on action.

Before You Read

KWL Chart: Alcohol and Your Health
Create a KWL chart, as shown below, to map what you know, what you want to know, and what you have learned about the effect of alcohol on your health.

| K
What you Know | W
What you Want to know | L
What you have Learned |
|---|---|---|
| | | |

A lcohol use has a number of negative consequences for a person's health. In fact, excessive alcohol use is the third leading lifestyle-related cause of death in the United States, and the third leading cause of disease and injury worldwide.

This lesson examines the effects of alcohol use on health. This lesson also examines the very serious consequences of underage drinking.

Alcohol Use, Accidents, and Violence

driving under the influence (DUI)
a legal offense that occurs when a person has driven with a blood alcohol concentration at or over 0.08; a criminal offense in most states; also known as driving while intoxicated (DWI)

Alcohol slows down the central nervous system, which leads to a number of effects on the body. These include a decrease in reaction time, difficulty coordinating movements, and a decreased ability to plan and use good judgment (Figure 10.8).

One of the most serious physiological effects of alcohol is that it impacts a person's ability to process information. This means that people are not very good at planning, using good judgment, or thinking about the consequences of their behavior while drinking alcohol. This is one reason why people who have been drinking are more likely to engage in unsafe behaviors.

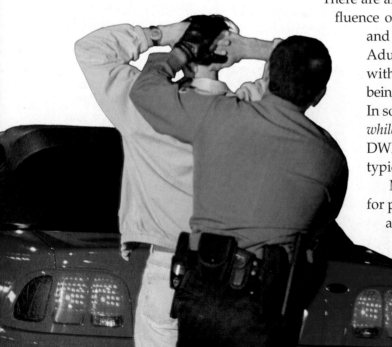

Motor Vehicle Accidents

Some of the most serious consequences of alcohol use result from people driving after drinking alcohol. In the United States, over 1.4 million drivers are arrested for driving under the influence of alcohol or drugs every year. Driving after alcohol use also leads to many deaths in the United States. Over 10,000 people die each year in alcohol-related motor vehicle crashes.

There are also legal consequences for driving under the influence of alcohol or drugs. For people 21 years of age and older, the legal BAC limit is 0.08 when driving. Adults who drive under the influence of alcohol with a BAC level of 0.08 or higher are at risk for being charged with *driving under the influence (DUI)*. In some states, this may also be referred to as *driving while intoxicated (DWI)*. If a driver receives a DUI or DWI, his or her license may be suspended. Penalties typically increase for repeat offenders.

Many states, however, follow a *zero-tolerance policy* for people younger than 21 years of age caught with any level of alcohol in their system while driving. Under zero-tolerance laws, there is no acceptable BAC level for people younger than 21 years of age. Penalties for violating a zero-tolerance policy vary from state to state.

Other Types of Accidents

Alcohol use is also associated with other types of accidents and injuries. People who have been drinking have higher rates of falls, burns, homicides, suicides, unintentional firearm injuries, electrical shocks, and incidents of near drowning. Alcohol use even increases the likelihood of death while bicycling and swimming.

Violence

People who have been drinking are more likely to behave violently than those who have not been drinking (Figure 10.9). About 35% of victims of some type of violent attack report that the person who assaulted them was under the influence of alcohol. Alcohol use is also associated with many cases of violence within families, including child abuse and neglect, and violence between romantic partners.

Binge Drinking and Alcohol Poisoning

Binge drinking is the consumption of large amounts of alcohol in a short period of time. For women, binge drinking refers to having four or more drinks during a single occasion. For men, binge drinking refers to having five or more drinks on a single occasion.

Binge drinking is much more common in men than women. It is also more common among young people than older adults. The majority of alcohol consumed by underage drinkers is in the form of binge drinks.

Binge drinking is associated with very dangerous consequences. One of the most serious short-term consequences of excessive alcohol use is alcohol poisoning.

Alcohol poisoning is a medical emergency that occurs when a high BAC suppresses the central nervous system. Loss of consciousness, low blood pressure and body temperature, and difficulty breathing can result

binge drinking
the consumption of a large amount of alcohol in a short period of time

alcohol poisoning
a medical emergency in which a person has consumed enough alcohol to suppress his or her central nervous system, and which is characterized by unconsciousness, low blood pressure and body temperature, difficulty breathing, and possible death

Figure 10.9

Alcohol's effect on a person's judgment often leads to violence. *Why do you think some people tend to become violent after drinking?*

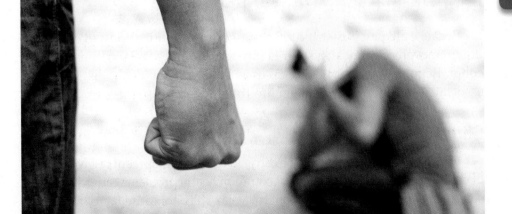

Rates of Binge Drinking by Age

Although 17% of all Americans report that they have engaged in binge drinking, the rate of binge drinking changes considerably across the life span (see table at right).

Why are there such differences in rates of binge drinking by age? One factor is that younger adults are less able than older adults to recognize the health, social, and legal consequences of their actions. They may be more comfortable with engaging in risky and potentially dangerous behaviors, which could include excessive alcohol use.

Analyzing Data

1. Which portion of the population engages in binge drinking the least?
2. Describe the general trend in the rate of binge drinking as a person ages.

Age Groups	Percent Who Have Engaged in Binge Drinking
18–24	28%
25–34	28%
35–44	19%
45–64	13%
65 and older	4%

from alcohol poisoning. Extreme levels of alcohol consumption—meaning a blood alcohol concentration of 0.40 or higher—can lead to permanent brain damage and death.

Signs of alcohol poisoning include

- mental confusion, stupor, coma, or unconsciousness;
- vomiting;
- seizures;
- slow or irregular breathing; and
- hypothermia (low body temperature), bluish skin color, and paleness.

Given the serious consequences of alcohol poisoning, you should know the danger signs and seek help immediately by calling 911 if you suspect a person is experiencing alcohol poisoning.

Long-Term Health Consequences

Because alcohol is distributed throughout the entire body, every single organ and physiological system is impacted when a person consumes alcohol. Regular consumption of excessive amounts of alcohol is, therefore, associated with serious and even life-threatening consequences.

Chronic Diseases

Excessive alcohol use over time can lead to the development of several types of chronic diseases. One of the most common health problems caused by excessive alcohol use is liver damage. High levels of alcohol cause fat to build up in the liver, which blocks blood flow. Eventually this lack of blood flow can cause *cirrhosis*, a buildup of scar tissue in the liver (Figures 10.10A & B on the next page). Cirrhosis is one of the 15 leading causes of death in the United States.

cirrhosis
a buildup of scar tissue in the liver; often leads to death

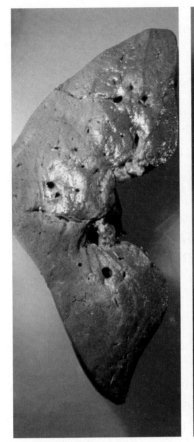

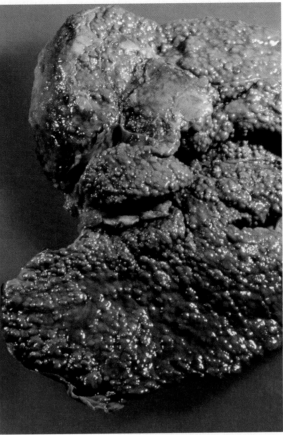

A. Healthy Liver

B. Liver Damaged by Cirrhosis

Figure 10.10

Repeated sessions of heavy drinking without time for the body to recover will damage the body's organs. Among the most common diseases caused by alcohol abuse are liver diseases. The cells in the liver shown in B died and hardened due to fat buildup from excessive drinking.

Heavy drinking can also lead to the development of other serious health problems, including

- cardiovascular problems, including an irregular heartbeat, high blood pressure, and heart attacks;

- gastrointestinal problems, including damage to the stomach and pancreas; and

- some types of cancer.

Brain and Cognitive Functioning

Excessive alcohol use can also have negative effects on the brain and cognitive functioning, which involves thinking. People who consume large amounts of alcohol on a regular basis can experience neurological problems, including dementia, stroke, memory problems, disorientation, and drowsiness.

Alcohol and Pregnancy

When a pregnant woman drinks, the alcohol she consumes passes from her bloodstream to the bloodstream of the fetus. Women who drink during pregnancy risk giving birth to babies with *fetal alcohol syndrome (FAS)*, a set of lifelong physical and mental birth defects. These defects include

- poor growth (both in the womb and after birth);

fetal alcohol syndrome (FAS)

term for a group of serious physical and mental birth defects caused by a woman's consumption of alcohol while pregnant

- decreased muscle tone and poor coordination;
- delayed development and problems with thinking, speech, movement, and social skills;
- heart defects; and
- facial defects.

Women who are pregnant, or even trying to become pregnant, should not consume any alcohol at all.

Consequences of Underage Drinking

Although it is illegal in all states for people younger than 21 years of age to drink, underage drinkers account for 11% of all alcohol consumed in the United States. Alcohol is the most commonly used and abused drug among youth in the United States.

Immediate Effects

Teenagers who drink alcohol, especially those who binge drink, are at greater risk of experiencing health problems, such as the following. These problems can affect teenagers' quality of life and athletic performance.

- *Physical problems.* Hangovers, illnesses, and injuries can result from alcohol consumption. These physical problems can interfere with school, work, and social relationships.

- *School problems.* Teenagers who consume alcohol may experience more school absences, difficulty focusing in class, and declining or failing grades. These consequences can have a negative impact on future educational plans.

- *Family and social problems.* Alcohol use can cause strained relationships with family and friends (Figure 10.11). Feelings of guilt and fear may result from disappointing loved ones. Teens may also withdraw from sports, clubs, or other extracurricular activities.

- *Legal problems.* Alcohol use is illegal for those younger than 21 years of age. Teenagers face legal consequences for alcohol consumption, which may include a suspended license for driving with any level of alcohol in their system.

Underage drinking is also associated with risky sexual behavior, which can have serious consequences. People who consume alcohol are more likely to engage in risky sexual behaviors, including unprotected sex and sex with multiple partners. These behaviors can result in unintended pregnancy, sexually transmitted infections, or HIV/AIDS. People who have

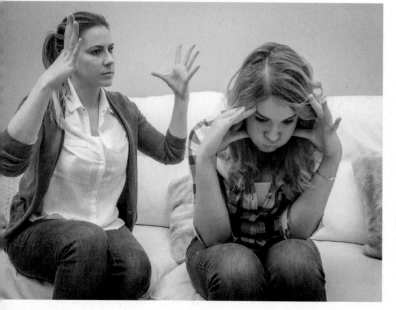

been drinking are also at a higher risk of experiencing sexual assault. Sexually risky behavior can cause feelings of guilt, fear of being caught, and fear of earning a bad reputation.

Long-Term Effects

Teenagers who start drinking also face serious lifelong consequences. Alcohol use during the teenage years can lead to changes in brain development and disrupt normal growth and sexual development. One recent study found that teenagers who binge drink show permanent changes in the brain, including problems with learning and memory (Figure 10.12).

Alcohol use can also lead to unsafe behaviors that can have long-term effects. Teenagers who drink alcohol are more likely to start abusing other drugs. Even drinking small amounts during the teenage years can lead to long-term problems with alcohol. In fact, people who start drinking before 15 years of age are five times more likely to develop alcohol dependence than those who begin drinking as adults. Teenagers who drink alcohol are also more likely to commit suicide or homicide.

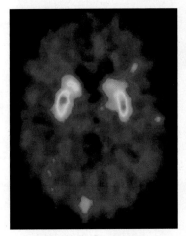

Alcoholic Damage   Normal

Figure 10.12

These PET scans illustrate the difference between a normal-functioning brain and a brain damaged by alcoholism. The red areas on these scans indicate normal mental and motor functioning. *Assume these are before and after PET scans. How much mental deterioration has resulted from alcohol abuse?*

Lesson 10.2 Review

Know and Understand Assess

1. Describe how alcohol impacts the central nervous system, and how these effects may lead to increased accidents and violence.
2. Define *binge drinking*.
3. Describe alcohol poisoning.
4. List at least four long-term consequences that can result from regular consumption of excessive amounts of alcohol.

Analyze and Apply

5. Why is it critical for pregnant women to avoid alcohol during their pregnancy?
6. Analyze how underage drinking can interfere with your personal relationships, school and work responsibilities, and physical health.
7. Write a paragraph advocating for athletes to abstain from alcohol use.

Real World Health

Imagine a new law has just been passed, which states that one must obtain a "drinking license" to legally drink alcohol. Your job is to determine the rules for obtaining a drinking license. Use the prompts below to outline your drinking license proposal and describe your reasons for each response. After considering these prompts, explain whether you believe this would be a successful law.

What should the minimum age be for obtaining a drinking license?

Will special alcohol education classes be required? If so, how many and how often?

Will the soon-to-be drinker be required to earn a certain GPA in school to be eligible for this license?

A driver's license can be taken away as a punishment for irresponsible driving—can your drinking license be suspended for irresponsible alcohol consumption?

Reasons People Use and Abuse Alcohol

Key Terms 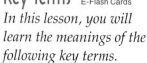 E-Flash Cards

In this lesson, you will learn the meanings of the following key terms.

alcoholics
alcoholism
moderate drinking
problem drinking

Lesson Objectives

After studying this lesson, you will be able to

- differentiate between levels of alcohol consumption, including moderate and problem drinking;
- recognize alcoholism as a disease and identify characteristics of alcoholism;
- explain the roles of biology and genetics in the development of alcoholism; and
- assess the influence of an individual's environment in the formation of attitudes and beliefs about alcohol.

Before You Read

Lesson Prediction

In a chart like the one shown below, write the first heading you see in this lesson and the first sentence under that heading. Then write at least 5 predictions you have about what content may be covered in this lesson.

Heading and first sentence	5 predictions

Warm-Up Activity

Word Swap

List the following terms—alcoholic, enabler, binge drinking, Alcoholics Anonymous, drug use, drug abuse—on a sheet of paper, leaving space next to each term, as shown below. Write the first thing you think of when you hear each term. Then switch your paper with as many students as you can in the time allotted by your teacher. Write something new for each term on your classmates' papers; do not repeat any comments from previous students. When the time is up, get your own paper back and read what your classmates wrote. Share your notes with the class.

alcoholic	
enabler	
binge drinking	
Alcoholics Anonymous	
drug use	
drug abuse	

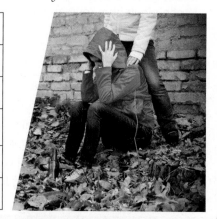

M ost adults drink alcohol at least occasionally. Some are considered regular drinkers. This means they have had at least 12 drinks in the past year.

Some people are more likely to be regular drinkers than others. Men are more likely than women to drink. Additionally, more college graduates are regular drinkers, compared with people who did not graduate high school.

Even if someone drinks alcohol, he or she does not necessarily *abuse* alcohol. Alcohol abuse occurs when alcohol use leads to problems with physical, mental, and social health, and interferes with personal responsibilities. Biological, genetic, and environmental factors can all lead people to use and abuse alcohol.

Alcohol Use versus Abuse

Moderate drinking, also called *social drinking,* is defined as no more than one drink per day on average for women, and no more than two drinks per day on average for men. People who drink moderately do not lose control of their drinking or experience alcohol-related problems that interfere with health, job responsibilities, or personal relationships. Although some adults are able to safely drink moderate amounts of alcohol, others experience major problems with alcohol use.

Problem Drinking

People who engage in **problem drinking** experience negative consequences as a result of their alcohol use. These consequences could include failing to complete projects for school or work, fighting with friends and family members about drinking, or having legal problems (Figure 10.13). Problem drinkers are *psychologically dependent* on alcohol, meaning they feel they need to drink in particular situations, such as when they are at a party or are feeling nervous. Problem drinkers are not *physically* addicted to alcohol, but alcoholics are. Problem drinking can lead to alcoholism.

Alcoholism

In contrast to problem drinkers, people who are **alcoholics** are both psychologically and physically addicted to alcohol. **Alcoholism**, or complete dependency on alcohol, is recognized as a disease by the Centers for Disease Control and Prevention (CDC). Physical addiction to alcohol occurs when a person needs to consume alcohol so he or she can function "normally."

People do not suddenly become alcoholics. Instead, people generally follow the stages of substance abuse, which you learned about in Chapter 9.

moderate drinking
the consumption of no more than one alcoholic drink per day for women or no more than two alcoholic drinks per day for men

problem drinking
the consumption of enough alcohol that a person experiences problems in his or her daily life; often characterized by psychological but not physical dependence on alcohol

alcoholics
people who are psychologically and physically addicted to alcohol

alcoholism
a disease in which a person is completely dependent on alcohol

Figure 10.13

Alcohol use can negatively affect a person's relationships, and his work and school performance. *How would using alcohol affect the relationships in your life right now?*

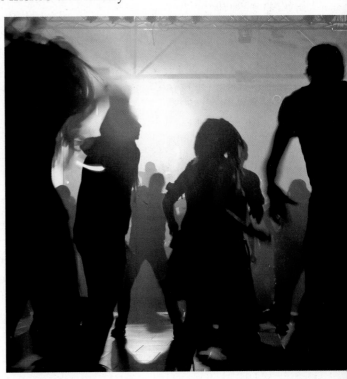

The first stage of substance abuse is *experimentation*. Experimentation with alcohol can lead to the second stage of substance abuse, *regular use*. Some people may stop at this stage.

People who become alcoholics, however, enter the third stage of substance abuse—*tolerance*. Gradually, the user consumes larger amounts of alcohol to feel the same effects. The tolerance stage of alcohol abuse resembles problem drinking.

The final stage of substance abuse, *dependence and addiction*, occurs when the user is psychologically and physically dependent on alcohol. Some health professionals refer to this as *late-stage alcoholism*.

Alcoholics show a number of symptoms, which include

- having a very high tolerance for alcohol;
- experiencing periods of memory loss (*blackouts*) after drinking; and
- experiencing withdrawal symptoms such as hallucinations, impaired motor coordination, and cognitive disruption when they stop drinking.

Alcoholics also continue to drink even when their alcohol use causes serious problems with their physical health, mental health, social health, and family or job responsibilities.

Biological, Genetic, and Environmental Factors

Biological and genetic factors may contribute to alcohol abuse. To examine the impact of biological factors on alcohol use, researchers compare the influence of biology with the influence of the environment. There are two ways of conducting this type of comparison. One way is to compare rates of alcohol abuse in identical twins—who share all their genes—to fraternal twins—who share half their genes. Researchers can also compare the alcohol use of adopted children with alcohol use of both their biological parents and their adoptive parents. These methods help determine whether alcohol abuse comes from genetics or from the environment.

Research using these methods provides important information about biological and environmental factors that lead to alcohol use and abuse.

The Contribution of Biology

Research has shown that biological factors do contribute to alcohol abuse. If one member of a twin pair has a problem with alcohol, an identical twin is twice as likely as a fraternal twin to also have a problem with alcohol. Similarly, an adopted child with an alcoholic biological parent is four times more likely to become a problem drinker than an adopted child whose biological parent is not an alcoholic. Regardless of the environment in which a person grows up, a person's biological makeup impacts whether he or she will have a problem with alcohol.

The Role of Genetics

Some research suggests that people with specific genes have a greater risk of developing problems with alcohol use. Having these genes does not mean that a person will definitely become an alcoholic, but the genes do increase the likelihood.

How exactly does genetic makeup influence whether people will develop a problem with alcohol? One theory is that certain genetic factors may cause some people to experience fewer negative consequences of alcohol use. For example, people with a particular gene may be less sensitive to the effects of alcohol. After consuming a set amount of alcohol, these people feel less influenced and show less impairment than other people. Typically, the negative consequences of drinking alcohol act as a signal to stop drinking. People who feel less influenced by alcohol, however, may drink even more alcohol. This pattern could lead to a dependence on, or addiction to, alcohol.

The Role of Environment

People's beliefs about alcohol use are influenced by their environment, including their culture, community, social relationships, and family. Certain people in an individual's environment, including parents, siblings, peers, and media figures, can influence that individual's beliefs and expectations about alcohol. These are generally people that an individual considers important, and whose opinion he or she values.

Research in Action
The Hazards of Parental and Media Modeling of Alcohol Use

Researchers in one study asked 3- to 6-year-old children to pretend they were going shopping at a "pretend store" that the researchers created. The children were given one doll and the researcher had another doll. The researcher suggested the dolls go shopping to buy items they could use that evening. The researcher then recorded each item the child suggested they buy.

Of the 120 children participating in the study, 62% of them chose to buy some type of alcohol at the pretend store. Children whose parents consume alcohol at least once a month were three times more likely to choose wine or beer as children whose parents do not drink alcohol. In addition, children who had viewed movies with PG-13 or R ratings were five times more likely to choose wine or beer as children who had not seen such movies.

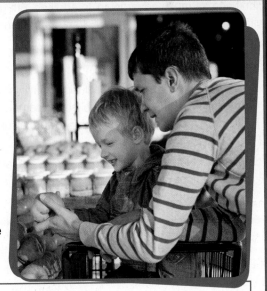

Thinking Critically

1. Why might children whose parents consume alcohol at least once a month be more likely to purchase alcohol at the pretend store?
2. What conclusions could you draw from this study that relates media influence to alcohol use?

The Scary Impact of Alcohol Advertisements

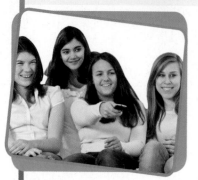

Think about the last time you saw an advertisement for alcohol. What images were shown in this ad? Alcohol advertisements are designed to show young, attractive people drinking in appealing settings and having a good time. Advertisements do not show the consequences of excessive alcohol use, including engaging in embarrassing and risky behavior, feeling sick, and getting into trouble with the law.

Greater exposure to such advertisements increases drinking in teenagers. In one study, researchers conducted in-school surveys with nearly 2,000 6th graders. Researchers asked these students how many times they had seen some type of advertisement for alcohol through various forms of media. One year later, researchers asked the same students, who were now 7th graders, whether they were currently drinking alcohol and whether they planned to drink alcohol in the future. Students who saw more alcohol advertisements during 6th grade were more likely to report planning to drink alcohol than those who didn't see as much advertising. In addition, 6th graders with frequent exposure to alcohol advertisements were twice as likely to report drinking a year later.

Thinking Critically

1. Based on this study, what conclusion could you draw about the relationship between alcohol advertisements and the attitudes of middle school students toward alcohol?

2. Do you remember seeing or hearing alcohol advertisements as a child? Do you believe these advertisements influenced your perceptions of alcohol? Why or why not?

Family. Families and cultures have their own attitudes, beliefs, and rules about alcohol use, which influence their children's attitudes toward alcohol. Children who have parents with very permissive attitudes toward alcohol are more likely to engage in excessive drinking when they become adults. Unfortunately, children whose parents have permissive attitudes are also more likely to experience problems caused by alcohol both in their current and future households.

Children also learn about the factors that lead to alcohol use by watching their parents' drinking habits. For example, children might see the following situations as reasons to drink alcohol:

- having a cocktail to relax after a stressful day at the office

- celebrating with a champagne toast at a college graduation

- socializing while drinking with friends at a party

Through these examples, children could learn that people drink alcohol to cope with negative emotions, such as tension and anxiety, as well as to enhance positive emotions, such as excitement.

Adopted children raised in a home with adoptive parents who have a drinking problem often show problems with alcohol use. For example, adopted children raised in families with alcoholic parents are more likely to develop alcoholism than adopted children raised in families without alcoholic parents. This means that the home environment also has a significant influence on forming alcohol attitudes and habits.

Friends. Friends are a factor that influences an individual's alcohol use. People tend to drink more alcohol when they have friends who drink. Pressuring friends into an activity they may be uncomfortable with is called *peer pressure.* Aggressively pressuring someone to drink alcohol is a form of bullying.

Watching people drink alcohol creates the belief that alcohol use is appropriate and desirable. People drink more when they are part of a group than when they are alone, especially when they are with people who are drinking heavily. Researchers in one study found that teenagers whose friends posted photographs of themselves consuming alcohol on social media sites were likely to drink themselves. Viewing pictures of peers drinking alcohol is an indirect form of peer pressure.

High school and college students are often misinformed, however, regarding how much other people actually drink. In fact, both high school and college students are often uncomfortable with drinking alcohol themselves, but believe that others are comfortable with that behavior. Most college students believe that there is too much alcohol use on campus. These college students also believe that other students are comfortable with the amount of alcohol use on campus. People who believe that their peers drink large amounts of alcohol may develop positive attitudes about drinking and, over time, drink more themselves (Figure 10.14).

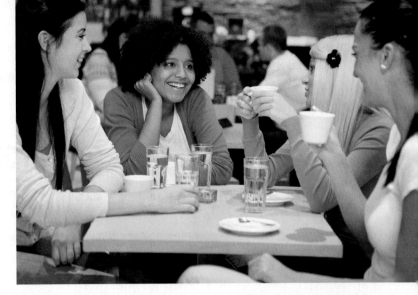

Figure 10.14

Despite what many high school and college students think, most students do not drink and are even uncomfortable with drinking. *How many people in your school do you think use alcohol?*

Media. Media is another factor that may contribute to alcohol use. Children form attitudes about alcohol use by watching television and movies as well as seeing advertisements for alcohol products. Alcohol use is frequently shown even in films marketed to children. Children who see drinking in movies tend to view alcohol use more positively. These children are also more likely to plan on drinking alcohol as adults.

It appears that seeing alcohol used in movies can also increase teenage drinking. In one study, more than 6,000 teenagers from across the United States completed surveys asking about their drinking behavior, movies they had seen, and their home environment. The researchers then examined whether the movies the teenagers had seen contained scenes of alcohol use. Teenagers who had seen the most movies including alcohol use were twice as likely to report drinking alcohol. These teenagers were also more likely to engage in binge drinking.

Lesson 10.3 Review

Know and Understand Assess

1. Define *alcoholism* and *alcoholic*.
2. List three signs or symptoms of alcoholism.
3. How do genetics affect a person's likelihood for becoming an alcoholic?
4. Name three environmental factors that contribute to the development of a person's attitudes and beliefs about alcohol.

Analyze and Apply

5. Explain the difference between moderate and problem drinking. What are signs that indicate problem drinking?

6. Why do researchers analyze biological, genetic, and environmental factors when determining the likelihood of developing alcoholism? Make a case for studying one factor more than the others.

Real World Health

People die for many different reasons every day, including alcohol-related reasons. Brainstorm as many reasons as you can to explain why there are more alcohol-related deaths on holidays. Consider the issues of problem drinking and alcoholism, which you read about in this lesson, as you come up with your answer.

Strategies for Preventing and Treating Alcohol Abuse

Key Terms 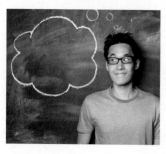 E-Flash Cards

In this lesson, you will learn the meanings of the following key terms.

detoxification

enabling

support groups

Before You Read

Your Anti-Drug

Drinking heavily can damage your health and lead to alcoholism. People who are emotionally healthy and have goals and hobbies are much less likely to drink heavily. These people can also be positive influences on others. On a separate sheet of paper, list a hobby, person, or goal that you can focus on as your anti-drug. This should be something or someone who inspires you not to drink. Write a paragraph about how your chosen anti-drug can keep you on a healthy path.

Lesson Objectives

After studying this lesson, you will be able to

- evaluate the importance of alcohol prevention strategies;

- outline detoxification, medications, support groups, and self-management as treatment strategies for recovering alcoholics; and

- recognize healthy and unhealthy ways of supporting someone who has a problem with alcohol.

Warm-Up Activity

Agree or Disagree

Recreate the chart shown below on a separate piece of paper. Before reading the lesson, list whether you agree or disagree with each of the statements. When you have finished reading the lesson, consider the statements again based on any new information you may have read. In the final column, list whether you agree or disagree now, and check to see whether your opinion has changed based on new evidence.

Before Reading	Statements	Page #	After Reading
1.	1. Alcohol use in teenagers can cause problems with brain development.		
2.	2. Learning good refusal skills is an effective technique to avoid alcohol when offered a drink by your peers.		
3.	3. One of the most effective ways a government tries to decrease alcohol abuse is to set a drinking age.		
4.	4. Increasing the cost of alcohol by 10% led to a 50% decrease in deaths caused by alcohol use.		
5.	5. The first step needed for an alcoholic to recover is detoxification.		
6.	6. Alcoholics Anonymous (AA) has 10 distinct steps a person must follow to recover from alcoholism.		
7.	7. Figuring out why a person drinks is essential for them to stop abusing alcohol.		
8.	8. Covering up someone's drinking is called enabling.		

Preventing alcohol use in adolescents is especially important because this behavior can lead to changes in brain development and long-term dependence on alcohol later in life. This lesson describes strategies for preventing alcohol abuse and treating alcoholism. The lesson also examines strategies you can use if someone you know is abusing alcohol.

Preventing Alcohol Abuse

There are very serious short- and long-term consequences of *any* alcohol use by teenagers, and of excessive alcohol use by adults. Fortunately, there are a number of strategies that can help prevent alcohol abuse and improve health and well-being.

Education and Refusal Skills

High schools and colleges have developed many education programs to decrease risky drinking, especially in underage drinkers. These programs include information about the short- and long-term consequences of alcohol use, such as physical, social, and mental consequences. This information might mention the physical effects of alcohol use on the body, the hazards of drinking and driving, strained personal relationships, and the legal consequences of possessing alcohol.

Even if you are aware of the many negative consequences of alcohol use and have made the decision not to drink, alcohol may still be present in your environment. Developing and practicing refusal skills can help when you are offered alcohol (Figure 10.15). Effective strategies for refusing alcohol could include the following:

- Just say no: "I don't drink," or "I don't have to drink to have fun."
- Blame not drinking on a health problem: "Drinking makes me sick," or "I'm on a medication that means I can't drink any alcohol at all."

SKILLS FOR HEALTH AND WELLNESS

Preventing Alcohol-Related Problems

The strategies listed below can help prevent you from experiencing alcohol-related problems.

- Practice what you could say to resist pressure to drink alcohol, such as "If I get caught, I'll be grounded," or "No, thanks, I don't drink."

- Make a list of reasons why you think it is a good idea not to drink alcohol.

- Avoid situations in which you think alcohol might be available. Simply being at a party with alcohol, even if you choose not to drink yourself, could lead you to get in trouble with your parents or the police. You are also putting yourself at risk of being injured or assaulted by someone who is drinking.

- Surround yourself with friends who will encourage and support your healthy decisions.

- If you have a friend who is having problems with drinking, talk to your parents, guidance counselor, or the school nurse. A national hotline or organization such as Al-Anon can also provide you with help and information.

- Never get into a car with a driver who has been drinking, even if the person claims to feel able to drive. Drinking while under the influence may lead to accidents or fatalities. Get a ride from someone who has not been drinking, or call your parents or other trusted adults.

- Mention other responsibilities you have: "I can't drink because I need to be in the best condition for the basketball game. I can't let the team down."

- Blame not drinking on another person: "My coach will be really mad," or "My parents will kill me."

Many studies with both high school and college students show that most teenagers do not drink and wish there was less drinking in their environment. Some colleges give new students information showing that many of their fellow students are also uncomfortable with how much drinking occurs on campus. These fellow students also do not drink very much alcohol themselves. Encouragingly, students who receive such information report drinking less alcohol than students who do not receive this information.

Government Approaches

One of the most obvious and effective government approaches to reducing alcohol abuse is setting the minimum legal drinking age at 21. Forbidding people who are younger than 21 years of age from purchasing alcohol makes it more difficult for teenagers to have access to alcohol. Similarly, making it illegal to use a fake ID to purchase alcohol reduces alcohol use by teenagers.

Other public policy approaches are also used to limit the purchase of alcohol, or at least make it more costly, in an effort to decrease problem drinking. For example, in some states alcohol is not sold on Sundays or in grocery and convenience stores. Raising the sales tax on alcohol, which makes buying alcohol more expensive, is another effective strategy that states use to discourage the use of alcohol.

Other drinking prevention programs focus on the negative effects of alcohol abuse. You have probably seen television and magazines ads that portray the negative consequences of drunk driving. Public policies may also place limits on alcohol advertisements, including the hours in which such ads can appear on television and what they can include.

detoxification
a necessary step in defeating addiction that means complete withdrawal from a substance; may cause intense anxiety, tremors, and hallucinations

Figure 10.15

Refusal skills are essential to turning down the offer of alcohol. *What refusal skills do you use in other areas of your life?*

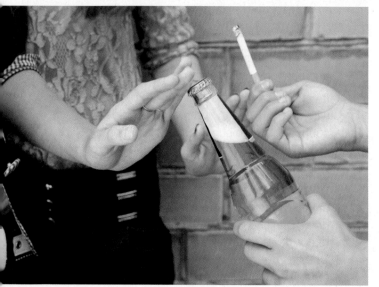

Strategies for Treating Alcoholism

People who are alcoholics are physically and psychologically addicted to drinking. Although breaking this addiction is difficult, there are a number of strategies that can help people quit drinking.

Detoxification

One of the first steps in recovery for all alcoholics is *detoxification*. Because alcoholics are physically addicted to alcohol, a necessary step in recovering from this addiction is completely withdrawing from alcohol. This "drying out" process may take up to a month. Detoxification can include severe symptoms, such as intense anxiety, tremors, and hallucinations. Some medications can be used to help the person cope with the symptoms of alcohol withdrawal.

Medications

Various medications can be used to help people stop drinking, such as *Antabuse*, which needs to be taken every day. If someone consumes alcohol while taking this drug, he or she will experience unpleasant side effects, such as extreme nausea. The goal of this approach is for alcoholics to connect drinking alcohol with feeling sick.

Other drugs can also be taken to help alcoholics stop drinking. These drugs work in various ways to help people who are addicted to alcohol. One drug helps restore the chemical balance in the brain that is disrupted by alcoholism. Another drug decreases alcohol cravings.

Support Groups

Community support groups can also be a helpful tool for those overcoming alcoholism. **Support groups** are groups of people with a common problem who share struggles and examples of getting through that problem. Alcoholics Anonymous (also known as *AA*) is the most well-known and widely used self-help program for alcohol abuse. The goal of AA is to help alcoholics change how they think about drinking. This program involves going through 12 distinct steps, which are a set of guiding principles designed to help people recover from addiction.

support groups
groups of people who communicate about their struggles and progress in battling a shared problem

The AA philosophy is based on two basic ideas:

- People who abuse alcohol are alcoholics and will remain that way for life, even if they never drink again.
- Taking even a single drink after having quit for an extended time period can set off an alcoholic binge.

According to AA, when a person who is an alcoholic consumes even a small amount of alcohol, the presence of alcohol in the bloodstream leads to an irresistible craving for more alcohol. Thus, the goal for alcoholics is to never drink any alcohol again.

During AA meetings, group members share alcohol-related problems they have experienced with other group members, which may help them stop drinking. People who are trying to stop drinking attend frequent AA meetings—even daily when they are first trying to quit drinking (Figure 10.16).

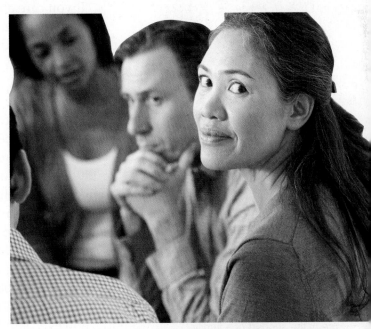

AA meetings bring together people who have stopped drinking to share their experiences.

Self-Management Techniques

Many programs that help people with a drinking problem also teach self-management skills. First, these programs focus on helping people become aware of why they drink. Understanding the motivations that lead someone to drink is an important first step in learning how to avoid alcohol abuse.

Next, people develop skills for managing the situations that lead them to want to have a drink. These skills include

- avoiding situations where alcohol is present;
- responding in new ways to these situations;
- learning new strategies for handling stress; and
- developing strategies for refusing alcohol.

These types of self-management skills can be used in combination with other strategies for recovering from alcohol addiction, including attending AA meetings or taking medication.

enabling
encouraging an addict's destructive behaviors, either intentionally or unintentionally

What Can You Do If Someone You Know Has a Problem with Alcohol?

It can be very difficult to love and care about someone who has a drinking problem, because you worry about that person and want him or her to be happy and healthy. Many people who care about someone with a drinking problem experience varied emotions, including shame, anger, fear, and guilt. Other people feel so overwhelmed by their loved one's problem with alcohol that they just deny the problem and pretend that nothing is wrong.

If you care about someone who has a problem with alcohol, the first step you need to take is finding a way to get the support you need. Try to find an adult you can talk openly and honestly with about the problem, such as a family member, guidance counselor, religious leader, or coach (Figure 10.17).

Some people who have a loved one with a drinking problem feel they should try to solve or fix the problem. They may try to punish, threaten, or bribe their loved one to stop drinking. They may beg their loved one to stop drinking, and try to make the person feel guilty about his or her alcohol use. The first step to alcohol recovery, however, is for the addicted person to recognize that he or she has a problem and wants to change. It is important to remember that you cannot force a person to stop drinking.

People who have a loved one with an alcohol problem may also try to keep other people from finding out about this problem. They may cover up the problems caused by the person's drinking or hide evidence of the drinking. These attempts to cover up evidence of the person's drinking, however, simply help the person avoid the natural consequences of their behavior, and can enable this behavior to continue. Encouraging an addict's unhealthy behaviors, either intentionally or unintentionally, is called *enabling*.

Many teenagers who have family members struggling with alcoholism find it helpful to join support groups for family members of alcoholics.

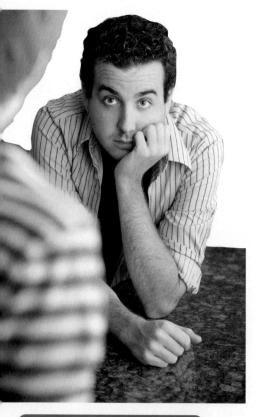

Figure 10.17

If you suspect your friend has an alcohol problem, the first thing you should do is seek the support of a family member, counselor, coach, or religious leader. *Why do you think trying to fix your friend's alcohol problem on your own is not an effective strategy?*

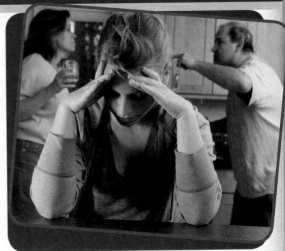

Casey is 14 years old and a freshman in high school. For as long as Casey can remember, her father has had a drinking problem. He has a couple shots of whiskey after he returns home from work and drinks several glasses of beer with dinner.

Casey has stopped having friends over in the evenings because she is embarrassed by her father's poor behavior. He speaks loudly and is clumsy when he helps clear the table.

When driving home from a work party recently, Casey's father was arrested for driving under the influence. Casey overheard her parents arguing about his arrest, and heard her mother worrying that Casey's father would be fired from his job.

Thinking Critically

1. List some signs that indicate alcoholism in the actions of Casey's father.

2. Assume that Casey's father is ready to quit drinking alcohol. What strategies could be used to help him stop abusing alcohol?

3. What advice would you give to Casey and other teenagers who find themselves in her situation? What steps could Casey and her family take to help cope with her dad's alcoholism?

These groups can help people with an alcoholic family member learn how to cope with the difficulties alcoholism causes for family members and friends of an alcoholic. Support groups can also be comforting for family members because they show that other people are facing the same challenges. Support groups for family members of alcoholics include Al-Anon and Alateen.

Lesson 10.4 Review

Know and Understand Assess

1. List two government approaches that restrict drinking among people younger than 21 years of age.

2. Identify four strategies for treating alcoholism.

3. Describe the process of detoxification.

4. Define *enabling*.

Analyze and Apply

5. Explain how refusal skills can help you turn down alcohol in a social situation. Give at least one example of how you could respond to an offer for alcohol.

6. Research community support groups that might be helpful for family members of alcoholics.

Real World Health

Addiction affects not only the addict, but the entire family. Create a poster with the following cast of characters: the addict, the chief enabler, the hero, the forgotten child, the mascot, and the scapegoat. Research all of these roles and draw a representation of each family member on your poster. Explain what role each person plays in trying to restore the balance lost by the addict's drinking.

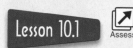

 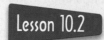
How Does Alcohol Impact Your Body

Key Terms

alcohol

blood alcohol
concentration (BAC)

depressant

hangover

inhibition

metabolize

Key Points

- Alcohol, a depressant, impacts the brain by reducing the ability to process information, walk steadily, and coordinate other body movements.
- Because the liver can only metabolize alcohol at a certain rate, blood alcohol concentration (BAC) level builds in the body and can lead to substantial physical and mental impairments, including death.
- Dehydration is a main cause of hangovers, which result in many unpleasant symptoms.
- Rate of intake, body weight, gender, food consumption, and ethnicity are factors that influence the effects of alcohol in individuals.

Check Your Understanding

1. *True or false?* One alcoholic drink equals 10 ounces of beer, malt liquor, wine, or distilled spirits.

2. Alcohol is a _____, or a type of drug that slows down the central nervous system.
   - A. vasopressin
   - B. stimulant
   - C. depressant
   - D. hormone

3. Alcohol can negatively impact the cerebral _____, which controls thought processing and consciousness.
   - A. cortex
   - B. cerebellum
   - C. hypothalamus
   - D. medulla

4. Once alcohol is consumed, it stays in the body until the liver can break down, or _____ the alcohol.
   - A. inhibit
   - B. metabolize
   - C. depress
   - D. suppress

5. **Critical Thinking.** How can alcohol, a liquid, dehydrate the body?

The Effects of Alcohol on Health

Key Terms

alcohol poisoning

binge drinking

cirrhosis

driving under the influence (DUI)

fetal alcohol syndrome (FAS)

Key Points

- The effects of alcohol lead to an increase in accidents, fatalities, and violence.
- Binge drinking occurs when large amounts of alcohol are consumed in a short period of time, which can lead to alcohol poisoning.
- Long-term health consequences of alcohol use include cardiovascular problems, gastrointestinal problems, some forms of cancer, and neurological and cognitive functioning problems.
- Short-term consequences of alcohol use include physical, social, family, school, and legal problems.
- Alcohol use by teenagers can result in changes in brain development.

Check Your Understanding

6. *True or false?* There is a relationship between alcohol use and the number of accidents and violence incidents in the United States.

7. _____ is a medical emergency caused when a high blood alcohol concentration suppresses the central nervous system and can result in loss of consciousness, low blood pressure, low body temperature, and difficulty breathing.
   - A. Binge drinking
   - B. Alcohol poisoning
   - C. Cirrhosis
   - D. Zero-tolerance policy

8. The buildup of scar tissue in the liver is called _____.
   - A. neurology
   - B. alcohol poisoning
   - C. cirrhosis
   - D. dementia

9. Which of the following describes a possible symptom of fetal alcohol syndrome?
   - A. decreased muscle tone and poor coordination
   - B. delayed development and problems with thinking, speech, movement, and social skills
   - C. heart defects
   - D. All of the above

10. **Critical Thinking.** Why is alcohol use especially dangerous for adolescents?

 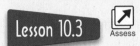

Reasons People Use and Abuse Alcohol

Key Terms

alcoholics

alcoholism

moderate drinking

problem drinking

Key Points

- Alcoholism is a disease that results from a person being physically and psychologically addicted to alcohol.
- Biological factors and genetic factors can contribute to a person's risk factor for developing an addiction to alcohol.
- Environmental factors, such as family, friends, and media, also contribute to a person's attitudes and habits relating to alcohol use.

Check Your Understanding

11. _____ describes a drinking pattern in which a female consumes no more than one drink per day on average and a male consumes no more than two drinks per day on average.
    A. Problem drinking
    B. Moderate drinking
    C. Alcoholism
    D. Alcoholic

12. *True or false?* People who are moderate drinkers continue to drink even when their use of alcohol causes serious problems with their physical, mental, and social health, and family or job responsibilities.

13. Which of the following is a sign of alcoholism?
    A. experiencing blackouts
    B. developing a high tolerance for alcohol
    C. experiencing alcohol-related problems that interfere with physical, mental, and social health
    D. All of the above.

14. *True or false?* Most high school and college students believe that other students are comfortable with drinking alcohol, when in reality, many are uncomfortable with alcohol.

15. **Critical Thinking.** How does the media influence children's views and attitudes toward alcohol?

 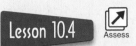

Strategies for Preventing and Treating Alcohol Abuse

Key Terms

detoxification

enabling

support groups

Key Points

- Practicing refusal skills and assessing the physical, social, and mental consequences of alcohol use are types of alcohol prevention strategies.
- Government alcohol prevention strategies include banning the sale of alcohol to people younger than 21 years of age, raising taxes, and promoting alcohol-free lifestyles.
- Treatment methods for alcoholism include detoxification, medications, support groups, and self-management techniques.
- Family members and friends of alcoholics are affected by actions of the alcoholic and may also need help and support.

Check Your Understanding

16. Assume that you tell a friend who is offering you alcohol that you simply don't want to drink it. This is an example of _____ skills.

17. *True or false?* One strategy the government uses to reduce the rate of alcoholism is to reduce the taxes for purchasing alcohol.

18. Which of the following is *not* a strategy for treating alcoholism?
    A. enabling
    B. detoxification
    C. medications
    D. support groups

19. The process of completely withdrawing from alcohol is called _____.
    A. enabling
    B. disabling
    C. hallucination
    D. detoxification

20. **Critical Thinking.** When helping a person with an alcohol addiction, why is trying to fix the problem for the alcoholic *not* recommended?

Health and Wellness Skills

21. **Analyze Influences.** Find an ad for an alcoholic product. Analyze the ad and describe it to your class. Explain why you think that the ad would or would not persuade people to buy this product.

22. **Communicate with Others.** Your teacher will divide you into groups. Each group will develop a 10-line rap about the effects of alcohol use and abuse on society using information you learned from the chapter. The rap must include different types of alcohol, the effects of alcohol, and reasons to stay away from alcohol. Each group will perform its rap for the other members of the class.

23. **Comprehend Concepts.** Draw an outline of the human body on a large piece of paper. Identify at least five effects of alcohol on the body, either short-term or long-term, and then draw those effects in a creative way in the appropriate places on your outline of the body.

24. **Reduce Health Risks.** Imagine that you have received a DUI, and it is now your job to write the news report about your DUI that will be published in the local paper. Make sure to include all of the facts of the incident, including your BAC. Was anyone hurt in the accident? When will you go to trial? Get a quote from the arresting officer about what happened. After writing the story, write a personal reflection about the ways in which this imagined incident and article would affect you. Include at least three researched facts about a DUI arrest in your reflection. Also include strategies that you could have used to prevent this incident from happening in the first place.

Hands-On Activity
Drinking Age on Trial

As you read in this chapter, one of the government's methods of reducing alcohol abuse is setting the minimum legal drinking age at 21. This makes it difficult for teenagers to have access to alcohol, reducing alcohol abuse among minors. Some people, however, think that the drinking age should be changed. This activity will simulate a courtroom environment where you can argue the case for changing the drinking age.

Steps for this Activity

1. Your teacher will divide the class into two groups. One group will be the prosecution in a court trial trying to convince a jury to change the legal drinking age. The other group will represent the defense, which wants to keep the drinking age at the current level.

2. In your group, pick a lead prosecutor or lead defense attorney, depending on which side you are on, and then pick three assistant attorneys. The remaining members of the group will be expert witnesses.

3. The prosecutor and the defense attorney will lead the investigations and present the team's findings to the jury. The assistant attorneys will conduct research to find as much evidence as possible to support their case. This research should include interviewing the expert witnesses—who will be acting as local politicians, students, and adults—to get their opinions.

4. The expert witnesses will be the local politicians, students, and adults being interviewed. It is the job of each expert witness to "become" one of these people by doing research regarding what their assigned person might think. The expert witnesses will be expected to testify on the day of the trial.

5. On the day of the trial, eight jurors will be chosen at random by the teacher from the pool of expert witnesses, who will turn over all of their research to their fellow team members and take their places on the jury.

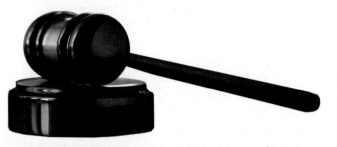

Core Skills

Math Practice

The following table represents the average number of alcohol-attributable deaths each year caused by excessive alcohol use in males and females. Analyze the information and answer the following questions.

Cause of Death	Average number of deaths in males	Average number of deaths in females
Alcohol poisoning	1,264	383
Motor vehicle traffic accidents	9,764	2,696
Homicide	6,221	1,535
Suicide	6,460	1,719

25. Which type of alcohol-attributable death is highest among males?
    A. alcohol poisoning
    B. motor vehicle traffic accidents
    C. homicide
    D. suicide

26. Which type of alcohol-attributable death is lowest among females?
    A. alcohol poisoning
    B. motor vehicle traffic accidents
    C. homicide
    D. suicide

27. What is the total average number of homicides attributable to excess alcohol use each year?
    A. 1,535
    B. 6,221
    C. 6,460
    D. 7,756

28. Of the average number of deaths related to alcohol poisoning each year, what percentage of deaths occurs in males?
    A. 77%
    B. 50%
    C. 37%
    D. 23%

29. Which type of alcohol-related death is most common?
    A. alcohol poisoning
    B. homicide
    C. motor vehicle traffic accidents
    D. suicide

Reading and Writing Practice

Read the passage below and then answer the questions.

People who have a loved one with an alcohol problem may also try to keep other people from finding out about this problem. They may cover up the problems caused by the person's drinking or hide evidence of the drinking. These attempts to cover up evidence of the person's drinking, however, simply help the person avoid the natural consequences of their behavior, and can enable this behavior to continue. Encouraging an addict's unhealthy behaviors, either intentionally or unintentionally, is called enabling.

30. What does the word *enable* mean?
    A. stop
    B. avoid
    C. encourage
    D. discourage

31. What is the author's main point in this paragraph?
    A. An alcoholic's loved ones may intentionally or unintentionally enable the consumption of alcohol.
    B. An alcoholic's loved ones should enable the consumption of alcohol.
    C. An alcoholic's loved ones should cover up problems caused by his or her drinking.
    D. An alcoholic always experiences the consequences of his or her drinking.

32. According to the passage, covering up evidence of the alcoholic's drinking _____.
    A. is healthy for the alcoholic
    B. is healthy for the family member
    C. helps the alcoholic avoid consequences
    D. is recommended behavior by support groups

33. Handing an alcoholic a drink is an example of _____.
    A. disabling
    B. enabling
    C. engaging
    D. helping

34. How might a family member of an alcoholic enable him or her to continue drinking? How might enabling an alcoholic be damaging to him or her? Write a brief paragraph identifying examples of enabling behavior, other than the example mentioned in the passage.

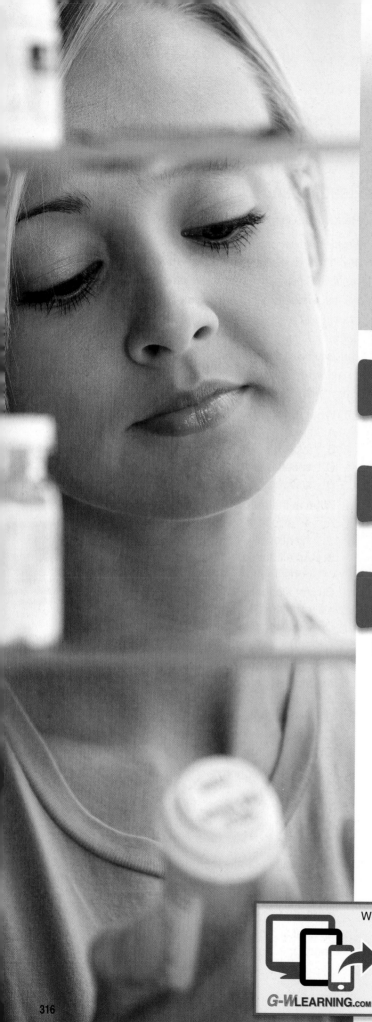

Chapter 11

Medications and Drugs

Lesson 11.1

Medications

Lesson 11.2

Drugs

Lesson 11.3

Drug Abuse and Addiction

While studying this chapter, look for the activity icon ⬀ to:

- **review** vocabulary with e-flash cards and games;
- **assess** learning with quizzes and online exercises;
- **expand** knowledge with animations and activities; and
- **listen** to pronunciation of key terms in the audio glossary.

G-WLEARNING.com

www.g-wlearning.com/health/

What's Your Health and Wellness IQ?

Take this quiz to see what you do and do not know about drug abuse and addiction and how using drugs can affect health. If you cannot answer a question, pay extra attention to that topic as you study this chapter.

1. *Identify each statement as* True, False, *or* It Depends. *Choose* It Depends *if a statement is true in some cases, but false in others.*

2. *Revise each* False *statement to make it true.*

3. *Explain the circumstances in which each* It Depends *statement is true and when it is false.*

Health and Wellness IQ Assess

1. Over-the-counter and prescription medications cannot be abused like other drugs, such as cocaine or heroin.	True	False	It Depends
2. Some medications can have different effects depending on whether they are taken with food, alcohol, or other medicines.	True	False	It Depends
3. More people die each year from drug overdose due to the misuse of prescription drugs than from other drug use.	True	False	It Depends
4. People only suffer serious consequences if they use a drug many times or over a long period of time.	True	False	It Depends
5. People who are addicted to a drug must take larger and larger amounts of it to experience the same effect.	True	False	It Depends
6. People who are addicted to drugs can stop using drugs relatively easily whenever they choose to do so.	True	False	It Depends
7. Because marijuana is a gateway drug, it is not dangerous.	True	False	It Depends
8. A person who uses inhalants just once can die.	True	False	It Depends
9. A person's environment is a risk factor for whether he or she will abuse or become addicted to drugs.	True	False	It Depends
10. Drug addiction is a relatively easy problem to treat, as long as the person wants to stop using drugs.	True	False	It Depends

Setting the Scene

Chances are, your experiences with medications are mostly positive—after taking them, your symptoms lessened or disappeared and you felt better. People sometimes use medications in ways that hurt their health, however. For example, some people may take more than the prescribed amount of a medication or another person's medication to experience different sensations. Some people use drugs for this same reason. Medication and drug abuse can have devastating results on a person's health.

In this chapter you'll learn how medications, when taken properly, can improve health. You'll also learn about the ways in which both medications and drugs can be abused. This chapter will also review some strategies for the prevention and treatment of medication and drug abuse and addiction.

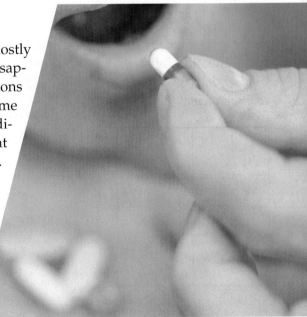

Medications

Key Terms E-Flash Cards

In this lesson, you will learn the meanings of the following key terms.

analgesics

euphoria

medication

medication abuse

medication misuse

opiates

opioids

over-the-counter (OTC) medications

prescription medications

Before You Read

Medicinal Knowledge

Create a 4-square organizer like the one shown below and place the word medicine *in the middle. Record 4 facts you know or think you know about medicine.*

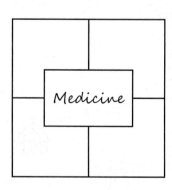

Lesson Objectives

After studying this lesson, you will be able to

- identify the main reasons people use medications;
- differentiate between over-the-counter and prescription medications;
- describe different ways to take medications;
- summarize common health risks associated with taking medications; and
- list safe strategies for using medications.

Warm-Up Activity

Explaining Medication

On a separate sheet of paper, list 5 specific reasons why someone may need to take medications. What kinds of diseases and disorders might require a medication? If you know of someone who is taking medication, is that person using an over-the-counter product or a prescription product?

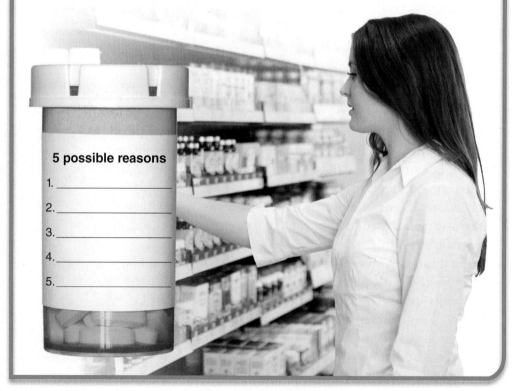

5 possible reasons

1. _____
2. _____
3. _____
4. _____
5. _____

In this lesson you will learn about medicine and how, when used safely, it can be an effective way to improve health. You'll learn about different types of medicines and the ways they can be taken. Health risks involved with taking medicines will also be reviewed. Finally, you will learn safe strategies for taking medicines.

Uses for Medications

A *medication* (also called *medicine*) is a substance used to treat disease or relieve pain. Sometimes people use medications to help them function in daily life. There are four main reasons people use medications:

- *treat* symptoms of an illness;
- *cure* a disease;
- *manage* a disease; or
- *prevent* a disease.

Types of Medications

In the United States, companies developing new medications must run tests to prove the medications are safe before selling them. These tests are called *clinical trials*. After a company tests a new medication, the *Food and Drug Administration (FDA)* must then approve it. The FDA is a government agency that is responsible for making sure medications are safe to use, effective, and secure from tampering.

Before determining whether medications are ready to be approved for use by the public, the FDA reviews the company's evidence about the chemicals in the medication, the side effects, and the medication's ability to impact the condition it is designed to treat. The FDA also decides whether a medication should be sold with or without a doctor's prescription.

Over-the-Counter Medications

Over-the-counter (OTC) medications are sold to people without a doctor's prescription. Over-the-counter medications are generally safe to use without specific instructions from a doctor or pharmacist. These medicines can easily be purchased at local stores and pharmacies (Figure 11.1).

OTC medications are used to treat the symptoms of many relatively minor health conditions. The most commonly used OTC medications are *analgesics* (pain relievers), such as aspirin, acetaminophen, and ibuprofen.

medication
a substance used to treat a disease or relieve pain

over-the-counter (OTC) medications
medications that are sold without a doctor's prescription

analgesics
medications that relieve pain

Figure 11.1

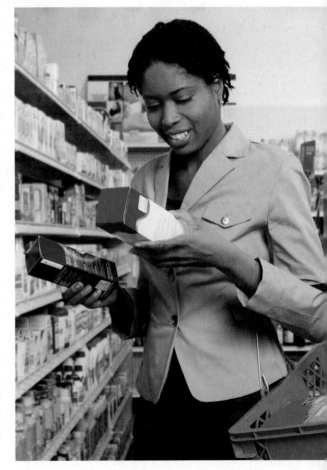

Over-the-counter medications can be purchased at a local drugstore with or without a prescription. *Which over-the-counter medications do you occasionally use?*

Prescription Medications

Prescription medications can only be sold to a person with a prescription from a doctor or other licensed healthcare professional. The doctor will determine how much of the medication a patient needs for treatment. The prescribed medication is obtained through a licensed pharmacist. A person cannot get more of the prescribed medication without an approval for a refill from the healthcare professional. Different types of prescription medications have different functions:

- *Antibiotics* kill or slow the growth of bacteria.
- *Anesthetics* eliminate or reduce pain.
- *Vaccinations* work with the body's natural immune system to reduce the risk of developing an infection or disease.

With many prescription medications, doctors will routinely check therapeutic medication levels by ordering blood tests to see how much of the medicine is in the body. If therapeutic levels are too high or too low, then the medication could either produce harmful results or not be effective at all.

Figure 11.2

Many different methods are used to deliver medicine into the body: taking pills, applying cream, or drinking a medicine in liquid form. *Why do you think there are so many different ways to take medicine?*

Ways to Take Medications

Medications are delivered, or taken, in many different ways (Figure 11.2). Medications that come in the pill, tablet, capsule, or liquid forms can be swallowed. Liquid medications can also come in drop form—drops are applied to a particular part of the body. For example, a liquid antibiotic to treat an eye infection may be applied to the eye using a dropper.

Medications in cream, gel, or ointment forms are rubbed on a particular part of the body. Transdermal patches have a specific dosage of medication on a patch that is placed on the skin, which absorbs the medication into the bloodstream. If you have asthma or allergies, you may treat your symptoms with medications you inhale into your nose or mouth. Medications may also be injected directly into the body.

Health Risks of Taking Medications

Taking over-the-counter and prescription medications can be beneficial for your health. Using these medications, however, can also carry some risks.

Side Effects

All medications, even OTC medications, can have side effects. For example, many medications used to treat cold symptoms may cause drowsiness. In some cases, medications can have more serious side effects, such as hallucinations, dizziness, and stomach bleeding and ulcers.

Over-the-counter medications can even cause life-threatening problems. *Reye's syndrome* is a rare but potentially fatal disease in children. Because some evidence suggests that aspirin can trigger this disease, children under 18 years of age should never be given aspirin.

Medication Interactions

Some medications cause health risks by interacting with other medications, dietary supplements, foods, or drinks. Many medications should not be taken with alcohol because alcohol use can reduce the medication's effectiveness and produce side effects.

Medication Sensitivities

Sometimes the same medication can have different effects on different people, which can cause further health risks. One person might experience a benefit from using only a small amount of a medication while another requires a larger amount.

Allergic Reactions

People can experience an adverse reaction to medication. In some cases these reactions can be relatively minor, such as vomiting, nausea, or a rash. In other cases, these reactions can be much more serious and even life-threatening. People are most often allergic to antibiotics.

Treat Symptoms, Not Causes

A drawback of using OTC medications is that they typically relieve the symptoms of a health problem but do not treat the underlying cause of these symptoms. A *symptom* is something that is experienced by an individual, such as a headache, sore throat, or nausea. Sometimes symptoms can clearly indicate the cause of a health problem.

In other cases, however, symptoms are not so clearly linked with their cause. If you have pain in your muscles, the cause of this pain may be difficult to determine. For example, muscle pain could be caused by an injury resulting from exercise. It could also be caused by an infection or disorder, such as lupus.

When the cause of a symptom is not clear, you should make it a priority to see a health professional. A professional can consider the symptoms and the different factors that might be causing these symptoms.

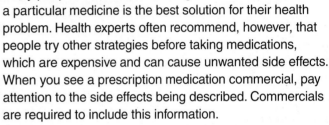

Health in the Media

The Media and Prescription Medication Use

In the United States and New Zealand, commercials and advertisements for prescription medications are common and legal. In other countries, however, these types of advertisements are illegal.

Marketing messages for prescription medications lead many people to believe that taking a particular medicine is the best solution for their health problem. Health experts often recommend, however, that people try other strategies before taking medications, which are expensive and can cause unwanted side effects. When you see a prescription medication commercial, pay attention to the side effects being described. Commercials are required to include this information.

Thinking Critically

1. Do you think commercials for prescription medications should be legal or illegal in the United States? Explain your answer.

2. Do you think consumers should be skeptical about ads promoting prescription medications? Why or why not?

Drug labels give instructions regarding how a medication should be used and warn of possible side effects associated with the drug. *Look at prescription drug labels to see if you can identify the types of information called out in the example at the right.*

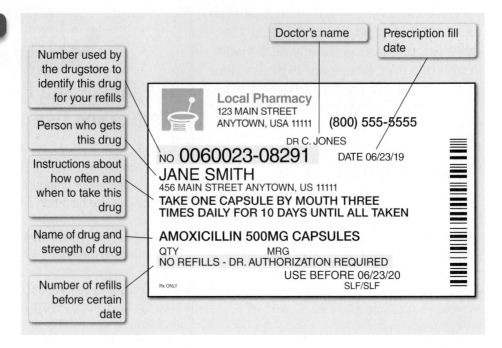

Number used by the drugstore to identify this drug for your refills

Person who gets this drug

Instructions about how often and when to take this drug

Name of drug and strength of drug

Number of refills before certain date

Doctor's name

Prescription fill date

Local Pharmacy
123 MAIN STREET
ANYTOWN, USA 11111   (800) 555-5555
DR C. JONES
NO 0060023-08291   DATE 06/23/19
JANE SMITH
456 MAIN STREET ANYTOWN, US 11111
TAKE ONE CAPSULE BY MOUTH THREE TIMES DAILY FOR 10 DAYS UNTIL ALL TAKEN

AMOXICILLIN 500MG CAPSULES
QTY   MRG
NO REFILLS - DR. AUTHORIZATION REQUIRED
                USE BEFORE 06/23/20
Rx ONLY   SLF/SLF

medication misuse
any use of medicine that does not follow the medicine's instructions

medication abuse
the intentional use of medicines for reasons other than the prescribed purpose

One in 10 teenagers have reported abusing cough medicine.

Suppose you take medication to relieve the pain of a sore throat. Although this medication will temporarily reduce the pain of swallowing, it will not actually treat the bacteria or virus causing your sore throat. If you have strep throat, you will need to see a doctor and will probably be prescribed an antibiotic.

Medication Misuse

Medication misuse involves not following a medication's instructions. Following the exact instructions will help you avoid many potential health risks. People may misuse medication unintentionally because they forgot or do not understand what their doctor told them. They might misunderstand the label or instructions for taking the medication. Medication misuse includes instances in which people stop taking a medication before they should. It is important to carefully read the labels on both OTC and prescription medications before taking them (Figure 11.3). Otherwise, medications may not be effective and increased health risks, such as unpleasant side effects, may result.

Medication Abuse

Medication abuse involves the intentional use of medications for purposes other than those intended by the prescribing doctor (Figure 11.4). You may be surprised to learn that more people die in the United States each year from overdoses caused by prescription medications than from the use of drugs. The most commonly abused prescription medications are opioids, depressants, and stimulants.

Opioids. *Opiates* are substances originating from the poppy plant, which contains opium. *Opioids* (synthetic opiates) are prescription medications typically prescribed to relieve pain (Figure 11.5). They include hydrocodone, codeine, morphine, and oxycodone. Examples of opioid medication include Vicodin®, OxyContin®, Percocet®, Kadian®, and Avinza®.

Using opioids causes people to feel euphoric, which is one reason these medications are misused and abused. A person may be prescribed an opioid by a doctor to relieve pain. Over time, the person may become psychologically and physically dependent on the medication. Continued opioid use leads the nerve cells in the brain to stop producing endorphins, which are natural painkillers. This leads the person to become physically dependent on taking opioids to relieve pain.

Opioid use can lead to numerous side effects, including drowsiness, dizziness and weakness, nausea, impaired coordination, confusion, sweating and clammy skin, and constipation.

Taking opioids is dangerous because they slow breathing and decrease a person's pulse and blood pressure. Opioid abuse is a growing problem in the United States. A person who abuses opioids can become unconscious and even die. People who combine opioids with alcohol or other depressants are at increased risk of experiencing a fatal drug overdose.

Depressants. *Depressants*, which are also called *sedatives* or *tranquilizers*, are used to reduce anxiety and increase a person's ability to relax and stay calm (Figure 11.6). Examples of depressant medication include Valium®, Xanax®, Ambien®, Lunesta®, Nembutal®, and Mebaral®. These medications are also used to help people sleep. A slang term for depressants is *downers*. Depressants include anti-anxiety medications, sleep medications, and *barbiturates*, which are more frequently used for surgical procedures or seizure disorders.

Depressants slow the central nervous system, causing a person's rate of breathing and heart rate to decrease. Depressant use can lead to side effects that include drowsiness and sleepiness, slowed and slurred speech, poor concentration, lack of coordination, confusion, and lowered inhibitions.

A person who takes relatively small amounts of a sedative may experience only a feeling of relaxation. Taking larger amounts, however, can dangerously decrease the heart rate and breathing, causing a person to lose consciousness and even die.

Stimulants. Stimulants are medications used to increase energy, alertness, and attention (Figure 11.7). Slang terms for stimulants include *speed*, *uppers*, and *vitamin R*. They are available both with a prescription and over the counter. People who have attention deficit hyperactivity disorder (ADHD) are often prescribed stimulants. Examples of OTC stimulants include energy pills and appetite suppressants. Using OTC stimulants can be extremely dangerous and even life threatening.

Common stimulants, such as *amphetamines*, increase the level of dopamine in the brain, producing *euphoria* (intense happiness). Although the brain naturally produces dopamine, stimulant use leads to a rapid increase in dopamine levels, which increases the likelihood of becoming addicted over time. Side effects of stimulant use are listed in Figure 11.8 on the next page.

opiates
substances that come from the poppy plant

opioids
synthetic opiates that are prescribed for pain relief

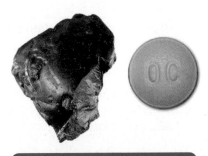

Figure 11.5

Opium (above left), often found in prescription medications such as OxyContin (right), is a substance that relieves pain.

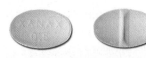

Figure 11.6

Prescription drugs such as Xanax, which contain depressants, slow the body's central nervous system and may lead to drowsiness.

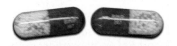

Figure 11.7

Prescription drugs that contain stimulants, such as these amphetamines, increase dopamine levels in the brain and lead to alertness and concentration.

euphoria
a feeling of intense happiness caused by high levels of dopamine in the brain

Figure 11.8   Prescription Medications and Their Side Effects

Drug	Side Effects	Long-Term Consequences
opioids (hydrocodone, codeine, morphine, and oxycodone)	drowsiness, dizziness, weakness, nausea, vomiting, impaired coordination, confusion, sweaty and clammy skin, constipation	dependence, tolerance, slower breathing rates, low blood pressure, unconsciousness, coma, death (especially when combined with alcohol or other depressants)
depressants and sedatives (antianxiety medications, sleep medications, and barbiturates)	drowsiness and sleepiness, slowed and slurred speech, poor concentration, lack of coordination, confusion, lowered inhibitions	dependence, tolerance, depression, chronic fatigue, breathing problems, difficulty sleeping, coma, death (often by overdose)
stimulants or amphetamines (ADHD medication, energy pills, weight-loss supplements)	increased blood pressure and heart rate, decreased quality of sleep, decreased appetite (possibly leading to malnutrition), apathy, depression	dependence, tolerance, feelings of hostility and paranoia, increased body temperature, irregular heartbeat, increased risk of heart attack and stroke

Personal Profile

Are You at Risk of Abusing Drugs?

These questions will help you assess your risk of using drugs.

I carefully read the instructions before taking any type of medication. **yes no**

I never take a medication prescribed for someone else. **yes no**

I tell a doctor or pharmacist about any medications or supplements I'm taking. **yes no**

I do not have family members who regularly misuse or abuse some type of medication or drugs. **yes no**

I do not have friends who regularly misuse or abuse some type of medication or drugs. **yes no**

I do not take risks because I am more concerned about the consequences. **yes no**

I avoid going to parties where drugs are present. **yes no**

I feel confident that I could refuse a friend's offer to try drugs. **yes no**

Add the number of no answers to assess your risk of developing problems related to drug use. The more no answers you have, the greater your risk.

Safe Strategies for Using Medications

Carefully reading and following OTC and prescription medication usage instructions can help avoid misuse and abuse of medications and reduce health risks (Figure 11.9). The instructions should be provided on the medication label, or with the medication box or container. The instructions should include the following:

- how much of the medication to take
- how to take the medication (by mouth, through injection, by inhalation)
- how to store the medication
- how long to wait before taking more medication
- possible side effects, such as dizziness or drowsiness
- whether you should take this medication with food or drink
- whether this medication interacts with other substances that should therefore be avoided

Talking to your doctor or pharmacist before taking any medication is important as well. You need to let them know if you are taking other medications regularly, including OTC medications and even herbal supplements. You also need to let them know if you have any allergies to medications. Other strategies for using medications safely include the following:

- Never use a medication prescribed for someone else or let someone else use medication prescribed for you. Prescriptions are given specifically for one person, based on that person's symptoms, age, weight, and height, and cannot be used safely by anyone else.
- Never take more than the recommended dosage of a medication. This can lead to accidental overdosing and other serious problems.
- Do not give OTC medications intended for adults to infants or children. There are OTC medications specifically intended for children's use.
- Store medications safely in their original containers and keep them away from where pets or younger children might reach them.
- Check expiration dates and safely discard any medications that have expired.

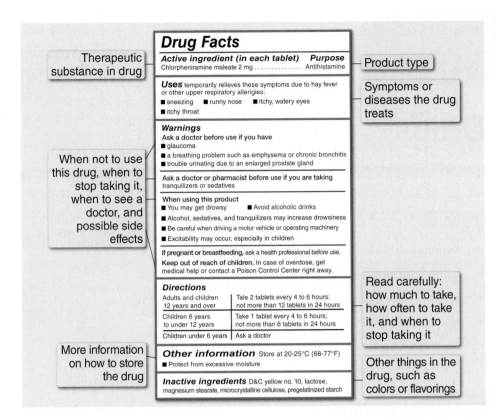

Drug Facts

Active ingredient (in each tablet) **Purpose**
Chlorpheniramine maleate 2 mg . . . . Antihistamine

Uses temporarily relieves these symptoms due to hay fever or other upper respiratory allergies:
■ sneezing   ■ runny nose   ■ itchy, watery eyes
■ itchy throat

Warnings
Ask a doctor before use if you have
■ glaucoma
■ a breathing problem such as emphysema or chronic bronchitis
■ trouble urinating due to an enlarged prostate gland

Ask a doctor or pharmacist before use if you are taking tranquilizers or sedatives

When using this product
■ You may get drowsy   ■ Avoid alcoholic drinks
■ Alcohol, sedatives, and tranquilizers may increase drowsiness
■ Be careful when driving a motor vehicle or operating machinery
■ Excitability may occur, especially in children

If pregnant or breastfeeding, ask a health professional before use.
Keep out of reach of children. In case of overdose, get medical help or contact a Poison Control Center right away.

Directions

Adults and children 12 years and over	Tale 2 tablets every 4 to 6 hours: not more than 12 tablets in 24 hours
Children 6 years to under 12 years	Take 1 tablet every 4 to 6 hours; not more than 6 tablets in 24 hours
Children under 6 years	Ask a doctor

Other information Store at 20-25°C (68-77°F)
■ Protect from excessive moisture

Inactive ingredients D&C yellow no. 10, lactose, magnesium stearate, microcrystalline cellulose, pregelatinized starch

Therapeutic substance in drug

When not to use this drug, when to stop taking it, when to see a doctor, and possible side effects

More information on how to store the drug

Product type

Symptoms or diseases the drug treats

Read carefully: how much to take, how often to take it, and when to stop taking it

Other things in the drug, such as colors or flavorings

Figure 11.9

Over-the-counter medication drug labels include information such as which diseases the medication treats, what the correct dosage is, and possible side effects.

If a health problem does not go away after using OTC medication, see a healthcare professional. Let your doctor know right away if you feel worse after taking a medication, or if you start to develop symptoms such as a rash, vomiting, or difficulty breathing. These symptoms may indicate that you are having an allergic reaction to the medication and need to immediately seek emergency medical care.

Lesson 11.1 Review

Know and Understand Assess

1. List four main reasons people use medications.
2. Which government agency is responsible for making sure medications are safe to use?
3. What are the three most commonly abused prescription medications?
4. List three side effects that may occur as a result of stimulant use.

Analyze and Apply

5. Differentiate between over-the-counter and prescription medications. Give an example of each.
6. Compare medication misuse and medication abuse.

Real World Health

Did you know that, in the United States, many people die each day from opioid overdose? In small groups, visit the website of the Centers for Disease Control and Prevention (CDC) to read about the epidemic of opioid overdose. What are the most common types of opioids abused? What can people do to prevent opioid overdose deaths? What programs and resources exist to battle this epidemic? After conducting your research, discuss your findings in class.

Drugs

Key Terms 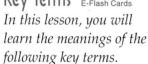 E-Flash Cards

In this lesson, you will learn the meanings of the following key terms.

bath salts

club drugs

cocaine

crystal meth

drug abuse

drug overdose

drugs

hallucinogens

heroin

hypoxia

inhalants

marijuana

Before You Read

Sticky Notes

Your teacher will pass out sticky notes. As you read this lesson, mark the text with sticky notes to indicate points of interest, confusion, or a place where you remembered a connection to something you already know. When you have finished the lesson, discuss the concepts you have selected with a fellow student.

Lesson Objectives

After studying this lesson, you will be able to

- name common types of drugs;

- identify side effects caused by different types of drugs;

- summarize the impact of drugs on the brain; and

- describe negative consequences people who abuse drugs often experience.

Warm-Up Activity

Media Versus Reality

Take a few minutes to think about how drugs are portrayed in the media and what you know about drugs in your environment. Pick three or four examples from both the media and your environment and describe them briefly in a chart like the one shown below. Do not mention names or places in your descriptions of the real instances of drug use.

Compare your examples and form a conclusion as to whether or not the media realistically portrays drug use. Write a paragraph stating your conclusion. Include specific examples from your chart that support your conclusion.

Media Examples
Realistic Examples

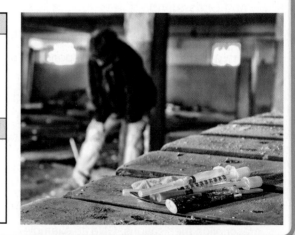

The word *drugs* refers to substances that cause a physical or psychological change in the body. Most drugs are illegal and can be very dangerous. In this lesson you will learn about some common types of drugs and the harmful effects they can have on the body.

Marijuana

Marijuana is the most commonly used illegal drug in the United States, according to the National Survey on Drug Use and Health. **Marijuana** is a drug made up of dried parts of the Cannabis plant (Figure 11.10). Although marijuana is usually smoked as a cigarette (a joint) or in a pipe, it can also be brewed into tea or mixed into food and eaten. Slang terms for marijuana include *weed*, *pot*, *Mary Jane*, and *grass*.

The active ingredient in marijuana is a chemical called *delta-9-tetrahydrocannabinol (THC)*. Upon entering the bloodstream, this chemical is carried to the brain and other organs. THC affects the parts of the brain that control pleasure, memory, thinking, concentration, sensory and time perception, and movement.

Side Effects

People who use marijuana experience a number of impairments, including distorted perceptions, poor coordination, difficulty thinking and solving problems, and problems with learning and memory. The effects of marijuana on learning and memory can last for days or weeks after the acute effects of the drug wear off.

Marijuana use can also lead to cardiovascular problems. People who use marijuana show a substantial increase in heart rate. Research has shown that a person's risk of experiencing a heart attack in the first hour after smoking marijuana is five times higher than their usual risk.

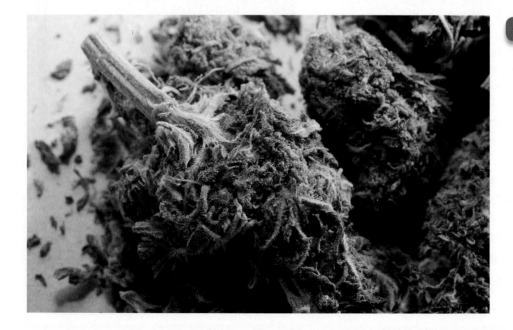

Figure 11.10

Marijuana comes from the dried part of the Cannabis plant and is usually smoked in a cigarette.

People tend to ingest marijuana by smoking it, so they are susceptible to the same respiratory problems that afflict tobacco smokers. Minor respiratory problems include daily cough, more frequent chest illnesses, and an increased risk of lung infection.

Like tobacco smoke, marijuana smoke contains carcinogens, or cancer-causing substances. Marijuana smoke damages people's DNA (genetic makeup) in ways that may increase the risk of developing cancer.

Legalization of Marijuana

Until recently, marijuana has been illegal to sell, buy, and use across the United States. Today, a number of states and the District of Columbia allow adults with a doctor's prescription to legally buy and use marijuana. The THC in marijuana, which is an FDA-approved medication, helps ease the symptoms of various medical conditions, including the nausea cancer patients experience during chemotherapy. In 2014, Colorado was the first state to allow citizens over the age of 21 to buy a limited amount of marijuana for recreational or nonmedical use. During the 2016 election, California, Nevada, Maine, and Massachusetts also legalized recreational marijuana use and sale. The majority of Americans who use marijuana, however, do so illegally.

Local and Global Health
Rates of Illegal Drug Use around the Country

The rates of illegal drug use vary by state. For each state, the rate of illegal drug use is the proportion of people in the state who use illegal drugs. This is the ratio of the number of people who use these drugs in the state to the total population of the state. According to the color-coded maps shown here, some states have more illegal drug use than others. Drug overdoses are also more common in some states than in other states. Use these color-coded maps to answer the following questions.

Thinking Critically

1. In which states do 9.36% or more of the population report using some type of illegal drug?

2. In which states do fewer than 7.39% of the population report using illegal drugs?

3. Which states report the highest rate of deaths by drug overdoses? Which states report the lowest rate?

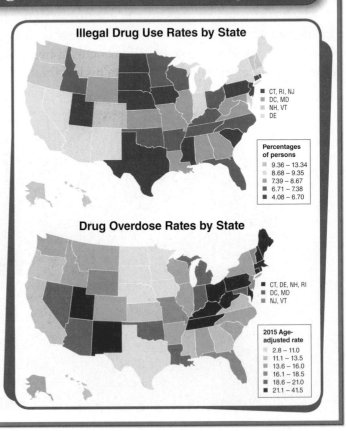

Although the THC in marijuana is approved by the FDA, the marijuana plant is not. The use of marijuana even for medicinal purposes can still pose health risks. Therefore, there is much debate on both federal and state levels of government about whether marijuana should be legalized. Research about medicinal uses for marijuana is ongoing.

Marijuana is commonly called a *gateway drug* because people who use it are more likely to abuse other, more potent and dangerous illegal drugs.

Cocaine

Cocaine, a stimulant, is a white powder that comes from the leaves of a coca plant. Cocaine can be snorted through the nose, dissolved in water and injected, or smoked. This illegal drug can also be processed into a solid substance known as *crack cocaine*, which can be smoked or injected. Slang terms for cocaine include *blow, coke, crack, candy, rock*, or *snow*.

Like amphetamines, cocaine stimulates the central nervous system by raising levels of the neurotransmitter dopamine in the brain. The increased level of dopamine makes users feel more energetic and mentally alert and less fatigued.

Cocaine can have both short- and long-term negative effects on many different body systems. These side effects include increased body temperature, heart rate, and blood pressure; headaches; abdominal pain and nausea; and paranoia. Cocaine use can also lead to sudden death due to a heart attack or stroke.

cocaine
a stimulant made of white powder that comes from the leaves of coca plants

Crystal Meth

Crystal meth, a manufactured form of methamphetamine, consists of clear crystal chunks (Figure 11.11). This drug is usually smoked, but it can also be snorted into the nose, injected directly into the bloodstream, or swallowed. Slang terms for this drug include *meth, ice, crank, crystal*, or *speed*. Crystal meth is a very powerful and extremely addictive illegal drug. People who use this drug quickly become physically and psychologically addicted to its use.

crystal meth
a manufactured drug that acts as an amphetamine and looks like clear crystal chunks

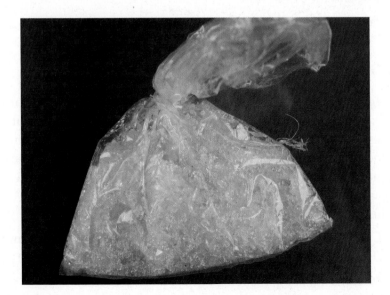

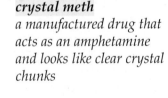

Figure 11.11

Crystal meth is an extremely addictive illegal drug that causes erratic behavior and severe anxiety. *Why do you think people use drugs like crystal meth, which are so dangerous?*

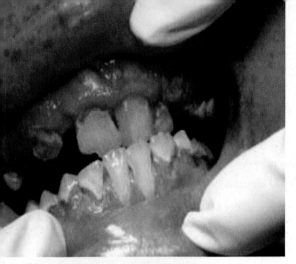

Figure 11.12

One of the more visible side effects of abusing crystal meth is damaged, blackened teeth.

bath salts
manufactured drugs that include the stimulant methylenedioxypyrovalerone (MDPV) and are often found in insect repellent, incense, or plant feeder

hallucinogens
drugs that cause hallucinations and alter a person's sense of reality

Crystal meth has many short-term side effects, which are similar to those of cocaine. These side effects include

- erratic and violent behavior;
- mood swings;
- increased blood pressure and irregular heart rate;
- homicidal and suicidal thoughts;
- tooth decay and cracked teeth (Figure 11.12);
- hallucinations;
- severe anxiety and paranoia; and
- difficulty sleeping.

Long-term use of crystal meth can lead to brain damage, coma, stroke, and death.

Bath Salts

Bath salts are manufactured drugs that contain a stimulant called *methylenedioxypyrovalerone (MDPV)*. These drugs are not to be confused with bathing products. Bath salts, which are chemically similar to amphetamines, often come in a white or brown crystalline powder and are marketed as different products, such as incense, plant feeder, or insect repellent. Some people ingest, snort, or inject bath salts. Slang terms for this drug include *cloud nine*, *ivory wave*, *vanilla sky*, *bliss*, or *blue silk*.

Using bath salts can lead to serious side effects, including

- paranoia;
- chest pains;
- headaches and nausea;
- hallucinations;
- increased heart rate and blood pressure;
- suicidal thoughts; and
- death.

Hallucinogens

Hallucinogens are drugs that change a person's perception of reality. After taking this type of drug, people see, hear, or feel things that are not real. These drugs can be manufactured chemically or created from plants. Hallucinogens can be swallowed as pills or capsules, applied to absorbent paper and dissolved in the mouth, and mixed in foods or beverages. These drugs can also be snorted or smoked.

Some of the most commonly known hallucinogens are

- *LSD* (lysergic acid diethylamide), a drug created from a fungus (Figure 11.13A);
- *Mescaline*, a drug created from the peyote cactus;

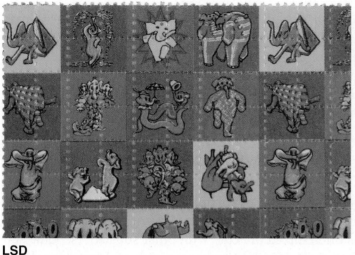

LSD

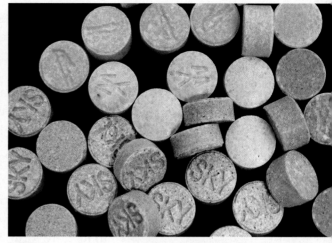

MDMA

Figure 11.13

(A) LSD is often added to absorbent paper divided into small squares with images printed on them. A square is one dose. (B) MDMA is usually distributed in the form of colorful tablets. Like many street drugs, MDMA tablets often contain ingredients users do not expect. Tablets such as these may be marketed as Ecstasy, but contain other dangerous drugs.

- *Psilocybin* (4-phosphoryloxy-N, N-dimethyltryptamine), which is found in certain types of mushrooms;

- *PCP* (phencyclidine), a drug initially developed for use as an anesthetic; and

- *MDMA* (3,4-methylenedioxymethamphetamine), meth, "Molly" or "ecstasy," a manufactured drug (Figure 11.13B).

Researchers believe that hallucinogens work, by temporarily disrupting the function of neurotransmitters in the body. Hallucinogens impact many natural processes, including hunger, mood, sexual behavior, aggression, sleep, learning, memory, pain, and sensory perceptions. People who use hallucinogens experience a variety of negative side effects, including

- increased heart rate and blood pressure;

- profuse sweating;

- tremors and uncoordinated movements;

- muscle weakness and numbness;

- sleep disturbances;

- anxiety;

- loss of appetite, nausea, and vomiting;

- confusion;

- delusions and hallucinations, and an inability to discern fantasy from reality;

- mood disturbances, increased anxiety and depression; and

- panic reactions and paranoia, including severe, terrifying thoughts and feelings of despair, fear of losing control, or fear of insanity and death.

Long-term abuse of hallucinogens can have even more serious consequences. These include memory loss; difficulties with speech and thinking; seizures; loss of balance; blurred vision; and a decrease in blood pressure, pulse rate, and respiration. Flashbacks, or recurrences of certain effects of the drugs, such as visual disturbances, may also occur. These flashbacks can happen suddenly, without warning, within a few days or more than a year after using the drug.

In some cases, even a single use of a hallucinogen can lead to death. Hallucinogen use can cause the blood vessels in the heart and brain to narrow, which can result in a heart attack or stroke. Elevations in blood pressure, heart rate, and body temperature can contribute to brain damage. Hallucinogens can also cause a severe drop in the level of sodium in the blood, which can cause brain swelling and seizures.

Heroin

The drug known as *heroin* is an opiate derived from morphine—a naturally occurring substance found in poppy plants (Figure 11.14). Heroin, in its pure form, is often mixed or "cut" with other substances. Some substances used to cut heroin may be toxic or poisonous. Heroin can be injected, snorted, or smoked. Slang terms for heroin include *blacktar*, *big H*, and *brown sugar*.

People who use heroin often develop a dependency on the drug and find it very difficult to stop using it. Also, people who use heroin do not know how much of the drug they are consuming in its pure form, which can be especially dangerous.

Heroin users report an initial feeling of pleasure or euphoria, known as a *high*, as the drug enters the brain. Many less positive effects soon follow, however, including dry mouth, severe itching, difficulty thinking, drowsiness, nausea, and vomiting.

Taking heroin and other opiates is dangerous because these drugs slow breathing and decrease a person's pulse and blood pressure. Someone who abuses opiates can become unconscious and even die.

Club Drugs

The term *club drugs* refers to several different types of drugs that may be abused by teenagers and young adults at parties, bars, and concerts. These drugs include Flunitrazepam (Rohypnol, or *roofies*) and gamma-hydroxybutyrate (GHB), ketamine, MDMA (ecstasy, or Molly), LSD, and other methamphetamines. Club drugs are often taken as a liquid, or in powder form mixed with a liquid. Some types may also be ground up and snorted or injected into the body.

Depending on the drug, side effects can include memory loss, impaired attention, delirium, intense drowsiness, coma, and death. These drugs can also be addictive, so people who attempt to stop using a club drug may experience unpleasant withdrawal effects, such as anxiety, nausea, and tremors.

In some cases, depressants or sedatives are given to people without their knowledge, which is dangerous and illegal. *Date rape drugs* are sedatives that can be slipped into someone's food or drink to make him or her drowsy and less able to resist unwanted sexual advances. Drugs that are commonly used for this purpose include "roofies" and GHB.

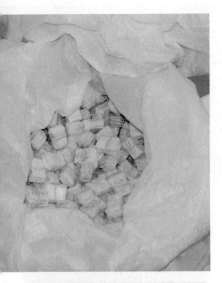

Figure 11.14

Above is a bag of raw heroin decks (bricks) that was confiscated during a drug bust. The illegal operation, called a *heroin mill*, generated millions of dollars from the sale of the drug.

heroin
an opiate drug derived from morphine and often mixed with sugar, powdered milk, or other drugs

club drugs
a category of drugs that are often used at parties, bars, or concerts; include LSD, ecstasy, GHB, and Flunitrazepam (roofies)

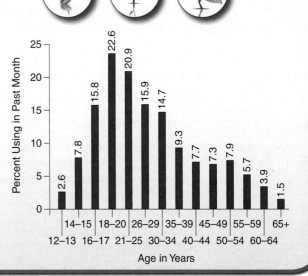

Rates of Illegal Drug Use by Age

Drug use is much more common among people in certain age groups. The bar graph at the right shows the percentage of people, by age group, who used illegal drugs in a particular month.

Analyzing Data

1. Which three age groups are especially at risk of using illegal drugs?
2. Why do you think drug use increases with age until the late teens and early 20s, and then starts to decrease?

Anabolic Steroids and PEDs

Some people use anabolic steroids to treat medical conditions. Other people use anabolic steroids illegally to help them gain strength and increase muscle size (Figure 11.15). Slang terms are not common, but they can include *roids* or *juice*.

Some side effects of steroid use are specific to gender and age. Men experience shrinking of the testicles, reduced sperm count, infertility, baldness, development of breasts, and increased risk of prostate cancer. Women experience growth of facial hair, baldness, changes in or disruption of the menstrual cycle, and a deepened voice. Adolescents experience stunted growth (caused by premature maturation of the skeleton and accelerated pubertal changes), which leads to a risk of not achieving expected height.

Anabolic steroids are a class of performance-enhancing drugs (PEDs). Other PEDs include *human growth hormone (HGH)*, which works in a way similar to anabolic steroids, increasing muscle mass, endurance, and strength. Synthetic or manufactured *erythropoietin (EPO)* is a drug used to increase the production of red blood cells. EPO increases the flow of oxygen to muscles and reduces muscle fatigue. *Beta-blockers* slow down the heart and relax the muscles, which can improve performance in sports that require steady hands, such as golf, archery, and gymnastics. Finally, several types of stimulants increase energy, alertness, and attention. All PEDs can lead to undesirable side effects, and the use of PEDs is banned by high schools, colleges, and professional sporting leagues. Thus, PED use can have very severe consequences.

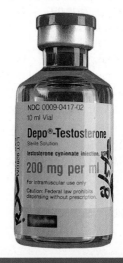

Figure 11.15

Anabolic steroids can be taken orally, injected, or applied as a gel or cream.

Inhalants

Inhalants are chemicals that people breathe in to experience some type of high. These chemicals are inhaled into the nose or mouth in several ways. Chemical fumes may be sniffed or snorted from a container, which is

inhalants
chemicals that people breathe in to experience some type of high

Figure 11.16 Illegal Substances and Their Side Effects

Drug	Side Effects	Long-Term Consequences
marijuana (weed, pot, Mary Jane, grass)	distorted perceptions, poor coordination, difficulty with thinking and problem solving, learning and memory problems	cardiovascular and respiratory problems
cocaine (blow, coke, crack, candy, rock, snow)	increases in body temperature, heart rate, and blood pressure; headaches; abdominal pain; nausea; paranoia	highly addictive; heart attacks, respiratory failure, strokes, and seizures; in rare cases, sudden death during or immediately after first use
crystal meth (meth, ice, crank, crystal, speed)	increased wakefulness; decreased appetite; mood swings; increased blood pressure and body temperature; irregular heart rate; hallucinations, severe anxiety, and paranoia; homicidal and suicidal thoughts	dependence, tolerance, tooth decay and cracked teeth, malnutrition, skin sores caused by scratching, brain damage, coma, stroke, death
bath salts (cloud nine, ivory wave, vanilla sky, bliss, blue silk)	paranoia, chest pains, headaches, nausea, hallucinations, increased heart rate and blood pressure, suicidal thoughts	dependence, tolerance, suicidal thoughts, death
hallucinogens (LSD, peyote, psilocybin, PCP, MDMA, ecstasy)	delusions and hallucinations; increased heart rate and blood pressure; extreme anxiety; profuse sweating; cramping, tremors, and uncoordinated movements; muscle weakness and numbness; sleep disturbances; paranoia	memory loss; difficulty speaking and thinking; seizures; loss of balance; blurred vision; drops in blood pressure, pulse rate, and respiration; flashbacks
heroin (blacktar, big H, brown sugar)	feelings of euphoria; dry mouth, nausea, and vomiting; severe itching; difficulty thinking; drowsiness	highly addictive, cardiovascular problems, spontaneous abortion, death
club drugs (GHB, Rohypnol, ketamine)	impaired attention, learning ability, and memory; amnesia, delirium, and hallucinations; sleep problems	dependence, tolerance, impaired motor function, seizures, coma, death
anabolic steroids (roids, juice)	acne, oily hair, swelling of the legs and feet, persistent bad breath	addictive; increased risk of developing heart disease, stroke, and cancer; high blood pressure; liver damage; severe mood swings and anger; hallucinations; paranoia
inhalants (liquids, aerosols, gases, nitrites)	slurred speech; memory problems; lack of coordination, muscle spasms, and tremors; lightheadedness and dizziness; hallucinations and delusions	hypoxia; hearing loss; damage to the brain, central nervous system, liver, and kidneys; death

called *huffing.* Chemicals can also be sprayed directly into the nose or mouth. Because the euphoria produced by the chemicals lasts just a few minutes, people tend to use inhalants repeatedly to maintain the feeling. Commonly abused inhalants include substances often found in the home, such as liquids (paint thinners, gasoline, felt-tip markers, and glue); aerosols (spray paints, hair or deodorant sprays, sprays used to protect fabrics, and vegetable oil sprays); gases (butane lighters and whipped cream canisters); and nitrites (products used for medical purposes, such as butyl and amyl nitrites).

When these chemicals are inhaled they enter the lungs and can cause hypoxia (Figure 11.16). *Hypoxia* is a condition that occurs when the supply of oxygen needed by the body is depleted. This results in widespread cell damage. Brain cells are particularly affected by a lack of oxygen. Over time,

hypoxia
a condition in which cells and tissue are deprived of oxygen; often results in severe cell damage

Luke is 16 years old and a junior in high school. He enjoys hanging out with friends and going to parties on the weekends. Most of Luke's friends share his view that using drugs is a bad idea. A couple of his friends, however, started huffing.

Luke did not think huffing was a big deal because it involved products he could easily buy. He would try it the next time his friends invited him to join them. Then Luke heard about a teenage girl in a nearby town who died from *Sudden Sniffing Death Syndrome (SSDS)*. She died after she tried huffing for the first time and her heart stopped beating. Luke agonized for some time but finally decided he would not try huffing—even one time. He also urged his friends to stop.

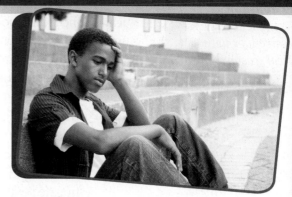

Thinking Critically

1. What are some factors that might have led Luke's friends to try inhalants?

2. What are some strategies Luke can use to avoid the temptation or pressure to use inhalants?

inhalants reduce the ability of nerve fibers to carry messages throughout the body.

Other side effects of using inhalants include slurred speech, memory problems, lack of coordination, muscle spasms and tremors, lightheadedness and dizziness, and hallucinations and delusions.

Inhalant use can also cause serious, permanent side effects. These include hearing loss and damage to the brain, central nervous system, liver, and kidneys. Using inhalants—even once—can cause death due to heart failure or suffocation.

The Impact of Drugs on the Brain

The brain naturally produces the chemicals dopamine and endorphins. *Dopamine* influences the parts of the brain that control movement, emotion, motivation, and feelings of pleasure. *Endorphins* increase feelings of happiness. When you do something you enjoy, your brain releases these chemicals, giving you a pleasurable sensation. This is why people feel good after being physically active, eating chocolate, or listening to music. All of these activities are natural ways of increasing the level of endorphins in your body, which lifts your mood.

Drugs contain chemicals that change the way nerve cells in the brain send, receive, and process information. Many drugs cause cells in the brain to release abnormally large amounts of dopamine. The brain then reduces its production of the natural chemicals. The person then becomes dependent on drug use for positive feelings. Moreover, the body develops a *tolerance* to a given level of the drug. Larger and larger amounts of the drug are required to achieve the same good feelings. This contributes to drug abuse.

Drug Abuse

drug abuse
the act of using drugs excessively or without medical reason

Drug abuse occurs when a person uses a drug excessively or without medical justification. The term *substance abuse* is sometimes used interchangeably with *drug abuse*. Substance abuse, however, is a broader term that includes the abuse of other substances—such as tobacco and alcohol—in addition to drugs.

People who abuse drugs often experience many negative health consequences. They also experience other types of negative consequences. These are likely to include the following:

- *Engaging in unsafe behaviors*—Because drug use impairs the ability to think clearly and carefully, people under the influence of drugs are at increased risk of engaging in risky, unsafe behaviors such as unsafe sexual behavior.
- *Contracting an infectious disease*—People who use drugs that are injected with a needle are at increased risk of contracting serious infectious diseases, such as hepatitis or HIV.
- *Being involved in an accident*—Drugs change brain functions and can impair a person's ability to drive safely.
- *Overdosing*—A **drug overdose** is caused by ingesting more of a drug than the body can properly process, or break down, at one time. A person who overdoses on a drug may do so intentionally or accidentally.

drug overdose
the ingestion of more of a drug than the body can successfully process at one time

In addition to these negative consequences, people who abuse drugs also experience other problems. For example, these people may also have

- legal problems, such as getting arrested;
- academic problems, such as being suspended or expelled from school;
- work problems, such as absenteeism, failing drug tests, and getting fired;
- financial problems; and
- social problems, such as losing friends.

Lesson 11.2 Review

Know and Understand

1. What are *drugs*?
2. Which illegal drug is a manufactured form of methamphetamine?
3. List two commonly known hallucinogens.
4. Which drug is an opiate derived from morphine?
5. What is *hypoxia*?
6. List three negative consequences experienced by people who abuse drugs.

Analyze and Apply

7. Explain why marijuana is commonly called a *gateway drug*.

8. Write a short public service announcement advocating for athletes not to use PEDs.

Real World Health

Imagine that while driving under the influence of marijuana, you caused a severe, life-altering injury to a close friend who was a passenger in your car. Your counselor suggests that you write a letter to your friend expressing your feelings about what happened. Think about your reasons for using marijuana and why you chose to drive with impaired judgment and reflexes. Also think about how the accident has affected your friend's hopes, dreams, and goals for the future, as well as your own. Then write your letter.

Lesson 11.3

Drug Abuse and Addiction

Lesson Objectives

After studying this lesson, you will be able to

- distinguish between physical and psychological addiction;
- describe risk factors for drug abuse and addiction;
- identify strategies for refusing drugs;
- summarize how drug abuse impacts families, friends, and society;
- describe ways to prevent and treat drug abuse and addiction; and
- determine how to help someone who is addicted to drugs.

Key Terms E-Flash Cards

In this lesson, you will learn the meanings of the following key terms.

drug addiction

self-medication

Warm-Up Activity

Motivation and Drugs

What behaviors do you associate with drug addiction? On a separate piece of paper, list these behaviors and then find a partner and combine your lists. As you read this lesson, categorize each behavior as a result of either psychological addiction, physical addiction, or both in a chart like the one shown below. Then, compare answers with your partner and discuss areas where you disagree.

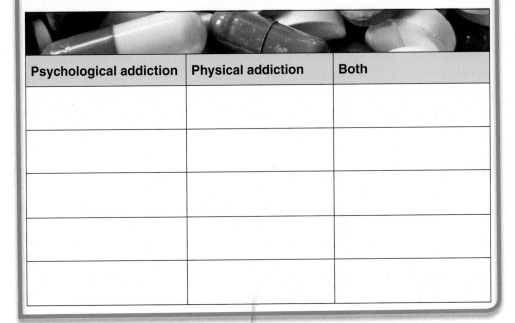

Psychological addiction	Physical addiction	Both

Before You Read

Abuse and Addiction

Create a Venn diagram and use it to compare and contrast drug abuse and drug addiction. What do they share? What is unique to each condition?

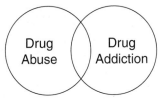

I n the first lesson of this chapter you learned about misuse and abuse of over-the-counter and prescription medications. (These medications are also commonly referred to as *OTC* and *prescription drugs*.) In the second lesson you learned about the abuse of other drugs, such as cocaine and heroin. People who abuse OTC drugs, prescription drugs, and other drugs are at risk of becoming addicted. Therefore, the use of the terms *drug abuse* and *drug addiction* in this lesson will include OTC and prescription drugs as well as other drugs.

No one who starts using drugs plans to become an addict. Unfortunately, many people who use drugs become addicted and spend years trying to break their habit. In this lesson you'll learn what people can do to avoid becoming addicted to drugs. You'll also learn how people can get help to treat a drug addiction.

What Is Drug Addiction?

drug addiction
a chronic disease characterized by the continued use of a drug regardless of its harmful consequences

Drug addiction is a chronic disease that involves the continued use of a drug regardless of any harmful or negative consequences that may result. People with a drug addiction may experience a physical or psychological addiction to the drug.

Physical Addiction

People often think it is harmless to experiment with drugs, but this is very untrue. Experimentation can lead to regular use, which often results in developing a tolerance for a drug. After people develop a tolerance to a drug, they often become physically addicted.

When people are physically addicted to a drug, their bodies require that drug to function normally. People become used to, or dependent on, having the sensations caused by that drug. If they reduce the amount they take, they experience a strong craving for the drug. They also experience *withdrawal*, or unpleasant physical side effects, when they try to stop taking the drug. These negative feelings make it particularly hard to stop using a drug.

The symptoms of withdrawal vary depending on the specific drug used. They can include vision problems, digestion problems, irritability, difficulty concentrating, sleeplessness, seizures, fatigue, hallucinations, aches and pains, muscle tremors, decreased appetite, and anxiety and depression.

Psychological Addiction

People who are psychologically addicted to a particular drug feel an intense need or desire for that drug. They feel they need that drug to function normally, and can become distressed if they are unable to use it. For example, someone who is used to taking caffeine pills to stay up writing a paper will feel anxious if the pills are not available the next time an assignment is due.

Risk Factors for Drug Abuse and Addiction

Although anyone can abuse and become addicted to a drug, experts point to certain risk factors that could increase a person's chances of becoming addicted.

Biological Makeup

A person's genetic makeup influences whether he or she will become addicted to drugs. People whose parents have addiction problems are at greater risk of becoming addicts themselves. Experts believe that people's genes account for about half of their risk of becoming addicted to drugs.

A person's biological makeup can also influence his or her personality. Some people have a cautious personality and are averse to risk taking. These people may be reluctant to use drugs due to their concerns about the consequences. Other people are more curious and likely to take risks. Unfortunately, a willingness to take risks and use drugs can lead to addiction.

Mental Health Problems

People who have mental health problems, such as depression or anxiety, may use drugs to cope with their symptoms. The use of drugs by an individual to treat problems and symptoms not diagnosed by a medical doctor is called *self-medication*. People who self-medicate do not get the professional help they need to successfully diagnose and treat their condition. Self-medicating also puts people at risk of developing addictions and more severe mental health problems.

self-medication
the use of drugs to treat symptoms that have not been diagnosed by a medical professional

Stage of Development

The earlier a person begins using a drug, the more likely he or she is to abuse and become addicted to that drug (Figure 11.17). Teenagers are at particular risk of becoming addicted to drugs. This is partly because the

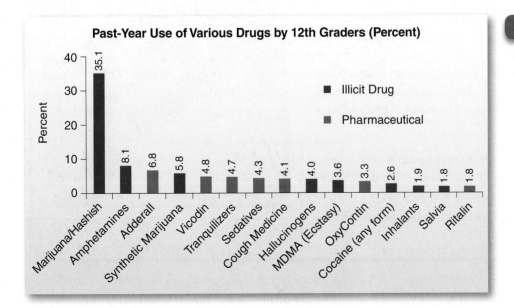

Past-Year Use of Various Drugs by 12th Graders (Percent)

- Illicit Drug
- Pharmaceutical

Marijuana/Hashish 35.1, Amphetamines 8.1, Adderall 6.8, Synthetic Marijuana 5.8, Vicodin 4.8, Tranquilizers 4.7, Sedatives 4.3, Cough Medicine 4.1, Hallucinogens 4.0, MDMA (Ecstasy) 3.6, OxyContin 3.3, Cocaine (any form) 2.6, Inhalants 1.9, Salvia 1.8, Ritalin 1.8

Figure 11.17

What information in this chart most suprises you? Which piece of information most concerns you?

brains of teenagers are still developing in the areas that govern decision making, judgment, and self-control.

Environment

The environment in which people live has an impact on their potential exposure to drugs and whether they feel pressured to use drugs. Environment includes a person's community, culture, school, family, and peers. For example, teens may feel pressured to try drugs if they attend parties where drugs are present.

A person's environment also includes social institutions, such as the media, that reflect and reinforce social values. Some research suggests that teenagers who see drug use in movies are more likely to experiment with drugs themselves. Another study found that half of high school students surveyed believed that seeing professional athletes use steroids influenced their friends' decisions to use steroids.

Choosing to live a drug-free lifestyle can be challenging for teens, especially when teens' environments expose them to drugs and the pressures of trying them. There are strategies, however, that teens can use to refuse drugs.

Research in Action

Can Listening to Music Be Bad for Your Health?

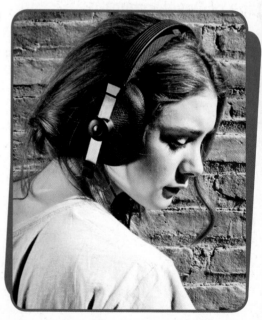

Research shows the typical teenager hears 84 references to alcohol and drug use in music every day—over 30,000 references each year. Researchers in one study looked for references to alcohol and drug use in the lyrics of 279 of the most current popular songs. They found that

- marijuana use is mentioned in about 14% of the songs;
- alcohol use is described in 24% of the songs; and
- other substances are mentioned in another 12% of the songs.

Even more alarming, many of the lyrics linked drug use with positive outcomes. The lyrics described people using drugs as being glamorous and wealthy with increased creativity and social status.

Thinking Critically

1. Does listening to suggestive lyrics have an impact on how you and other teenagers behave? Why or why not?

2. Do artists have a responsibility to create products that promote positive instead of negative behaviors? Please explain your answer.

Strategies for Refusing Drugs

Knowing how to respond and what to say if someone offers you drugs can help you avoid them. For example, one good strategy for refusing drugs is to be direct and say in a firm, but polite way, "No thanks, I don't use drugs." Another strategy is to provide an excuse, such as "I don't want to try drugs because my parents will kill me if I do."

If you continue to be pressured to use drugs, you might ask the person pressuring you why it is so important to him or her that you use drugs. After all, you have already expressed your lack of interest. Remember that people respect each others' choices in healthy relationships. Let the person know that you need him or her to respect your decision to not try drugs. If the person refuses to accept this, you may need to stop spending time with that person.

You may feel pressured to use drugs because it seems like everyone is doing it, but this is not true. Many teens have never tried drugs and have committed to living a drug-free lifestyle. A good rule is to make friends with people who share your values. You may want to make new friends by getting involved in activities that promote health and wellness.

The Broader Impact of Drugs

People who abuse drugs or are addicted to drugs obviously hurt themselves. The problems of drug abuse and addiction, however, also negatively impact their friends, family, and society.

People who are addicted to drugs often put their own need to use drugs above the needs of their families and friends. Drug abuse and addiction are costly for society—approximately $215 billion each year in the United States (Figure 11.18). These costs include the expense of healthcare services that treat drug abusers, as well as the victims of their accidents and criminal activities. The criminal justice system is burdened with tracking down, prosecuting, and jailing people involved in drug-related crimes. Businesses also suffer as a result of productivity loss, absenteeism, and theft. Unemployment and homelessness are other potential issues that stem from drug abuse and addiction.

Prevention of Drug Abuse and Addiction

Drug addiction is a preventable disease. People who never try drugs cannot abuse them and become addicted to them. Unfortunately, many people do not understand how quickly drug abuse can lead to addiction. Learning about and identifying risk factors for drug abuse and addiction, and educating people about the hazards of drug use can help prevent drug abuse and addiction.

Many schools have established substance abuse prevention programs to help educate students about the dangers of using tobacco, alcohol, and drugs. School policies and regulations exist to eliminate drug use on school property.

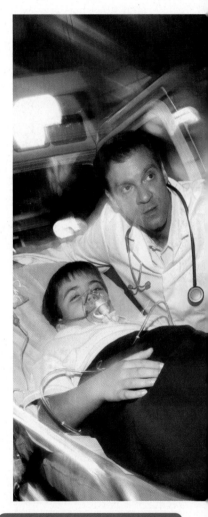

Figure 11.18

Drug abuse can lead to soaring healthcare costs. *What other costs result from drug abuse?*

Avoiding the Abuse of Medications and Other Drugs

The strategies listed below can help you avoid misusing and abusing medications and other drugs.

- Before you use a medication, make sure to carefully read all of the instructions.

- Understand the side effects of all medications before you take them.

- Understand the short- and long-term consequences of abusing different types of drugs.

- Develop strategies for handling offers or pressure from other people to try drugs.

- Avoid going to places where other people may be using drugs.

Community outreach programs are also available to help prevent substance abuse among teens and others. Reliable online sources provide information specifically for teens about drug abuse and prevention.

Treatment for Drug Abuse and Addiction

Drug addiction is a disease just like any other. People with a drug addiction cannot just fix themselves—they need the help of family, friends, and professionals, such as counselors, to end their dependence on drugs and return to their normal lives. Even after breaking the addiction to drugs, many people struggle with managing their addiction throughout their lives. The following programs are available to help treat drug abuse and addiction:

- *Residential treatment programs.* The goal of residential treatment programs is to help people get through the early stages of breaking an addiction in an inpatient environment with lots of support and relatively few distractions. Treatment programs often begin with a process called *detoxification*, which clears all drugs from a person's body. Medications may be needed to help suppress the withdrawal symptoms that occur. These programs may last for weeks or for months.

- *Outpatient treatment programs.* These programs vary in the types of services they provide. Some may only provide drug education. Others provide services similar to those offered in residential treatment programs. Many outpatient treatment programs provide group counseling.

- *Skills-training programs.* These programs help people recognize and avoid situations that lead them to use drugs. People are able to learn alternative ways of dealing with peer pressure and how to handle stressful life events without relying on drugs.

- *Support groups.* People who are trying to overcome a drug addiction come together and discuss the challenges they face. Narcotics Anonymous is an example of a support group for drug abuse.

- *Sober living communities.* Sober living houses or communities are alcohol- and drug-free living environments for people who are trying to abstain from substance use. These environments reduce some of the temptation and pressure to use alcohol and drugs and provide social support for abstaining.

Helping Someone Who Is Addicted to Drugs

If you know someone who is addicted to drugs, here are some ways you can help that person.

- Express your concern about the person's health. Knowing that you care and are concerned about him or her can help the person understand the seriousness of the problem (Figure 11.19).
- People with an addiction can feel alone and isolated. Assure this person that you care about him or her and will be available when help is needed.
- Offer to help the person find someone to talk with about the addiction.
- Offer to go with the person to a meeting with a counselor.
- Attend a meeting of a group that provides support to relatives and friends of someone with a drug addiction.
- Give your friend the number of a hotline he or she can call.

Remember that it is not your responsibility to help other people stop abusing drugs. They must want to break their addiction, and have to be willing to make an effort to do so. You may need to wait for them to admit they have a problem and want help in treating their addiction.

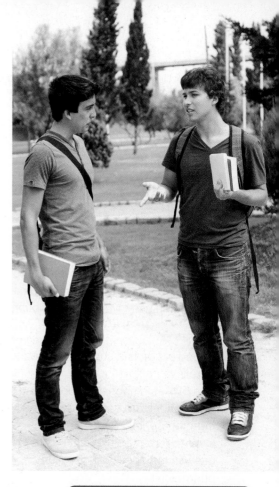

Figure 11.19

It is not easy to confront a friend about what you believe is your friend's serious, even dangerous, problem with drugs. Sometimes, however, the more difficult option is the best option.

Lesson 11.3 Review

Know and Understand
Assess

1. What is *drug addiction*?
2. List five symptoms of withdrawal.
3. List four risk factors that could increase the chances of a person becoming addicted to drugs.
4. Identify three ways in which drug abuse and addiction are costly for society.
5. How can people help prevent drug abuse and addiction?

Analyze and Apply

6. Explain how building up a tolerance for a drug can lead to addiction.

7. Analyze strategies for refusing drugs and identify which strategy would be most effective for you.

Real World Health

You have learned about the negative effects of drug and medication misuse and abuse on health and well-being. Now consider the positive effects of abstaining from a life of drug use. With a partner, share about your career goals, relationships, personal aspirations, and desires. Predict how abstaining from drug use will benefit your future lifestyle and research school and community resources that could help you abstain from drug use.

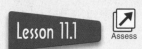

Medications

Key Terms

analgesics
euphoria
medication
medication abuse
medication misuse

opiates
opioids
over-the-counter (OTC)
medications
prescription medications

Key Points

- A medication is a substance used to treat disease or relieve pain.
- The FDA is responsible for making sure medications are safe to use, effective, and secure from tampering.
- Over-the-counter medications are generally safe to use without specific instructions from a doctor or pharmacist.
- Using over-the-counter and prescription medications carries some risks.
- Following safe strategies for using medications can help you avoid medication misuse and abuse.

Check Your Understanding

1. The most commonly used OTC medications are _____.
   A. sleeping pills
   B. analgesics
   C. anti-diarrheal medications
   D. anti-fungal creams

2. _____ kill or slow the growth of bacteria.
   A. Analgesics
   B. Anesthetics
   C. Antibiotics
   D. Vaccinations

3. *True or false?* A transdermal patch is a type of medication that is rubbed on a particular part of the body.

4. Mistakenly taking two pills instead of one is an example of _____.

5. *True or false?* Medication misuse includes instances in which people stop taking a medication before they should.

6. The intentional use of medications for purposes other than those intended by the prescribing doctor is called _____.

7. Prescription medications typically prescribed to relieve pain are called _____.
   A. sedatives
   B. depressants
   C. opioids
   D. stimulants

8. What does *euphoria* mean?

9. *True or false?* Prescriptions given specifically for one person can also be used safely by other people.

10. **Critical Thinking.** Describe the functions of opioids, depressants, and stimulants.

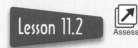

Drugs

Key Terms

bath salts
club drugs
cocaine
crystal meth
drug abuse
drug overdose

drugs
hallucinogens
heroin
hypoxia
inhalants
marijuana

Key Points

- Drugs are substances that cause a physical or psychological change in the body.
- Most drugs are illegal and can be very dangerous.
- Drugs cause many harmful side effects, including death.
- Drugs contain chemicals that change the way nerve cells in the brain send, receive, and process information.
- People who abuse drugs often experience many negative health consequences.

Check Your Understanding

11. _____ is a drug made up of dried parts of the Cannabis plant.
    A. Cocaine
    B. Crystal meth
    C. Marijuana
    D. Mescaline

12. Cocaine stimulates the central nervous system by raising levels of the neurotransmitter _____ in the brain.

13. *True or false?* Tooth decay and cracked teeth are examples of common side effects from taking bath salts.

14. LSD is a drug created from _____.
    A. the coca plant
    B. the cannabis plant
    C. a fungus
    D. the peyote cactus

15. Flashbacks may occur with the long-term abuse of _____.
    A. cocaine
    B. bath salts
    C. marijuana
    D. hallucinogens

16. The drug known as _____ is an opiate derived from morphine—a naturally occurring substance found in poppy plants.
    A. cocaine
    B. GHB
    C. heroin
    D. MDMA

17. Chemicals that people breathe in to experience some type of high are called _____.
    A. hallucinogens
    B. anabolic steroids
    C. inhalants
    D. bath salts

18. Being physically active is a natural way of increasing the level of _____ in the body, which lifts a person's mood.

19. A drug _____ is caused by ingesting more of a drug than the body can properly process at one time.

20. **Critical Thinking.** Research and analyze how drug abuse and addiction affect success in the workplace. What could happen if a person fails a drug test? How do drug abuse and addiction impact workplace safety?

Lesson 11.3

Assess

Drug Abuse and Addiction

Key Terms

drug addiction

self-medication

Key Points

- People may experience a physical or psychological addiction to a drug.
- Certain risk factors, such as biological makeup and environment, can increase the chances of a person becoming addicted to drugs.
- Developing strategies for refusing drugs can help people know how to respond if pressured to use drugs.
- People who abuse or are addicted to drugs hurt themselves and negatively impact their families, friends, and society.
- Drug addiction can be prevented by encouraging people to never try drugs.
- Treatment programs are available to help treat drug abuse and addiction.

Check Your Understanding

21. People who have a(n) _____ addiction to a drug feel that they need a drug to function normally.

22. The use of drugs by an individual to treat problems and symptoms *not* diagnosed by a medical doctor is called _____.

23. *True or false?* People who are addicted to drugs often put the needs of their families and friends above their own need to use drugs.

24. Treatment programs for drug addiction often begin with a process called _____, which clears all drugs from a person's body.

25. Narcotics Anonymous is an example of a(n) _____ for drug abuse.

26. Long- or short-term programs that treat people with a drug addiction in an inpatient setting for weeks or months are called _____.
    A. outpatient treatment programs
    B. skills-training programs
    C. residential treatment programs
    D. support groups

27. *True or false?* To stop abusing drugs, a person must first admit that he or she has a problem and wants help in treating the addiction.

28. **Critical Thinking.** Compare physical and psychological addiction.

Health and Wellness Skills

29. **Make Decisions.** Suppose you get invited to a party. When you show up, you see a bowl of pills on the table and are asked to take a handful. Having just learned about the dangers of participating in these types of activities, you must make a choice: join the crowd or refuse the risk. Use the steps in the "DECIDE" model below to determine what you will do, then explain and compare your reasoning with your classmates' ideas.
    - Define the problem
    - Explore the alternatives
    - Consider the consequences
    - Identify your values
    - Decide and act
    - Evaluate the result

30. **Access Information.** Search your school's website for your school's drug and alcohol policy. What are the penalties for students having illegal substances in their possession or being under the influence of an illegal substance on school grounds? What are the penalties for a second violation? Write a reflection on what you think a student's attitude toward drugs might be if he or she resorts to using or selling drugs at school.

31. **Reduce Health Risks.** Take the survey below for yourself and a friend to see if you or your friend has a problem with drugs. Do you think you or your friend should discuss your responses with a teacher, a counselor, or your parents?
    - Have we missed school due to drinking alcohol or using drugs?
    - Do we use drugs to feel more comfortable, forget about worries, or build self-confidence?
    - Do we use substances alone?
    - Do we ever feel guilty because of substance use?
    - Have we ever been in trouble at home or school for substance use?
    - Have we ever borrowed money to get the substance?
    - Do we feel a sense of power when using substances?
    - Have we lost friends due to substance use?
    - Are we hanging out with a substance-abusing crowd?

Hands-On Activity
Consequences of Addiction

Drug addiction can have many negative consequences beyond health problems, including trouble with the law, loss of a job, or strained relationships with loved ones. Follow the steps listed below to create a scenario in which an addicted individual deals with these consequences.

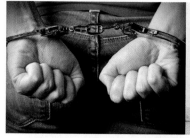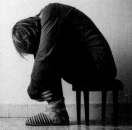

Steps for this Activity

1. Create a story about a fictional teenager who is negatively affected by drugs or addiction. Use six storyboard-style comic strip boxes to create a Public Service Announcement (PSA) warning about the dangers of drug use. Perhaps your strip would include your renderings of images such as the ones shown below. Using information in your textbook, from the Internet, and in class notes, gather information on marijuana, inhalants, heroin, cocaine, and prescription pill abuse. In your PSA, address one of the following topics: strained relationships with boyfriend, girlfriend, friends, or parents; trouble with the law; overdose or death; or inability to pursue goals and dreams.

2. In 1 or 2 paragraphs, briefly explain what is happening in your comic strip. How does it warn teens about the dangers of drug use?

Core Skills

Math Practice

As you may recall, *opioids* (synthetic opiates) are commonly abused prescription medications typically prescribed to relieve pain. The following graph shows deaths from opioid pain relievers by age group, beginning at 15 years of age. Study the graph and then answer the questions.

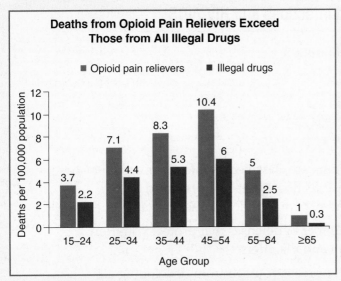

Deaths from Opioid Pain Relievers Exceed Those from All Illegal Drugs

32. Which of the following combined age groups has the highest number of deaths caused by opioid pain relievers?
    A. 15–24, 25–34, and 55–64
    B. 25–34 and 45–54
    C. 15–24 and 45–54
    D. 45–54 and 55–64

33. What is the average number of illegal drug deaths among all age groups?
    A. 3.45
    B. 6.25
    C. 4.75
    D. 5.45

34. What is the approximate ratio of deaths caused by opioid pain relievers for 45–54 year olds as compared to 15–24 year olds?
    A. 2 to 1
    B. 3 to 1
    C. 4 to 1
    D. None of the above

Reading and Writing Practice

Read the passage below and then answer the questions.

In the United States, companies developing new medications must run tests to prove the medications are safe before selling them. These tests are called clinical trials. After a company tests a new medication, the Food and Drug Administration (FDA) must then approve it. The FDA is a government agency that is responsible for making sure medications are safe to use, effective, and secure from tampering.

Before determining whether medications are ready to be approved for use by the public, the FDA reviews the company's evidence about the chemicals in the medication, the side effects, and the medication's ability to impact the condition it is designed to treat. The FDA also decides whether a medication should be sold with or without a doctor's prescription.

35. What is the author's main idea in this passage?
    A. Medications are available at low and high strengths.
    B. Side effects of medications are harmful.
    C. The FDA must determine whether medications are safe for public consumption.
    D. Medications are either prescription or over-the-counter.

36. In this passage, the term *prescription* means _____.
    A. a written message from a doctor
    B. a medication or drug
    C. a certificate from the FDA
    D. a chemical in a medication

37. Analyze how the author uses specific word choices to shape the meaning in this passage. Then rewrite the paragraphs using your own word choices. Read your paragraphs in class.

38 Conduct research online to learn more about drug safety information provided by the Food and Drug Administration (FDA). Gather the relevant information and write a one-page summary of your findings to share with the class. Be sure to use your own words and cite your sources.

Unit 5 | Diseases and Disorders

Big Ideas

- Diseases and disorders are classified as infectious or noncommunicable. Infectious diseases are caused by microorganisms and noncommunicable diseases are not.

- Your body has a number of defenses that protect you from developing diseases and disorders.

- Although you can't prevent yourself from developing all diseases and disorders, you can take steps to lower your risk of getting many of them.

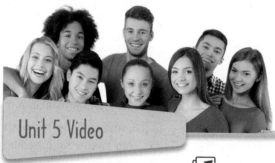

Unit 5 Video

"No Big Deal," or Is It?

Some teenagers make unhealthy choices that raise their risk of developing diseases and disorders. They believe that their choices and behavior do not put them at risk. Their beliefs, however, are based on misconceptions.

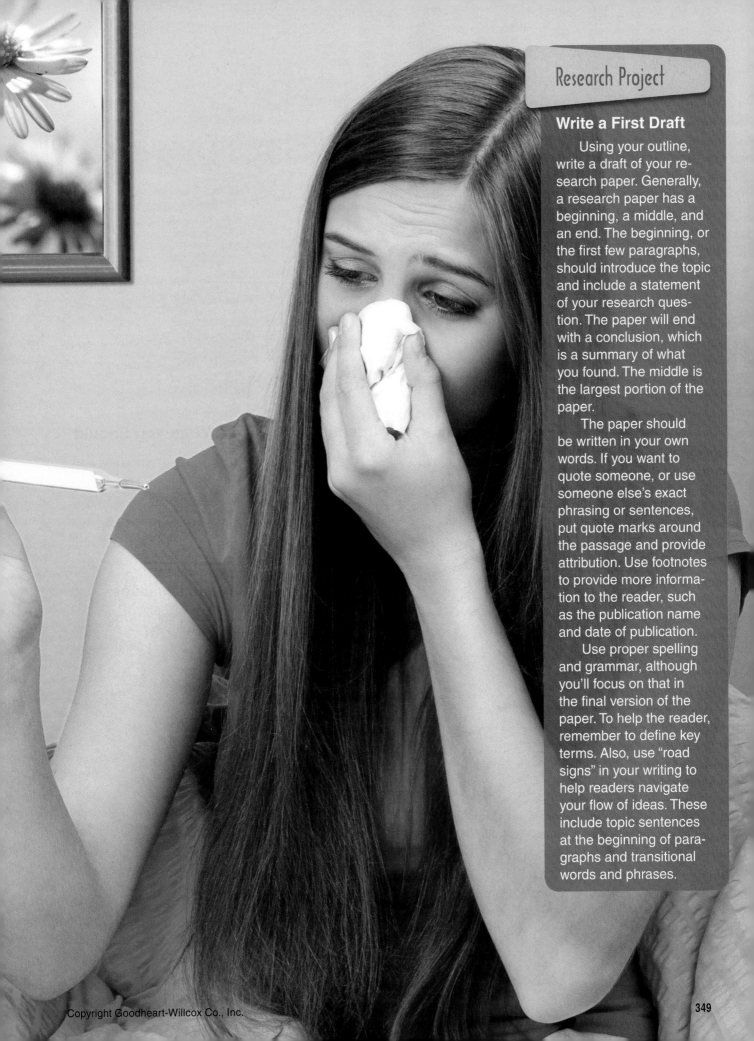

Write a First Draft

Using your outline, write a draft of your research paper. Generally, a research paper has a beginning, a middle, and an end. The beginning, or the first few paragraphs, should introduce the topic and include a statement of your research question. The paper will end with a conclusion, which is a summary of what you found. The middle is the largest portion of the paper.

The paper should be written in your own words. If you want to quote someone, or use someone else's exact phrasing or sentences, put quote marks around the passage and provide attribution. Use footnotes to provide more information to the reader, such as the publication name and date of publication.

Use proper spelling and grammar, although you'll focus on that in the final version of the paper. To help the reader, remember to define key terms. Also, use "road signs" in your writing to help readers navigate your flow of ideas. These include topic sentences at the beginning of paragraphs and transitional words and phrases.

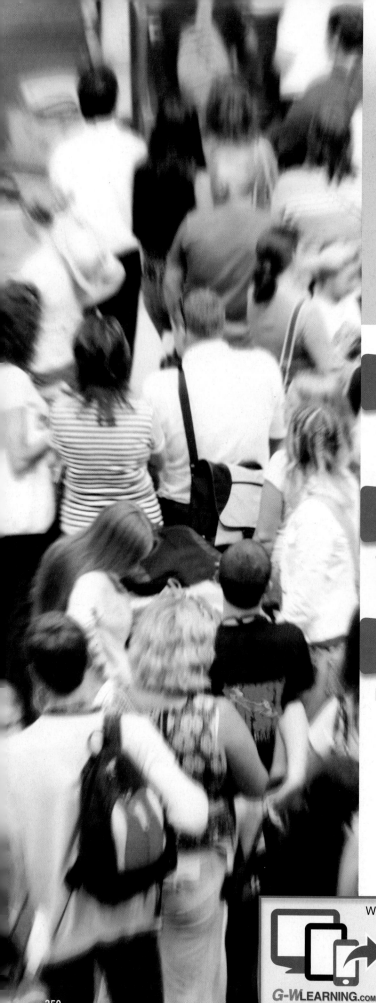

Chapter 12
Infectious Diseases

Lesson 12.1

Infectious Diseases: What You Should Know

Lesson 12.2

Transmission, Treatment, and Prevention of Infectious Diseases

Lesson 12.3

Immunity to Infection

While studying this chapter, look for the activity icon  to:
- **review** vocabulary with e-flash cards and games;
- **assess** learning with quizzes and online exercises;
- **expand** knowledge with animations and activities; and
- **listen** to pronunciation of key terms in the audio glossary.

G-WLEARNING.com

www.g-wlearning.com/health/

Take this quiz to see what you do *and* do not know about infectious diseases. If you cannot answer a question, pay extra attention to that topic as you study this chapter.

1. *Identify each statement as* True, False, *or* It Depends. *Choose* It Depends *if a statement is true in some cases, but false in others.*

2. *Revise each* False *statement to make it true.*

3. *Explain the circumstances in which each* It Depends *statement is true and when it is false.*

Health and Wellness IQ [Assess]

	True	False	It Depends
1. All bacteria cause disease.	True	False	It Depends
2. Fevers are harmful.	True	False	It Depends
3. Antibiotics can cure the flu.	True	False	It Depends
4. There is no way to prevent infectious diseases.	True	False	It Depends
5. The flu is just a serious form of the cold.	True	False	It Depends
6. Food and water can transmit infectious diseases.	True	False	It Depends
7. Viruses are just very small bacteria.	True	False	It Depends
8. Fungi normally do not cause disease.	True	False	It Depends
9. You can't get an infectious disease just by touching someone or something.	True	False	It Depends
10. Vaccines work by causing a mild form of an infectious disease.	True	False	It Depends

Setting the Scene

Malaria, a dreaded illness that causes flu-like symptoms, high fevers, and chills, was once a mystery to people. The word *malaria* means "bad air" because people thought the disease was caused by exposure to the still, warm air around stagnant water and swamps. People now know that malaria is caused by a parasite, which is carried by mosquitoes that breed in water. The mosquitoes transmit the parasite to humans, and humans become infected with malaria.

Today people know that infectious diseases like malaria are caused by living things that are too small to see with the naked eye. Modern understanding of infectious diseases opened the door to science-based, effective methods of prevention and treatment.

Still, each year infectious diseases kill 17 million people worldwide and take their toll in other ways. For example, each year US children miss more than 38 million days of school due to influenza. This chapter will help you learn the causes of infectious diseases and how they are transmitted, prevented, and treated.

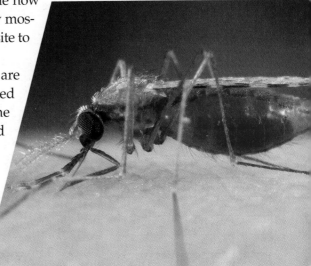

Infectious Diseases: What You Should Know

Key Terms   E-Flash Cards

In this lesson, you will learn the meanings of the following key terms.

bacteria
clinical stage
convalescent stage
germ theory
incubation period
infectious disease
mycosis
opportunistic infection
parasite
protozoa
virus

Before You Read

Questions of Note

Make a list of three to four questions that you expect to be answered while reading this lesson. After reading the lesson, revisit your questions. Were they answered in the lesson? Do you need to do some more research on your own?

My questions	My answers
1.	
2.	
3.	
4.	

Lesson Objectives

After studying this lesson, you will be able to

- differentiate between infectious and noncommunicable diseases;
- compare signs with symptoms for detecting the presence of disease;
- understand how infections affect the body;
- summarize the stages of infection in the body; and
- compare the various microorganisms that can infect the body.

Warm-Up Activity

What Would a Pathogen Do?

In this lesson, you will learn that a type of microorganism known as a pathogen (see below) causes infectious diseases. Before reading the lesson, work in small groups to develop a brief description of the ways in which you think a pathogen might go about creating a disease. Tell where the pathogen comes from, how it goes about its work, what it eats, what it's afraid of, and how long it lives. Compare descriptions in a short class discussion.

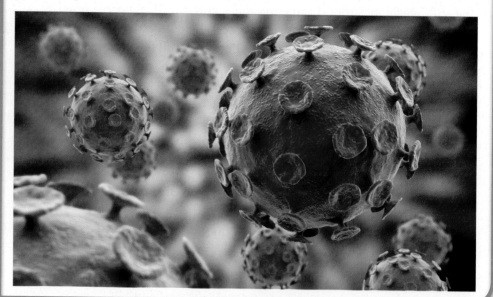

Common living things that people can see are called *organisms.* Many living things, however, are too small to be seen with the naked eye. These tiny organisms, called *microorganisms,* are composed of single cells that can only be seen with a microscope.

Late in the nineteenth century, scientists developed new tools that opened the door to a whole new world of living things to study. These tools included improved microscopes, stains for viewing bacterial cells, and methods for growing microorganisms in the laboratory. As a result, the germ theory was born.

The *germ theory* is a scientific concept stating that specific microorganisms cause specific diseases. With the invention of the new tools mentioned above, scientists could view microorganisms, study them in the lab, and determine their relationship to human disease. This new understanding of infectious diseases revolutionized medicine and continues to make an enormous impact on human health.

germ theory
a scientific theory, which states that specific microorganisms cause specific diseases

What Are Infectious Diseases?

Infectious diseases are caused by microorganisms living in or on humans, animals, or plants. The microorganisms that cause these diseases are known as *pathogens,* which were named for Greek words meaning "to cause suffering." Pathogenic microorganisms include certain bacteria, viruses, fungi, protozoa, and worms.

Infectious diseases, also called *communicable diseases,* are caused by pathogens that can be transmitted from one living thing to another. Some pathogens require a "middle man"—such as a mosquito or contaminated food—to be transmitted to humans. Diseases not caused by pathogens are known as *noncommunicable diseases* (Figure 12.1).

infectious disease
a disease caused by microorganisms or pathogens that can be transmitted from one person, animal, or object to another

Signs and Symptoms of Disease

The presence of a disease is detected by observing signs or symptoms. *Signs* are evidence of disease that can be outwardly observed or measured. Signs include fever, an abnormal pulse, changes in skin color, or altered breathing rate.

Figure 12.1 Comparing Two Types of Disease

	Disease	Cause
Communicable	pneumonia	bacteria and viruses
	influenza (flu)	virus
	strep throat	bacteria
Noncommunicable	diabetes	genetics, diet, lifestyle
	lung cancer	genetics, tobacco smoking
	heart disease	genetics, diet, lifestyle

A doctor or nurse can see or measure these signs during a physical exam. Signs are *objective evidence* for the presence of a disease, because signs can be observed and measured by anyone.

Symptoms are evidence of disease sensed by the sick person. Symptoms may include pain, shortness of breath, itching, and headache. Patients need to report symptoms to a nurse or doctor because symptoms cannot be easily seen or measured by other people.

Symptoms are called *subjective evidence* for a disease. They are called *subjective* because the evidence is based on feeling instead of outwardly measurable indicators of illness.

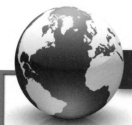

Local and Global Health
The Unequal Burden of Infectious Disease

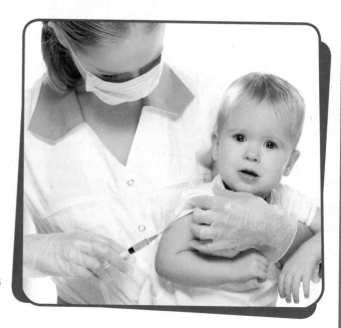

Vaccines prevent about two to three million deaths worldwide each year. While an increasing number of people have access to vaccines, the World Health Organization reports that about 1.7 million children younger than five years of age still die each year from preventable diseases. Clearly, there is still room for improvement.

The story of measles is a story of the unequal burden of infectious disease. A highly contagious viral disease, measles is well known for its fever and rash. Its complications include pneumonia, swelling of the brain, and death, but measles can be prevented with a vaccine. The number of measles cases in the United States has dropped 99% since the vaccine was introduced in 1963. Worldwide, however, measles causes 134,000 deaths each year. Most of these cases occur outside the United States and Europe.

Measles Deaths Reported to the World Health Organization for One Year	
Region	**Number of Deaths**
Worldwide	134,200
Africa	61,600
Southeast Asia	54,500
Eastern Mediterranean	15,900
Western Pacific	2,100
Europe	80
Americas	0

Thinking Critically

1. Why do you think so many more deaths occur from measles in Southeast Asia and African countries compared with the Americas and Europe?

2. What factors might affect whether people are being vaccinated in these regions?

3. How would you reduce the number of measles infections and deaths in Southeast Asia and African countries?

How Do Infections Cause Illness?

After pathogens enter the body, they grow, reproduce, and produce toxins that cause the familiar symptoms and signs of illness. Certain bacterial toxins cause fever. *Salmonella* bacteria make toxins that disrupt the intestine's ability to absorb water, leading to the diarrhea associated with *Salmonella* food poisoning.

Bacteria also cause disease when they trigger the immune response and cause inflammation, pain, and the formation of pus in infected tissues. Many pathogens cause disease indirectly, through no action of their own. In these instances, signs and symptoms result mainly from the body's immune response to the infection. For example, influenza is well-known for its muscle aches and pains, sore throat, headache, and fatigue. These symptoms result from the body's immune response to the virus growing inside the body's cells rather than the virus itself.

The Predictable Course of Infections

Infections often follow stages in a recognizable pattern. It is helpful to know something about these stages so you will know what to expect if you have an infection. You will also be able to identify the stages during which you are most likely to spread the disease and take action to avoid infecting others.

incubation period
the time between a pathogen's entrance into the body and the first symptoms of disease

Incubation Period

First a pathogen enters the body at a specific site. For example, influenza viruses enter the respiratory system when a person swallows or inhales droplets of mucus from an infected person.

Next, the pathogen begins to grow and reproduce inside the body, usually in a specific organ or tissue. The *incubation period* is the time between the pathogen's entrance into the body and the first appearance of symptoms (Figure 12.2). A person exhibits mild or no symptoms during the incubation period. The infected person may, however, be contagious, or capable of spreading the pathogen to other people during this period.

Incubation periods vary from disease to disease. For example, influenza viruses attach to cells lining the upper respiratory tract, invade these cells, and begin reproducing inside them. Influenza's incubation period is about two days. Adults with influenza are contagious one day before they experience symptoms and continue to be contagious for about one week after they become sick. Children tend to be contagious longer—up to 10 days. This is important to know because it suggests that people can spread the virus for many days after becoming sick. They should stay home from work or school until they are no longer contagious.

Figure 12.2

To study pathogens, scientists often grow the microorganisms in Petri dishes. These *Streptococcus pyogenes* colonies are in the incubation period.

Clinical Stage

After the incubation period, the infection moves to the most severe stage, the *clinical stage*, in which signs and symptoms characteristic of the disease arise. During this stage, the pathogen produces toxins, or the immune response reaches its height, causing familiar signs of illness. Influenza lasts about three to five days for otherwise healthy people. Unfortunately, symptoms like coughing and fatigue can sometimes linger for up to two weeks, even though the virus is no longer present.

Convalescent Stage

Finally, if the immune system successfully destroys the pathogen, the illness enters the *convalescent stage*, during which signs and symptoms fade. Usually a person is no longer contagious during this stage.

Each infectious disease progresses through these stages. Each disease differs, however, in the length of its incubation period, its window of contagiousness, and in the duration and severity of its clinical stage. For example, strep throat likely progresses through the stages differently than another infection would (Figure 12.3).

Figure 12.3 Profile of an Infection: Strep Throat		
Incubation Period	**Clinical Stage**	**Convalescent Stage**
1–3 days after exposure to bacteria	Signs and symptoms last 4–5 days if not treated. These include sudden sore throat, fever, swollen lymph nodes at throat, red throat interior with white or yellow patches. You are contagious if not treated.	no longer contagious 1 day after beginning antibiotics

Microorganisms

Microorganisms are diverse, specialized, and sophisticated living things. They are found everywhere and are typically invisible to the naked eye. While most people are unfamiliar with microorganisms, these organisms influence human lives in countless ways. They include bacteria, viruses, fungi, and parasites.

Bacteria

Bacteria are single-celled organisms living in nearly every possible place that can sustain life. The good news about bacteria is that most are helpful and few of them cause disease. Very large amounts of bacteria live on the body's surfaces and in the digestive tract. Helpful bacteria in the digestive tract hold back the growth of pathogens and provide essential

---

clinical stage
the stage in which the signs and symptoms of a disease arise and are most prominent

convalescent stage
the stage during which signs and symptoms of a disease fade and a person is no longer contagious

bacteria
single-celled organisms that grow and reproduce in and outside of the body, and can be helpful or harmful to body function

Personal Profile

What's Your Risk for Infectious Disease?

These questions will help you assess your risk for acquiring and transmitting infectious diseases.

I get my flu vaccine each year. **yes no**

I wash my hands before I eat or handle food. **yes no**

I use "respiratory etiquette" when I sneeze and cough. **yes no**

I get enough sleep each night. **yes no**

I eat regular nutritious meals. **yes no**

I understand how colds, flu, and common infections are transmitted. **yes no**

I do not share food or drinks with people. **yes no**

I understand how to store and prepare food safely. **yes no**

Add up your number of yes answers to assess your risk for acquiring or transmitting infectious diseases. The more no answers you have, the higher your risk of infection.

services such as producing vitamin K and aiding digestion. So many bacteria live in the body that, of the several trillions of cells that make up your body, 90% are bacterial cells. The bad news is that certain bacteria cause disease, ranging from minor to deadly illnesses.

Each bacterium is composed of a single tiny cell, which is about 10 to 100 times smaller than many of your body's cells. Bacteria are quite different from the cells contained in your body in several other ways as well. Bacteria cannot be seen without a microscope, and they have a relatively simple cell structure enclosed by a sturdy cell wall. Bacteria are defined by their lack of a nucleus, which is present within most other cells.

Each kind of bacterial cell has a specific shape, habitat, and nutritional needs. Most bacteria can grow independently outside of your cells. Bacteria can be found growing on your skin, in your intestines, or in your blood and tissues. Some bacteria actually reside within your cells. Their numbers are kept in check by your immune system.

Some species of bacteria may be familiar to you. Scientists assign a unique two-part name to each species of organism, including bacteria. You may have read about *Escherichia coli* (*E. coli*), a bacterium that resides in animal and human intestines and causes food poisoning (Figure 12.4). Another common bacterium is *Staphylococcus aureus*. Carried by many people in their nasal passages, *S. aureus* causes serious skin infections called *staph infections*, MRSA, abscesses, pneumonia, bone infections, and other serious diseases.

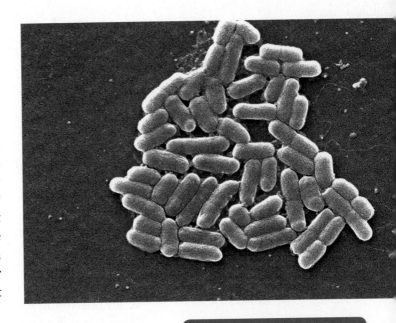

Figure 12.4

E. coli is a bacterium that causes food poisoning in humans and animals. *What kinds of foods contain E. coli?*

Viruses

Everyone knows about the common cold and influenza, which are notorious viral diseases. Lesser-known but important viral diseases include measles, chicken pox, West Nile virus, and mumps. Few people know the nature of viruses themselves.

A **virus** differs significantly from bacteria and your body's cells. Viruses do not grow or reproduce independently, have no metabolism, and do not use energy as all other cells do. Completely incapable of doing anything cells can do on their own, viruses depend entirely on other cells for reproduction and growth. In fact, every virus must live inside a cell and use that cell's resources and energy to grow and reproduce. For this reason, scientists do not consider viruses to be living organisms.

Viruses are much smaller than bacteria, and are so small they cannot be seen with ordinary microscopes used to study cells. Only powerful *electron microscopes* specialized for viewing the smallest of structures can study viruses. Exceptionally simple, viruses are composed only of viral genetic material wrapped in a protein coat, sometimes further surrounded by a

virus
a pathogen that infects cells and uses their energy because it cannot reproduce or grow on its own

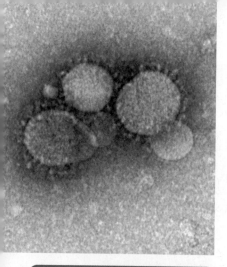

The MERS virus causes a respiratory illness by instructing cells to make more viruses. *What viruses are common in your community?*

mycosis
a fungal infection that usually attacks damaged tissues or weakened people

opportunistic infection
a disease that takes advantage of a body's weakened immune system

parasite
an organism that must live inside or on another living organism to draw upon that organism's strength and energy for survival

protozoa
single-celled organisms that are larger and more complex than bacteria, and which may cause disease

fatty membrane. Essentially, viruses are made of specially packaged genes that direct cell machinery to make more viruses (Figure 12.5).

Fungi

Fungi (singular—*fungus*) are much more complex than bacteria and viruses. Fungi are built from larger cells that resemble animal cells far more than bacterial cells. Fungi include mushrooms, molds, and yeast. A typical fungus contains cells specialized for feeding; cells that anchor the organism to surfaces like soil particles, leaves, or body tissues; and other cells that produce spores for reproduction.

Like bacteria, few fungi cause disease, and many are beneficial. The mold *Penicillium notatum* makes the life-saving drug penicillin, an antibiotic that controls bacterial infections. Both organisms—fungi and bacteria—are also indispensable decomposers, breaking down dead and decaying matter and recycling nutrients in soil.

Other fungi, however, damage crops and can spoil stored food. A few fungi cause disease in humans. A fungal infection is called a **mycosis**. Mycosis usually attacks damaged tissues or people weakened by other infections. People with poor immunity, which can result from cancer chemotherapy, are especially susceptible to mycoses. Because fungi usually infect people with low disease resistance, mycoses are described as **opportunistic infections**.

Some fungi are composed of many cells just like animals and plants, and are considered *multicellular organisms*. Familiar multicellular fungi include mushrooms and molds. Other fungi are composed of only a single cell and are called *single-celled organisms*. The single-celled fungi include yeasts.

Athlete's foot and ringworm are common fungal infections that take advantage of some imbalance or damage in the tissues. More serious opportunistic infections plague individuals with compromised immunity. These include *Pneumocystis jirovecii*, which causes pneumonia, and *Cryptococcus neoformans*, which causes dangerous brain infections.

Parasites: Protozoa and Worms

Protozoa and worms are grouped together, not because they are closely related, but because doctors refer to them collectively as *parasites*. **Parasites** are organisms that must live inside or on another living thing, where they cause damage and disease.

Parasitic worms and protozoa infect an enormous number of people. Worldwide, nearly one-third of all people are infected with the intestinal roundworm *Ascaris lumbricoides*, and more than one-fifth have intestinal hookworms. Recent estimates suggest that each year about 200 million people are infected with the malaria parasite (a protozoan parasite), resulting in around one million deaths.

Protozoa. **Protozoa** are single-celled organisms, different from bacteria in that they possess a nucleus and other complex structures and are larger. Protozoa live nearly everywhere and only a few cause disease. Many kinds of protozoa form the basis of food chains, providing nutrients for other organisms.

Certain protozoa, however, cause some of the world's most feared diseases, among them malaria and *dysentery*, a severe intestinal infection. Another protozoan called *Cryptosporidium* causes diarrhea and is transmitted in contaminated water.

Worms. Unlike protozoa, parasitic worms are multicellular organisms with specialized tissues and organs. Parasitic worms can be transmitted to humans in water or food that has been contaminated with human waste, or in undercooked meat and fish.

The eggs of the large intestinal roundworm *Ascaris lumbricoides*, for example, can be found in water or food contaminated with human waste. After ingestion, these eggs grow into adult worms that absorb nutrients from the intestine, causing malnutrition and anemia. These worms can grow so large and numerous that they block the intestine, even tearing holes in it.

Hookworms and pinworms attach to the intestine wall, feeding on blood. Flukes and tapeworms can be transmitted in undercooked fish, pork, or beef (Figure 12.6). These worms also live in the intestine but can migrate to the liver or brain where they cause serious harm. *Trichinella* worms, which are ingested in undercooked pork, damage muscles and other organs. Fortunately, *Trichinella* worms have been virtually eliminated from domestic pigs in the United States.

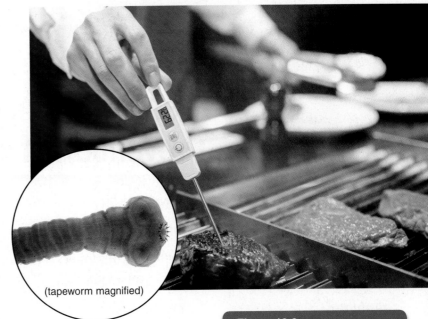
(tapeworm magnified)

Figure 12.6

Parasitic tapeworms can enter a person's digestive system when that person eats uncooked or undercooked meat, such as this steak. *Do you know the minimum internal temperatures for cooking various types of meat? Where do you think you could find this information?*

Lesson 12.1 Review

Know and Understand

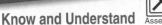
Assess

1. What advancements in the late nineteenth century made development of the germ theory possible?

2. List five types of pathogens that can cause infectious disease.

3. Inflammation, pain, and the formation of pus are indications of a response from the body's _____.

Analyze and Apply

4. Compare fungi and protozoa.

Real World Health

Divide a sheet of paper into four parts, or quadrants. Label each quadrant with the name of a microorganism mentioned in this lesson: *bacteria*, *viruses*, *fungi*, or *parasites*. Research each type of microorganism. Within each quadrant, draw a general picture of each microorganism and include a short definition. Though some of these microorganisms are generally helpful, they can also cause disease. In each microorganism's quadrant, list two diseases caused by that microorganism, along with the method of treatment for each disease.

Transmission, Treatment, and Prevention of Infectious Diseases

Key Terms 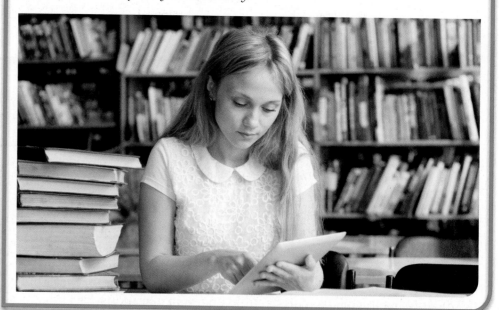 E-Flash Cards

In this lesson, you will learn the meanings of the following key terms.

antibiotic
antibiotic resistance
endemic
epidemic
MRSA (methicillin-resistant Staphylo-coccus aureus)
pandemic
pasteurization
respiratory etiquette
vaccine
vector
zoonosis

Before You Read

3-2-1 Chart

While you are reading, think about information you discover, concepts you find interesting, and what you still question within the lesson. After you finish reading, list three pieces of information you discovered, two that you found interesting, and one that you still question.

3 discovered	2 interesting	1 question

Lesson Objectives

After studying this lesson, you will be able to

- differentiate between methods of disease transmission;
- explain the various patterns of infectious disease occurrence;
- practice effective methods of infectious disease prevention; and
- compare treatments for bacterial and viral infections.

Warm-Up Activity

What Do You Touch?

List all the objects you touch each day. Then pair up with a classmate and compare lists. Highlight those objects that your lists have in common. It is likely these objects are touched by others as well. Touching these items increases the likelihood for contact with pathogens, and the chances that they could enter your body. With your partner, brainstorm ways to avoid contracting an infectious disease from the surfaces you touch daily.

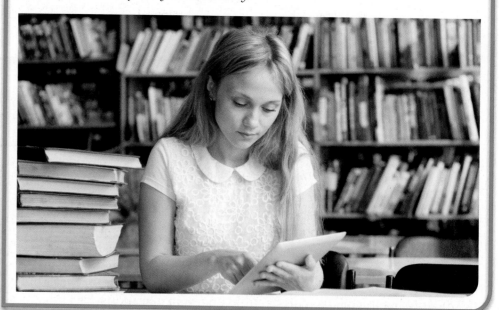

U ntil Ronald Ross' scientific breakthrough in malaria research in 1897, there was little hope for preventing malaria because no one knew how it was transmitted. Ross' experiments showed that mosquitoes transmit the malaria parasite, which transformed understanding of the disease. Finally the way to break the chain of infection was understood. Understanding how diseases are transmitted is the single most important key to prevention.

Methods of Transmission

Mosquitoes transmitting malaria is an example of disease transmission. A *method of transmission* is simply the way a disease gets from one organism to another. Methods of transmission are classified as either direct or indirect, depending on how the transmission occurs.

Direct Transmission

Direct transmission is the exchange of infectious material from its origin to a susceptible individual. This transmission can occur through direct contact or by droplet spread (Figure 12.7 and Figure 12.8 on the next page).

Direct Contact. When microorganisms are passed during physical intimacy or contact, the mode of transmission is considered *direct contact*. Infections transmitted by direct contact between people include sexually transmitted infections, skin infections, and respiratory diseases. When a person contracts a hookworm after contact with soil that is home to such parasites, it is also considered direct contact.

Droplet Spread. *Droplet spread* transmits infection when an individual is within a few feet of an infected person who is coughing, sneezing, or simply speaking. These droplets are so large they cannot remain suspended in the air for long. Droplet spread is considered direct transmission because it requires the recipient to be in close proximity to the carrier.

Coughing, sneezing, and talking can produce an enormous number of small respiratory droplets that contain pathogens. In close quarters, these contaminated droplets can be inhaled or swallowed. These droplets can also land on hands or other objects that move microorganisms to the mouth or nose. Respiratory droplets are known to transmit the common cold, influenza, strep throat, meningitis, measles, mumps, pneumonia, and tuberculosis.

Indirect Transmission

Indirect transmission is the exchange of infectious material to a susceptible person by a source that acts solely as a carrier. The distinction is that the infectious material does not originate in the carrier. The carrier is simply moving the infectious material from one source to another.

Figure 12.7

Direct transmission of infection can occur in two basic ways: through droplets when an infected person sneezes or coughs and through various types of direct contact.

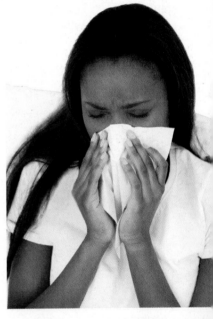

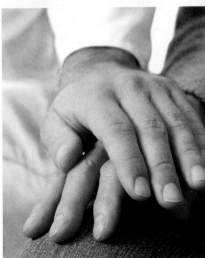

Figure 12.8 Direct Transmission

Select Diseases Transmitted by Direct Contact

Disease	Cause	Signs and Symptoms	Treatment	Prevention
athlete's foot, jock itch, ringworm	fungi	itching, burning, redness of infected skin	over-the-counter antifungal cream	Keep skin clean and dry; do not share towels or combs in the gym.
MRSA	*Staphylococcus aureus* bacteria that are resistant to antibiotics	red, swollen, oozing wounds that do not heal	antibiotics; requires doctor attention	Wash hands following athletic events, using workout equipment and mats, and after visiting hospitalized patients; do not share towels.
impetigo	*Staphylococcus aureus* bacteria	red, crusty sores below nose and on face; forms blisters, dries, and itches	antibiotic cream	Wash hands regularly and avoid touching face; common in preschool and elementary school age children; also occurs among athletes.
pinkeye (conjunctivitis)	bacteria or viruses	red, itching eyes; if bacterial infection, pus	antibiotic eye drops (prescription) for bacterial infection	Wash hands, especially when handling contact lenses; contagious—if infected stay home from school.

Select Diseases Transmitted by Respiratory Droplets

Disease	Cause	Signs and Symptoms	Treatment	Prevention
cold	viruses: rhinovirus, coronavirus, adenovirus	nasal and sinus congestion, sneezing, sometimes a cough	no cure; relieve symptoms with decongestants; warm liquids; rest	respiratory etiquette and hand hygiene
influenza	influenza viruses	headache, fever, dry hacking cough, muscle aches and pain, extreme fatigue	no cure; treatment for severe cases includes a prescription medication that controls the virus in the body; otherwise, treat headache and body aches with pain medicine, rest	vaccines are available each year; respiratory etiquette and hand hygiene
meningitis	bacteria	high fever, stiff neck, painful headache, vomiting, exhaustion, possible rash	medical emergency that requires doctor's attention; will prescribe antibiotics and anti-inflammatory medications	respiratory etiquette and hand hygiene; "Hib" vaccine in infants; "Meningococcal" vaccine is available for others
mono (infectious mononucleosis)	virus	sore throat, extreme fatigue, low fever, spleen may become swollen; symptoms may last a month or more	no specific treatment; rest, fluids, and good nutrition	respiratory etiquette and hand hygiene
pneumonia	bacteria and viruses	fever, chest congestion and pain, cough, fatigue	antibiotics for bacterial infections; must consult doctor	vaccine for one bacterial cause is recommended for elderly and people with respiratory problems like asthma
strep throat (pharyngitis)	bacteria	painful, sore, red throat with white or yellow patches of pus; fever	antibiotics, rest	respiratory etiquette and hand hygiene

By Animal. Sometimes pathogens use animals as transportation to a human victim. *Vectors* are animals such as mosquitoes, flies, ticks, fleas, and lice that transmit diseases from one living thing to another. For example, Lyme disease is a bacterial infection transmitted by ticks (Figure 12.9A). Vectors transmit many infectious diseases: mosquitoes transmit malaria, West Nile virus, and encephalitis; and fleas transmit plague.

Other pathogens cause disease in animals, do not normally infect people, and are not transmitted from person to person. These pathogens can, however, cause animal infections that the animal then transmits to humans. The resulting infection is called *zoonosis*. A well-known example of a zoonosis is the viral disease *rabies*, a nervous system infection that can affect all warm-blooded animals, including raccoons, foxes, bats, dogs, and cats (Figure 12.9B). The rabies virus can be transmitted to humans through the bite of an animal that has been infected by the virus.

By Contaminated Objects. Some infections are transmitted indirectly to people by objects that are contaminated with pathogens. For example, pathogens can be transmitted in water or food, and by contaminated medical instruments, shared hypodermic needles, blood, and other objects.

Food and water are common sources of infection, transmitting some of the world's most notorious pathogens, including the bacterial infection called *cholera*. It was not until the nineteenth century that cholera was linked to water contaminated with human waste. Until this discovery, there was no effective way to prevent this horrible disease that literally wastes the body through severe diarrhea and dehydration.

The development of food and water sanitation has significantly improved the quality of human life. When systems break down, however, infections inevitably flare up. The leading cause of food- and waterborne infections remains contamination by human and animal waste.

Food crops can become contaminated during irrigation with contaminated water or by fertilization with animal waste that has not been correctly composted to kill pathogens. Crops also become contaminated by the people who handle the food during harvest, storage, and processing.

vector
an animal that transmits a disease from one living thing to another

zoonosis
an infection transferred from an animal to a human

Figure 12.9

Vectors such as the deer tick (on the left) and the raccoon can transmit infections from animals to humans. Humans are usually infected from the bite of an infected animal. *How can you tell if an animal is infected? What should you do if you see an infected animal?*

A. Deer Tick

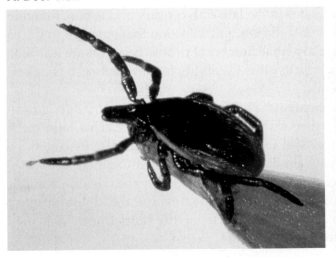

B. Raccoon

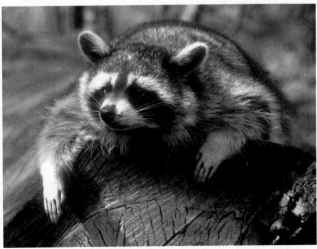

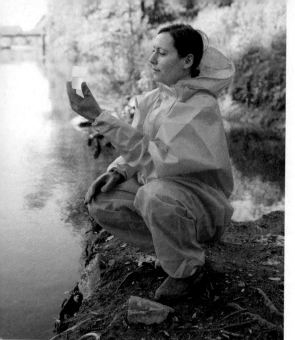

Figure 12.10

Scientists must continually test and analyze our water supply to make sure that it is safe for human consumption. *What are some diseases that could be spread through contaminated water?*

epidemic

an outbreak of a disease that occurs in unexpectedly large numbers over a geographic area

pandemic

a widespread epidemic that affects an enormous number of people and spreads between countries and across the world

endemic

a disease that naturally occurs in low numbers in a certain area

Bacteria from animal intestines can contaminate meat during butchering and processing. That is why eating undercooked meat has been linked to illness. In many cases, the main concern is food poisoning with bacterial pathogens, including *E. coli*, which grow in animal intestines and are naturally found in animal waste.

Water transmits not only pathogens from animals, but also those found in human waste. Water sources include natural lakes, reservoirs, and wells, all of which may become contaminated with sewage containing human waste, especially during floods and in rain runoff. Human diseases transmitted in water include *E. coli*, hepatitis, typhoid, cholera, and other parasitic infections (Figure 12.10).

By Airborne Means. Pathogens also "hitch rides" on dust particles or droplets much smaller than those included in direct transmission. These tiny carriers can remain suspended in the air for extended periods. When a carrier makes contact with a human, the pathogen has found its next opportunity to spread infection.

Occurrence of Infectious Disease

Diseases and other infections follow patterns, and there are several ways to describe these patterns. For example, an *epidemic* infection occurs in unexpectedly large numbers over a particular area. In some years, influenza is epidemic. A *pandemic* infection affects an enormous number of people and spreads from one country to much of the world. In the years 1918 and 1919, for example, an influenza pandemic killed about 40 million people around the world. In contrast, an *endemic* infection is one that naturally occurs at low levels in a particular area. The common cold and strep throat are examples of endemic infections in the United States. Yellow fever and malaria do not occur in the United States, but they are endemic to certain tropical countries.

Emerging infectious diseases are diseases that are new or increasing unexpectedly. West Nile virus, a brain infection spread by mosquitoes, first occurred in the United States in the late 20th century and is now found in most states. Avian flu, or *bird flu*, is a bird infection that emerged in China and has caused influenza in a small number of people. Scientists are watching the virus closely. If avian flu evolves the ability to move between people, it could become a pandemic.

Another infection scientists have been watching is bovine spongiform encephalopathy (BSE), also known as *mad cow disease*. This fatal cattle disease destroys brain tissue. In its present form, this disease cannot be transmitted to humans. A similar, rare disease called *Creuetzfelt-Jakob disease (CJD)* already occurs in humans. CJD also damages the brain and is fatal. Scientists are concerned that BSE may evolve the ability to infect humans, too. For this reason, BSE-infected cattle cannot be sold as food and must be destroyed.

Scientists are also concerned about Zika virus. The Zika virus originated in Africa and has spread widely in South America. Zika infections appeared in the United States in 2016. The Zika virus is transmitted by infected mosquitoes and through sexual contact with an infected partner. The virus causes a few mild symptoms, but results in serious brain damage to the developing fetus of an infected mother. Scientists are testing vaccines to prevent Zika.

Prevention of Infectious Diseases

During most wars before WWII, infections killed far more people than sabers, bullets, and bombs did. Helpless doctors could only watch soldiers die from wound infections. Since then, medical science has developed preventive measures that reduce the incidence of infectious diseases and limit the suffering and death caused by them.

Hand Washing

Hand washing is universally acknowledged to be the most important method of preventing many infectious diseases. Practiced regularly and correctly, hand washing dramatically reduces the occurrence of infectious diseases that are transmitted by respiratory droplets, blood, or direct skin contact.

Figure 12.11 lists occasions to wash your hands. Other situations also call for hand washing. For example, always wash your hands before and after visiting a person in the hospital and after visiting your doctor.

Alcohol-based hand rubs are very effective when soap and water are unavailable. Visibly dirty hands, however, need to be washed first for the alcohol rubs to work. Alcohol-based sanitizer dispensers are often located in stores and other public places.

Respiratory Etiquette

From November through March each year, colds and the flu spread quickly. These infections spread rapidly because infected people disperse the cold and flu viruses in respiratory droplets. Droplets inevitably coat an infected person's hands and make their way to the nose and mouth of another person, spreading the infection.

Figure 12.11 When to Wash Your Hands

Be sure to wash your hands

- after using the bathroom;
- after blowing your nose;
- after changing a diaper;
- after handling waste or trash;
- before preparing and eating food;
- after handling uncooked meat and fish;
- following contact with blood or body fluids; and
- when your hands are visibly dirty.

Doctors recommend that people practice ***respiratory etiquette*** to prevent spreading diseases (Figure 12.12). You should cover your nose and mouth with a tissue when coughing or sneezing. Don't reuse or store the tissue; throw the tissue in the trash after use. If you have no tissues, do not cough or sneeze into your hands. Instead, cough or sneeze into your upper arm, sleeve, or elbow. Wash your hands after using a tissue, or sneezing and coughing into your hands.

Food Sanitation

Consumers in the United States enjoy a relatively safe and sanitary food supply. You can adopt certain safeguards and food safety practices to maintain the safety of the food you handle and eat. The goal of food sanitation is to prevent contamination during food processing, storage, and preparation.

Avoid Nonpasteurized Drinks. ***Pasteurization*** kills pathogens in milk, juices, and other food products. This is done by heating the food item to a certain temperature for a time and then quickly cooling it. Pasteurization also prolongs the food's storage life and improves its quality. Never drink unpasteurized milk, juice, or cider. These unpasteurized drinks have been linked to outbreaks of *E. coli*.

Refrigerate and Freeze Perishables. Refrigeration and freezing are effective methods of food storage that slow or stop the growth of microorganisms. Food that can spoil should be kept cold or frozen to slow the spoiling process. Remember, however, that these methods do *not* kill microorganisms. For example, a refrigerated or frozen turkey may contain *Salmonella* bacteria, a cause of food poisoning. While a turkey stands at room temperature, the bacteria will reproduce and, if undercooked, the turkey will still contain bacteria.

Cook Meat Thoroughly. Cooking meat thoroughly will kill pathogens. You should not consume rare hamburger because the undercooked meat will not have reached a high enough temperature to kill. Instant meat thermometers have a scale noting safe temperatures for various types of meat (Figure 12.13). Always use a meat thermometer or cook meat until its juices no longer run pink. Wash your hands with soap and water before and after handling meat.

Wash Vegetables and Fruits. Vegetables and fruits must be washed before eating and unused, prepared portions must be refrigerated. Spinach has transmitted *E. coli*; raspberries have transmitted *Cyclospora*, a protozoan that causes food poisoning; and cantaloupes have caused an outbreak of *Listeria*, a severe bacterial food poisoning. Fruits you peel or cut open should be washed before cutting because the peels or rinds can be contaminated. If you were to cut contaminated fruit, the knife would spread microorganisms into the flesh intended for eating.

Use Safe Drinking Water. The United States draws its water supply from natural lakes, reservoirs, and wells. Most city water is treated in some way to remove pathogens. Filtration, ozone treatment, and chlorination are well-established, safe, and effective methods for treating city water supplies.

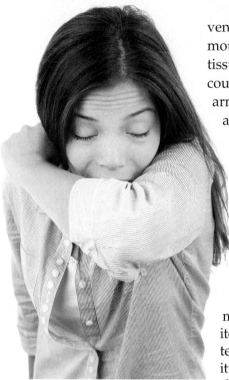

Figure 12.12

Covering your mouth and nose when you cough or sneeze is good respiratory etiquette, and can help prevent the spread of disease. *What precautions do you take when you sneeze or cough?*

respiratory etiquette
the practice of covering your mouth and nose with a tissue while coughing or sneezing, or sneezing into your sleeve

pasteurization
the process of heating and then quickly cooling liquids to kill pathogens

Wells are often naturally filtered because water entering a well passes through layers of rock and sand. Even so, well water should be tested regularly to confirm its safety.

Never drink water from a natural lake, river, or reservoir without first filtering or boiling the water. These natural water sources can be contaminated with rain runoff containing animal and human waste and, therefore, can transmit bacterial and parasitic diseases.

Vaccines

Vaccination is the only proven method of successfully eradicating an infectious disease. For example, the highly contagious, deadly viral infection *smallpox* was eliminated by vaccination. In the next few years vaccines will probably conquer *polio*, which has caused paralysis in many people throughout history.

A *vaccine* contains either a dead pathogen or a nontoxic component of a pathogen, such as part of a bacterial cell wall or the coating of a virus. When injected into a person, the vaccine provokes an immune response. The injected person's body produces white blood cells, proteins, and chemicals that fight infections. The dead pathogen or pathogen component is incapable of causing an illness.

If the real, disease-causing pathogen is ever encountered, the immune system, revved up by the encounter with the pathogen's components in the vaccine, responds strongly and quickly. It produces many white blood cells and antibodies, often destroying the pathogen before symptoms of the disease begin. Because vaccination activates the immune system, it is also called *immunization*. Vaccines are safe and effective, and they have transformed public health through prevention.

Several vaccines are required before a child may begin attending school. These vaccines include the MMR vaccine, which prevents the viral infections measles, mumps, and rubella. You may also have had vaccines for chicken pox, polio, hepatitis B, and hemophilus (ear infections and meningitis). Children also receive the DTP vaccine, which prevents diphtheria, tetanus, and pertussis (whooping cough). Other vaccines are administered as needed and under special circumstances. For example, army recruits receive vaccines for diseases they could encounter in deployment or that could arise through *biological warfare* (the use of pathogens as weapons).

Each year a vaccine is offered to prevent the flu, and while not required by schools, it is encouraged because it can prevent flu outbreaks. Some vaccines are effective for nearly a lifetime, others for many years. Some vaccines require follow-up injections called *boosters* to restimulate the immune system.

Treatment for Infectious Diseases

Until the 1940s, there were no antibiotics to treat bacterial infections. Today, medical science has developed effective treatments that have decreased suffering and death caused by infectious disease. In some cases, an infection overwhelms the body's defenses. When that happens, you

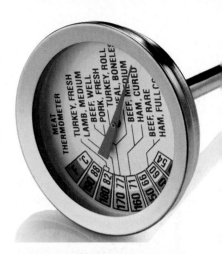

Figure 12.13

You can use a meat thermometer to determine whether meat has been thoroughly cooked and is safe to eat.

vaccine
a dead or nontoxic part of a pathogen that is injected into a person to train his or her immune system to eliminate the live pathogen

Health across the Life Span

Prevent Infections throughout Your Life

The immune system remains undeveloped during the first months of life. Therefore, infants are susceptible to contagious diseases, including infections passed through the respiratory system. As a result, infants easily contract colds, the flu, ear infections, and throat infections.

The digestive system also protects people from infections. The intestines contain an enormous number of bacteria that keep pathogens out, slow their growth, and stimulate the immune system. An infant's intestines have poorly developed populations of bacteria, making the child susceptible to infections that cause vomiting and diarrhea.

Infants rely completely on their caretakers to help prevent infectious disease. The following steps reduce an infant's risk for infectious disease:

- **Breast-feeding**: Breast milk contains cells and antibodies that fight infections.
- **Hand washing**: People should wash their hands before handling babies or babies' food.
- **Sanitizing bottles**: Caretakers should clean baby formula bottles and rinse them in boiling water.

- **Vaccinating**: Babies should receive certain necessary vaccines.

During childhood and adolescence, growth and development produce a robust immune system that is capable of fighting many infections. Late in life, however, immunity declines and people become susceptible to infectious diseases again. From childhood on, people can take the following steps to prevent infectious disease:

- **Hand washing**: Wash hands before eating or preparing food, and after using the restroom.
- **Vaccination**: Visit a doctor regularly and keep vaccinations up to date.
- **Food safety**: Learn how to prepare and store food safely.
- **Rest, exercise, nutrition**: Get enough of each to keep the immune system strong.

Thinking Critically

1. List the ways you avoid catching or transmitting infectious diseases during a typical day at school.
2. List the ways you prevent infectious diseases at home.
3. If you have the cold or the flu, what can you do to prevent spreading the infection to other people?

---

can take certain medications that will kill the infection-causing pathogens. Such medications also shorten the disease's duration, reducing the chance that a disease will cause lasting damage.

Treating Bacterial Infections

antibiotic
a substance that targets and kills pathogenic bacteria

Naturally made by fungi and helpful bacteria, ***antibiotics*** are substances that target and kill pathogenic bacteria. Antibiotics are effective against many kinds of pathogenic bacteria, but it is important to know that they are ineffective against viruses, fungi, and parasites.

Most antibiotics, such as penicillin, erythromycin, and amoxicillin, are prescription medications. A doctor must order these for a patient to buy from a pharmacist. These antibiotics are typically taken as pills or capsules. For some serious infections, antibiotics might be injected or infused directly into veins. These are called *intravenous* or *IV antibiotics*.

A few antibiotics are available "over-the-counter"—they can be purchased at drugstores without a doctor's prescription. Examples include creams with bacitracin or neomycin for treating minor cuts and scrapes.

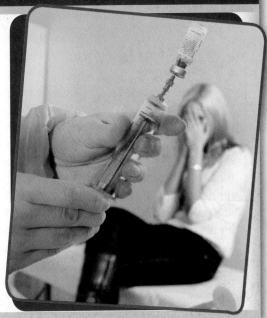
Unfortunately, several strains of bacteria have developed *antibiotic resistance*. An antibiotic resistant bacterium cannot be killed by antibiotics. These strains of bacteria are extremely difficult, if not impossible, to treat because the antibiotics once used are no longer effective. For example, *MRSA (methicillin-resistant* **Staphylococcus aureus***)* is a strain of ordinary *S. aureus* that cannot be controlled with many antibiotics.

Antibiotic resistance is both a personal and public health problem. It can be avoided by taking the following precautions:

- Use antibiotics only when prescribed.
- Do not share antibiotics.
- Do not take antibiotics for viral infections.
- Take the entire dose for the length of time prescribed by your doctor.

antibiotic resistance
a pathogen's ability to fight back against an antibiotic; develops over time and as a result of contact with certain antibiotics

MRSA (methicillin-resistant **Staphylococcus aureus***)*
a strain of S. aureus *that is resistant to antibiotics*

Treating Viral Infections

There are few treatments for viral infections. Most medications target the symptoms and do not attack the virus. In many cases, medicines treat the signs and symptoms of disease, with the goal of making you more comfortable. That is the purpose of medicines like acetaminophen, which reduces fever, aches, and pains associated with influenza. Cough medicines, decongestants, anti-inflammatories, and antihistamines treat various symptoms, but provide no cures.

For infections such as genital herpes, hepatitis, and severe influenza, drugs can reduce the severity of the infection, but do not cure these viral infections. In these cases, the drugs keep the virus under control while the body fights back. Rest, good nutrition, and fluids strengthen the body and help it fight the virus.

There are also several drugs that control and cure infections caused by worms and protozoan parasites.

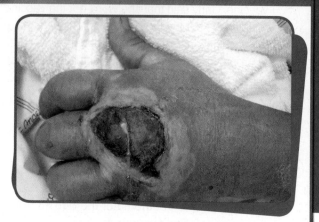

Bacteria possess *antibiotic resistance* if they cannot be killed with an antibiotic. In any population, some bacteria have mutations that permit them to survive in the presence of antibiotics. The antibiotics kill susceptible or weak bacteria, leaving behind those with resistance. In this way, an antibiotic-resistant population of bacteria evolves. The solution has been to switch to other effective antibiotics, but it appears that more bacteria are developing resistance to more antibiotics.

One such bacterium is MRSA (methicillin resistant *Staphylococcus aureus*), a strain that cannot be treated with most antibiotics. An area of skin or wound infected with MRSA is very dangerous and may kill up to 5% of those infected. Resistance has also been detected in strains of the bacterium *Streptococcus pyogenes*, the cause of strep throat and ear infections.

For several years, it has been known that strains of bacteria causing tuberculosis had developed resistance to several antibiotics. These strains cause multidrug resistant (MDR) tuberculosis. Early in 2012, totally drug resistant (TDR) tuberculosis was identified in India. There is no treatment for this strain. People infected with this strain are no better off than individuals with tuberculosis in the nineteenth century.

The World Health Organization and the US Centers for Disease Control and Prevention have made antibiotic resistance a top public heath priority.

Thinking Critically

1. Antibiotics are also found in over-the-counter creams and lotions. How do these fit into the problem of antibiotic resistance?

2. Most sore throats and coughs are caused by viruses, not bacteria. Why should you not take an antibiotic for most sore throats or coughs?

Lesson 12.2 Review

Know and Understand

1. What are the two classifications used to organize methods of infectious disease transmission?

2. List three examples of vectors and the diseases each vector transmits.

3. Explain how food can become a method of transmitting infectious disease.

4. What is the most important method of preventing infectious disease?

5. What does a vaccine contain that provokes the immune response in the body?

6. Do antibiotics help cure diseases caused by a virus? Explain.

Analyze and Apply

7. Explain why a physician is unlikely to prescribe an antibiotic for a patient with the flu (influenza).

8. Compare zoonosis with disease transmission by a vector.

Real World Health

In this lesson, you learned the spread of infectious disease can be prevented by washing your hands. In this activity, you will practice this important method of prevention. With a partner, review the proper methods for hand washing. Wash your hands using warm, soapy water for at least 20 seconds. (Singing "Happy Birthday" twice takes roughly 20 seconds.) Discuss alternative methods to use when water is not available.

Immunity to Infection

Lesson Objectives

After studying this lesson, you will be able to

- explain how the immune system protects the body;
- identify the key components for each line of defense;
- summarize each component's role in fighting infection; and
- understand how the immune system's "memory" works.

The Body as a Fortress

The body is like a fortress in that it has many ways of defending itself against disease-causing intruders:

A. *walls to keep intruders out;*

B. *warriors to fight intruders should they get in;*

C. *substances (acids and enzymes) to dissolve intruders;*

D. *heat to weaken or kill intruders;*

E. *a sticky substance to trap intruders and small finger-like projections to carry them out; and*

F. *liquids to flush out intruders.*

With a partner, find and print out an image of a human body with major organs identified, or copy the image shown above. Determine a place on the human body where each defense (A–F) is used. Draw a line from that place to a label A, B, C, D, E, and F. As a class, compare drawings, making additions or correction as needed.

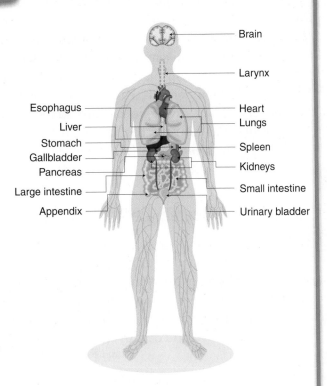

Key Terms E-Flash Cards

In this lesson, you will learn the meanings of the following key terms.

antibody

B cell

cilia

fever

inflammation

mucous membrane

mucus

phagocyte

T cell

Before You Read

Immunity Mindmap

Create a mindmap like the one shown below to connect facts in the text with your prior knowledge. In the center of your mindmap, write Immunity to Infection. *Then brainstorm as much information as you know now about your body's three lines of defense.*

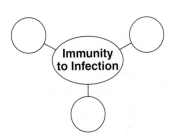

The immune system continually defends the body against infection. Such vigilance is vital to your health and survival. The importance of the immune system becomes apparent when you see what happens if it breaks down. An inherited disease called *severe combined immunodeficiency (SCID)* wipes out a person's immune system. A child with SCID is vulnerable to attacks from all types of pathogens, which a healthy immune system would easily combat. SCID results in repeated and serious infections, and it is fatal without treatment. The body's immune system has a number of different ways to protect itself from infectious diseases.

The First Line of Defense against Infection

The internal and external body surfaces are always in contact with microorganisms that could include pathogens. Fortunately, the body's surfaces are protected against invasion.

Integumentary System Defenses

The body's outermost skin is composed of many layers of scaly, overlapping cells that form a nearly impenetrable physical barrier to pathogens. The skin is also dry. Microorganisms thrive in moist environments and will not grow on skin where little water is available. Sweat secreted onto the skin contains salt, which blocks the growth of bacteria by dehydrating them. Skin oils make the body's outer surface acidic, which knocks out bacterial metabolism, keeping bacterial growth under control.

The body's inner surfaces also have protection. The internal surfaces of the respiratory, digestive, and urinary systems are lined with a ***mucous membrane*** that forms a barrier against microorganisms. Mucous membranes produce ***mucus***, a thick, watery substance that shields the body from invading pathogens.

Respiratory System Defenses

Mucus protects the respiratory system and covers the surfaces of the nasal passages, trachea, and inner air passages of the lungs. In addition, the respiratory system includes many microscopic ***cilia***—fine, short, hair-like appendages that move mucus up and away from the lungs. In this way, bacteria and other harmful particles that become lodged in mucus move up to the throat where they are swallowed and destroyed by the acid in your stomach (Figure 12.14).

Digestive System Defenses

In the digestive system, mucus coats the inner surfaces of the mouth, throat, esophagus, stomach, intestines, and rectum to repel pathogens.

Additionally, microorganisms not killed by stomach acid may be digested in the intestine by the body's digestive enzymes. Many millions of helpful bacteria normally occupy the large intestine and work to inhibit the growth of pathogens.

mucous membrane
a barrier lining the body cavities and passages that open to the outside world

mucus
a thick, watery substance that shields the body from pathogens

cilia
small, hair-like appendages that move mucus and fluids within the body

Figure 12.14

The "good" kinds of bacteria in your stomach help to digest swallowed microorganisms that may be harmful to your health.

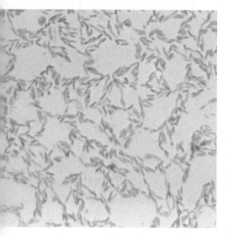

Urinary System Defenses

Normally, a few bacteria make their way into the urinary system through the opening of the *urethra*, the small tube that carries urine out of the body from the urinary bladder. The regular flow of urine usually flushes microorganisms from the urinary system.

The Second Line of Defense against Infection

What happens if microorganisms bypass or break through the first line of defense? For example, certain bacteria cling tightly to the inside of the urethra and do not get flushed out by urine. Other bacteria possess toxins that help them invade the lining of the urethra.

What happens if microorganisms gain access to the body's tissues or blood? A simple accident such as cutting your finger with a knife, for example, allows microorganisms to pass through the skin into the body's tissue.

In spite of the barriers provided by the first line of defense, microorganisms do invade the body's tissues. When this happens, the body activates a number of mechanisms in response. Pathogens entering the blood or tissues face a second line of defense that includes phagocytes, inflammation, and fever.

Phagocytes

Numerous phagocytes reside in the body's tissues, lymph nodes, spleen, and blood. A ***phagocyte*** is a white blood cell that specializes in engulfing and destroying microorganisms, especially bacteria (Figure 12.15). A phagocyte surrounds the bacteria, pulls them inside, and digests them—it is almost as if the phagocytes "eat" the bacteria. Phagocytes act as another defense against any bacteria that evaded the body's first line of defenses.

Inflammation

A clear indication that the second line of defense is working is the presence of inflammation. ***Inflammation*** is a response to infection or injury, which prepares the body to control and remove pathogens. Inflammation is characterized by four key signs: redness, heat, swelling, and pain.

During inflammation, chemicals released by injured tissues cause increased blood flow to the site, which causes the observed redness and heat. Increased blood flow also brings more pathogen-combating phagocytes to the area. The smallest blood vessels become leaky, permitting more fluids and phagocytes to leave the blood and enter the tissues. As fluids enter the inflamed area, swelling occurs, which may press on nerves and cause pain. Inflammation helps remove pathogens, and the phagocytes recruited to the area also engulf damaged body cells and debris, which promotes healing.

phagocyte
a white blood cell that engulfs and destroys microorganisms

inflammation
increased blood flow to an injured or diseased area of the body, causing redness, hurt, swelling, and pain

Figure 12.15

Phagocytes engulf foreign bacteria to fight infection and keep the body healthy.

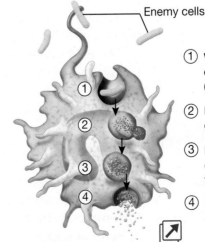

Enemy cells

① White blood cell engulfs enemy cell (bacteria, dead cells)

② Enzymes start to destroy enemy cell

③ Enemy cell breaks down into small fragments

④ Indigestible fragments are discharged

Animation

Fever

Fever may accompany infection or inflammation. During *fever*, the body's temperature rises above its normal level of about 98°F (37°C). The higher body temperature stimulates phagocytes and other white blood cells important for immunity. Fever also blocks the growth of bacteria because bacteria cannot reproduce well at higher temperatures. Although it can cause discomfort, fever is a protective and helpful body function. A doctor should be consulted regarding a high fever that lasts more than a few days.

The Third Line of Defense against Infection

Pathogens can, and sometimes do, overcome even the body's second line of defense. Fortunately, invading pathogens then encounter the third and most remarkable set of the body's defenses. This final defense system, comprised of specialized cells and chemicals, is capable of attacking and remembering specific pathogens. At the heart of this system are white blood cells called *T cells* and *B cells*, and chemicals called *antibodies*.

T Cells

T cells reside in the blood, lymph nodes, and spleen, where they play several roles. One type of T cell, called a *T-helper cell*, coordinates and stimulates the immune response. T-helper cells activate other T cells, B cells, and phagocytes, turning on the immune system in response to infections. T cells act as captains in the army, giving orders to other cells and assigning them defensive tasks. T cells also fight infections using their own weapons. Without the fighting leadership of T cells, the immune system becomes disorganized and ineffective.

Another type of T cell, the *T-cytotoxic cell*, attacks and kills cells in your body that have been infected with viruses. This stops cells from reproducing viruses and helps control viral infections. Some T cells kill tumor cells and fungi, too.

B Cells and Antibodies

B cells also reside in the blood, lymph nodes, and spleen, where they make special chemicals called *antibodies*. An **antibody** is capable of binding to pathogens or parts of pathogens called *antigens*. For example, the coating of a virus and the wall of a bacterial cell can be antigens (Figure 12.16).

An antibody sticks to a pathogen, labeling it as foreign to the body. This makes it easier for phagocytes to find and engulf the pathogens. Other antibodies "cloak" viruses, preventing them from attaching to cells and reproducing. Antibodies also stick to bacterial toxins and render them harmless.

Immune System "Memory"

The truly amazing aspect of immunity is its memory. The B cells and T cells of the immune system remember encounters with pathogens. Since they remember pathogens, they can respond quickly to later exposures to these same pathogens.

---

fever
a rise in the body's temperature, which stimulates white blood cells and blocks pathogen reproduction

T cell
a cell that coordinates the body's immune response and attacks cells that have been infected by a virus

B cell
a cell that produces antibodies

antibody
a molecule that attaches to and marks a pathogen as foreign, signaling white blood cells to destroy it

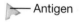

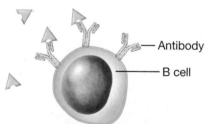

Figure 12.16

Antibodies attach to antigens to mark them as foreign bodies, thus alerting phagocytes to potential infection.

Promoting Resistance to Infection

Resistance to infectious diseases depends on a healthy immune system and a healthy body. There are many steps you can take to promote health.

- **Eat well**. Give your body a balanced diet with plenty of fruits, vegetables, and fiber. Reduce intake of empty calories from sodas and sweets.
- **Practice food sanitation**. Prepare, store, and cook your food safely.
- **Establish healthy habits**. Wash your hands regularly and practice respiratory etiquette.
- **Get enough sleep**. A tired body has a weak immune system and is vulnerable to infection. Manage your time and balance your activities.
- **Reduce stress**. Develop strategies for managing stress. The immune system can be suppressed by stress.
- **Get plenty of exercise**. Physical activity stimulates the immune system.
- **Avoid alcohol and tobacco**. Use and abuse of alcohol and tobacco reduce resistance to infection. Cigarette smoke destroys the cilia lining the respiratory tract, which normally sweep bacteria and debris from the lungs. Smokers develop more respiratory infections than nonsmokers.
- **Avoid illegal drugs**. These substances are toxic to overall health and immunity. Contaminated needles used for injecting drugs transmit a number of bloodborne infectious diseases.
- **Get regular checkups with your doctor**. Catch developing diseases early and be sure your vaccines are up-to-date.

The first time your body is invaded by a pathogen, you often become sick. The immune response to later encounters can, however, be so strong that you may not become ill at all. This is the scientific basis for vaccinations. A vaccine introduces the body to antigens from a pathogen.

Each of immunity's three lines of defense benefits from good nutrition and exercise, which provide the energy and building blocks for the immune system's cells and chemicals. Some lifestyle choices suppress immunity. Smoking interferes with the respiratory system's defenses by paralyzing the cilia. Stress produces chemicals that suppress the action of white blood cells. Quitting smoking and reducing stress will restore immune system resistance to infections.

Lesson 12.3 Review

Know and Understand

1. List three barriers the integumentary system provides that protect against invasion by pathogens.
2. How do cilia help to prevent infection?
3. Explain how the inflammation response and phagocytes work together to fight infection.
4. What infectious disease prevention method relies on the immune system's "memory" to be effective?

Analyze and Apply

5. Individuals who are fighting infections often have elevated white blood cell counts. Based on what you've learned in this lesson, why do you think this happens?

Real World Health

Vaccines, or *immunizations*, introduce the body to antigens from a pathogen. The immune system responds and retains memory of that chemical. If the body is later exposed to that pathogen, the immune system remembers it and knows how to fight it. As a student, you must receive certain vaccines to attend school. Obtain a copy of your "Shot Chart." Make a table of the immunizations you have received, the disease each immunization prevents, and your age at the time of immunization. Research to find any additional vaccines you might need in the future and add this information to your table. If you plan to attend college or the military after high school, will you need to get additional immunizations? Research and chart these as well.

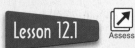
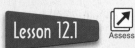

Lesson 12.1

Infectious Diseases: What You Should Know

Key Terms

bacteria	mycosis
clinical stage	opportunistic infection
convalescent stage	parasite
germ theory	protozoa
incubation period	virus
infectious disease	

Key Points

- Infectious diseases can be transmitted from one living thing to another.
- Evidence of disease can be either objective or subjective.
- Pathogens cause illness either directly or indirectly.
- Most infections follow a similar progression.
- Microorganisms are everywhere and can have either positive or negative effects on your health.

Check Your Understanding

1. _____ is a scientific concept stating that specific microorganisms cause specific diseases.

2. *True or false?* Infectious diseases are caused by microorganisms known as pathogens.

3. List five types of pathogenic microorganisms.

4. _____ are evidence of disease sensed by the sick person.
   A. Symptoms
   B. Signs
   C. Prognoses
   D. Complications

5. *True or false?* A person is usually still contagious during the convalescent stage of infection.

6. Which of the following statements is true of fungi?
   A. Fungi are less complex than bacteria and viruses.
   B. Most fungi cause disease.
   C. Mushrooms, molds, and yeast are fungi.
   D. Both A and C are true statements.

7. *True or false?* Symptoms are subjective evidence for presence of a disease.

8. *True or false?* Viruses are able to grow and reproduce independently.

9. Which of the following statements is true about protozoa?
   A. Protozoa are parasites.
   B. Protozoa are very similar to bacteria.
   C. Certain protozoa cause dysentery and malaria.
   D. Both A and C are true.

10. **Critical Thinking.** Compare and contrast bacteria and viruses.

Lesson 12.2

Transmission, Treatment, and Prevention of Infectious Diseases

Key Terms

antibiotic	pandemic
antibiotic resistance	pasteurization
endemic	respiratory etiquette
epidemic	vaccine
MRSA (methicillin-resistant	vector
Staphylococcus aureus)	zoonosis

Key Points

- Infectious disease-causing material may be spread either directly from its origin to a susceptible individual, or indirectly through a carrier.
- Occurrences of infectious disease usually follow one of several patterns.
- Medical science has developed a number of effective preventive measures to reduce the incidence of infectious disease.
- Effective treatments for infectious diseases vary based on the type of infection.

Check Your Understanding

11. Which of the following is classified as direct transmission of infectious disease?
    A. droplet spread
    B. vector
    C. zoonosis
    D. contaminated food

12. *True or false?* A pandemic infection affects an enormous number of people and spreads from one country to much of the world.

13. List four preventive measures that reduce the incidence of infectious disease.

14. Doctors recommend people practice _____ to prevent spreading diseases.
    A. vector
    B. antibiotic resistance
    C. respiratory etiquette
    D. zoonosis

15. Which of the following statements is true about vaccines?
    A. Vaccines contain live pathogens.
    B. Vaccines provoke an immune response in the body.
    C. Vaccines are also called antibiotics.
    D. Vaccines are responsible for eradicating chicken pox.

16. *True or false?* Antibiotics are used to kill pathogenic viruses.

17. Which of the following precautions are recommended to avoid antibiotic resistance?
    A. Use antibiotics only when prescribed.
    B. Take the entire dose for the length of time prescribed by your doctor.
    C. Take antibiotics for viral infections.
    D. Both A and B.

18. Identify each of the following as direct (D) or indirect (I) transmission of infectious disease.
    A. Hookworm infection after a day spent gardening.
    B. Food poisoning after eating a hamburger at a restaurant.
    C. Lyme disease from a tick bite.
    D. Influenza symptoms after the ill student sitting next to you in class sneezes and fails to cover her mouth.

19. **Critical Thinking.** Differentiate between direct and indirect transmission of infectious disease.

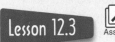

Lesson 12.3
Assess

Immunity to Infection

Key Terms

antibody
B cell
cilia
fever
inflammation

mucous membrane
mucus
phagocyte
T cell

Key Points

- The body's outer and inner surfaces provide a variety of barriers to prevent disease-causing pathogens from invading.
- The body activates additional mechanisms to fight pathogens that succeed in invading blood or tissue.
- Specialized cells and chemicals are the body's final defense against pathogens.

Check Your Understanding

20. The thick, watery substance that shields the body from invading pathogens is called _____.
    A. *cilia*
    B. *mucus*
    C. *phagocyte*
    D. *antigen*

21. Which of the following describes the skin's defenses against infection?
    A. Mucus coats the inner surfaces, repelling pathogens.
    B. Many layers of scaly, overlapping cells form a physical barrier to pathogens.
    C. Skin oils make the surface acidic, which controls bacterial growth.
    D. Both B and C are true.

22. *True or false?* Bacteria in the large intestine act to block the growth of pathogens.

23. Which of the following statements is true about phagocytes?
    A. Phagocytes are pathogens that "eat" healthy tissue.
    B. Phagocytes reside in the body's tissues, lymph nodes, spleen, and blood.
    C. Phagocytes are part of the body's first line of defense against infection.
    D. Phagocytes are leaky blood vessels.

24. Explain how fever helps fight infection from pathogens.

25. *True or false?* B cells coordinate an organized and effective immune system.

26. List three ways antibodies work to fight infection.

27. *True or false?* Stress is capable of suppressing your immunity.

28. **Critical Thinking.** Analyze the role of inflammation in health.

Health and Wellness Skills

29. **Access Information.** Imagine that you are experiencing cold or flu-like symptoms and need medicine for relief. Your parents are out of town, and you must decide which over-the-counter (OTC) medicines to purchase. Visit a local pharmacy. After reading the labels of available cold and flu medicines, make a list of questions to ask the pharmacist so you can make an informed decision.

30. **Advocate for Health.** Working in small groups, create a public service announcement (PSA) about the importance of getting a flu shot. Your group's PSA can be in the form of a radio, television, or print ad. Your television or radio ad should be sixty seconds or less in duration, and your print ad should be one letter-size page of paper. Your message should be attention-getting, clear and concise, and include current information that creates an emotional awareness amongst your audience.

31. **Practice Health Behaviors.** Help prepare a meal at home. Be observant of proper sanitation to help prevent foodborne illnesses: wash hands often, especially after handling raw meat; avoid cross-contamination by storing meats separate from vegetables and fruits; keep surfaces clean; use a meat thermometer to cook meats to the proper temperatures; and keep foods refrigerated. After helping with the meal, create a digital presentation or a poster that reflects the steps you took to avoid foodborne illnesses.

32. **Communicate with Others.** Imagine it is cold and flu season. In this lesson, you learned that one way to prevent the spread of these diseases is hand washing. You have observed that many students at your school don't wash their hands properly or often enough. You want to get the word out about how important hand washing is! Working in small groups, consult the CDC website and gather information on washing hands. With the information that your group finds, write a song or a rap that emphasizes the importance of hand washing. Each group will share their composition with the rest of the class.

Hands-On Activity
The Spread of Infectious Disease

This activity will show how infection can spread from person-to-person contact. The liquid in the cups will simulate respiratory secretions that can be produced by coughing, sneezing, or talking. Do *not* drink the liquid in the cups.

Materials Needed
- plastic cups, water, lemon juice, Bromothymol blue pH indicator (Bromo Blue)

Steps for this Activity

1. Your teacher will give you a cup of water filled halfway. One person will have "infected" water (two teaspoons of lemon juice for every two cups of water).

2. "Interact" with a classmate by "sharing" the liquid in your cup. (Don't drink the liquid.) Pour all your liquid into your classmate's cup, and then she will pour all her liquid back into yours. You will then pour half of the liquid from your cup back into your classmate's cup.

3. Repeat this process with several other classmates.

4. Form a circle. Your teacher will drop a few drops of Bromothymol blue in each student's cup. The liquid in any "infected" cups will turn yellow. The liquid in the cups that have not been infected will turn blue.

5. Consider and discuss the following questions: How many cups were infected? Were you able to tell if your cup was infected just by looking at it? Predict the outcome if more rounds of "interactions" had been done.

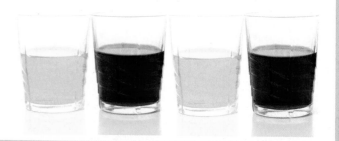

Core Skills

Math Practice

Use the information presented in the pie graph to answer the questions that follow.

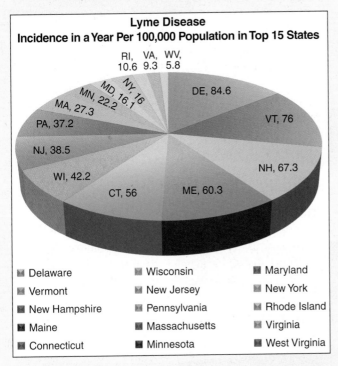

Lyme Disease
Incidence in a Year Per 100,000 Population in Top 15 States

RI, 10.6   VA, 9.3   WV, 5.8
NY, 16
MD, 16.1
MN, 22.2
MA, 27.3
PA, 37.2
NJ, 38.5
WI, 42.2
CT, 56
ME, 60.3
NH, 67.3
VT, 76
DE, 84.6

- Delaware
- Vermont
- New Hampshire
- Maine
- Connecticut
- Wisconsin
- New Jersey
- Pennsylvania
- Massachusetts
- Minnesota
- Maryland
- New York
- Rhode Island
- Virginia
- West Virginia

33. How many more incidences of Lyme disease per 100,000 did Vermont experience compared to Connecticut?
    A. 20
    B. 15.7
    C. 2
    D. 8.7

34. Incidence of Lyme disease per 100,000 in New Hampshire are _____ the incidence in Minnesota.
    A. less than
    B. greater than
    C. less than or equal to
    D. equal to

35. What percentage of the pie graph does the Vermont incidence of Lyme Disease represent?
    A. 13%
    B. 76%
    C. 7.6%
    D. 1.3%

Reading and Writing Practice

Read the passage below and then answer the questions.

This final defense system, comprised of specialized cells and chemicals, is capable of attacking and remembering specific pathogens. At the heart of this system are white blood cells called T cells and B cells, and chemicals called antibodies.

T cells reside in the blood, lymph nodes, and spleen, where they play several roles. One type of T cell, called a T-helper cell, coordinates and stimulates the immune response. T-helper cells activate other T cells, B cells, and phagocytes—turning on the immune system in response to infections. T cells act as captains in the army, giving orders to other cells and assigning them defensive tasks. T cells also fight infections using their own weapons. Without the fighting leadership of T cells, the immune system becomes disorganized and ineffective.

Another type of T cell, the T-cytotoxic cell, attacks and kills cells in your body that have been infected with viruses. This stops cells from reproducing viruses and helps control viral infections. Some T cells kill tumor cells and fungi, too.

36. What is the author's main idea in this passage?
    A. B cells are not necessary for an effective immune response.
    B. T cells are necessary for an organized and effective immune response.
    C. T cells attack and kill cells in your body.
    D. T cells are solely responsible for fighting infection.

37. Which of the following best exemplifies the role of T cells in the immune response?
    A. to turn on the immune system in response to infections
    B. to kill tumor cells and fungi
    C. to fight infections using their own weapons
    D. to stop cells from reproducing viruses

38. In this passage, the phrase "captains in the army" was used to describe T cells. How would you describe T cells? Write a brief paragraph explaining your description.

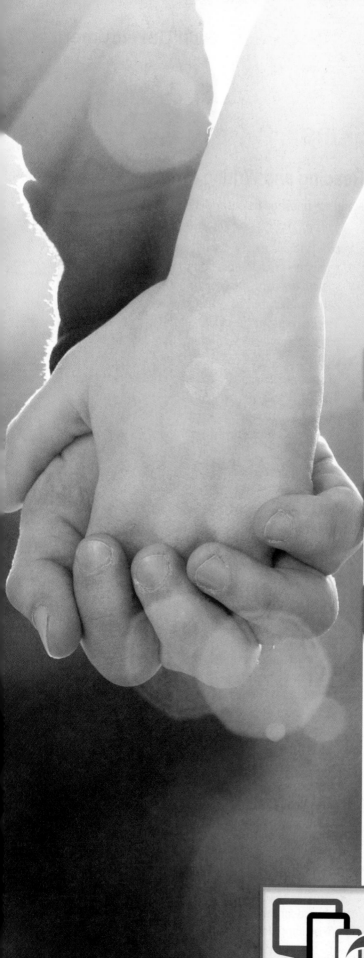

Chapter 13

Sexually Transmitted Infections and HIV/AIDS

Lesson 13.1

Sexually Transmitted Infections: What You Should Know

Lesson 13.2

Common STIs

Lesson 13.3

HIV/AIDS

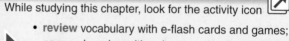

While studying this chapter, look for the activity icon to:
- **review** vocabulary with e-flash cards and games;
- **assess** learning with quizzes and online exercises;
- **expand** knowledge with animations and activities; and
- **listen** to pronunciation of key terms in the audio glossary.

G-WLEARNING.com

www.g-wlearning.com/health/

What's Your Health and Wellness IQ?

Take this quiz to see what you do *and* do not *know about STIs and HIV/AIDS. If you cannot answer a question, pay extra attention to that topic as you study this chapter.*

1. *Identify each statement as* True, False, *or* It Depends. *Choose* It Depends *if a statement is true in some cases, but false in others.*
2. *Revise each* False *statement to make it true.*
3. *Explain the circumstances in which each* It Depends *statement is true and when it is false.*

Health and Wellness IQ Assess

1. Young people rarely get STIs.	True	False	It Depends
2. People know when they are infected with an STI because they will notice symptoms.	True	False	It Depends
3. STIs are fatal.	True	False	It Depends
4. There is no way to prevent STIs.	True	False	It Depends
5. Abstinence is the only method that is 100% effective in preventing STIs.	True	False	It Depends
6. Women who are not treated for chlamydia can lose their ability to have children.	True	False	It Depends
7. There is a vaccine available to help prevent cervical cancer.	True	False	It Depends
8. The human papillomavirus is the most common STI.	True	False	It Depends
9. Kissing transmits HIV.	True	False	It Depends
10. A person with HIV also has AIDS.	True	False	It Depends

Setting the Scene

In the previous chapter you studied different types of infectious diseases. In this chapter you will learn about *sexually transmitted infections* (*STIs*), which are diseases transmitted specifically during sexual activity. These infections are also referred to as *STDs* (sexually transmitted diseases).

Like many people, you may be curious about STIs, but feel uncomfortable or embarrassed discussing them. Some people find it difficult to ask questions at all. Others don't know whom to ask, or even which questions to ask.

Should people be concerned about STIs? What should people know about STIs? This chapter will provide answers to these and many more questions.

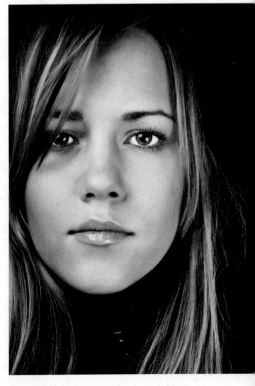

Sexually Transmitted Infections: What You Should Know

Key Terms 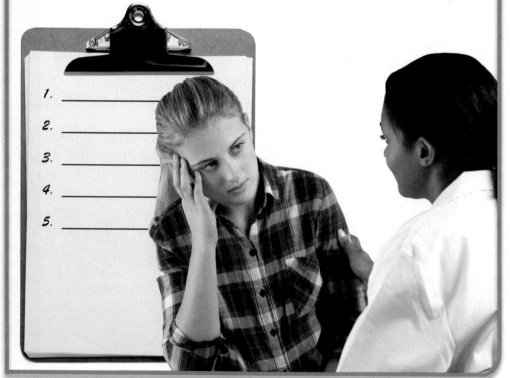 E-Flash Cards

In this lesson, you will learn the meanings of the following key terms.

abstinence

asymptomatic

latex condom

sexually transmitted infections (STIs)

Before You Read

Preliminary Questions

Many STIs are asymptomatic, *meaning they exhibit no visible symptoms. How do you think this might affect an infected person's health? What roles do symptoms play in motivating people to seek treatment? How do you think asymptomatic infections can be diagnosed? On a separate sheet of paper, answer these questions. As you read this lesson, add new information to your answers.*

Lesson Objectives

After studying this lesson, you will be able to

- explain how people can contract STIs;
- describe what happens when a person contracts an STI;
- list the three critical components for effective treatment of an STI;
- identify the most effective way to prevent STIs; and
- determine resources available for people dealing with STIs.

Warm-Up Activity

Health Predictions

Before you read this lesson, make predictions and list at least five ways that STIs could negatively impact a person's health.

I nfections spread from one person to another during sexual activity are called ***sexually transmitted infections (STIs)***. When discussing STIs, many young people ask the question, "Am I at risk of contracting an STI?" The answer is *no* if they do not engage in sexual activity. The answer is *yes*, however, if they are sexually active. This lesson will discuss health problems associated with STIs, as well as treatment and prevention for these conditions.

sexually transmitted infections (STIs)
infections that are transmitted by sexual contact, and are caused by bacteria, viruses, or protozoa that live in and on reproductive organs

How People Contract STIs

STIs are infectious diseases caused by certain microorganisms such as bacteria, viruses, and protozoa (Figure 13.1). These microorganisms live in and on the surfaces of the reproductive organs. Depending on the type of STI, these microorganisms may also reside in the mouth, rectum, blood, semen, and other bodily fluids of an infected person.

Engaging in sexual activity one time with just one infected sexual partner is all it takes to contract an STI. People with more sexual partners have greater chances of getting an STI (Figure 13.2 on the next page). Although it is possible for a person with certain oral STIs to transmit the infection by kissing, other STIs cannot be transmitted by kissing (the next lesson includes specific examples). Casual contact with an infected person, such as using the same toilet seat, does not transmit STIs.

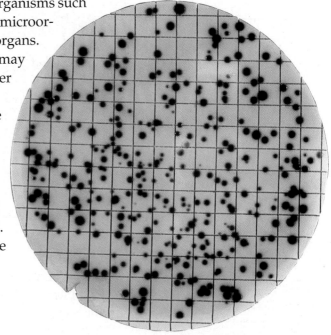

STIs Cause Serious Health Problems

STIs are caused by infectious microorganisms, which cause many health problems. Bacteria produce toxins that damage organs, and most infectious microorganisms trigger inflammation. *Inflammation* is the body's reaction to infection. When inflammation occurs, a body part may become red, warm, swollen, or painful. Inflammation often occurs in body parts affected by an STI.

People with STIs are often ***asymptomatic***, which means they exhibit few or no symptoms of infection. Asymptomatic people with STIs do have the infection, however, and they do carry the bacteria or viruses. This means they can also transmit the disease to others primarily through sexual acts. Additionally, having no symptoms does not mean that health problems are not occurring in an infected person.

While some STIs cause little or no discomfort, these diseases can still damage the reproductive organs and cause *infertility*, the inability to conceive and have children. For example, two of the STIs you will read about in the next lesson can scar the *fallopian tubes*, which normally deliver fertilized eggs to the uterus. In fact, people can develop infertility or other permanent health problems even if they have been cured of an STI.

Figure 13.1

STIs are caused by harmful microorganisms. The colonies of *N. gonorrhoeae* shown above can infect a person with gonorrhea. *What do you already know about microorganisms? How are microorganisms spread?*

asymptomatic
the quality of exhibiting no recognizable signs or symptoms of disease

Figure 13.2 Exposure to Sexually Transmitted Infections

If Person A has this number of sexual partners...	and if each of Person A's sexual partners has the same number of sexual partners as Person A, Person A is exposed to this many people	
1		(1)
2		(4)
3		(9)
4		(16)
5		(25)
6		(36)
7		(49)
8		(64)
9		(81)
10		(100)

If left untreated, STIs can damage not only the reproductive organs, but also the brain, heart, liver, and other internal organs. Worse, a few STIs are incurable, some cause cancer, and some are fatal. Sadly, it is possible for a pregnant woman with an STI to transmit the infection to her baby during pregnancy, birth, or breast-feeding. Some of the problems caused by the STI transmission may be seen in the baby at birth. Some effects, however, may not be visible for months or years after birth.

STIs Can Be Treated

Many STIs are easily treated, especially in their early stages. For example, bacterial STIs are treatable, even curable, with antibiotics prescribed by a physician. Being cured does not mean, however, that people develop immunity. Any subsequent exposure to the STI can lead to another infection.

Viral infections cannot be treated with antibiotics, but they can be controlled with a number of antiviral medications. These infections are not curable, however. Antiviral medications simply control the virus, sometimes greatly reducing the severity and frequency of symptoms.

Effective treatment of STIs includes three critical components. First, treatment from a doctor must begin as soon as possible. Early treatment controls microorganisms more easily and can prevent complications such as infertility. To be effective, all medications must be taken exactly as prescribed by the doctor. Second, all sexual partners of the infected individual must be notified, tested, and treated. Otherwise, a person can get reinfected by his or her partner. Third, an infected person must abstain from sexual activity until a doctor determines that the disease is cured or no longer able to be transmitted.

abstinence
the decision and practice of refraining from sexual activity

STIs Can Be Prevented

The good news is that certain STIs (chlamydia and gonorrhea for example) are curable. The bad news is that even some curable infections can leave a person with serious health problems. Even worse, certain infections remain incurable. The most effective way to deal with STIs, therefore, is to prevent them.

Two methods commonly used to help prevent STIs are practicing abstinence and using latex condoms. Other methods are simply ineffective. For example, the birth control pill (*the pill*) can help prevent pregnancy, but it has no effect on STIs. A woman using only the pill must abstain from sex or insist that her partner use a latex condom if she wants to prevent STIs.

Abstinence

The most effective way to prevent STIs is to practice abstinence. Sexual *abstinence* is the decision to refrain from sexual activity. Abstinence is the only method that is 100% effective in preventing STIs. The decision to abstain from sex is not difficult to make, but abstinence can prove challenging in practice. Barriers that can prevent people from practicing abstinence may include pressure from a partner or fear of rejection, peer pressure, societal and commercial media influences, alcohol or drug use, or a desire for intimacy.

Anticipating Challenges to Abstinence. Healthy intimate relationships require honest communication and should include communication about sex. When a person makes a commitment to sexual abstinence, he or she must be ready to explain this commitment to a boyfriend or girlfriend (Figure 13.3 on the next page). A commitment to abstinence becomes easier when a person's romantic partner understands and respects the decision.

A person's first major challenge may arise if a girlfriend or boyfriend disagrees with the commitment to abstinence. In that case, a person should be prepared to avoid risky situations and refuse sexual advances. A person may need to reevaluate his or her relationship if a partner continues to apply unwanted pressure to engage in sexual activities.

Alcohol and drug use poses many health risks to young people, including the increased possibility of engaging in sexual activity. Alcohol and drugs impair judgment and inhibition (feelings of restraint), so their use is an important factor in early and unwanted sexual activity. By avoiding risky situations that may include drugs and alcohol, a person can make responsible decisions involving his or her choice to maintain abstinence.

Developing Refusal Skills. Planning and even practicing skills for refusing sex, drugs, and alcohol can help people become familiar with words and actions they can use if risky situations do arise. For example, consider the words you might use if you find yourself at an unsupervised party, or

Personal Profile

Can You Avoid Risky Situations?

These questions will help you assess how well you deal with difficult situations.

I refuse to attend unsupervised parties. **yes no**

I refuse to try drugs or alcohol even if pressured by my peers. **yes no**

I know what to say and which actions to take when I am at an event where alcohol or drugs may be present. **yes no**

I am committed to sexual abstinence. **yes no**

I have openly and honestly explained my commitment to sexual abstinence to my boyfriend or girlfriend. **yes no**

I know what to say or which actions to take when pressured by my boyfriend or girlfriend to engage in sexual activity. **yes no**

I am willing to end a relationship if my boyfriend or girlfriend refuses to accept my commitment to sexual abstinence. **yes no**

I feel comfortable talking to a parent or another trusted adult about the pressures I am facing. **yes no**

The more yes answers you have, the more confident you are at handling difficult situations.

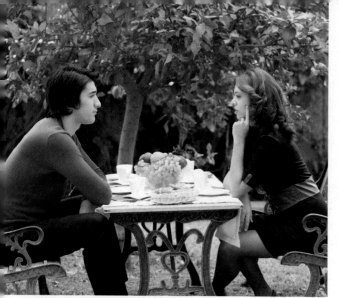

if you are invited to an event where alcohol or drugs may be present, and your boyfriend or girlfriend is pressuring you to have sex. How would you respond? Sometimes verbally refusing may not be enough. You may need to walk away from the situation. Remember that you do not need to face this stress and pressure alone. Guidance for handling specific situations may be available from a friend, parent, teacher, counselor, or other trusted adult.

Other Methods

Although abstinence is the most effective method for preventing STIs, a correctly used latex condom can also reduce the chances of contracting STIs. A *latex condom* is a birth control device that provides a barrier to microorganisms that cause STIs.

To be effective, a latex condom must be applied correctly, must fit well, must be used for each sex act from beginning to end, and must be removed correctly. A condom can be used only once; a new one must be used each time a person has sex. Any condom that has expired, has holes or tears, or has dried out must be discarded because it will not work. In fact, a person should only use condoms he or she has recently purchased or has received from a reliable source, such as a clinic nurse. Condoms may become damaged if stored in places that become very cold or hot, as in a car, or where they could be crushed, like in a wallet.

As mentioned previously, abstinence is the only 100% effective method for preventing STIs. Latex condoms are *not* 100% effective in eliminating the risk of pregnancy or STI transmission. It is also important to know that

Figure 13.3

Couples should talk about their expectations and boundaries regarding sex and abstinence. *Should a person be willing to compromise regarding his or her sexual boundaries? Why or why not?*

latex condom

a birth control device that provides a barrier to semen and microorganisms that cause STIs

---

SKILLS FOR HEALTH AND WELLNESS

Anticipating Challenges to Abstinence: Words, Action, and Preparation

When you make a commitment to abstain from sexual activity, you are likely to receive challenges to your choice. These may come from your boyfriend or girlfriend, or friends in various risky situations. Knowing what words to use, what actions to take, and how to prepare can help in these situations.

Make your *WORDS* count. Say *no* in a firm and clear voice if you are

- asked or pressured to have sex;
- invited to an unsupervised party;
- offered alcoholic drinks; or
- offered any kind of drugs.

Take *ACTION*. Be prepared to leave when

- someone does not respect your refusal to have sex;

- you learn that a party is not supervised by responsible adults;
- you are pressured to drink alcohol;
- you are pressured to take illegal drugs;
- you are in unfamiliar surroundings with people you do not know; or
- you feel unsafe or uncomfortable.

PREPARE. Think about and discuss

- your commitment to abstinence;
- your decision to avoid alcohol and drugs;
- your decision to avoid risky situations; and
- who can offer you advice, such as a parent, teacher, counselor, coach, or trusted adult.

Figure 13.4 Fact and Fiction about Preventing STIs

Method of Prevention	Can this method prevent STIs?
abstaining from sex	YES Sexual abstinence is 100% effective.
using latex condom	MAYBE Latex condoms are highly effective when used properly and when used every time.
taking birth control pill	NO The pill only prevents conception. It cannot prevent disease.

non-latex condoms, such as *lambskin condoms*, can reduce the risk of pregnancy, but will not prevent STIs (Figure 13.4).

STI Resources

If a person suspects he or she might have an STI, community resources are available to help. Doctors can provide testing, counseling, and treatment. Public health departments often provide diagnosis, treatment, and prevention programs. Private and nonprofit organizations may also be available to offer assistance.

People can learn more about resources available to them through the Internet or yellow pages, or by asking a doctor or nurse. Sometimes additional emotional support may be needed. Counseling services and support groups can help meet this need. Friends and family can also be a source of support. Getting help when necessary is a good way to promote overall health and well-being.

Lesson 13.1 Review

Know and Understand Assess

1. What are STIs?
2. What does *asymptomatic* mean?
3. List three critical components for effective treatment of STIs.
4. Name two methods commonly used to help prevent STIs.

Analyze and Apply

5. Compare and contrast treatments of bacterial STIs and viral infections.
6. Explain how alcohol and drug use can increase a person's risk for contracting an STI.

Real World Health

Chris and Stacy have been dating for three months, and Chris just asked Stacy to the prom. The relationship is starting to get serious, and they have even said they love each other and want to possibly attend the same college. Lately, Chris has been pressuring Stacy for sex, but she does not feel ready to take this step in the relationship. Stacy is excited about prom, but she does not want the night to be ruined by Chris pressuring her. Write a dialogue between Chris and Stacy in which Stacy firmly, yet fairly, communicates her feelings to Chris. She should use good refusal skills against all of Chris's pressuring tactics.

Common STIs

Key Terms 🔗 E-Flash Cards

In this lesson, you will learn the meanings of the following key terms.

cervical cancer

chlamydia

genital herpes

genital warts

gonorrhea

human papillomavirus (HPV)

oropharyngeal cancer

pelvic inflammatory disease

syphilis

trichomoniasis

Before You Read

Roll the Dice

Roll a die six times. Each time you do so, record the number you get on a piece of paper. After the sixth time, circle any 5s or 6s you have rolled. Each 5 you rolled represents contracting an STI. Each 6 you rolled represents a pregnancy. These numbers illustrate the gamble of having sex, especially unprotected sex. Now, write a short paragraph about what you want to learn in this lesson.

Lesson Objectives

After studying this lesson, you will be able to

- identify six common STIs;
- describe the signs and symptoms of STIs; and
- explain ways in which STIs are diagnosed and treated.

Warm-Up Activity

Agree or Disagree?

Read the statements in the chart shown below. In a similar chart on a separate piece of paper, circle agree *or* disagree *for each statement before you read this lesson. When you have finished reading this lesson, consider the statements again based on any new information you may have read. Decide again whether you agree or disagree. Have any of your opinions changed?*

Before Reading	Statements	Page #	After Reading
Agree/Disagree	1. Chlamydia infections are the most reported STI in the United States.		Agree/Disagree
Agree/Disagree	2. Ectopic pregnancies can be fatal.		Agree/Disagree
Agree/Disagree	3. There is no cure for bacterial infections.		Agree/Disagree
Agree/Disagree	4. Syphilis is fatal if not treated.		Agree/Disagree
Agree/Disagree	5. Herpes blisters can appear on the mouth as well as the genitals.		Agree/Disagree
Agree/Disagree	6. Herpes can be cured with antibiotics.		Agree/Disagree
Agree/Disagree	7. Almost all sexually active people carry human papillomavirus at one time or another.		Agree/Disagree
Agree/Disagree	8. Human papillomavirus can cause cervical cancer in women.		Agree/Disagree

T his lesson will discuss six of the most commonly reported STIs (Figure 13.5). These include chlamydia, gonorrhea, syphilis, trichomoniasis, genital herpes, and human papillomavirus (HPV). You will learn about the signs, symptoms, diagnoses, and treatments for each of these STIs. HIV/AIDS will be addressed in the next lesson.

Figure 13.5 New Cases of Sexually Transmitted Infections Reported in the United States Each Year	
all STIs	about 20,000,000
chlamydia	2,860,000
gonorrhea	820,000
syphilis	74,000
trichomoniasis	1,090,000
genital herpes	776,000
HPV	14,000,000
HIV/AIDS	39,500

Chlamydia

According to the Centers for Disease Control and Prevention (CDC), more than 1,500,000 *chlamydia* infections are reported per year in the United States. Caused by a bacterium, chlamydia is also known as a *silent disease* because it has few or no symptoms. Due to its lack of symptoms, many cases of chlamydia are never diagnosed. The CDC estimates that the actual number of people infected each year is over 2,800,000.

Chlamydia poses a serious threat to the reproductive health of women. Young women are especially susceptible to chlamydia because their bodies are not yet fully developed. The "silent" nature of the disease allows it to quietly progress to an infection of the fallopian tubes and the pelvic cavity. This condition is called *pelvic inflammatory disease*, which causes infertility (Figure 13.6 on the next page).

If a woman with pelvic inflammatory disease does become pregnant, she may develop *ectopic pregnancy*. This is a life-threatening condition in which a fertilized egg implants outside the uterus. The fertilized egg cannot develop properly unless it implants in the uterus. An egg implanted elsewhere, such as the fallopian tube, could rupture the tube and cause serious bleeding and a dangerous pelvic infection.

Signs and Symptoms

Symptoms for chlamydia are often mild or absent in both men and women. If symptoms do arise, men may experience burning during urination, itching at the opening of the penis, and a watery discharge from the penis. Rectal and oral infections may also occur.

chlamydia
an almost asymptomatic STI that may cause pelvic inflammatory disease if not treated

pelvic inflammatory disease
an infection of the fallopian tubes and pelvic cavity, which occurs as the result of an STI and often causes infertility

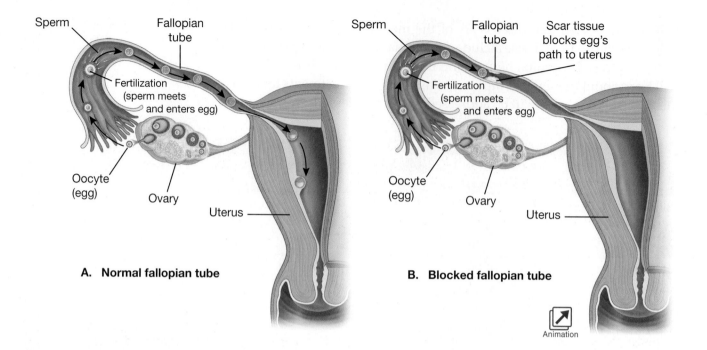

Sperm
Fallopian tube
Fertilization (sperm meets and enters egg)
Oocyte (egg)
Ovary
Uterus

A. Normal fallopian tube

Sperm
Fallopian tube
Scar tissue blocks egg's path to uterus
Fertilization (sperm meets and enters egg)
Oocyte (egg)
Ovary
Uterus

B. Blocked fallopian tube

Animation

Figure 13.6

Normal and blocked fallopian tubes. A) A fertilized egg moves through a woman's fallopian tube to her uterus, where it implants and grows into a new life. B) When a woman has pelvic inflammatory disease, scar tissue can form in the fallopian tube, blocking the path of the fertilized egg to the uterus. This results in infertility and in ectopic pregnancy, if the egg implants in the fallopian tube.

A woman may experience abnormal vaginal discharge and a burning sensation during urination. The bacteria associated with chlamydia can infect the cervix, which connects the vagina to the uterus. If the infection spreads past the cervix to the fallopian tubes, a woman may still have no symptoms. She may, however, experience nausea, abdominal pain, and fever, as well as abnormal bleeding between menstrual periods.

A pregnant woman with chlamydia may deliver her baby prematurely. A baby born to a mother with chlamydia can develop pneumonia, conjunctivitis (pinkeye), or *trachoma*, a chlamydial eye infection that leads to blindness.

Diagnosis and Treatment

Chlamydia can be diagnosed simply, quickly, and painlessly with a urine test, or with a laboratory test of a sample swabbed from an infected site such as the penis or cervix. Test results are often available within one day. If a person tests positive for chlamydia, he or she can be treated and cured with antibiotics.

As with other STIs, all sexual partners of an individual with chlamydia need to be notified so they can be tested and treated. To prevent spreading chlamydia or any STI, an infected person should abstain from sex until a doctor determines that the infection is cured and no longer able to be transmitted to others.

Gonorrhea

gonorrhea
a bacterial STI that causes burning or itching of reproductive parts, and can cause infertility or even death if not treated

Gonorrhea is a bacterial infection that primarily affects the reproductive tract, rectum, and throat. According to the CDC, gonorrhea is a very common STI—an estimated 820,000 people becoming infected with gonorrhea each year. The highest rates of gonorrhea occur among young men and women aged 15 to 24.

Point-of-Care Tests for STIs

STI screening and testing are an essential part of diagnosing and treating STIs, especially when so many people with STIs are asymptomatic. The Johns Hopkins University Center for Point-of-Care Tests for Sexually Transmitted Diseases currently researches and tests diagnosis methods for STIs.

One current study involves determining what patients want in an STI *point-of-care test* (POCT). Point-of-care devices, such as a home pregnancy test, allow for rapid testing and diagnosis. Point-of-care tests can be performed in the home, in ambulances, physicians' offices, clinics, or hospitals.

To find out what patients want in a POCT, researchers established five focus groups of people attending state-specific STI and adolescent health centers. The focus groups met over a period of a year and discussed the following topics:

- advantages and disadvantages of a POCT
- potential problems with using a POCT at home or in a clinic setting
- priorities for developing STI-specific POCTs
- characteristics of an ideal POCT

The results from these focus groups determined that people are in favor of rapid, easy-to-read, and simple-to-use diagnostic tests. Advantages of

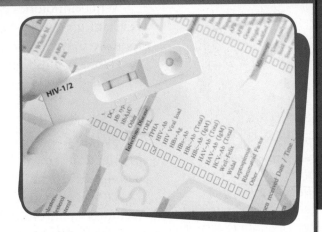

at-home testing options include better confidentiality, privacy, and convenience. Testing in a clinic setting was also viewed favorably with a major advantage being accuracy of results and immediacy of treatment.

Thinking Critically

1. What do you think would be advantages and disadvantages of a POCT?
2. What problems might occur with using a POCT at home?
3. Research the at-home tests that are currently available for STIs. What STI-specific POCTs are currently most needed?

Signs and Symptoms

Like chlamydia, gonorrhea causes mild or no symptoms in many people. Symptoms do, however, arise in some cases of gonorrhea. In men, the urethra burns during urination and produces yellow or white pus. Sometimes the testicles swell.

Women with gonorrhea may experience mild burning or itching that seems like a vaginal yeast infection. In addition, women might have pelvic pain, abnormal bleeding between menstrual periods, and abnormal vaginal discharge. Women may also develop chronic pelvic and lower back pain.

If left untreated, gonorrhea can cause pelvic inflammatory disease and infertility. Gonorrhea can also infect the blood and spread throughout the body, a potentially fatal complication.

Diagnosis and Treatment

Men with gonorrhea symptoms can be diagnosed by swabbing and examining discharge from the urethra for the gonorrhea bacteria under a microscope. Gonorrhea in females can be diagnosed with a urine test or by swabbing an infected body part for laboratory analysis.

While antibiotics can successfully treat and cure gonorrhea, antibiotic-resistant gonorrhea bacteria have been found. Infections with these bacteria are more difficult to treat. Therefore, gonorrhea is often treated with two kinds of antibiotics.

Syphilis

Syphilis is a bacterial infection that causes extremely serious health problems and disability. Syphilis is fatal if untreated and, if contracted by a pregnant woman, can threaten the life of a developing fetus. Today, over 74,000 cases of syphilis occur each year. By comparison, recent flu seasons recorded about 40,000 cases of influenza. According to these numbers, syphilis is about as common as the seasonal flu.

Signs and Symptoms

Sexual activity can transmit syphilis bacteria. At the site of the infection, a sore, called a *chancre*, develops. Sometimes only a single sore develops on the penis, in the vagina, mouth, or rectum. If only one sore develops, it can easily be missed or go unrecognized. The sores are not painful, do not itch, and heal after a few weeks. This stage of syphilis is called *primary syphilis* (Figure 13.7A).

Days, weeks, or even months later, *secondary syphilis* develops (Figure 13.7B). In this stage, a red or copper-color rash appears, mainly on the palms and soles, but sometimes elsewhere. The rash does not itch and it could be so small that it goes unnoticed. This rash cannot transmit syphilis. Symptoms of secondary syphilis include swollen lymph nodes, fatigue, and mild fever. The signs and symptoms of secondary syphilis resemble those of

syphilis

a bacterial infection that causes a sore (or chancre), rashes, and internal infection in later stages, and can be fatal if untreated

Figure 13.7

During primary syphilis (A), painless chancres may develop on the genitals, rectum, or mouth. During secondary syphilis (B), a rash will appear on the palms or soles and may be accompanied by fever or fatigue. *If you notice a painless sore in your mouth, or on your genitals or rectum, what should you do?*

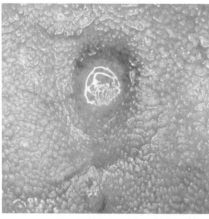

A

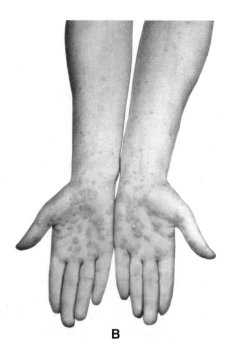

B

During a routine visit to her pediatrician's office, Malika sees a poster about the HPV (*human papillomavirus*) vaccine. The poster recommends that preteens and teenagers, 11 years of age and older, receive the HPV vaccine. Although she is 15 years old, Malika has not been vaccinated. She has not been sexually active and does not plan to be, so Malika does not feel she needs to be vaccinated.

Thinking Critically

1. What complications or symptoms can arise from HPV infection?
2. Do you think Malika should be vaccinated? Why or why not?
3. Boys can carry HPV, but usually do not get sick. Should boys be vaccinated? Why or why not?

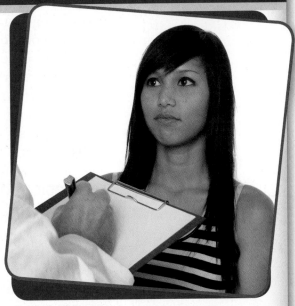

many other diseases, and so syphilis has been called the *great imitator*. The rash heals, but the person remains infected and enters latent (hidden) and late stages of the disease.

Late-stage syphilis is an internal infection that doesn't include obvious external signs. It is characterized by damage to the brain in the form of *dementia* (deteriorating mental function), paralysis, and fatal damage to the heart, liver, and blood vessels. A pregnant woman with syphilis often delivers a stillborn child, or a child who dies shortly after birth. Surviving children are born with *congenital syphilis*, a condition that causes severe physical and intellectual disabilities. Syphilis is most treatable during the early stages. Even if late-stage syphilis is cured, the damage remains permanent.

Diagnosis and Treatment

Syphilis can be diagnosed by using a special microscope to study a sample swabbed from syphilis sores. A blood test can also be used to detect antibodies the body makes in response to the syphilis bacteria. Both tests are easy and painless.

Pregnant women should talk to their doctor about a syphilis blood test to determine whether they have the disease. Early diagnosis is important because antibiotics can cure syphilis in its primary and secondary stages. The organ damage caused by late-stage syphilis cannot be reversed or repaired by antibiotics.

Trichomoniasis

Trichomoniasis is caused by a single-celled microorganism called a *protozoan* (Figure 13.8). This infection is more common among young women than men. Trichomoniasis is often asymptomatic and is also considered to be the most curable common STI. The CDC estimates that there are almost 4 million people in the United States who have this infection.

trichomoniasis
a curable STI, caused by a protozoan, which may cause burning or itching, but is usually asymptomatic

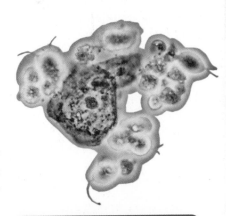

Figure 13.8

The protozoan *Trichomonas vaginalis* causes trichomoniasis, which is characterized by itching and burning of the genitals and by yellow-green vaginal discharge.

Signs and Symptoms

Most men with trichomoniasis have no symptoms, but some experience itching and burning in the urethra. In men, the symptoms tend to go away without treatment. Men can, however still carry the protozoa and infect their sexual partners.

In women, trichomoniasis primarily infects the vagina and causes few symptoms. If symptomatic, women have yellow-green vaginal discharge with a foul odor, and burning, itching, and pain during urination and sexual intercourse. Pregnant women with trichomoniasis often have babies with a low birth weight.

Diagnosis and Treatment

Trichomoniasis is difficult to diagnose in both men and women without a laboratory test. A doctor must examine a woman's vagina and cervix for small red sores. Trichomoniasis does not cause visible sores on the penis, but it can cause pain in the urethra or a discharge from the penis. Trichomoniasis is easily cured with prescription drugs. Because men often have no symptoms, their infection may go undiagnosed and untreated, making it easy to reinfect their partners. Therefore, both partners must be treated to control reinfection.

Genital Herpes

Two kinds of herpes simplex virus (HSV) cause infections. *HSV type 1* (HSV-1) causes cold sores on the mouth and lips. It also causes genital infections. HSV-1 can be transmitted by kissing or through sexual activity. *HSV type 2* (HSV-2) causes genital infections only and is transmitted only through sexual contact.

Genital herpes is primarily a herpes simplex virus infection of the genitals, mouth, or rectum. Genital herpes is very common in the United States among both men and women between 14 and 49 years of age. In fact, about one out of every six people has genital herpes.

genital herpes
an STI that infects the genitals, mouth, or rectum, and causes outbreaks of sores sometimes accompanied by fever

Signs and Symptoms

Usually a person infected with genital herpes has mild or no symptoms. Blisters arise at the site of infection, burst, and heal after a few weeks. Typically, these blisters repeatedly return, but in a milder form, perhaps with swollen lymph nodes and fever. This recurrence of genital herpes is called an *outbreak*.

Diagnosis and Treatment

Genital herpes can sometimes be diagnosed by a physical examination of the herpes sores along with lab tests on samples swabbed from the sores. If no sores are visible or if an individual is between outbreaks, a blood test can detect antibodies that indicate the presence of the herpes viruses.

No cure exists for herpes, but medication can control the frequency and severity of outbreaks. Newborns with herpes are seriously ill and may die. Treatment of pregnant women with herpes has improved and it is now uncommon to transmit the infection to developing babies. It remains possible, however, to transmit herpes to babies during vaginal delivery.

Human Papillomavirus

The *human papillomavirus (HPV)* is the most commonly contracted STI. HPV infects cells in skin and membranes, causing them to grow abnormally. At least 40 kinds of HPV are known to cause genital infections, and some types can cause cancer.

Signs and Symptoms

Almost all sexually active people carry HPV at one time or another. Luckily, most HPV infections do not cause health problems because the body fights and eliminates the viruses. Still, some types of HPV cause genital warts and some types can cause cervical and oropharyngeal cancer. *Genital warts* are abnormal growths on the skin and membranes around the genitals and anus. The growths range from small raised bumps to large, cauliflower shapes. *Cervical cancer* is an abnormal cancerous growth of the cervix. *Oropharyngeal cancer* affects the back of the throat, base of the tongue, and tonsils (Figure 13.9).

human papillomavirus (HPV)
the most common STI, which infects and causes cells to grow abnormally; can result in genital warts, cervical cancer, and oropharyngeal cancer

genital warts
abnormal growths on the skin and membranes around the genitals and anus

cervical cancer
a type of cancer in which the cells of the cervix grow abnormally

oropharyngeal cancer
a type of cancer in which the cells of the back of the throat, base of the tongue, and tonsils grow abnormally

Figure 13.9 Signs and Symptoms of STIs

STI	Signs and symptoms in females	Signs and symptoms in males
chlamydia	often asymptomatic; itching and burning in vagina during urination; watery vaginal discharge	often asymptomatic; itching and burning during urination; watery discharge from penis
gonorrhea	often asymptomatic; itching and burning in vagina during urination; vaginal discharge; pelvic pain	often asymptomatic; itching and burning during urination; yellow or white discharge from penis
syphilis	*Primary syphilis*: single painless sore in vagina, in mouth, on lips, or in rectum *Secondary syphilis*: painless copper or red rash on palms, soles, or trunk; swollen lymph nodes; fatigue; fever *Late stage syphilis*: internal organ damage including the brain, heart, and vessels	*Primary syphilis*: single painless sore on penis, in mouth, on lips, or in rectum *Secondary syphilis*: painless copper or red rash on palms, soles, or trunk; swollen lymph nodes; fatigue; fever *Late stage syphilis*: internal organ damage including the brain, heart, and vessels
trichomoniasis	often asymptomatic; foul vaginal discharge; itching and burning during urination	often asymptomatic; itching and burning during urination
genital herpes	sometimes asymptomatic; blisters form and burst in and around the vagina, mouth, and anus; recurring outbreaks of blisters	sometimes asymptomatic; blisters form and burst on the penis, in the mouth, and on the anus; recurring outbreaks of blisters
HPV	abnormal growths ranging from small raised bumps to cauliflower-sized growths around the vagina and rectum	abnormal growths ranging from small raised bumps to cauliflower-sized growths around the penis and rectum
HIV/AIDS	*Early*: fatigue, swollen lymph nodes, fever, weight loss *Late*: recurring opportunistic infections such as *Pneumocystis* pneumonia, tuberculosis, oral thrush, diarrhea, severe weight loss	

Diagnosis and Treatment

The genital warts associated with HPV infection can be diagnosed by a doctor's examination and a lab test. If a person develops visible genital warts, the doctor may prescribe skin treatments, prescription medication, or surgical removal. Oropharyngeal cancer is often detected through tests that examine the mouth and throat. Treatments vary depending on the severity and location of the cancer.

The *Pap test*, or *Pap smear* is normally used to screen for cervical cancer, which is also caused by HPV. In this test a swab of the cervix is examined under the microscope to look for abnormal cells. A doctor can perform an HPV test on the cells obtained in the Pap smear to determine the presence and type of HPV in the cervix. Routine Pap tests can detect cervical cancer early, which permits early treatment.

The risk for HPV infection can be reduced by a vaccine. The vaccine is recommended for girls and boys from 11 to 12 years of age. The vaccine is given in three shots over a six-month time period. If people do not get all of the vaccine at this age, they can still receive the vaccination between 13 and 26 years of age. Figure 13.10 summarizes information about the diagnosis and treatment of the most common STIs.

Figure 13.10 Diagnosis and Treatment of STIs

STI	Diagnosis	Treatment
chlamydia	blood test, swab infected site	antibiotics
gonorrhea	swab cervix or other infected area, microscopic exam of discharge from penis	two types of antibiotics
syphilis	microscopic exam of samples swabbed from sore on infected area, blood test	antibiotics
trichomoniasis	visual exam of infected area, blood test	metronidazole
genital herpes	swab sores on infected area, blood test	antiviral medication
genital warts/ HPV	Pap smear and HPV test	antiviral medication, surgical or medical removal of warts or tumor
HIV/AIDS	blood tests	anti-retroviral therapy (ART)

Lesson 13.2 Review

Know and Understand

1. List four common STIs.
2. Which STI is also known as a *silent disease*?
3. What is *pelvic inflammatory disease*?
4. Which STI is often treated with two kinds of antibiotics?
5. What occurs during a genital herpes outbreak?
6. Which STI can cause genital warts, cervical cancer, and oropharyngeal cancer?

Analyze and Apply

7. Explain what occurs during each stage of syphilis.

8. Compare and contrast the two kinds of herpes simplex virus (HSV).
9. Assume you are a research scientist. Explain which STI you have chosen to study and why.

Real World Health

On a sheet of paper, list 10 reasons why you might choose abstinence. On the back of that sheet, list 10 strategies you could use to remain abstinent while dating. Make the list of strategies specific to your likes, interests, and the support systems available to you. Put this list somewhere in your room where you can see it.

HIV/AIDS

Lesson Objectives

After studying this lesson, you will be able to

- differentiate between HIV and AIDS;
- explain how HIV is transmitted;
- list signs and symptoms of HIV/AIDS;
- explain how HIV/AIDS is diagnosed; and
- describe treatment methods for HIV/AIDS.

Warm-Up Activity

Staying HIV-Free

Many factors can distract you from your goals and ideals. This is why an important part of setting goals is identifying what situations or factors you might have to avoid to reach those goals. What behaviors, situations, or pressures might derail a person from remaining HIV-free? What strategies could a person use to avoid dangers? Organize your answers to these questions in a table like the one shown below.

Behaviors, situations, or pressures to avoid	Strategies to help avoid them

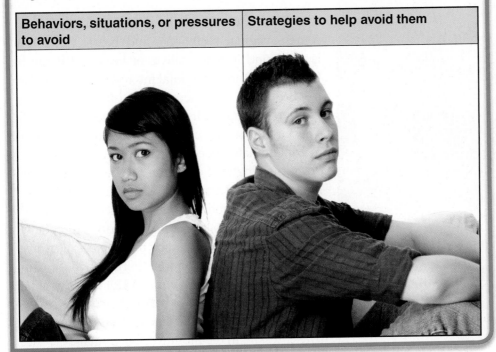

Key Terms E-Flash Cards

In this lesson, you will learn the meanings of the following key terms.

acquired immuno-deficiency syndrome (AIDS)

anti-retroviral therapy (ART)

HIV-positive

human immunodeficiency virus (HIV)

long-term non-progressors

Before You Read

Give One, Get One

Fold a piece of paper in half to make two columns. At the top of one column, write "Give One," and at the top of the other column write "Get One." Prior to reading the lesson, list five facts you know about HIV/AIDS under "Give One." Then walk around the room and exchange facts with your classmates. Write facts that you get from your classmates in the "Get One" column.

Give One	Get One

A lthough an intact immune system easily eliminates many infections, people with an immune system ravaged by HIV/AIDS cannot battle even minor infections caused by ordinary microorganisms. In spite of recently discovered medications that significantly extend and improve the quality of life for someone with HIV/AIDS, this disease remains incurable. The painful reality of AIDS is an eventual death from uncontrollable infections or numerous complications.

HIV/AIDS continues to be the leading infectious cause of death worldwide, killing about 2 million people per year. Studies show that HIV/AIDS does not discriminate and knows no national boundaries. HIV/AIDS affects men, women, and children of all ages and races, and people of all countries.

HIV and AIDS Defined

It is important to distinguish between HIV and AIDS. *Human immunodeficiency virus (HIV)* infects and kills cells, weakening the body's immune system (Figure 13.11). When the body can no longer fight infections and diseases, then HIV can lead to *acquired immunodeficiency syndrome (AIDS)*. AIDS can develop later, perhaps many years after HIV infection. In other words, HIV refers to the virus and AIDS refers to the disease. Therefore, people transmit HIV, not AIDS. The title of this chapter uses the term *HIV/AIDS* to recognize this relationship between HIV and AIDS.

A person is said to be *HIV-positive* if a laboratory test detects the presence of HIV antibodies in the person's blood. This means that the person is infected with HIV, but it does not necessarily mean that the person has AIDS.

Figure 13.11

Micrograph of HIV (green spheres). HIV weakens the body's immune system by killing and infecting cells.

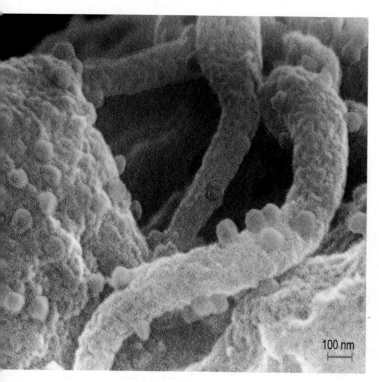

100 nm

HIV Transmission

HIV is found in bodily fluids, including blood, semen, vaginal secretions, and breast milk. HIV is *not* found in tears, saliva, or sweat. HIV can be transmitted through sexual intercourse. Babies born to HIV-positive mothers can become infected, and mothers can transmit the virus in their breast milk. The virus can also be transmitted in blood found in contaminated needles used for drugs, tattoos, or body piercings. At one time HIV was often transmitted in blood transfusions. In the United States, however, the blood supply is now screened for HIV, so transfusions no longer pose a serious threat.

HIV is *not* transmitted by mosquitoes or by kissing, spitting, shaking hands, sharing food, or using the same toilet seats (Figure 13.12). Healthy, intact skin provides an effective barrier to HIV infection. It is possible for HIV to be transmitted through open sores on skin, in the mouth, or on genitals.

Certain factors increase the risk for HIV transmission. As you know, just one sex act with one infected partner can transmit an STI. Therefore, it makes sense that sex with multiple partners increases the chance of getting an STI like HIV. People who abuse injected drugs are more likely than others to share hypodermic needles and potentially become exposed to HIV-positive blood. Having other STIs also increases the risk for becoming infected with HIV.

Remember that intact, healthy skin and membranes provide some barrier to HIV. Syphilis sores break that barrier, as does inflammation associated with herpes, chlamydia, gonorrhea, trichomoniasis, and genital warts. For example, if exposed to HIV, a person with syphilis has up to five times more risk of getting HIV than a person without syphilis. The reverse is also true: an HIV-positive person who has other STIs more easily transmits those STIs to sexual partners.

Figure 13.12 Fact and Fiction about HIV/AIDS Transmission

HIV/AIDS can be transmitted...	FACT or FICTION?
sharing injection drug needles	FACT
kissing	FICTION
shaking hands	FICTION
sweating	FICTION
sharing a water bottle	FICTION
having sexual intercourse	FACT
getting a tattoo with a used or unsterilized needle	FACT
from mother to child during birth	FACT
during breast-feeding	FACT
hugging	FICTION
using the same toilet seats	FICTION
sharing food	FICTION
coughing and sneezing	FICTION

Signs and Symptoms of HIV/AIDS

Following HIV infection, the infected person may develop minor symptoms that are not recognized. In some people, these symptoms do not arise for months. Early symptoms resemble a flu-like illness with fatigue and swollen, painful lymph nodes. HIV infection may not develop into AIDS for two years or more. AIDS develops when the immune system becomes disabled. This decline in immunity can be measured with blood tests that show a greatly reduced number of a key white blood cell called the *T-helper cell* or *CD4 cell*, which HIV specifically destroys (Figure 13.13 on the next page).

When the virus sufficiently disables the immune system, unusual or normally harmless microorganisms continuously assault the body, causing *opportunistic infections*. These infections take advantage of a weakened body and are

Figure 13.13 Sequence of Events from HIV Infection to Immune System Breakdown Due to AIDS

Phase 1	Phase 2	Phase 3
First six months	**Six months to 8-10 years**	**Ten years**
high amount of virus in blood	amount of virus in blood rapidly declines	amount of virus in blood rises steadily
normal level of T-helper cells in blood rapidly declines	T-helper cell level increases and then declines slowly and steadily	T-helper cell level becomes too low to mount immune responses to infections
No symptoms in some people, but others have a fever and swollen lymph nodes.	Some people have few serious symptoms. Many people develop yeast infections in the mouth, throat, and vagina. Viral infections develop.	Yeast infections affect the throat and lungs. Fungal infections cause pneumonia. Tuberculosis occurs. Viruses cause eye infections. Brain infections, meningitis, and blood vessel tumors (Kaposi's sarcoma) develop.

the cause of death in HIV/AIDS cases. One of these infections, a fungus called *Pneumocystis*, causes a form of pneumonia that healthy immune systems easily combat. A yeast infection of the mouth (called *thrush*) also takes advantage of the crippled immune system. *Tuberculosis*, a bacterial lung infection, is often associated with AIDS. Worldwide, about 1 in 4 people with AIDS die from tuberculosis. With collapse of the immune system, infections of the intestines, skin, and nervous system plague the body. In addition, people with AIDS are vulnerable to a blood vessel tumor called *Kaposi's sarcoma*. Other signs and symptoms of AIDS include severe weight loss, diarrhea, fever and chills, and nausea.

Medical research has found that HIV/AIDS develops differently and at different rates for all affected people. In some people, HIV infection quickly leads to AIDS, while others do not progress to AIDS for decades. HIV-positive people who progress to AIDS more slowly are **long-term non-progressors**. Long-term non-progressors are of interest to medical researchers because their physiology may help explain how the body successfully fights HIV. After developing AIDS, some people live a few years while others live a long life. Because of powerful drugs and medical intervention, today people can live 20–25 years after diagnosis.

long-term non-progressors
HIV-positive people whose infection progresses to AIDS slowly

Diagnosis

HIV/AIDS testing is critical for personal and community health. The HIV test examines a blood sample for the presence of antibodies to the virus. Weeks or months may pass before a person develops antibodies following exposure to HIV. Therefore, if a person gets a negative blood test, and they think they were exposed within the past three months, HIV testing should be repeated after three more months have passed.

Test results are available in a few days, or the rapid version of the test gives results in 20 minutes. Tests can be performed in a number of places besides doctors' offices and hospital labs. HIV test sites can be found online or by contacting the Centers for Disease Control and Prevention (CDC).

Local and Global Health
HIV/AIDS in Africa

In many ways the HIV/AIDS picture in developing nations contrasts starkly with the situation in North America and other developed nations. In South Africa, for example, 1 in 5 adults is living with HIV/AIDS, while in North America, 1 in 200 adults is living with HIV/AIDS. Incredibly, more than 68% of the world's 33.3 million people with HIV/AIDS live in African countries south of the Sahara desert. That means 22.5 million people with HIV/AIDS are concentrated in this sub-Saharan region, with devastating consequences.

So many adults in the region have died from AIDS that sub-Saharan African countries now have more than 15 million orphans. Developing African nations do not have the economic resources to care for these orphans or to control the AIDS epidemic. In fact, the entire world economy is unable to provide enough money to cope with the HIV/AIDS epidemic.

Recent annual HIV/AIDS spending reached $16 billion, but this falls $10 billion short of estimated yearly needs. Sadly, this means that only 37% of people in sub-Saharan Africa get the anti-retroviral therapy (ART) treatment they need, leaving 11 million people untreated.

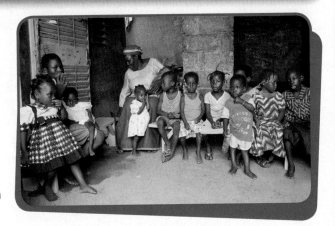

Thinking Critically

1. Why is the AIDS epidemic so severe in this region of Africa? The complex answer involves many aspects of life in sub-Saharan Africa. Discuss how each of the following might contribute to this AIDS epidemic:
   - availability and cost of ART
   - availability and cost of HIV tests
   - cultural practices
   - availability of accurate information about HIV/AIDS
   - availability and cost of latex condoms
   - nutrition and general level of health

Testing and results can be kept confidential if requested. A home version of the HIV test is available without a prescription at drug stores. The test is inexpensive, rapid, painless, and private. If the test is positive, the person should see a healthcare provider for a confirming test.

HIV testing permits diagnosis and treatment to begin, and is the key to controlling HIV/AIDS transmission within society. Sexually active people should be tested every year and every time they switch sexual partners. Sadly, the CDC estimates that 1 in 5 people with HIV do not know they are infected. If each affected individual knew he or she was HIV-positive, steps could be taken to prevent further transmission of the virus. Increased testing could significantly reduce HIV transmission.

HIV Test Results are Confidential and Private

The *Health Insurance Portability and Accountability Act (HIPAA)* is a federal law that requires confidentiality for HIV test results, just as it does

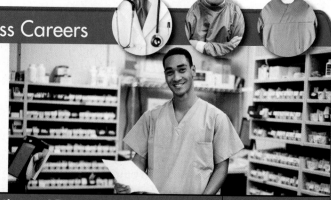

Sexual Health Careers

Many healthcare professionals encounter STIs in some way during their careers. Following are some of the careers in which workers are likely to deal with STIs.

Career	Typical Education and Training	Typical Job Duties and Demands	Career Resources
Medical Laboratory Technologist	Bachelor's degree and certification or licensure	Collection of samples and performing of tests to analyze patients' blood and tissue specimens. Should be able to be on feet for long periods and work in a fast-paced environment.	American Society for Clinical Laboratory Science
Health Information Technician	Associate's degree and/or certification	Organization, maintenance, and recording of patient health data. Reporting cases of STIs per guidelines. Should be able to work independently and respect confidentiality.	American Health Information Management Association
Community Health Workers	Associate's degree and/or certification	Conducting community outreach programs to educate people about health concerns, such as STI testing and prevention. Should be able to advocate for and communicate well with others.	American Public Health Association
Microbiologist	Bachelor's degree and/or master's degree or Ph.D.	Studying microorganisms, such as those that cause STIs, including their structure, function, genetics, growth, and reproduction. Should be able to follow strict safety procedures and meet deadlines.	American Society for Microbiology

Exploring Careers

1. Think about your interests, strengths, and weaknesses. With these in mind, which career described above appeals most to you? Which career does not interest you?

2. Do you know a person who works in one of these careers? If so, ask why the person chose this career and what he or she likes most and least about the work.

for other medical records. If a test is positive, healthcare providers must report the results to the state because the states track and study the number of cases. The results, however, are reported with no identifying personal information to protect the identity of the individual. Should anyone else know the HIV test results? Certainly, an HIV-positive person ought to notify sexual partners. In fact, some cities and states have partner-notification laws requiring HIV-positive individuals or their doctors to notify sexual partners (or needle-sharing partners).

Protecting HIV-Positive Individuals from Discrimination

Two important laws protect the rights of HIV-positive people. The *Americans with Disabilities Act (ADA) of 1990* and the *Rehabilitation Act of 1973* prohibit discrimination against people with HIV/AIDS. That is to say, people with HIV/AIDS cannot be denied jobs, benefits, education, services, or other rights because of their HIV/AIDS status. These laws also protect the families of people living with HIV/AIDS.

Treatment

The cornerstone of HIV/AIDS treatment is **anti-retroviral therapy (ART)**, so named because HIV is a type of virus known as a *retrovirus*. The specific aim of ART is to reduce the number of viruses in the body so that the immune system remains strong. ART also greatly reduces the likelihood that HIV will be transmitted. ART does not, however, cure HIV/AIDS (Figure 13.14).

ART consists of a mixture of three drugs, sometimes called *a cocktail of drugs*, each of which interferes with the reproduction of HIV inside the body. Inside the body, HIV can change its genes and develop resistance to a drug. This means that the drug becomes ineffective against the virus.

The ART cocktail is designed to prevent HIV from developing resistance to drugs. It may be unnecessary to begin ART immediately after exposure to HIV. Each circumstance differs and depends on how long a person has been HIV-positive and on their general health and immunity.

A similar ART cocktail called *Truvada* may prevent HIV infection. This treatment is called *pre-exposure prophylaxis* (*PrEP*). The pre-exposure treatment is intended for HIV/AIDS researchers who study the virus in a laboratory and for doctors and nurses who regularly work closely with HIV-positive patients.

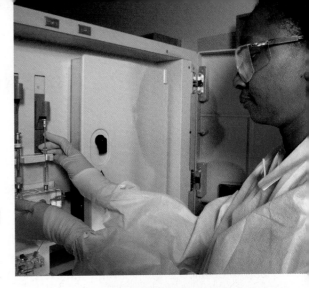

Figure 13.14

A researcher at the Centers for Disease Control tests samples of blood from HIV-positive people for drug resistance. Research such as this led to the creation of the ART cocktail.

anti-retroviral therapy (ART)
a treatment for HIV/AIDS in which a cocktail of three drugs is given to interfere with HIV reproduction

Lesson 13.3 Review

Know and Understand 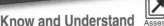 Assess

1. What does it mean when a person is said to be *HIV-positive*?

2. List three factors that can increase the risk for HIV transmission.

3. When does AIDS develop?

4. What are *opportunistic infections*? Give an example.

5. What is meant by the term *long-term non-progressors*?

6. How often should sexually active people be tested for HIV?

Analyze and Apply

7. Explain how HIV is transmitted.

8. Explain how HIV is treated.

Real World Health

Imagine that you have just tested positive for HIV. You also just recently became involved in a new dating relationship with someone you really like. At what point do you share this personal information with your new dating partner? Working with another class member, take turns role-playing the conversation you will have with your new dating partner.

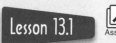

Sexually Transmitted Infections: What You Should Know

Key Terms

abstinence
asymptomatic
latex condom

sexually transmitted
infections (STIs)

Key Points

- Engaging in sexual activity only once with an infected sexual partner is all it takes to contract an STI.
- People with STIs are often asymptomatic.
- Any exposure to an STI can lead to another infection.
- Some STIs are curable while other infections remain incurable.
- Prevention is the most effective way to deal with STIs.

Check Your Understanding

1. *True or false?* People with more sexual partners have greater chances of contracting an STI.

2. *True or false?* STIs can be transmitted through casual contact with an infected person.

3. When _____ occurs, a body part may become red, warm, swollen, or painful.

4. What does infertility mean?

5. _____ STIs are treatable, even curable, with antibiotics prescribed by a physician.
   A. Viral
   B. Bacterial
   C. Antiviral
   D. Retroviral

6. Which of the following is 100% effective in preventing STIs?
   A. abstinence
   B. non-latex condoms
   C. latex condoms
   D. the birth control pill

7. **Critical Thinking.** How can a person develop skills for refusing sex, drugs, and alcohol? Give an example.

Common STIs

Key Terms

cervical cancer
chlamydia
genital herpes
genital warts
gonorrhea
human papillomavirus (HPV)

oropharyngeal cancer
pelvic inflammatory
   disease
syphilis
trichomoniasis

Key Points

- Six of the most common STIs are chlamydia, gonorrhea, syphilis, trichomoniasis, genital herpes, and human papillomavirus (HPV).
- Signs and symptoms vary for STIs and some people with an STI may be asymptomatic.
- Many STIs can be diagnosed by taking a lab sample or blood test.
- Bacterial STIs are curable by taking antibiotics while viral STIs are incurable, but symptoms are controllable by taking antiviral medications.

Check Your Understanding

8. Which of the following is an example of a bacterial STI that can be cured?
   A. genital herpes
   B. gonorrhea
   C. HPV
   D. trichomoniasis

9. _____ infections are the most commonly reported STI in the United States.

10. At the site of a syphilis infection, a sore, called a(n) _____, develops.

11. _____ is caused by a single-celled microorganism called a *protozoan*.
   A. Chlamydia
   B. Gonorrhea
   C. Syphilis
   D. Trichomoniasis

12. _____ is often called the *great imitator*.
   A. Chlamydia
   B. HPV
   C. Syphilis
   D. Genital herpes

13. _____ is primarily a herpes simplex virus infection of the genitals, mouth, or rectum.
    A. Chlamydia
    B. Genital herpes
    C. Gonorrhea
    D. Syphilis

14. _____ causes cold sores on the mouth and lips, and also causes genital infections.
    A. HSV type 1
    B. HSV type 2
    C. Secondary syphilis
    D. Late-stage syphilis

15. At least 40 kinds of _____ are known to cause genital infections.

16. **Critical Thinking.** Compare and contrast two STIs discussed in this lesson. Include information on signs, symptoms, diagnosis, and treatment.

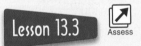

Lesson 13.3   Assess

HIV/AIDS

Key Terms

acquired
    immunodeficiency
    syndrome (AIDS)
anti-retroviral therapy (ART)
HIV-positive

human
    immunodeficiency
    virus (HIV)
long-term
    non-progressors

Key Points

- People with HIV/AIDS cannot battle even minor infections caused by ordinary microorganisms.
- HIV is found in bodily fluids, including blood, semen, vaginal secretions, and breast milk.
- Opportunistic infections take advantage of a weakened body and are the cause of death in HIV/AIDS.
- HIV develops differently and at different rates for all affected people.
- HIV/AIDS testing is critical for personal and community health.
- ART is the cornerstone of HIV/AIDS treatment.

Check Your Understanding

17. A person is said to be _____ if a laboratory test detects the presence of HIV antibodies in the person's blood.

18. HIV is found in bodily fluids, such as _____.
    A. saliva
    B. tears
    C. sweat
    D. blood

19. Babies born to HIV-positive mothers can become infected and mothers can transmit the virus in their _____.

20. *True or false?* Having any one of the many common STIs decreases a person's risk for becoming infected with HIV.

21. *True or false?* Opportunistic infections are the cause of death in HIV/AIDS cases.

22. HIV-positive people who progress to AIDS more slowly are called _____.

23. *True or false?* Any adult who is interested can take a home version of the HIV test only by obtaining a doctor's prescription.

24. The _____ is a federal law that requires confidentiality for HIV test results, just as it does for other medical records.
    A. *Americans with Disabilities Act (ADA) of 1990*
    B. *Health Insurance Portability and Accountability Act (HIPAA)*
    C. *HIV/AIDS Act*
    D. *Rehabilitation Act of 1973*

25. The cornerstone of HIV/AIDS treatment is _____ therapy.

26. ART consists of a mixture of _____ drugs, each of which interferes with the reproduction of HIV inside the body.
    A. two
    B. three
    C. four
    D. five

27. **Critical Thinking.** Explain the difference between HIV and AIDS.

Chapter 13 Skill Development

Health and Wellness Skills

28. **Make Decisions.** Think about how you want to live when you are 25 years of age. Where do you want to live? What type of housing do you want? Whom do you want to live with? What kind of transportation will you have? What job or career will you have, and what will you have done to get there? Now, consider how engaging in unprotected sex might affect your imagined life.

29. **Set Goals.** Construct a plan to help a young person avoid contracting HIV. The plan should have a clearly stated goal, at least four steps toward meeting the goal, and ways of evaluating progress. The plan should consider ways people can and cannot contract HIV, and what activities might put someone at risk for infection.

30. **Advocate for Health.** Design a one-page advertisement that will outline the dangers of unprotected sex and offer abstinence as a healthy alternative for high school students. Use slogans and pictures in your advertisement, and make your advertisement suitable for publication in a teen magazine.

31. **Comprehend Concepts.** In small groups, write a rap that is at least twelve lines long. The rap should include facts about the damage STIs can do to your body and life. It should include one line about how a person can say no to someone pressuring him or her to have sex.

32. **Analyze Influences.** Write a story about a teen who did not have a plan for remaining abstinent and ended up having unprotected sex. What might have happened to this teenager? What behaviors, situations, or pressures led the teenager to have unprotected sex? List all of the possible physical, social, and emotional consequences he or she may experience as a result of this decision.

Hands-On Activity

The AIDS Quilt

The AIDS quilt was started in San Francisco, California, during June of 1987. The purpose of the quilt is to commemorate the lives of people who died of AIDS. Each panel of the quilt is three feet wide and six feet tall, the size of a coffin. Each panel is decorated with the date of birth, date of death, photos, and various objects that best represent the person who has died of AIDS. In this activity, you and your classmates will each create a poster quilt of your own lives.

Materials Needed

- one sheet of poster board per student
- photos and objects that represent who you are and who you want to be
- staplers or tape

Steps for this Activity

1. Create a poster that represents who you are and celebrates your life. Include your date of birth and any photos or objects that highlight the most important relationships, activities, or experiences of your life.

2. Once everyone in your class is finished, tape or staple your posters together to make one "poster quilt."

3. Display the poster quilt and look at some of your classmates' posters.

4. As a class, reflect on the following questions:
    - What new facts did you learn about your classmates? Try to list one fact for each person.
    - Approximately 50 people die each day from complications due to AIDS. What kind of impact do you think this has on our society?
    - If your life, as it is represented on your poster, ended right now, what goals and aspirations of yours would remain unfulfilled?

5. Find the AIDS quilt website and view at least three panels. Write a paragraph about your thoughts and feelings regarding these panels. Does anything about these panels surprise you? Why or why not? How do these panels influence your perception of HIV and AIDS?

Core Skills

Math Practice

The following bar graphs show the number of cases of gonorrhea and chlamydia reported in one year, arranged according to age. Study the graphs and then answer the questions.

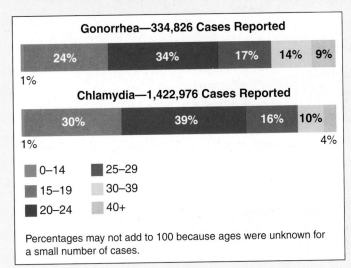

Gonorrhea—334,826 Cases Reported

| 24% | 34% | 17% | 14% | 9% |

1%

Chlamydia—1,422,976 Cases Reported

| 30% | 39% | 16% | 10% |

1%   4%

- 0–14
- 15–19
- 20–24
- 25–29
- 30–39
- 40+

Percentages may not add to 100 because ages were unknown for a small number of cases.

33. What is the ratio of total cases of gonorrhea to chlamydia?
    A. 1 to 4.25
    B. 1 to 3
    C. 2 to 5.25
    D. 2 to 4

34. How many more cases of chlamydia were reported for people between 20 and 24 years of age than for people between 15 and 19 years of age?
    A. 58,833
    B. 128,068
    C. 268,015
    D. 398,831

35. How many fewer cases of gonorrhea were reported for people between 15 and 19 years of age than for people between 20 and 24 years of age?
    A. 33,483
    B. 46,358
    C. 59,841
    D. 94,199

Reading and Writing Practice

Read the passage below and then answer the questions.

While some STIs cause little or no discomfort, these diseases can still damage the reproductive organs and cause infertility, *the inability to conceive and have children. In fact, people can develop infertility or other permanent health problems even if they have been cured of an STI.*

If left untreated, STIs can damage not only the reproductive organs, but also the brain, heart, liver, and other internal organs. Worse, a few STIs are incurable, some cause cancer, and some are fatal.

Sadly, it is possible for a pregnant woman with an STI to transmit the infection to her baby during pregnancy, birth, or breast-feeding. Some of the problems caused by STI transmission may be seen in the baby at birth. Some effects, however, may not be visible for months or years after birth.

36. In this passage, the term *transmission* means _____.
    A. process of sending electrical signals to something
    B. part of a vehicle
    C. process of spreading something from one person to another
    D. process of giving birth

37. In pregnant women, STIs are _____.
    A. transmittable during pregnancy, birth, or breast-feeding
    B. transmittable to the baby during pregnancy only
    C. not transmittable to the baby during birth
    D. always fatal for mother and baby

38. Analyze how the author introduces and develops key points and ideas in this passage. Write an essay describing your analysis and citing specific examples. Discuss your essay in class.

39. Working with a partner, write a public service announcement about the harmful effects of STIs on the human body. Include ways in which people can effectively protect themselves from contracting an STI.

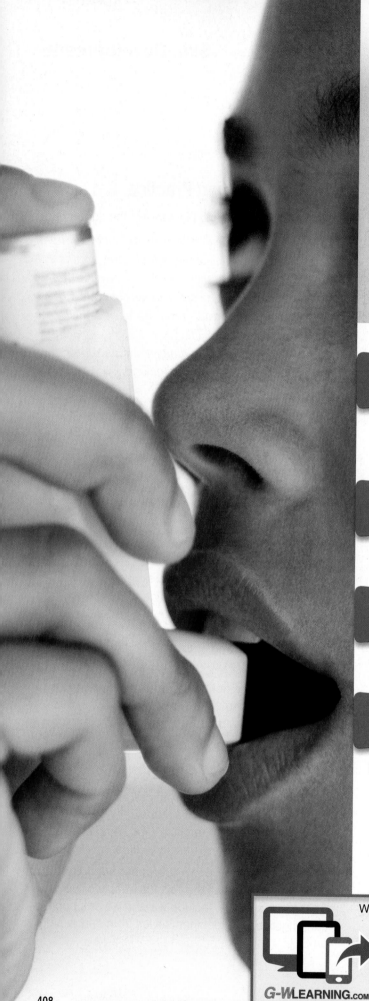

Chapter 14

Noncommunicable Diseases

Lesson 14.1

Noncommunicable Diseases: What You Should Know

Lesson 14.2

Diseases of the Blood Vessels and Heart

Lesson 14.3

Cancer: Cells out of Control

Lesson 14.4

Diabetes, Allergies, Asthma, and Arthritis

While studying this chapter, look for the activity icon to:
- **review** vocabulary with e-flash cards and games;
- **assess** learning with quizzes and online exercises;
- **expand** knowledge with animations and activities; and
- **listen** to pronunciation of key terms in the audio glossary.

G-WLEARNING.com

www.g-wlearning.com/health/

408

What's Your Health and Wellness IQ?

Take this quiz to see what you do and do not know about noncommunicable diseases. If you cannot answer a question, pay extra attention to that topic as you study this chapter.

1. *Identify each statement as* True, False, *or* It Depends. *Choose* It Depends *if a statement is true in some cases, but false in others.*

2. *Revise each* False *statement to make it true.*

3. *Explain the circumstances in which each* It Depends *statement is true and when it is false.*

Health and Wellness IQ Assess

1. Heart disease is inherited.	True	False	It Depends
2. A high-fat diet increases the risk for heart disease.	True	False	It Depends
3. Like other muscles, the heart muscle can function without oxygen for a period of time.	True	False	It Depends
4. Using tanning beds increases your risk for skin cancer.	True	False	It Depends
5. Smoking is the leading cause of lung cancer.	True	False	It Depends
6. All chemicals and radiation can cause cancer.	True	False	It Depends
7. Diabetes is caused by eating too much sugar.	True	False	It Depends
8. Children cannot get diabetes.	True	False	It Depends
9. Asthma is an acute disease of the nervous system.	True	False	It Depends
10. There is no cure for gout.	True	False	It Depends

Setting the Scene

Heart disease and cancer rarely affect young people, so you probably view these diseases as vague, distant threats to your health. Should you be concerned about heart disease and cancer, diseases that afflict mainly older adults? Should you worry about diabetes?

Before you answer, consider the rate of heart disease and cancer in the United States. Of the approximately 2.6 million deaths in the United States each year, nearly half are caused by heart disease and cancer. Does this mean that you have a 50% chance of dying from one of these diseases? Fortunately, the answer is no. The risk for developing heart disease or cancer is not written in stone—behaviors, habits, diet, and regular preventive health-care significantly affect your chances of developing these diseases. In this chapter you will learn about steps you can take to avoid certain diseases and improve the quality of your life.

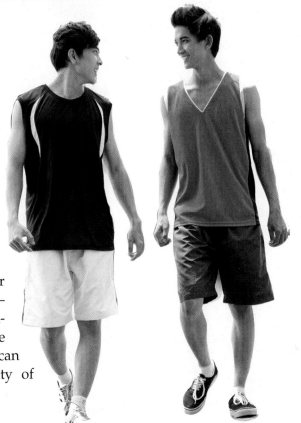

Noncommunicable Diseases: What You Should Know

Key Terms 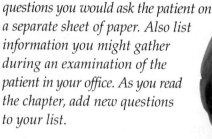 E-Flash Cards

In this lesson, you will learn the meanings of the following key terms.

complication

homeostasis

mutations

noncommunicable
   diseases

prognosis

relapse

remission

Before You Read

Brainstorming Risk Factors

On a separate sheet of paper, create a visual chart like the one shown below. Brainstorm risk factors that fall into the three categories and list them in your chart. After reading the lesson, add any knowledge you gained.

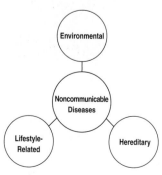

Lesson Objectives

After studying this lesson, you will be able to

- differentiate between infectious and noncommunicable diseases;

- explain homeostasis and how disease disrupts the body's internal balance;

- assess environmental factors, heredity, and lifestyle choices as risk factors for developing noncommunicable diseases; and

- analyze characteristics of and diagnosis methods for noncommunicable diseases.

Warm-Up Activity

Diagnosis Puzzle

Before a doctor can treat a patient's ailment, the doctor needs to diagnose the ailment, or determine what disease or disorder the patient has. The process of diagnosis is like piecing together a jigsaw puzzle from bits of information. Suppose you were a doctor and a patient came to you with the following symptoms: shortness of breath, pain in the chest and abdomen, and extreme fatigue. What information would you want from the patient to make a diagnosis? List questions you would ask the patient on a separate sheet of paper. Also list information you might gather during an examination of the patient in your office. As you read the chapter, add new questions to your list.

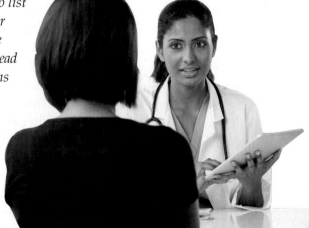

U nlike infectious diseases, ***noncommunicable diseases*** cannot be spread through person-to-person contact. Instead, noncommunicable diseases, also called *noninfectious diseases*, can be attributed to genes, diet, behavior, smoking, and other factors. These diseases include heart disease, stroke, cancer, high blood pressure, and lung diseases like asthma. Your choices impact your chances of getting these diseases (Figure 14.1).

Homeostasis

Homeostasis refers to the body's internal, steady state of balance. The body maintains homeostasis by regulating processes such as body temperature, the amount of sugar in the blood, blood pressure, and the oxygen level in tissues. When the body maintains homeostasis, the body is healthy. If the body departs from homeostasis, it will enter a state of disease (Figure 14.2).

Think of the thermostat that regulates the temperature in your home. When the temperature drops below the set level, the thermostat signals the furnace to turn on and heat the house. When enough heat has been generated to bring the temperature back up to the set level, the thermostat signals the furnace to shut off. If the thermostat and the furnace are working properly, your home is in a state of homeostasis. But if the furnace didn't turn on during a cold winter, the house would become very cold, possibly causing the water pipes to freeze and burst. In this situation your house would have departed from its homeostasis and become, in a way, very sick.

Risk Factors for Noncommunicable Diseases

Microorganisms cause infectious diseases, but the causes of noncommunicable diseases are more complicated. A combination of lifestyle choices, environmental factors, and genetics impact a person's overall risk for developing certain types of noncommunicable diseases.

Lifestyle and Environment

Lifestyle choices and the environment are key areas that indicate a person's risk factor for certain diseases. Unhealthy lifestyle choices include drug use, lack of physical activity, and a high-fat diet. Environmental risk factors include hazards in the home or work environment.

The origins of noncommunicable diseases can be traced to habits that typically began in youth (Figure 14.3). Noncommunicable diseases often develop in adulthood, following years of an unhealthy

Figure 14.1

You can reduce your risk of developing a noncommunicable disease by getting regular exercise.

noncommunicable diseases
diseases that are not caused by a pathogen and cannot be transmitted from one person to another; noninfectious diseases

homeostasis
the body's internal balance and stability; typically maintained despite changing conditions

Figure 14.2

When you are sick with a fever, your body attempts to lower your temperature and restore homeostasis by sweating.

Figure 14.3

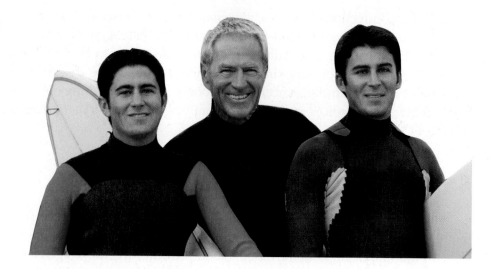

The genes you inherit from your biological parents can increase your risk of developing certain noncommunicable diseases. On the other hand, factors such as leading an active lifestyle can help lower your risk. *What other lifestyle factors can help lower your risk of developing many noncommunicable diseases?*

lifestyle or exposure to environmental risk factors. Unhealthy habits you begin now can cause damage that builds to the point of disease.

Heredity Interacts with Lifestyle

Scientists have identified genes, especially mutated genes, that increase the risk for developing certain diseases. *Mutations* are alterations in a gene's normal structure.

Although a certain disease may run in your family, you can reduce your risk for developing that disease by controlling exposure to other risks.

mutations
alterations of a gene's normal structure; can lead to disease

Characteristics of Noncommunicable Diseases

Understanding characteristics associated with noncommunicable diseases allows doctors to better treat their patients, and patients to better understand the disease affecting them.

Acute and Chronic Disease

Physicians can evaluate whether a disease is acute or chronic. *Acute* diseases occur suddenly and resolve fairly quickly, often without long-lasting effects. Influenza and the common cold are examples.

In contrast, many noncommunicable diseases are *chronic* illnesses—long-term diseases that may not heal for years and can cause permanent disability or health complications. Diabetes and asthma are examples.

Prognosis

A *prognosis* is the probable outcome of a disease. It includes the chances for full recovery, disability, or dying. A prognosis also predicts the duration and severity of a disease. Diseases that will end in death are described as *terminal*.

prognosis
the probable consequence of a disease (death or recovery, for example)

Remission and Relapse

Sometimes a disease enters *remission*, which is a period of time without signs and symptoms associated with that disease. Remission may last for weeks, years, or indefinitely. The term *relapse* refers to the recurrence of a disease, in which signs and symptoms return after a period of remission. Certain cancers can leave remission and recur in an even more severe way than before. *Exacerbation* describes the worsening of signs and symptoms.

Complication

A *complication* is a new problem or second disease that arises in a person already suffering from one disease. For example, a serious complication of diabetes is loss of eyesight.

remission
a period of time in which the signs and symptoms of a disease subside

relapse
the recurrence of a disease, in which signs and symptoms return after a period of remission

complication
a problem or secondary infection that results from or accompanies a disease

Diagnosing Noncommunicable Diseases

A *diagnosis* identifies the type of disease a person has. Once a diagnosis has been determined, a doctor can begin the correct treatment. To diagnose a disease, doctors use information from several sources.

A physical exam of the patient will uncover signs and symptoms. At this point, a doctor can measure weight loss, hear abnormal breathing sounds, or detect a fever.

Family history can indicate whether a certain disease is common in a patient's family. Doctors also learn from a patient's personal history, which includes past diseases, dietary patterns, and other behaviors.

Important information about disease also comes from laboratory tests. A wide variety of diagnostic technology is also used to visualize the structure and function of internal organs. Once a diagnosis becomes clear, treatment can begin.

Lesson 14.1 Review

Know and Understand Assess

1. Define *noncommunicable disease* and provide at least two examples.
2. How does your body maintain homeostasis?
3. Explain the difference between remission and relapse.
4. List four factors doctors assess to diagnose a disease.

Analyze and Apply

5. Are noncommunicable diseases acute or chronic illnesses? Explain.

6. How do heredity and lifestyle impact your risk factors for developing certain diseases?

Real World Health

Interview a healthcare professional who works with patients suffering from noncommunicable diseases. Prepare 10 thought-provoking, open-ended questions to ask. After the interview, give a presentation to the class that includes answers to your questions and a brief summary of what you learned.

Diseases of the Blood Vessels and Heart

Key Terms
E-Flash Cards

In this lesson, you will learn the meanings of the following key terms.

angina

aorta

arrhythmias

arteries

arteriosclerosis

atherosclerosis

blood pressure

blood vessels

capillaries

congestive heart failure

coronary arteries

coronary artery disease

heart attack

hypertension

stent

stroke

valves

veins

Before You Read

Risk of Heart Disease
Create a chart (see below) to show what you know about the lifestyle causes of heart disease.

Lesson Objectives

After studying this lesson, you will be able to

- explain how a healthy network of blood vessels functions in the body;
- describe four diseases related to blood vessels;
- differentiate between major diseases of the heart; and
- consider the risk factors and preventive measures for developing heart disease.

Warm-Up Activity

Blood's Journey Through the Body
Write a brief story entitled "A Day in the Life of Blood." Tell the story from the perspective of the blood moving through someone's circulatory system. Imagine that this person has a disease or disorder involving his or her heart or cardiovascular system. Where does the blood go first? What obstacles does it encounter along its way? What does it see, feel, and hear? Be creative and use at least 10 of the key terms from the chapter in your story.

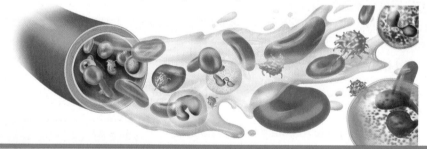

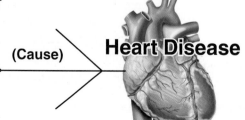

(Cause)   **(Cause)**   **Heart Disease**

T he heart, blood vessels, and blood comprise the body's *circulatory system*, also called the *cardiovascular system*. The heart adapts to the changing needs of your body, speeding up when your body requires more oxygen, and slowing down when your body is at rest. If blood vessels should fail in their task, an organ could be injured or die. Likewise, if the heart should fail in its task, the body may die.

Profile of Healthy Blood Vessels

Blood vessels are narrow tubes that run throughout the body and serve as the body's transportation system for blood, oxygen, and nutrients. There are three different types of blood vessels—arteries, capillaries, and veins. *Arteries* are large, muscular blood vessels that carry blood from the heart to the capillaries. *Capillaries* are tiny, thin blood vessels that deliver oxygen and nutrients to body tissues. Capillaries carry blood to the *veins*, larger blood vessels that return blood to the heart. Blood vessels work best when their inner walls are smooth and somewhat *elastic*, or capable of stretching and rebounding.

Diseases of the Blood Vessels

When the blood vessels are damaged or unhealthy, many diseases can result. Following are brief descriptions of some of the more common diseases.

Arteriosclerosis

Arteriosclerosis is a type of blood vessel disease in which the walls of the arteries thicken, harden, and become inflexible. The arteries cannot stretch as they should when the heart pumps blood into them, leading to high blood pressure and heart disease. Arteriosclerosis is caused by cigarette smoking and by atherosclerosis.

Atherosclerosis

Atherosclerosis describes the fatty deposits in the walls of arteries. These fatty deposits are dangerous if they build up in the arteries of the heart or brain because blood flow to these vital organs will be restricted (Figure 14.4 on the next page).

Fatty deposits can also become unstable, break away from the artery walls, and lodge in smaller arteries, completely blocking blood flow to part of the heart or brain. They stimulate the production of blood clots, which can block small arteries (Figure 14.4 on the next page). Atherosclerosis is caused by cigarette smoking, high blood pressure, and a high-fat diet.

Hypertension

Blood pressure is the force that blood exerts against the walls of arteries as the blood is pumped out of the heart. High blood pressure is called *hypertension*. Hypertension injures blood vessels by causing arteries to develop arteriosclerosis and atherosclerosis.

blood vessels
narrow tubes that transport oxygen, blood, and nutrients throughout the whole body; include arteries, capillaries, and veins

arteries
large, muscular blood vessels that transport blood from the heart to the capillaries

capillaries
small, thin blood vessels that carry oxygen and nutrients from the arteries to the body's tissues

veins
blood vessels that carry blood from the capillaries back to the heart

arteriosclerosis
a disease of the blood vessels in which arteries harden and become unable to stretch, leading to high blood pressure and heart disease

atherosclerosis
a disease in which fatty substances collect on the walls of the arteries and restrict blood flow

blood pressure
the force that blood exiting the heart exerts on the walls of the arteries

hypertension
a condition that is characterized by high blood pressure, which can lead to heart disease or stroke

Figure 14.4

Here you see the progression of atherosclerosis, leading ultimately to artery blockage and a heart attack. *What can you do to decrease the chances of this type of increased blockage occurring in your arteries?*

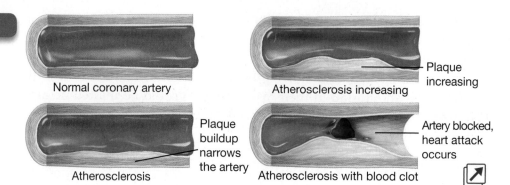

Normal coronary artery

Atherosclerosis increasing

Plaque increasing

Atherosclerosis

Plaque buildup narrows the artery

Atherosclerosis with blood clot

Artery blocked, heart attack occurs

Animation

Blood pressure is measured by a device called a *sphygmomanometer*, or blood pressure cuff (Figure 14.5). The pressure is recorded as millimeters of mercury (mmHg). The blood pressure measurement has two parts. The first number, called the *systolic pressure*, is the blood pressure that exists when the heart muscle is contracted. The second number is called the *diastolic pressure*, which records the blood pressure when the heart muscle is relaxed between contractions.

A healthy adult has systolic blood pressure no higher than 120 mmHg and a diastolic pressure no higher than 80 mmHg. Blood pressure higher than 140/90 mmHg in adults is hypertension. Systolic blood pressure ranging from 120 to 139 mmHg, or diastolic pressure ranging from 80 to 89 mmHg, is *prehypertension*, a condition that can develop into hypertension.

Hypertension produces few signs and symptoms. It silently causes problems in blood vessels and organs throughout the body and sets the stage for a heart attack or stroke. Monitoring blood pressure is important so hypertension can be detected and treated early.

Hypertension is most common among older adults, and is associated with a physically inactive lifestyle, excess weight and obesity, and excessive salt and alcohol consumption. Hypertension can also be genetic.

Stroke

stroke
an interruption of the blood flow to a section of the brain

Stroke is a disease that occurs when the blood flow to a part of the brain is interrupted, injuring or killing brain cells. A stroke can leave a person paralyzed, unable to speak, or mentally disabled.

There are two types of stroke. An *ischemic stroke* is the most common type of stroke. The term *ischemia* describes a condition in which no oxygen is available. Ischemic strokes are caused by narrowed or blocked blood vessels in the brain that disrupt the flow of oxygen. Some people experience *transient ischemic attacks* (TIAs), or *mini-strokes*, in which blood flow to a part of the brain temporarily stops. TIAs are sometimes called *warning strokes* and suggest that a person has a high risk factor for a stroke.

The second, less common type of stroke is called a *hemorrhagic stroke*. In a hemorrhagic stroke, a brain blood vessel bursts and fails to deliver oxygen to brain cells. These strokes arise when vessels become weakened after years of hypertension.

Risk factors for stroke include genetics and advanced age. Preexisting conditions, such as hypertension and atherosclerosis, are also risk factors.

Lifestyle risk factors include tobacco use, particularly smoking; a high-fat diet; obesity; and an inactive lifestyle.

A stroke comes on suddenly. Symptoms include numbness or weakness on one side of the body, face, arm, or leg; confusion; trouble speaking or understanding speech; vision problems affecting one or both of the eyes; dizziness, loss of balance or coordination, or trouble walking; and severe headache. Someone with these symptoms needs immediate medical attention. Bystanders should dial 911.

Profile of a Healthy Heart

The heart requires its own continuous supply of oxygen and nutrients, which is delivered by blood vessels called *coronary arteries*. These blood vessels are branches of the largest artery in the body, the *aorta*. The coronary arteries enter the heart muscle, form increasingly smaller branches, and eventually end as microscopic capillaries, where oxygen leaves the blood and enters the heart's muscle cells.

Other muscles in your body can function without oxygen for a period of time, but the cells in the heart muscle cannot. If its supply of oxygen becomes restricted or cut off, the heart's muscle cells die quickly. When its cells die, the heart muscle weakens and stops circulating blood.

Diseases of the Heart

Although the term *heart disease* is sometimes used to mean one disease, there are different types of heart disease. Heart disease arises from interactions among many factors, most of which you have read about throughout this text. They include genetics and family history, smoking, a high-fat and high-cholesterol diet, lack of physical activity, stress and anger, and inflammation.

Coronary Artery Disease

Coronary artery disease occurs when the coronary arteries become narrow or blocked, and reduce or stop blood flow to the heart muscle.

Signs and Symptoms of Coronary Artery Disease. *Angina*, or chest pain, is pressure or squeezing in the chest, or a dull or sharp pain. Some report pain or tingling sensations radiating to the left arm, shoulder, and jaw. Some people also sweat or become dizzy, nauseated, and short of breath.

Angina requires immediate medical attention because it could indicate a *heart attack.* A heart attack occurs when the coronary arteries become blocked. The heart beats irregularly and inefficiently, and pain arises partly because the heart is not receiving enough oxygen (Figure 14.6 on the next page).

A heart attack is a medical emergency. Immediate help can save lives and reduce the amount of heart damage. Cardiopulmonary resuscitation (*CPR*) can be used to help someone suffering from a heart attack. See the back of the book for CPR procedures.

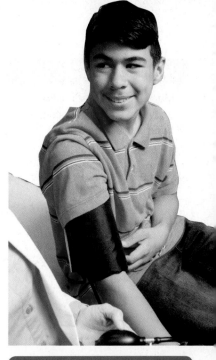

Figure 14.5

A blood pressure cuff, or *sphygmomanometer*, is used to check a person's blood pressure. The cuff is inflated to cut off circulation, and is then slowly deflated while a healthcare professional uses a stethoscope to listen for the sound of blood pulsing.

coronary arteries
blood vessels that deliver blood, oxygen, and nutrients to the heart

aorta
the largest artery in the body

coronary artery disease
a disease in which the arteries that carry blood to the heart become narrow or blocked

angina
a pressure, squeezing, or pain in the chest that is often a sign of heart disease or a heart attack

heart attack
a medical emergency in which the coronary arteries become blocked and restrict blood flow to the heart, causing the heart to beat irregularly and inefficiently

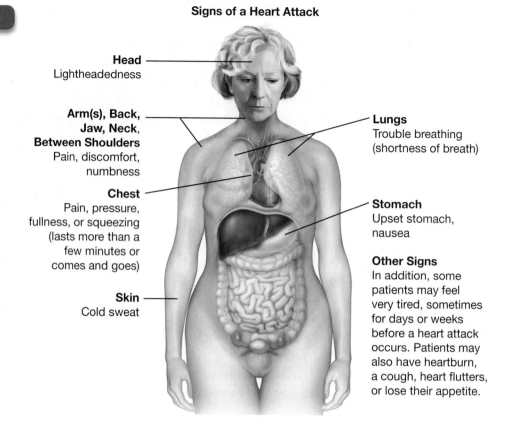

Figure 14.6

Many different parts of the body can signal an upcoming heart attack.

Signs of a Heart Attack

Head
Lightheadedness

Arm(s), Back, Jaw, Neck, Between Shoulders
Pain, discomfort, numbness

Chest
Pain, pressure, fullness, or squeezing (lasts more than a few minutes or comes and goes)

Skin
Cold sweat

Lungs
Trouble breathing (shortness of breath)

Stomach
Upset stomach, nausea

Other Signs
In addition, some patients may feel very tired, sometimes for days or weeks before a heart attack occurs. Patients may also have heartburn, a cough, heart flutters, or lose their appetite.

Causes of Coronary Artery Disease. Atherosclerosis is the leading cause of coronary artery disease. The reduced blood flow to the heart muscle stresses the heart or kills some of its cells.

Congestive Heart Failure

congestive heart failure
a condition in which the heart weakens due to strain and becomes unable to successfully pump blood

Congestive heart failure is a condition in which the heart is too weak to pump blood effectively. Heart failure results from chronic strain on the heart caused by pumping blood through narrow, stiff blood vessels. Over time, the heart weakens until it can no longer work. Coronary artery disease, atherosclerosis, arteriosclerosis, and many other heart diseases can strain the heart enough to cause congestive heart failure (Figure 14.7).

SKILLS FOR HEALTH AND WELLNESS

Commit to a Healthy Heart

Many people don't like changing routines and habits. The challenge each person faces is identifying and overcoming barriers to forming new, healthy habits.

For each heart-healthy habit listed below, identify barriers or difficulties you may face while trying to develop that habit. Then, describe your strategy for overcoming each difficulty.

1. Be physically active on a regular basis, or most days each week.
2. Reduce the fat in your diet.
3. Determine your body mass index (BMI) and maintain healthy body weight.
4. Increase the amount of fiber in your diet.
5. Eat several servings of fresh fruit and vegetables each day.
6. Reduce and cope with daily stress.
7. Do not smoke tobacco, or quit smoking.

Signs and Symptoms of Heart Failure. Signs and symptoms of heart failure include ankle swelling, shortness of breath, and fatigue. As the heart weakens, its pumping power diminishes and blood does not move through the blood vessels. Blood pools within blood vessels of the feet and hands, causing swelling. Fluid builds up in the lungs, interfering with breathing and the ability to obtain enough oxygen to supply the body's needs. People feel short of breath even when resting. At this point, some people exhibit blue-tinged skin and lips, a condition called *cyanosis.* This happens because blood in the skin's capillaries turns blue when it does not carry oxygen.

Normal   **Heart Failure**

Oxygen-rich blood is pumped to the body.

Left ventricle

Reduced volume of blood

Dilated ventricle

Animation

Figure 14.7

The heart muscle on the left is pumping more powerfully than the one on the right (as indicated by the arrows). *Assuming the person whose heart we see on the right has congestive heart failure, what caused her heart to pump less powerfully?*

Treatment of Heart Failure. Treating heart failure can reduce the severity of symptoms and slow progression of the disease. Medications include *diuretics,* which lower the blood pressure and relieve the heart's workload. Other medications strengthen the heart's pumping or reduce blood pressure.

The only cure for a failing heart is a heart transplant. This complicated surgery involves removing the diseased heart and replacing it with a heart donated by another person upon his or her death.

Disorders of Heart Rhythm

The heart muscle normally beats in a coordinated fashion and at a regular rate. Uncoordinated or irregular heartbeats pump blood inefficiently and strain the heart. Disorders of heart rhythm are called ***arrhythmias*** and can arise from abnormal communication within the heart muscle.

Arrhythmias include problems with the heart's rate of beating. *Tachycardia* is an abnormally fast heart rate of over 100 beats per minute (Figure 14.8). Tachycardia causes the heart to feel like it is racing even when the body is resting. In contrast, *bradycardia* is an abnormally slow heart rate of less than 50 beats per minute. Bradycardia means the heart rate fails to keep up with the body's demands for oxygen and nutrients. Both tachycardia and bradycardia could be signs of another heart disease.

Fibrillation is uncoordinated beating of heart muscle. When in fibrillation, the heart muscle quivers instead of contracts, and blood is not pumped from the heart. This condition is called *cardiac arrest,* a life-threatening emergency.

Signs, Symptoms, and Causes of Arrhythmias. People with an arrhythmia feel palpitations, as though their heart is fluttering, skipping beats, or quivering. These people also feel faint, lightheaded, and out of breath because they have poor blood circulation.

arrhythmias
disorders that cause an irregularity in a person's heart rhythm

Figure 14.8

Explain what tachycardia is by comparing the two electrocardiograms (ECGs).

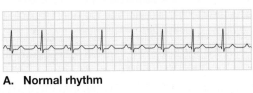
A. Normal rhythm

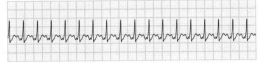
B. Tachycardia

valves
flaps of tissue that control blood flow in the heart

Causes of arrhythmia include coronary artery disease, heart attack, hypertension, and atherosclerosis. Smoking and drug abuse also cause arrhythmia.

Treatment of Arrhythmia. Some medications can control arrhythmia. If these medications are ineffective, doctors can use *cardioversion*, which involves application of electrical voltage to reset the heart's normal rate and rhythm. If cardioversion does not provide relief, the parts of the heart that are sending abnormal signals can be selectively destroyed, a procedure called *ablation*. Some people must have a pacemaker inserted, which electrically sets the pace of the heartbeat.

Diseases of the Heart Valves

The heart pumps blood in one direction. Blood flow begins at the *atria*, two chambers at the top of the heart that receive blood from the body. The atria pump blood into the two larger chambers called *ventricles* at the bottom of the heart. The ventricles pump blood out of the heart to the body. Flexible but sturdy flaps of tissue called **valves** control the movement of blood in this direction. There are several diseases that can affect the heart valves and impact their performance.

One type of heart valve disease is called *mitral valve prolapse*. The mitral valve controls blood flow from the left atrium to the left ventricle by blocking backward blood flow from the ventricle into the atrium. In mitral valve prolapse, however, blood *does* flow backward into the atrium because the valve is defective. In most cases, mitral valve prolapse causes few health problems. In some cases, a great deal of reverse blood flow occurs, stressing the heart muscle. A valve that functions poorly can be surgically repaired or replaced.

Diagnosis and Treatment of Heart Disease

Doctors need to determine the exact nature of a heart disease so they can begin the correct treatment. Figure 14.9 lists some methods of diagnosing heart disease.

Figure 14.9 Methods of Diagnosing Heart Disease

Method	Description
electrocardiogram (ECG)	detects the electrical rhythm of the heart muscle and determines if blood flow to an area of the heart is disrupted
stress test	an ECG performed while walking on a treadmill to determine how physical activity affects the heart's function
angiogram	dye injected into a vein circulates into the coronary vessels; an X-ray reveals narrowed or blocked coronary arteries
echocardiography	sound waves used to visualize the structure and motion of the heart
cardiac catheterization	a long, thin, hollow tube called a *catheter* is threaded through blood vessels into the heart to sample the blood in each chamber for oxygen content and pressure; used to determine how well the heart functions and to detect valve disorders

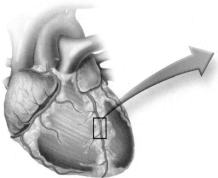

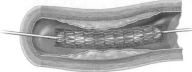

A. Cholesterol buildup partially blocking blood flow through the artery.

Figure 14.10

When buildup of cholesterol partially blocks blood flow through the artery (A), doctors often perform a *stent angioplasty procedure* by inserting a stent with balloon into the partially blocked artery (B). The balloon is then inflated to expand the stent (C). Once the stent is expanded, the balloon is removed and blood flow is restored in the partially blocked artery (D).

B. A stent with a balloon is inserted into the partially blocked artery.

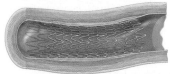

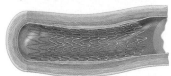

C. The balloon is inflated to expand the stent.

D. The balloon is then removed from the expanded stent.

One common treatment for blocked coronary arteries involves inserting a stent (Figure 14.10). A *stent* is shaped like a straw and is made of a fine mesh. Doctors insert the stent in a vein and guide it along blood vessels until it reaches the coronary arteries. The stent expands to push aside and crush the fatty buildup in the vessel, restoring blood flow. *Bypass surgery* may also repair blocked blood flow. In bypass surgery, a vein from the leg is inserted to conduct blood around the blocked sections of arteries. Coronary artery disease can also be treated with medicine. Blood-thinning medications and aspirin prevent the formation of blood clots. Diuretics lower blood pressure. Some medicines decrease the amount of cholesterol in the blood.

stent
a circular, hollow, wire mesh tube

Lesson 14.2 Review

Know and Understand Assess

1. Define *blood vessels.*
2. Describe blood pressure.
3. List three types of arrhythmias.
4. Name four methods doctors use to diagnose heart disease.
5. Describe the procedure that involves inserting a stent to treat blocked coronary arteries.

Analyze and Apply

6. Explain why arteriosclerosis and atherosclerosis are central to the development of heart diseases.

7. Compare the ways in which fast, slow, and irregular heartbeats can affect the heart.

Real World Health

In groups of three or four, research a major heart disease. Write two to three paragraphs on your chosen disease, including the following information:
- a brief explanation of the disease
- the disease's prevalence
- causes of the disease
- treatments for the disease

Create a poster that highlights this information and present your findings to the class.

Cancer: Cells out of Control

Key Terms E-Flash Cards

In this lesson, you will learn the meanings of the following key terms.

benign tumors
biopsy
cancer
chemotherapy
colonoscopy
malignant tumors
metastasis
proto-oncogenes
tumor
tumor-suppressor genes

Before You Read

Cancer Treatments

Create a visual chart like the one below to connect the content in this lesson with your prior knowledge and experience. List as much information as you know. After reading the lesson, add any extra knowledge you gained.

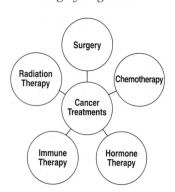

Lesson Objectives

After studying this lesson, you will be able to

- describe the development of cancer in the body, including the formation of benign tumors and malignant tumors;

- analyze how risk factors related to genetics, the environment, lifestyle choices, and infections contribute to the development of cancer;

- identify common signs and symptoms of cancer;

- assess common forms of cancer in the United States and risk factors linked to each form; and

- describe available cancer treatments.

Warm-Up Activity

Cancer: Signs and Symptoms

Your teacher will set a timer for one minute. During that time, you will list as many signs and symptoms of cancer as you can. As you read this lesson, add new signs and symptoms to your list. Put a check mark next to the signs and symptoms of cancer that you already knew. If any of your signs and symptoms are not covered in the lesson, research that sign or symptom and record in your chart whether it signals cancer.

Cancer sign or symptom	√ if covered by lesson	If not covered, what does your research say?

C ancer is rooted in interactions among genes, environment, and lifestyle. Although scientists do not completely understand cancer, they have worked out many parts of the puzzle.

Characteristics of Cancer

Cancer is a complex disease, with different forms of the disease having different characteristics. One characteristic that all forms of cancer share is an uncontrolled growth of abnormal cells. All cell reproduction occurs by division of cells, which is the basis for organ growth, tissue repair, and tissue development. Healthy cells control their growth, dividing only when needed. Cancerous cells divide rapidly and produce abnormal cells that do not function like normal cells.

Scientists call a mass of abnormal cells a *tumor*. Tumors fall into two categories. Malignant tumors are cancerous; benign tumors are not.

Benign tumors usually remain in the area of the body where they first develop and do not invade nearby tissues. Moles and skin calluses are examples of benign tumors (Figure 14.11). Because benign tumors remain localized within organs or tissues, they usually pose few health hazards and may not require treatment. If a benign tumor does cause health problems, it may be more easily removed than a cancerous tumor.

In contrast, *malignant tumors* invade the normal tissues around the area where they first develop. A key characteristic of malignant tumors is *metastasis.* This is the ability to spread to other parts of the body, where additional tumors then develop. Metastasis is possible because malignant cells can break away from the main tumor and enter blood vessels, which transport the malignant cells throughout the body (Figure 14.12).

Risk Factors for Cancer

Certain risk factors can increase your likelihood of developing cancer. The next two pages contain brief descriptions of these factors.

cancer
a disease characterized by a mass of abnormally growing cells that spread and can cause pain, illness, and death

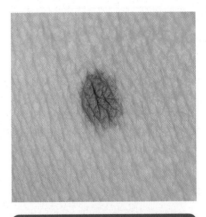

Figure 14.11

A mole is an example of a benign tumor. *What does the word* benign *mean?*

tumor
a growth of abnormal cells in the body's tissues

benign tumors
masses of abnormal cells that remain in the areas of the body where they first develop

malignant tumors
masses of abnormal cells that spread and invade other areas of the body

metastasis
the spread of abnormal cells from one part of the body (initial site) to another (secondary site)

Figure 14.12 Comparison of Benign and Malignant Tumors

	Benign (noncancerous) tumor	Malignant (cancerous) tumor
Location	localized; occurs in well-defined location	invasive; grows into surrounding normal tissue
Movement	remains at original site	metastasizes (spreads) to other organs
Size	usually remains small	may remain small, but can become large
Blood vessels	does not develop new blood vessels	causes formation of new blood vessels
Examples	moles, skin calluses, uterine fibroids	lung cancer, breast cancer, colon cancer, melanoma

Genetics

proto-oncogenes
genes that trigger division in cells

tumor-suppressor genes
genes that stop cell division when it is no longer necessary

Genes called ***proto-oncogenes*** are the cell's normal accelerators, which turn on cell division as needed. A cell with faulty proto-oncogenes divides much more rapidly than surrounding cells.

Tumor-suppressor genes stop cell division when it is no longer required. A cell with faulty tumor-suppressor genes cannot stop cell division. Uncontrolled cell division is the first step toward developing cancer.

For a cell to become cancerous, multiple genetic changes must occur. Certain genes in the body control whether cells remain in place, migrate within tissues, or move into the bloodstream. These genes must also be faulty for cells to become cancerous. Researchers cannot simply say that any single gene is the "cancer gene."

Environmental Influences

One environmental risk factor is a group of substances known as *carcinogens*. Carcinogens cause mutations in genes, leading to cancerous changes in cells.

Chemical carcinogens include substances like formaldehyde, asbestos, and tobacco smoke. Other chemical carcinogens include asbestos and radon gas (Figure 14.13).

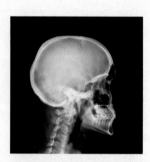
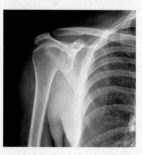

Figure 14.13 Carcinogens

Chemicals	Radiation
aflatoxin (fungus toxin) arsenic asbestos benzene formaldehyde radon gas soot tobacco smoke	gamma radiation ultraviolet radiation (sun) ultraviolet radiation (tanning lights and tanning beds) X-ray radiation

Carcinogens also include some types of radiation. One of the most common types of cancer in the United States is skin cancer, which is linked to ultraviolet (UV) radiation's carcinogenic effects on skin cells. In high doses, X-rays can also cause cancer. Doctors and dentists take care to avoid unnecessarily using X-rays on patients to limit their lifetime exposure to radiation (Figure 14.14).

Figure 14.14

An X-ray is a type of radiation that penetrates the body and leaves an image on film. In high doses, or with multiple exposures over time, X-rays can cause cancer. *What can people do to minimize their exposure to X-rays?*

Lifestyle

Choices you make and habits you form today affect your risk for developing cancer later in life (Figure 14.15). Smoking cigarettes is the leading preventable cause of lung cancer. Exposure to secondhand smoke can also increase your risk for developing lung cancer.

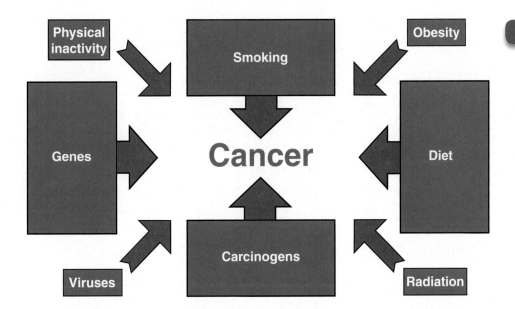

Figure 14.15

Many factors affect a person's risk for developing cancer. *Which of these factors can a person control? Which factors are beyond a person's control?*

Obesity and physical inactivity are known risk factors for cancer of the pancreas, esophagus, kidney, and *endometrium* (lining of the uterus). Over the past several years, death rates for cancers related to physical inactivity and obesity have risen. It is also harder for people who are obese or physically inactive to recover from cancer. An unbalanced diet can also contribute to cancer development.

Infections

Infectious microorganisms are also linked to certain cancers (Figure 14.16). Human papillomavirus (HPV), a sexually transmitted virus, is the leading cause of cervical cancer. Both the hepatitis B virus and hepatitis C virus are capable of causing liver cancer. Infection with human T-lymphotropic virus, Epstein-Barr virus, and HIV are linked with *lymphoma* (cancer of lymphatic tissue). Additionally, infection with the bacterium *Helicobacter pylori* can cause stomach ulcers and stomach cancer.

Figure 14.16 Microorganisms that Cause Cancer

Microorganism	Type of Cancer	Prevention
human papillomavirus (HPV)	cervical cancer	HPV vaccine; avoid sexual activity
hepatitis B virus (HBV)	liver cancer	HBV vaccine
hepatitis C virus (HCV)	liver cancer	HCV vaccine
Helicobacter pylori (bacteria)	stomach cancer	none; antibiotics are an effective treatment if infected
herpes virus type 8	Kaposi's sarcoma (blood vessel cancer associated with HIV infections)	abstinence or use of a latex condom
human T-lymphotropic virus type 1	adult leukemia	abstinence or use of a latex condom
Epstein-Barr virus	lymphoma and Hodgkin's lymphoma	unknown

Figure 14.17 Signs and Symptoms of Cancer—CAUTION

C	change in bowel or bladder habits
A	a sore that does not heal
U	unusual bleeding or discharge
T	thickening or lump in the breast or any part of the body
I	indigestion or difficulty swallowing
O	obvious change in a wart or mole
N	nagging cough or hoarseness

Common Cancers

Early detection of cancer permits early treatment and better chances for recovery and survival. There are common signs and symptoms of cancer, which can be summarized by the acronym C.A.U.T.I.O.N (Figure 14.17). Cancers of the skin, lung, breast, and colon are some of the most common types of cancer.

Skin Cancer

Skin cancer is caused by ultraviolet (UV) light, which is found in sunlight and in tanning beds. The UV light directly damages genes and triggers cancerous changes in skin cells.

There are three main types of skin cancer (Figure 14.18). Two of these types—*basal cell carcinoma* and *squamous cell carcinoma*—are common and curable. *Melanoma* is the most dangerous type of skin cancer because it spreads rapidly throughout the body, sometimes before the initial skin cancer is recognized. The use of tanning beds is associated with all three types of skin cancer.

Monitor your skin for possible signs of skin cancer. Use the *ABCDE method* to note any unusual changes in the skin.

A—asymmetry (one half of the mole looks different from the other)

B—border irregularity (the edges of the mole are jagged)

Figure 14.18

Three major types of skin cancer: A) basal cell carcinoma, B) squamous cell carcinoma, C) malignant melanoma. *Which type of skin cancer is the most dangerous?*

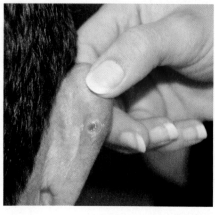

A

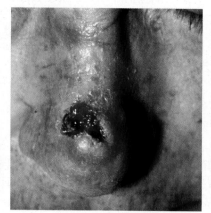

B

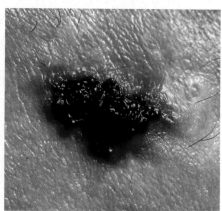

C

George and Randy spend many days at the beach each summer playing volleyball. Randy never gets a dark tan like George does. In fact, Randy sunburns easily.

As Randy pulled on his shirt after a game one afternoon, he felt a familiar itch on his shoulder. He'd had a mole on his shoulder for many years, but it had just begun to itch recently.

He asked George to look at the mole, and George noticed it was darkly colored, with a purple center and a ragged edge. George suggested that Randy see his family's primary care physician about the mole.

Thinking Critically

1. Why do you think that Randy is at risk for developing skin cancer?
2. Why did the mole worry George?
3. Are both boys at risk for skin cancer? Explain your answer.

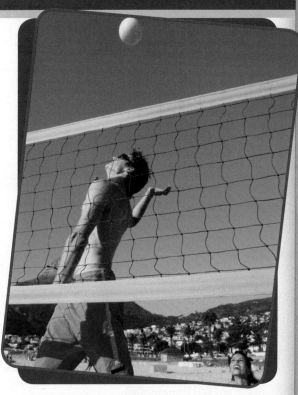

C—color, especially uneven color (for example, a purplish center in a black mole)
D—diameter (the mole grows bigger in size)
E—evolving (the mole changes by becoming bigger, red, itchy, or raised)

Lung Cancer

Most lung cancers begin in the lungs and spread to other organs, including the lymph nodes and the brain. A small percentage of lung cancers begin elsewhere in the body and spread to the lungs.

The chief risk factor for developing lung cancer is smoking tobacco. Exposure to radon gas or asbestos also causes lung cancer. Genetics and family history also influence a person's risk.

Signs and symptoms of lung cancer include a cough that gets progressively worse, chest pain, difficulty breathing, and coughing blood. Lung cancer also causes fatigue and weight loss.

Breast Cancer

Both women and men can develop breast cancer. Risk factors for breast cancer include genetics, age, and lifestyle choices. Generally, the risk for breast cancer increases with age. Breast cancer is also associated with family history, being overweight, and being physically inactive. The presence of breast cancer-related genes *BRCA1* and *BRCA2* also increase risk.

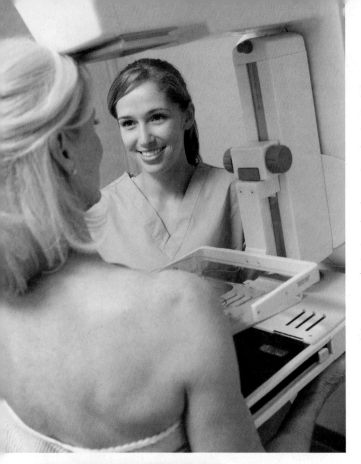

Signs and symptoms of breast cancer include a lump in the breast or armpit, as well as thickening, swelling, and irritation or pain in part of the breast tissue or nipple. People should be aware of any unusual changes in breast tissue and see their doctor if any signs or symptoms cause them concern.

Breast cancer prevention requires scheduling regular screenings, controlling weight, engaging in regular physical activity, limiting alcohol consumption, and researching family history. Scientists recommend that women have regular *mammograms* (X-ray of the breast) beginning at 40 years of age. A mammogram can detect cancer long before it becomes large enough to notice or feel (Figure 14.19). Self-exams—using the hands to feel changes in the breast tissue—can be done regularly at home. This screening method, however, is not as effective as a doctor's exam for detecting smaller cancers. A biopsy can confirm or rule out the presence of cancer. A **biopsy** is a sample of tissue removed from the body for further testing.

Figure 14.19

Mammograms, or X-rays of the breast, can detect breast cancer while it can be successfully treated. *At what age should women begin to have regular mammograms?*

biopsy
a sample of tissue removed from the body for microscopic study; also the procedure of removing a tissue sample from the body for testing

colonoscopy
a procedure used to examine the colon

Colon and Rectal Cancer

The colon (also called the *large intestine*) carries waste to the rectum, where it is stored before elimination. Cancer in the colon and rectum is called *colorectal cancer*, or simply *colon cancer*.

The majority of colon cancer cases appear in people 50 years of age or older. Genetics also play a role. Lifestyle risk factors for colon cancer include physical inactivity and being overweight or obese. A diet high in red meat but low in fruits, vegetables, and fiber are also risk factors.

Early stages of colon cancer cause no signs or symptoms. Later, colon cancer can be indicated by blood in the stool, stomach pain that does not go away, and unexplained weight loss. If cancer is suspected, the colon can be inspected by a **colonoscopy**, a procedure in which a flexible tube with a camera and small surgical instruments are inserted into the colon. A colonoscopy allows the doctor to see the lining of the intestine and remove tissue samples for lab tests.

Prevention of colon cancer requires regular screening, which usually involves a colonoscopy every two years beginning around 50 years of age. Screening for colon cancer is very effective. A balanced diet and regular physical activity can also decrease risks.

Cancer Treatment

A combination of treatments is often more effective than any treatment alone. Surgery is more likely to be effective if the cancer is confined to a small area and has not invaded any vital tissues that could be damaged by surgery.

Chemotherapy involves the use of medicines to kill cancer cells (Figure 14.20). Chemotherapy can also shrink cancerous tumors to a more manageable size for surgery. Side effects of chemotherapy include weight loss, hair loss, nausea and diminished diet, lowered resistance to infections, and bleeding.

Additional treatments include other types of therapy. *Hormone therapy* targets hormones to cut off favorable conditions that cancers need. *Immune therapy* stimulates the body's defenses to attack the cancer. *Radiation therapy* causes damage to cancer cells and triggers their death. Treatments are tailored to specific cancers and to the needs of individual patients since each patient and each type of cancer are different.

chemotherapy
a treatment in which medicines are administered to kill cancer cells

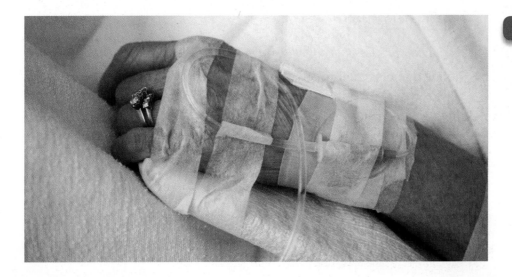

Figure 14.20

A cancer patient undergoes chemotherapy. *What are some of the possible side effects of chemotherapy?*

Lesson 14.3 Review

Know and Understand

1. Explain the activity of cancerous cells.
2. Explain the difference between a benign tumor and a malignant tumor.
3. Name four lifestyle habits that affect your risk factor for developing cancer.
4. Identify four common types of cancer in the United States.
5. List three types of therapy that can be used to treat cancer.

Analyze and Apply

6. What are the functions of proto-oncogenes and tumor-suppressor genes? What is the result if both proto-oncogenes and tumor-suppressor genes are faulty?

7. How is metastasis an indicator of malignant tumors?
8. Why is it important to be attentive to even one of the signs or symptoms listed in the C.A.U.T.I.O.N. acronym?

Real World Health

With a partner, contact one cancer-related organization and attend a meeting or event hosted by that organization. Ask questions about the organization and then write a report that covers the following information:

- What is the history of the organization?
- What activities is this organization involved in?
- How could a teen get involved in or contribute to the mission of this organization?

Diabetes, Allergies, Asthma, and Arthritis

Key Terms E-Flash Cards

In this lesson, you will learn the meanings of the following key terms.

acidosis

allergens

allergy

anaphylaxis

arthritis

autoimmune disease

diabetes mellitus

edema

gout

histamine

hyperglycemia

insulin

local allergies

osteoarthritis

rheumatoid arthritis

systemic allergies

type 1 diabetes mellitus

type 2 diabetes mellitus

Before You Read

KWL Chart: Diabetes
Create a KWL chart to map what you know, what you want to know, and what you have learned about diabetes.

Lesson Objectives

After studying this lesson, you will be able to

- define diabetes mellitus (DM) and explain how it is characterized;
- differentiate between type 1 and type 2 diabetes mellitus;
- analyze how allergies develop and the body's reaction to them;
- describe how asthma impacts the respiratory system; and
- explain osteoarthritis, rheumatoid arthritis, and gout as different forms of arthritis.

Warm-Up Activity

Myth or Fact?
Take a few moments to consider the following statements about diabetes:

1. *Diabetes is a disease resulting from the body's inability to regulate glucose.*
2. *Type 1 diabetes is more common than type 2 diabetes.*
3. *Type 1 diabetes may be caused by genetics or a viral infection.*
4. *Type 2 diabetes is initially caused by the pancreas not producing enough insulin.*
5. *Diabetes is the leading cause of amputation in the United States.*

Your teacher will place a piece of paper with the word Myth *on one side of the room and a piece of paper with the word* Fact *on the other side of the room. As your teacher reads a statement aloud, move to the Myth sign if you believe the statement is false, or to the Fact sign if you believe the statement is true. Discuss your choice with the other students who made the same choice. Select a spokesperson to explain your decision to the class.*

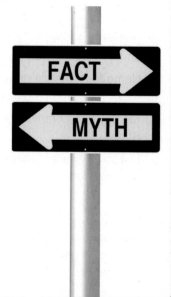

T oday, there are no cures available for diabetes, allergies, asthma, and arthritis. Scientists have, however, discovered much about how to manage the symptoms of these diseases, giving people a chance to live healthy, active lives.

Diabetes

Diabetes mellitus, commonly referred to as *diabetes*, is a disease resulting from the body's inability to regulate glucose (sugar). Diabetes is characterized by *hyperglycemia*, or high blood glucose, which has serious consequences for the entire body. Scientists recognize two types of diabetes, which differ in their underlying causes.

Type 1 Diabetes Mellitus

Type 1 diabetes mellitus is also known as *juvenile-onset diabetes* or *insulin-dependent diabetes*. The onset of type 1 diabetes usually occurs between 10 and 14 years of age. Type 1 diabetes develops because the immune system destroys insulin-producing cells in the pancreas. This abnormality may be genetic or may be triggered by viral infections.

In type 1 diabetes, the body is unable to make the hormone *insulin*. Insulin is normally produced by the pancreas and is needed to instruct cells to take in glucose from the blood. Without insulin, glucose remains in the blood, depriving cells of their main source of energy. Starving cells then seek their energy from fat and protein. Using fat for energy produces a great deal of acid, which builds to toxic levels in the blood. *Acidosis*, excess acid in the blood, is dangerous and can lead to coma and death if left untreated.

Some of the most common symptoms of type 1 diabetes include excessive urination, thirst, hunger, and weight loss (Figure 14.21). As glucose

diabetes mellitus
a disease in which the body is unable to regulate its levels of glucose

hyperglycemia
a condition characterized by dangerously high blood glucose levels

type 1 diabetes mellitus
a disorder in which the body cannot process glucose properly due to a lack of insulin-producing cells

insulin
a hormone that is produced in the pancreas and directs cells to consume blood glucose

acidosis
a condition characterized by dangerously high levels of acid in the blood

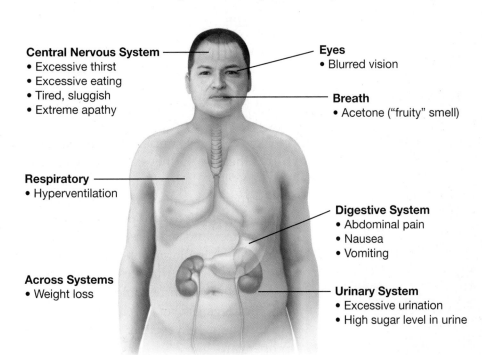

Central Nervous System
• Excessive thirst
• Excessive eating
• Tired, sluggish
• Extreme apathy

Eyes
• Blurred vision

Breath
• Acetone ("fruity" smell)

Respiratory
• Hyperventilation

Digestive System
• Abdominal pain
• Nausea
• Vomiting

Across Systems
• Weight loss

Urinary System
• Excessive urination
• High sugar level in urine

Figure 14.21

The major signs and symptoms of diabetes mellitus occur in different body systems.

accumulates in the blood, the kidneys excrete extra glucose in the urine. A large amount of water is also excreted with the glucose, which triggers thirst.

Type 1 diabetes must be treated with insulin, strict diet management, and regular physical activity. Insulin is administered by regular injections. Diabetics must monitor their own blood glucose using a needlestick method (Figure 14.22). Diabetics must also control the amount of sugar in their blood by controlling the amount of food and the sugars they eat. Regular, moderate physical activity also helps regulate blood glucose.

Type 2 Diabetes Mellitus

Type 2 diabetes mellitus is also called *adult-onset diabetes* or *insulin-independent diabetes*. Type 2 diabetes develops later in life and is associated with obesity. The underlying cause of type 2 diabetes is insulin resistance, meaning that the pancreas produces insulin normally, but the body's cells do not respond to the insulin. As type 2 diabetes progresses, the ability of the pancreas to make insulin becomes impaired. Another problem caused by type 2 diabetes is the production of extra glucose by the liver. The overall result is high blood sugar, low levels of insulin, and signs and symptoms similar to type 1 diabetes.

There are many risk factors for type 2 diabetes, and treatment options are available. Risk factors include a family history of diabetes, advanced age, obesity, a physically inactive lifestyle, high blood pressure, and high cholesterol. Treatment for type 2 diabetes includes modifying the diet, managing weight, and taking medications to assist cells with insulin usage. Some people also need insulin if they cannot control their diabetes with diet and weight loss.

type 2 diabetes mellitus
a disorder in which the body cannot process glucose properly due to the body developing insulin resistance

Figure 14.22

A glucometer, or blood glucose monitor, is used by people who have diabetes to monitor the level of glucose in their blood. *Why would monitoring blood glucose levels be important for diabetics?*

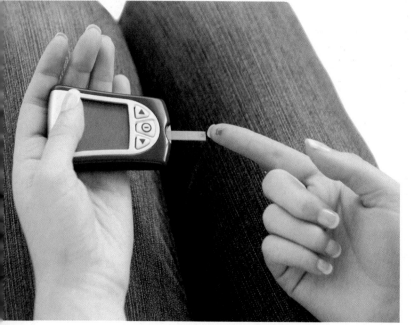

Health Complications Related to Diabetes

The long-term health consequences of diabetes stem from the effects of hyperglycemia on blood vessels. The excess sugar in the blood damages the lining of blood vessels, causing the vessels to become narrow and blocked. Similar injuries to small blood vessels of the eyes, kidneys, and nerves can lead to vision loss, kidney failure, and impaired nerve function. Vessels of the heart are also affected, leading to cardiovascular disease.

The feet and legs are especially vulnerable to the circulatory and nerve problems associated with diabetes. Diabetics are prone to severe, untreatable infections in the feet and legs that may require amputation. Amputation, however, is preventable with proper care.

Improved Diabetes Control

Diabetics must monitor and control blood glucose levels regularly to understand their condition and prevent complications. With the help of insulin pumps and easy-to-use glucose meters, monitoring blood glucose levels has become easier and less painful than before. Diabetics can administer steady levels of insulin and conveniently check their blood glucose with these new devices. Insulin pumps automatically give the proper dose of insulin through a tiny tube inserted into a vein. As a result of these innovations, there has been a large drop in lower-limb amputations among adult diabetics. Scientists attribute this to improved monitoring and insulin treatment.

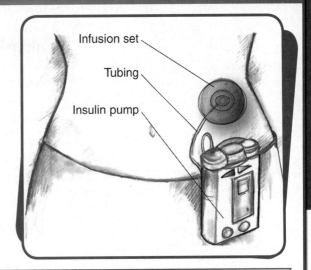

Infusion set
Tubing
Insulin pump

Thinking Critically

1. Why do diabetics need to monitor their blood sugar level?
2. How have insulin pumps and glucose meters helped reduce the number of amputations among diabetics?

Allergies

An *allergy* is an abnormal, destructive immune response with effects that can range from merely annoying to deadly.

Causes

An allergy is triggered by substances in the environment called *allergens*. An allergen can be a substance or food item such as plant pollen, mold, pet hair, dust, peanuts, or shellfish. An allergen typically enters the body through the mouth, nose, or skin. It then attaches to cells called *mast cells* that reside in these tissues (Figure 14.23 on the next page). Mast cells respond by releasing potent chemical signals, including *histamine*, a substance that causes blood vessels to leak fluids into the tissues. These fluids cause swelling known as *edema*. In the nasal passages, edema causes congestion, irritation, and a runny nose. On the skin, edema causes itchy red spots and bumps called *hives*.

Local and Systemic Allergies

Some allergies are restricted to specific organs, while other allergies affect the entire body. Allergies that affect a specific part of the body are called *local allergies*. For example, hay fever affects mainly the respiratory system and eyes.

allergy
an immune response in which the body reacts destructively to a harmless substance

allergens
substances that trigger allergic reactions in the body

histamine
a substance that causes blood vessels to leak fluids into body tissues, resulting in swelling

edema
the swelling of body tissues during an immune response

local allergies
allergies that affect a specific part of the body

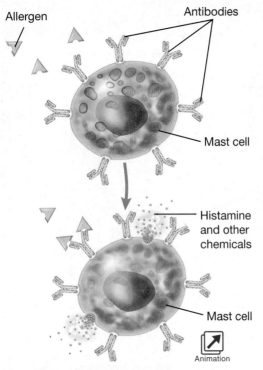

Allergen

Antibodies

Mast cell

Histamine and other chemicals

Mast cell

Animation

Figure 14.23

People who are allergic to a substance have antibodies for that substance. When the person is exposed to the allergen, certain cells in the body release histamines and other chemicals, which trigger an allergic reaction.

systemic allergies
allergies that affect the entire body

anaphylaxis
an allergic response in which fluid fills the lungs and air passages narrow, restricting breathing

arthritis
a condition in which the joints become inflamed, causing pain and stiffness

osteoarthritis
a type of arthritis in which the cartilage in joints wears down so that the bones touch

Allergies that affect the entire body are called *systemic allergies*. Examples of systemic allergies include the reaction to peanuts. Systemic allergies can cause *anaphylaxis*, a dangerous allergic response in which the lungs fill with fluids and the air passages constrict. Anaphylaxis causes a person to wheeze and can cause a person's blood pressure to drop to deadly levels.

People who have severe allergies to substances such as peanuts often carry an emergency supply of epinephrine preloaded in a needle called an *EpiPen®*. *Epinephrine* is a chemical that stimulates the heart to beat strongly so blood pressure can be restored.

Asthma

Asthma is a chronic disease of the respiratory system in which the air passages constrict and fill with mucus, making it difficult to breathe. Membranes in the airways swell, blocking airflow even more and trapping stale air in the lungs. This triggers the wheezing that is characteristic of asthma.

Causes of Asthma

Many scientists believe heredity and environment play a role in the development of asthma. People with asthma may also have allergies that can trigger asthma symptoms. Other causes of asthma include anxiety, exertion, infection, and exposure to airborne chemicals like those in perfumes. Heredity plays a role because asthma often runs in families.

Treating Asthma

Asthma cannot be cured, but medications can reduce the number and severity of attacks. In the midst of an asthma attack, people inhale certain medicines through *rescue inhalers* to quickly relax the airways. Other asthma medicines are used for long-term prevention of asthma.

Arthritis

Arthritis means inflammation of the joints. People with arthritis move slowly and stiffly. There are many types of arthritis, each with different causes, treatments, and outcomes.

Osteoarthritis

Osteoarthritis is the most common form of arthritis among older adults. It is caused by the wearing down of cartilage that normally pads the surfaces of bones that meet at the joints. The bones then come into contact with each other, triggering pain, swelling, and stiffness. Osteoarthritis can be treated with anti-inflammatory medicine, pain relievers, and mild exercises. Severely damaged joints may require surgery or replacement with an artificial joint.

Rheumatoid Arthritis

Rheumatoid arthritis occurs in adults of all ages and affects many joints, the eyes, and the heart. Rheumatoid arthritis is an *autoimmune disease*—a defect that causes the body's immune system to attack and damage the joints. The same joints often swell painfully on opposite sides of the body, and the pain and swelling often come and go, repeatedly becoming worse, then improving. Over time, the damage from this disease causes crippling deformities in the joints.

Treatment for rheumatoid arthritis includes anti-inflammatory medication, pain relievers, and mild exercises. Certain medications target the immune system and block its attack on the joint tissues.

rheumatoid arthritis
a type of arthritis in which the body's immune system attacks, damages, and eventually immobilizes the joints

autoimmune disease
a disease in which the immune system attacks and damages healthy body tissues

Gout

Gout is another type of arthritis that occurs in some aging adults. Gout causes sudden, painful swelling of joints, especially in the feet and big toe. The affected joint may make walking difficult.

A family history of gout increases a person's risk of developing the disease. Gout can also be caused by diets that are rich in purines (found in red meat, anchovies, and asparagus), and can be triggered by alcoholic beverages. There is no known cure for gout, but medications can significantly reduce the pain and swelling.

gout
a type of arthritis characterized by sudden, severe, and painful swelling of a joint

Lesson 14.4 Review

Know and Understand

1. Define *diabetes mellitus*.
2. Explain the difference between type 1 diabetes and type 2 diabetes.
3. Differentiate between local allergies and systemic allergies.
4. What physical reaction occurs in the airways that triggers the wheezing associated with asthma?
5. List three different types of arthritis.
6. Why are rescue inhalers used during an asthma attack?

Analyze and Apply

7. How do the causes of osteoarthritis and rheumatoid arthritis differ?

Real World **Health**

Using the Internet, research the common causes of hay fever in your area. What pollens are prevalent in your region? During which time of year are they most prevalent? How is hay fever diagnosed and treated? Create a PowerPoint® presentation to teach your classmates about the common environmental allergens in your community.

Lesson 14.1

Noncommunicable Diseases: What You Should Know

Key Terms

complication	prognosis
homeostasis	relapse
mutations	remission
noncommunicable diseases	

Key Points

- Noncommunicable diseases are not contagious.
- When homeostasis is not maintained, the body becomes diseased.
- Heredity, lifestyle choices, and environmental factors contribute to a person's risk for developing certain noncommunicable diseases.
- Characteristics of disease include a prognosis, remission and relapse, complications, and whether a disease is acute or chronic.
- To diagnose a disease, physicians evaluate a patient's signs and symptoms, physical exams, family history, and lab tests.

Check Your Understanding

1. Diseases that are *not* contagious are called _____ diseases.
   A. infectious
   B. communicable
   C. noncommunicable
   D. acute

2. Homeostasis refers to _____.
   A. a disease
   B. a bacteria
   C. X-rays and related technology
   D. the body's internal, steady state of balance

3. *True or false?* Lifestyle has no effect on a person's risk factors for developing certain noncommunicable diseases.

4. **Critical Thinking.** Your friend just discovered she has a family history of diabetes. What can your friend do to reduce her risk factors? What school and community resources are available to support early detection of diabetes?

Lesson 14.2

Diseases of the Blood Vessels and Heart

Key Terms

angina	congestive heart failure
aorta	coronary arteries
arrhythmias	coronary artery disease
arteries	heart attack
arteriosclerosis	hypertension
atherosclerosis	stent
blood pressure	stroke
blood vessels	valves
capillaries	veins

Key Points

- Blood vessel diseases include arteriosclerosis, atherosclerosis, hypertension, and stroke.
- The term *heart disease* includes many different types of diseases, such as coronary artery disease, congestive heart failure, heart rhythm disorders, and heart valve diseases.
- Treatment options for various forms of heart disease include a stent, surgery, medicines, cardioversion, and ablation.
- Risk factors for developing heart disease include genetics, environmental factors, unbalanced diet, lack of physical activity, smoking, high stress and anger, and inflammation.

Check Your Understanding

5. Which of the following is *not* a type of blood vessel?
   A. arteries
   B. capillaries
   C. veins
   D. arteriosclerosis

6. A condition in which the coronary arteries become narrow or blocked, and reduce or stop blood flow to the heart muscle, is called _____.

7. Identify six risk factors for developing heart disease.

8. **Critical Thinking.** Explain the difference between a stroke and a heart attack.

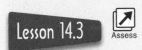
Lesson 14.3   Assess

Cancer: Cells out of Control

Key Terms

benign tumors   malignant tumors
biopsy   metastasis
cancer   proto-oncogenes
chemotherapy   tumor
colonoscopy   tumor-suppressor genes

Key Points

- Cancer develops on a molecular level with changes occurring in the cells.
- Genetic, environmental, infectious, and lifestyle conditions and choices are risk factors for the development of cancer.
- Common cancers include skin, lung, breast, and colon cancers.
- Treatment options include surgery and various types of therapy.

Check Your Understanding

9. A _____ tumor usually remains in the area of the body where it first developed and does not invade nearby tissues.

10. *True or false?* Carcinogens cause mutations in genes, leading to cancerous changes in cells.

11. Which of the following health problems is a sign or symptom of cancer?
    A. change in bowel or bladder habits
    B. unusual bleeding or discharge
    C. a sore that does not heal
    D. All of the above.

12. **Critical Thinking.** How can early detection of cancer improve recovery and survival rates?

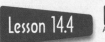
Lesson 14.4   Assess

Diabetes, Allergies, Asthma, and Arthritis

Key Terms

acidosis   allergy
allergens   anaphylaxis

arthritis   insulin
autoimmune disease   local allergies
diabetes mellitus   osteoarthritis
edema   rheumatoid arthritis
gout   systemic allergies
histamine   type 1 diabetes mellitus
hyperglycemia   type 2 diabetes mellitus

Key Points

- Diabetes mellitus results from the body's inability to regulate glucose.
- Type 1 diabetes develops during youth when the body is unable to produce insulin.
- Type 2 diabetes develops later in life as a result of insulin resistance.
- An allergy develops when the immune system has an abnormal, destructive response to a normally harmless substance.
- Although the causes of asthma are unknown, asthma can be treated and asthma attacks can be minimized.
- Osteoarthritis, rheumatoid arthritis, and gout are different forms of arthritis.

Check Your Understanding

13. The hormone _____ is needed to instruct cells to take in glucose from the blood.
    A. insulin
    B. acidosis
    C. hyperglycemia
    D. pancreas

14. A chronic disease of the respiratory system in which the air passages constrict and fill with mucus, making it difficult to breathe, is called _____.

15. Which of the following is *not* a type of arthritis?
    A. rheumatoid
    B. osteoarthritis
    C. gout
    D. anaphylaxis

16. **Critical Thinking.** Why might a person with a systemic allergy carry an *EpiPen*® at all times?

Health and Wellness Skills

17. **Advocate for Health.** 600,000 people die of heart disease every year in the United States. Many of those deaths could be prevented if people made simple lifestyle changes. Create a pamphlet explaining the risk factors for heart disease and how people can reduce their risk. Include information about a person's diet, exercise habits, and smoking habits. Include both text and visuals in your pamphlet. Arrange to distribute this pamphlet through a local organization such as a community health center, senior center, or library.

18. **Analyze Influences.** To effectively guard against noncommunicable diseases, you need to know what influences your risk for disease. Create a diagram of your family tree that includes your siblings, parents, grandparents, and great-grandparents. Then, interview your family members to determine what genetic, environmental, and lifestyle-related risk factors have contributed to disease in your family. Include these risk factors on your family tree diagram.

19. **Make Decisions.** Imagine that a family friend is over and he is acting strangely. He is sweating even though the room is cool, seems short of breath, and is complaining of pain in his left arm. Use the DECIDE process to determine what course of action you should take.

    Define the problem. Identify your values.
    Evaluate the options. Decide and act.
    Consider the Evaluate the outcome.
    consequences.

20. **Practice Healthy Behaviors.** Create a plan of action for maintaining a healthy heart. List the behaviors you already practice to reduce your risk of developing heart disease. What steps could you take to further protect your heart? Write a specific and detailed plan and schedule for at least one behavior you could engage in to reduce your risk of heart disease.

Hands-On Activity

Liquid Sugar

Eating and drinking large amounts of sugar has been linked to an increased risk of developing type 2 diabetes. This activity will examine just how much sugar is in some popular soft drinks.

Materials Needed

- four to six empty drink containers with visible nutrition labels
- small digital scales
- bowls
- small snack bags
- three or more pounds of sugar
- permanent marker
- poster board

Steps for this Activity

1. For this activity, gather in groups of four to six students. Decide who will bring the required materials.

2. The World Health Organization recommends that adults obtain less than 5% of their daily calories from sugar. This equals about 25 grams of sugar for the average adult. Use a scale to measure out 25 grams of sugar. Then, place the sugar in a snack bag and label it *WHO recommendation for daily sugar intake, 25g.*

3. In your groups, compare the drink containers that you brought. Without looking at the nutrition labels, predict the grams of sugar in each drink and rank them from least sugary to most sugary.

4. Next, look at each drink's nutrition label to determine how many grams of sugar are in each bottle. Multiply the grams of sugar by the number of servings listed, if needed. Measure out the grams of sugar contained in each drink, and place the sugar into snack bags with labels for each drink.

5. Compare each drink's sugar content with the WHO-recommended daily sugar intake. Are there any drinks that contain a greater amount of sugar than the WHO recommends for daily consumption?

6. Discuss the following questions in your group:
   - How accurate were your predictions? Explain.
   - Based on the WHO recommendation for daily sugar intake, which drinks should be avoided?

Core Skills

Math Practice

The following graph demonstrates the rates of stomach cancer per 100,000 people in the United States over a span of 35 years. Analyze the graph and answer the following questions to interpret the data presented.

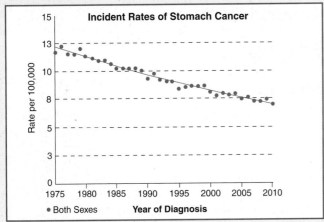

21. What has been the overall trend in the rates of stomach cancer?
    A. The number of incidences has decreased.
    B. The number of incidences has increased.
    C. The number of incidences has been inconsistent; there is no trend.
    D. The number of incidences has decreased, increased significantly, and decreased again.

22. In what year did the rate of stomach cancer incidences peak?
    A. 2010
    B. 1993
    C. 1981
    D. 1976

23. What was the approximate rate of stomach cancer incidents per 100,000 during the year that data was last collected?
    A. 15
    B. 10
    C. 7
    D. 3

24. What is the approximate difference in incident rates per 100,000 from the time data was first collected in this study to the time data was last collected?
    A. 15
    B. 10
    C. 7
    D. 5

Reading and Writing Practice

Read the passage below and then answer the questions.

Sometimes a disease enters remission, *which is a period of time without signs and symptoms associated with that disease. Some cancers enter remission after treatment and stay in remission for weeks, years, or indefinitely. The term* relapse *refers to the recurrence of a disease, in which signs and symptoms return after a period of remission. Certain cancers can leave remission and recur in an even more severe way than before. Exacerbation describes the worsening of signs and symptoms.*

25. What is the meaning of *remission*?
    A. The recurrence of signs and symptoms.
    B. A period of time without signs and symptoms.
    C. The worsening of symptoms.
    D. A disease that has been cured.

26. What is the author's main point in this paragraph?
    A. Signs and symptoms of cancer enter remission, but never relapse.
    B. Signs and symptoms of cancer relapse, but never enter remission.
    C. Sometimes signs and symptoms of a disease enter remission and then relapse.
    D. A disease's signs and symptoms are often exacerbated by treatment.

27. According to the passage, the worsening of signs and symptoms when a disease relapses is called _____.
    A. cancer
    B. remission
    C. relapse
    D. exacerbation

28. Compare the etymological structure (word origins) and definitions for *relapse*, *remission*, and *recurrence*. Based on these three terms, you can deduce that the prefix *re-* means _____.
    A. to happen again
    B. to happen only one time
    C. near
    D. far

29. What is the difference between *remission* and *relapse*? Write a brief paragraph illustrating the difference between remission and relapse.

Unit 6 Mental and Emotional Health and Wellness

Big Ideas

- Your emotional and intellectual health impacts the other dimensions of your health.

- Learning how to recognize and manage your emotions, including your reactions to stress, will help you improve your health and wellness.

- Mental illnesses and disorders are like physical illnesses and disorders—they can be diagnosed and treated, often successfully.

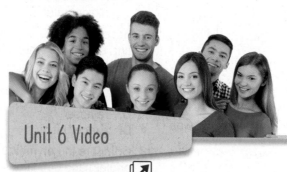

Unit 6 Video

Stressed Out Videos

The night before an important exam, a teenager panics when she discovers she misplaced her study notes. Like other teenagers, she struggles to find time for her activities and responsibilities—from homework and college applications to extracurricular activities and hanging out with friends. She asks for and gets help.

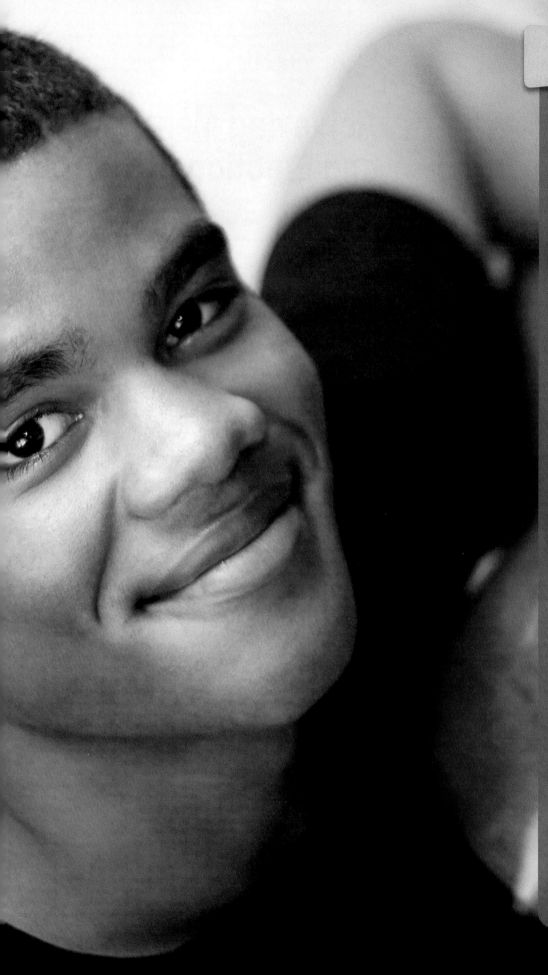

Receive Feedback

Share a paper or electronic copy of your draft with each member of your group. As people read the draft, they should ask themselves the following:

- What do you like about the work? Is there anything you don't like?
- Is the research question expressed clearly?
- Does the organization of the draft make sense?
- Does the body of the draft present information that addresses the question? Is there extraneous material that should be cut?
- Are there key terms or concepts you don't understand? What can the author do to clarify them?
- Does the author use his or her own words?
- Is there a conclusion and does it make sense?

After reading, the group should come together to share their feedback with the author. First discuss ground rules for the discussion, which should include showing courtesy and respect to others. The author should take notes as people speak and thank them for their feedback.

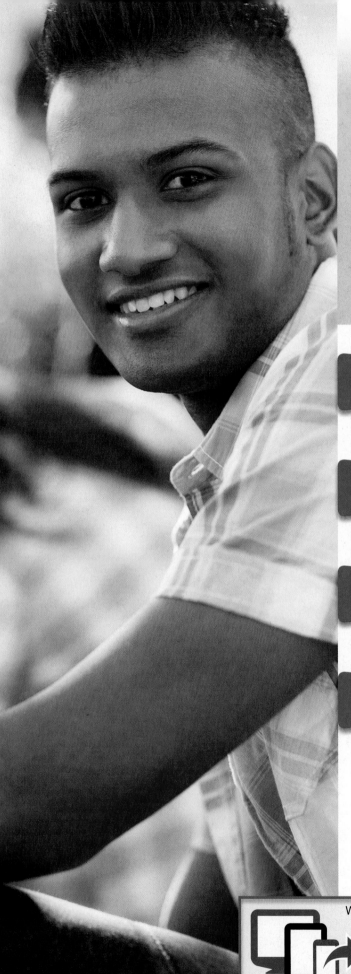

Chapter 15

Achieving Mental and Emotional Health

Lesson 15.1

Making Sense of Your Emotions

Lesson 15.2

Establishing Your Identity

Lesson 15.3

Understanding Self-Esteem

Lesson 15.4

Improving Your Mental and Emotional Health

While studying this chapter, look for the activity icon  to:

- **review** vocabulary with e-flash cards and games;
- **assess** learning with quizzes and online exercises;
- **expand** knowledge with animations and activities; and
- **listen** to pronunciation of key terms in the audio glossary.

 G-W LEARNING.com

www.g-wlearning.com/health/

Take this quiz to see what you do *and* do not *know about mental and emotional health. If you cannot answer a question, pay extra attention to that topic as you study this chapter.*

1. *Identify each statement as* True, False, *or* It Depends. *Choose* It Depends *if a statement is true in some cases, but false in others.*
2. *Revise each* False *statement to make it true.*
3. *Explain the circumstances in which each* It Depends *statement is true and when it is false.*

Health and Wellness IQ Assess

1.	People with good mental and emotional health spend time developing and maintaining close relationships.	True	False	It Depends
2.	People with good mental and emotional health never experience disappointments or failures.	True	False	It Depends
3.	Most teenagers regularly experience mood swings.	True	False	It Depends
4.	Many teenagers have a distinct identity and clear sense of who they are.	True	False	It Depends
5.	Once people establish their identity, it remains set for their lifetime.	True	False	It Depends
6.	If you are experiencing unpleasant emotions, it is best to distract yourself and not think about what is causing them.	True	False	It Depends
7.	People with good mental and emotional health also have good physical health.	True	False	It Depends
8.	Having fun is an important part of maintaining good mental and emotional health.	True	False	It Depends
9.	People with high self-esteem are often boastful and conceited.	True	False	It Depends
10.	Gender identity is more important for boys than girls.	True	False	It Depends

Setting the Scene

Researchers describe mental health as "a state of well-being in which the individual realizes his or her own abilities, can cope with the normal stresses of life, can work productively, and is able to make a contribution to his or her community."

Intellectual health is a concept related to mental and emotional health. Intellectually healthy people think clearly and critically. They enjoy exploring new ideas and learning new facts. They face challenging problems head-on and work through them in a positive way. Intellectually healthy people can adapt to an ever-changing world. People with good mental, emotional, and intellectual health feel good about themselves and the future.

In this chapter, you will learn about emotions and how to manage them. You will learn how identity and self-esteem affect mental and emotional health and well-being. You will also learn strategies you can use to improve your mental, emotional, and intellectual health.

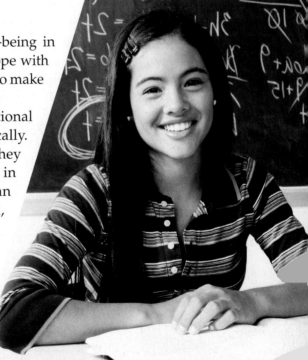

Making Sense of Your Emotions

Key Terms 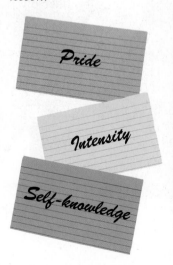 E-Flash Cards

In this lesson, you will learn the meanings of the following key terms.

emotional intelligence
emotions
empathy
optimism
resilience

Lesson Objectives

After studying this lesson, you will be able to

- recognize common unpleasant emotions;
- recognize common positive emotions;
- describe how to manage emotions and express feelings in a healthy way; and
- identify characteristics of people who have good emotional intelligence.

Before You Read

New Vocabulary

Scan this lesson for words that you do not recognize or understand. Write each unfamiliar word on a piece of paper. Consider these words additions to the Key Terms list, which you will learn while reading this lesson.

Pride

Intensity

Self-knowledge

Warm-Up Activity

Tally Your Emotions

Evaluate how you feel throughout the course of a single school day. Using a chart like the one shown below, check off the various ways you feel each hour. If a way you feel is not listed, write it in the box marked other. *You may check off more than one emotion during a particular hour. After you complete the chart for one day, consider the emotions that you have marked. How did your emotions affect your mind and body?*

Try repeating this activity for each of the next four school days. Then compare the five tables and look for patterns. Write a paragraph describing your findings. For example, does a particular emotion tend to occur at a particular time of day? If so, why do you believe this emotion occurs at that time?

Day of the week: _____								
How You Feel	**8:00**	**9:00**	**10:00**	**11:00**	**12:00**	**1:00**	**2:00**	**3:00**	**4:00**
Lonely									
Pessimistic									
Optimistic									
Sad									
Happy									
Angry									
Annoyed									
Bored									
Tired									
Other									
_____									

M any teenagers feel happy during some parts of the day, but can quickly shift to feeling angry, sad, and lonely. These *mood swings*, which are a normal part of the teenage experience, are caused in part by chemical changes in the body. Mood swings can also be caused by the increasing pressure that many teenagers face as they try to balance family relationships, homework, extracurricular activities, peer relationships, and overall physical health.

In this lesson you will learn about different types of feelings people experience. You will also learn some strategies for recognizing and managing these feelings and using them in a constructive way.

Understanding Emotions

Your *mental and emotional health* has to do with your internal life—your feelings and thoughts. This encompasses who you believe you are, how you feel about yourself and others, and how skilled you are at identifying and managing your thoughts and emotions. Your **emotions** are the moods or feelings you experience.

emotions
moods and feelings that you experience

The same event or experience can often lead to different feelings. This can make understanding your emotions challenging. For example, the end of the school year might cause you to feel happy because you will not have to do homework, but sad because you will not see some of your friends every day.

Figuring out which emotions you feel and why can be difficult. This is because one emotion sometimes masks or hides another emotion. If you try out for a sports team and are not chosen, you might feel angry at the coach for not selecting you. This feeling of anger might be hiding your feelings of sadness, however, because you really wanted to be a part of the team.

People experience many different emotions, some of which are unpleasant. Unpleasant emotions are a normal part of life, which everyone experiences at one time or another. Unpleasant emotions are not unhealthy, especially when you learn effective ways to manage them. Some of the most common unpleasant emotions experienced by teenagers include loneliness, anxiety, anger, jealousy, guilt, stress, and depression.

Fortunately, positive emotions are a part of normal daily life, too. Many teenagers experience positive emotions such as joy, gratitude, love, pride, and interest on a regular basis.

Health in the Media

The Rapid Spread of Negative Emotions

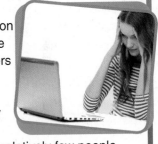

A study was conducted to examine how emotions shared on social media can spread from one person to another. The researchers in this study examined how the emotions one person posted impacted the emotions posted by others in that person's friendship network. Researchers found that relatively few people passed on emotions of sadness or disgust. These seem to be emotions that people are not interested in sharing with others. People did, however, pass on joyful emotions, especially to close friends.

Anger was the emotion that was most likely to be spread. In fact, people who posted something angry were much more likely to have that emotion shared with others, both within their social network and beyond to other social networks.

Thinking Critically

1. Do you agree or disagree that anger is more likely to be shared than other emotions? Explain your answer.

2. How does time spent on social media sites positively affect mental and emotional health? negatively?

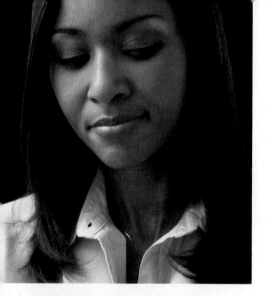

Figure 15.1

Identifying what emotions you are feeling and why you are feeling them is a critical step in managing your emotional well-being. *What do you think this teenager is feeling? What factors or events might cause you to feel this way?*

Managing Emotions

Learning how to manage your emotions can have a positive effect on your mind and body. Try the following steps to manage your emotions and express your feelings in a healthy way.

Identify What You Are Feeling

First, identify what emotion or emotions you are feeling. It can be confusing to separate feelings of sadness and fear or happiness and love. Think about the factors that might be triggering the emotion, which can help you determine the actual emotion you are experiencing.

Jennifer started the day angry at the world (Figure 15.1). At lunch, Jennifer was tempted to wallow in her anger, but instead she reflected on her bad mood. After considering this question, Jennifer remembered something that happened a few days ago. Her mother mentioned that she was applying for a new job, and that it may entail Jennifer moving to a new school. By identifying the cause of her angry mood, Jennifer is now better prepared to work through her emotions.

Acknowledge Your Feelings

Once you identify your feelings, try to accept and acknowledge them. Sometimes people try to cover up or deny their emotions and hope those feelings will just go away. It is important to allow yourself to experience your emotions. Burying emotions deep inside can increase the intensity of emotions and have a negative effect on your mind and body.

After Jennifer understood that she was feeling anxious about potentially moving, it did not make this feeling go away. It did, however, help her understand why she was feeling so angry. Just accepting and acknowledging your feelings can help you handle those feelings in a healthy, positive way.

Express Your Feelings

The third step is to express your emotions, which helps you release them. You can share your feelings with another person or release them by writing in a journal. You can also express your emotions by crying if you feel sad or running if you feel angry.

It is important to remember to not hurt someone, or yourself, when expressing emotions. Try talking with the person who hurt you or caused you to feel a certain emotion without hurting him or her or being negative. Suppose Jennifer decided to talk calmly with her mom and explain how she is feeling about the potential move. Talking with her mom could give Jennifer more information about the situation and help her calm down.

In other cases, directly confronting the person who caused you to feel a certain way can make the situation worse. If you are angry at your friend for telling another person something you shared in confidence, it might be

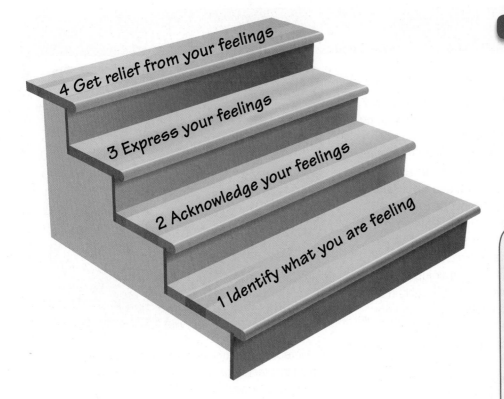

4 Get relief from your feelings

3 Express your feelings

2 Acknowledge your feelings

1 Identify what you are feeling

Figure 15.2

Identifying, acknowledging, and expressing your feelings are all steps in eventually gaining relief from your feelings. *Which of the "steps" described in this section are most difficult for you? Why?*

Personal Profile

How Resilient Are You?

How well can you cope with difficult and stressful events in your life? Answer the following questions to assess your level of resilience.

I feel proud when I accomplish my goals. **yes no**

I usually view disappointments optimistically. **yes no**

I am determined. **yes no**

I have self-discipline. **yes no**

I can usually find something that causes me to laugh and makes me happy. **yes no**

I can usually find my way out of a difficult situation. **yes no**

My belief in myself gets me through difficult times. **yes no**

I believe my life has meaning. **yes no**

Add the number of yes answers to assess your own resilience. The more yes answers, the more resilient you are.

better to wait until you cool off before talking about your feelings. By waiting, you can manage your emotions and express them in a more positive way when you are not so angry. You are allowing yourself time to work through your feelings of anger.

Get Relief from Your Feelings

Finally, find a way to make yourself feel better (Figure 15.2). Some people find it most helpful to spend time with friends and family members who can provide much-needed love and support during difficult times. Other people find it more helpful to have a distraction from what they are feeling. Some distractions may include walking outside, taking a long shower or bath, or watching a funny movie or television show.

Develop Resilience and Coping Skills

Unfortunately, disappointments, rejections, and mistakes are a normal part of life for everyone. Feeling sad, anxious, and frustrated during these times is normal. Developing coping skills can help you get through the more difficult times.

You may know some people who seem better able to cope with difficulties. These people have *optimism*. They keep a positive outlook and know they will eventually feel better. They are flexible and adapt, change, and grow as they encounter different life experiences. People who cope well with problems also show *resilience*, or the ability to recover from traumatic and stressful events. Having resilience helps people work through their emotions in positive ways.

optimism
the ability to keep a positive outlook

resilience
the ability to recover from traumatic or stressful events

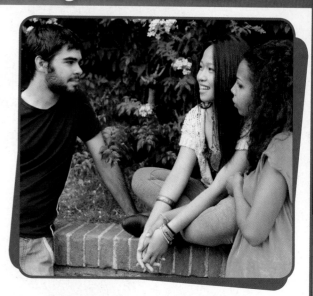

Should schools teach emotional intelligence? To test this question, researchers provided training sessions in emotional intelligence to a group of 300 students. The 24 one-hour sessions took place over a two-year period. These training sessions included games, role-playing, art, and discussions that focused on recognizing emotions in different settings. The sessions also included training in building empathy and managing problems. A comparison group of teenagers did not receive any training. Six months after the training ended, researchers examined psychological health in both groups of teenagers—those who did and did not receive the emotional intelligence training.

The students who received the training showed higher levels of mental and emotional health, and lower levels of anxiety, depression, and social stress than those who did not receive training. These findings show that training teenagers to understand, manage, and express their emotions benefits their psychological well-being.

Moreover, research from other studies has revealed that teenagers who are mentally healthier may engage in fewer risky health behaviors and more positive health behaviors. In this way, teaching emotional intelligence in schools could lead to substantial benefits for students' psychological and physical well-being.

Thinking Critically

1. Why do you think training in emotional intelligence helps reduce anxiety and depression? Do you think this type of education would show similar benefits in your own school? Why or why not?

2. This study only examined the effects of training on emotional intelligence in high school students. What would you expect if researchers did the same study with younger children? Would they find the same benefits of this type of education? Why or why not?

3. Some people believe that schools should focus only on providing traditional education in core subjects, such as math, English, history, and science. Other people believe that providing training in emotional intelligence is also very important. Do you believe schools should provide training in emotional intelligence? Defend your answer.

---

emotional intelligence
the skill of identifying one's own emotions and understanding the emotions of others

empathy
the ability to imagine yourself in someone else's place, and to understand someone else's wants, needs, and point of view

Emotional Intelligence

Do you know people who sense that you are feeling down, even before you say anything to them? People with this ability have high **emotional intelligence**—they are skilled at identifying the emotions they feel. They are also skilled at understanding the emotions other people are feeling.

People who have high emotional intelligence have high levels of **empathy**, or the ability to put themselves in someone else's shoes. They understand others' wants, needs, and points of view. As a result, they are better able to support their friends when they are in need. In this way, they develop strong, healthy relationships.

People who have high emotional intelligence are also able to express their emotions in healthy, positive ways. They can openly share their feelings with friends. For example, suppose someone begins a dating relationship that becomes more and more serious. As a result this person does not spend as much time with his or her old friends as before. Some of these friends may begin to feel neglected and become angry. If one of these friends is high in emotional intelligence, however, he or she might speak to the unavailable friend about the situation instead of becoming angry.

People who have high emotional intelligence exhibit other characteristics, including the following:

- *self-awareness*—they understand their emotions and how those emotions impact people around them. They also feel comfortable relying on their intuition, and have a good sense of their own strengths and weaknesses.

- *self-regulation*—they can control their feelings and impulses and act with careful deliberation and integrity.

- *motivation*—they are willing to work on challenging tasks and are highly productive.

- *social skills*—they work well with other people, help build and maintain relationships, and resolve conflicts in constructive ways.

People who have high emotional intelligence tend to be more successful in school, work, and interpersonal relationships. They also experience greater mental and emotional health. Therefore, developing skills in emotional intelligence can help you succeed in all aspects of your life.

Lesson 15.1 Review

Know and Understand  Assess

1. List five common unpleasant emotions.
2. List five common positive emotions.
3. What does it mean when people have high *emotional intelligence*?
4. What does *empathy* mean?
5. List four characteristics exhibited by people who have high emotional intelligence.

Analyze and Apply

6. Explain why making sense of your emotions can be difficult.

7. What steps can you take to manage your emotions and express your feelings in a healthy way?

Real World | Health

Interview a guidance counselor at your school to learn effective strategies for managing emotions. After completing the interview, compile a detailed list of the suggestions and strategies recommended by the guidance counselor. Implement these strategies over the course of the next few days. Then, write a summary describing how these strategies helped you manage your emotions.

Establishing Your Identity

Key Terms 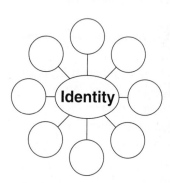 E-Flash Cards

In this lesson, you will learn the meanings of the following key terms.

androgynous
ethnicity
gender identity
gender roles
gender stereotypes
identity

Before You Read

Mindmap

Complete a mindmap for the physical, active, social, and psychological parts of your identity. For each mindmap, identify specific examples of traits that would fall under each main topic. For example, height and weight would fall under physical identity.

Identity

Lesson Objectives

After studying this lesson, you will be able to

- describe the different parts of a person's identity;
- summarize how gender and ethnicity influence a person's identity;
- describe how adolescents show changes in the way they think about moral decisions; and
- identify the primary task for adolescents according to Erik Erikson.

Warm-Up Activity

Who Are You? Collage

Construct a "Who Are You?" collage on a piece of card stock. Completely cover the front of the card stock with pictures, words, and quotes that describe who you are. With permission from your teacher, you can create your collage online using a social media tool. Once you have finished your collage, answer the following questions in as much detail as possible.

Past
- *Which people have had the biggest effect on your life?*
- *What meaningful places have you visited?*
- *What past experiences have had an effect on your life?*

Present
- *What do you think of yourself at this very moment?*
- *What activities do you enjoy?*
- *What makes you happy?*
- *What interests you?*

Future
- *What do you want to do in your life?*
- *What are your goals and dreams?*
- *What profession would you choose if you had no limitations, hurdles, or barriers to stand in your way?*

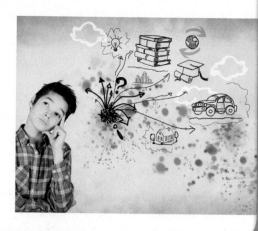

The teenage years are typically a period of self-exploration, which often includes testing out different interests, values, and beliefs as part of learning more about who you are. You might hang out with different friends, experiment with fashion and music, or join clubs as a way of discovering more about yourself.

People with good mental and emotional health recognize their skills, abilities, interests, and goals. They know what they like and what they do not like, and what makes them feel uncomfortable. They know their *core values*, which are their fundamental beliefs and ideals about the attitudes they hold and how they want to act. Through self-exploration you will be able to develop this type of self-knowledge, too.

Forming an Identity

As a teenager, one of the most important challenges you face is figuring out your *identity*, or who you are (Figure 15.3). Your identity has different parts, which include

- *physical identity*—gender, race, age, and physical characteristics, such as height, weight, and hair color;
- *active identity*—engagement in particular activities and interests, such as sports, music, and community service;
- *social identity*—connection to other people, including family members, friends, and group members; and
- *psychological identity*—internal thoughts and feelings.

People often focus on different parts of their identities at different ages. Before they become adolescents, children typically define themselves in terms of the physical and active aspects of their identity. Young children often describe themselves in terms of their height, hair and eye color, and activities in which they are involved.

As children enter adolescence, their focus often shifts to social identity (Figure 15.4 on the next page). A person's social identity can include his or her cultural or religious group, friendship networks, or family relationships. Young adolescents may feel their own identity is influenced by the people in their friendship group—are they popular, athletic, musical, or studious? Their identity may also be influenced by whether they have a boyfriend or girlfriend.

During high school, adolescents may begin to focus more on their unique personal or psychological identity. This identity is made up of internal thoughts and feelings, including personal values, beliefs, and attitudes. Your psychological identity may include how you prefer to spend your time, religious beliefs, attitudes about political parties, and your career goals. It could also include personality traits, such as whether you are extroverted or introverted. Your psychological identity can be a combination of many views, which often change throughout life.

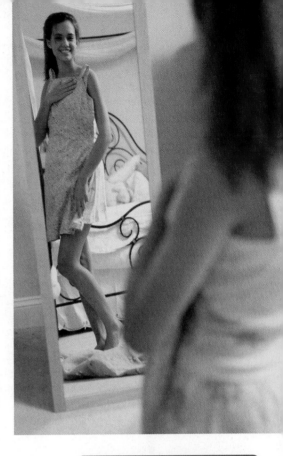

Figure 15.3

During this time in their lives, teenagers may try out different styles of clothing to see which best fits their identity.

identity
who you are, which includes your physical traits, activities, social connections, and internal thoughts and feelings

Figure 15.4

Your social identity consists of your connection to other people, and is formed by your background, activities, and relationships. *If you had to represent your social identity with one photo or piece of art, what image would you choose?*

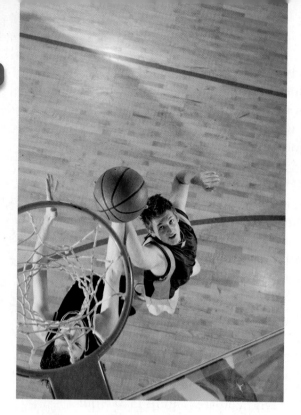

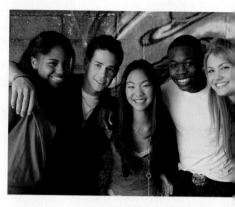

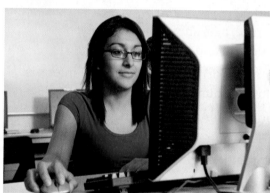

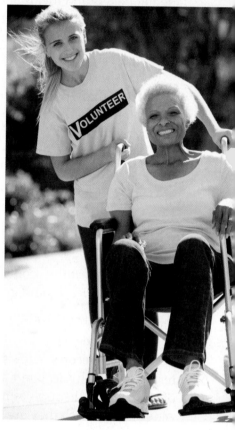

The *role models* in your life, or the people whose behaviors you particularly admire, influence your identity formation. Parents, teachers, other adults, or even older students may be your role models. You might decide to pursue a particular career because a person you respect is in that career. Your role models can also affect your attitudes, such as your beliefs about political issues, sports teams, and music. Perhaps most importantly, your role models can influence your behavior.

Gender Identity

gender identity
a person's biological makeup—male or female—and how a person experiences or expresses that makeup

Gender identity describes not just whether people are biologically male or female—based on their genetic makeup and body parts—but also how people feel about and express their gender. This includes the clothes they wear and their physical appearance.

By three years of age, children usually know whether they are a boy or a girl. Soon after, young children also learn *gender roles*—the "appropriate" types of attitudes and behaviors for someone of their gender. Gender roles are influenced by a person's environment, which includes parents, siblings, peers, other adults, and even media, such as television and movies.

Gender identity is influenced in part by a person's culture. Society typically associates certain traits with *femininity* (being female) and *masculinity* (being male). Society may use certain words to describe feminine traits and other words to describe masculine traits. Societal perceptions of feminine and masculine traits, however, are unrealistic. This is because women may have some masculine traits and men may have some feminine traits. *Androgynous* is a term that refers to people who exhibit feminine and masculine traits equally.

These culturally-defined assumptions about females or males are called *gender stereotypes.* Believing that only girls should play with dolls or only boys should play with trucks is gender stereotyping. Another example is thinking that all women are emotional or all men are aggressive. Gender stereotypes influence how people view themselves and others, and can lead to unfair treatment of a specific gender.

Ethnic Identity

Another factor that influences a person's identity is ethnicity. A person's *ethnicity* describes his or her connection to a particular social group that shares similar cultural or national ties. People may define their ethnicity through traditions, language, religious practices, or cultural values. These aspects of identity can help people feel connected to a particular group that shares their experiences. Ethnic identity can be a very important part of identity formation.

According to Jean Phinney, a developmental psychologist, ethnic identity emerges in stages during adolescence. The following are Phinney's stages:

- *unexamined (or diffused) ethnic identity*—teenagers do not think about the meaning of their ethnic identities.

- *identity search/moratorium*—teenagers actively search for information about the meaning of their ethnicity. The search can include researching their group's history, learning the group's language, and participating in cultural activities associated with their ethnic group.

- *achievement*—teenagers feel secure in their sense of ethnic identity. They see this identity as an important aspect of who they are.

Identity Changes throughout Life Stages

One of the most famous figures in psychology, Erik Erikson, believed that people go through a series of eight stages in life. In each stage, people focus on accomplishing different goals. For example, young children learn how to get dressed and brush their teeth. Being able to master these tasks allows young children to become more independent and less reliant on parents. Setting and accomplishing the particular goals that are most

gender roles
attitudes and behaviors that a society considers "appropriate" for males or females

androgynous
a term that describes a person who exhibits feminine and masculine traits equally

gender stereotypes
culturally defined assumptions about what it means to be male or female

ethnicity
a person's connection to a cultural or national social group

Health across the Life span

Goals throughout the Life Stages

As you can see in the chart below, the particular issues and tasks that people are working on change across the life span. This makes sense because the goals and challenges that must be accomplished change with age.

Analyzing Data

1. Do you think these stages are the same across all cultures? Why or why not?
2. What do you think causes life tasks to change with age? Is this due to nature (meaning biology) or nurture (meaning environment)? Defend your answer.

Erikson's Life Stages	
Stage	**Goal**
Stage 1 (birth to 1 year of age)	*Trust versus mistrust*—Children develop a sense of trust when they have caregivers who provide consistent care. Children who do not receive this type of nurturing develop mistrust in others.
Stage 2 (1 to 2 years of age)	*Autonomy/independence versus doubt/shame*—Children need to develop a sense of control and an ability to act on their own. Children who are successful in these tasks develop a sense of independence. Those who fail develop a sense of shame and doubt.
Stage 3 (2 to 6 years of age)	*Initiative versus guilt*—Children initiate control over their environment, which gives them a sense of purpose. Children who are not succesful at this task feel guilty over their continued dependence on others.
Stage 4 (6 to 12 years of age)	*Competence/industry versus inferiority*—Children need to feel confident about their ability to manage social and academic demands. Children who fail to develop this ability feel inferior to their peers.
Stage 5 (12 to 18 years of age)	*Identity versus role confusion*—Teenagers develop a sense of their own personal identity. Teenagers who fail to do this experience confusion about their identity.
Stage 6 (19 to 40 years of age)	*Intimacy versus isolation*—Young adults form close, intimate relationships with other people. Those who are unable to form such relationships feel isolated and alone.
Stage 7 (40 to 65 years of age)	*Generativity versus stagnation*—Adults feel a sense of usefulness and accomplishment in their families, community, or work. People who do not develop this feel a lack of contribution to the world.
Stage 8 (65 years of age to death)	*Integrity versus despair*—Older adults look back on their lives and feel proud of what they have accomplished. Older adults who feel they have failed to lead fulfilling lives experience a sense of regret, bitterness, and despair.

important during a certain life stage help people feel good about themselves and maintain good mental and emotional health.

According to Erikson, the primary task for you and other adolescents is to form a sense of your own unique identity, meaning who you are as a distinct individual. Perhaps most importantly, Erikson believed that people must develop a sense of who they are before they are ready to join with another person in an intimate relationship. By exploring and testing different interests, values, and beliefs now, you will learn more about who you are. It is important to remember, however, that your identity will likely grow and change further as you mature and develop new interests over time.

Emotional and Social Changes

During adolescence, many teenagers experience changes in their emotions and social relationships. These are all normal changes that occur in part due to the development of greater maturity. These changes can include

- having more interest in dating relationships;
- showing more independence from parents;
- developing a greater capacity to care about others and form more intimate relationships;
- spending more time with friends and less time with family members; and
- feeling more intense emotions, including sadness or depression (Figure 15.5).

Moral Development

Adolescents also show changes in how they think about moral decisions. At the start of early adolescence, around 11 to 13 years of age, most teenagers can engage in abstract reasoning. This ability leads them to question rules and standards from authority figures. By the time they reach high school, teenagers have typically formed their own sense of moral code in terms of what behavior they believe is right and what behavior they believe is wrong.

Teenagers often face difficult moral decisions and can use this code to decide how to act. Suppose you have a friend who tells you she is thinking of cutting herself, but has made you promise that you will not share the secret with anyone else. You have a difficult decision to make. You have to weigh whether it is more important to keep a promise or to seek help in preventing your friend from hurting herself. Teenagers who have a strong moral code understand that some moral principles are more important than others, and that getting a friend help is more important than keeping a promise.

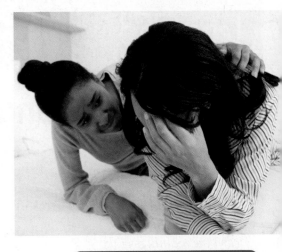

Figure 15.5

One big change that teenagers experience is more intense emotions. *Have you noticed any new, emotional changes in yourself as you've grown?*

Lesson 15.2 Review

Know and Understand Assess

1. List the four different parts of a person's identity.
2. What does *androgynous* mean?
3. Give an example of a way people might define their ethnicity.
4. What are the three stages of ethnic identity that emerge during adolescence?
5. According to Erikson, what is the primary task for adolescents?

Analyze and Apply

6. Differentiate between gender identity and gender roles.

7. Describe how adolescents show changes in the way they think about moral decisions. Do this by creating a story in which 10-year-old and 17-year-old siblings react to a moral dilemma.

Real World Health

Research a published article about gender stereotypes. After finding an article, write a fully developed opinion paper on the topic. Whether you agree or disagree with different parts of the paper, you must state your opinion clearly and provide detailed reasons to support your opinion. Be sure to provide specific examples and details from the article in your paper.

Understanding Self-Esteem

Key Terms
E-Flash Cards

In this lesson, you will learn the meanings of the following key terms.

self-actualization

self-esteem

self-image

Lesson Objectives

After studying this lesson, you will be able to

- distinguish between self-image and self-esteem;
- describe different types of self-esteem;
- identify factors that can affect a person's self-esteem;
- summarize Maslow's hierarchy of human needs; and
- recognize characteristics of people who are achieving self-actualization.

Before You Read

Assess Your Needs

Create a hierarchy of your personal needs using Maslow's Hierarchy. Draw or print a blank copy of the model, as shown below, and fill in each level based on which needs you believe fall in each category.

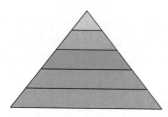

Warm-Up Activity

Understanding Self-Esteem

Choose two people you know who appear to have high self-esteem. Identify which characteristics these people possess that show they have high self-esteem. List these characteristics in a chart like the one shown below.

The characteristics you list may include aspects of physical appearance, such as the person's grooming, hygiene, and dress. Characteristics may also include aspects of social health, such as a person's friendships, or involvement in clubs, sports teams, or other social activities. You may also note your observations about behavior and emotional state. For example, is the person often smiling, pleasant, and friendly?

Using your chart, compare the lists of characteristics for the two individuals. Which characteristics, if any, appear for both of them? What conclusions can you draw from your findings?

Individual #1	Individual #2

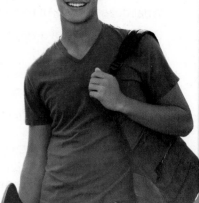

Many teenagers feel good about some aspects of themselves and their lives, but feel dissatisfied about other aspects. These sometimes complex feelings are a normal part of adolescence, when many people are still struggling to figure out what they think of themselves.

In this lesson you will learn about different factors that influence how people think about themselves. You will also learn why the thoughts you have about yourself really matter, and some strategies for trying to become the best person you can be.

Defining Self-Image and Self-Esteem

Do you generally like yourself and feel good about who you are? Answering this question can give you a sense of your self-image. Your *self-image* is your mental picture of yourself, which includes how you look, your skills and abilities, and your weaknesses. You are not born with a self-image. It forms gradually over time, starting in childhood, and it is influenced by your life experiences and interactions with others. As you experience different events and interact with different people, your self-image may change.

Self-esteem is closely related to self-image. *Self-esteem* describes how you feel about yourself. People vary considerably in terms of how they feel about themselves. Self-esteem also changes with life experiences and new understanding.

self-image
your mental picture of yourself

self-esteem
your feelings of self-worth

Types of Self-Esteem

People who like themselves have *high self-esteem*. If you have high self-esteem, you feel good about yourself—including your skills and abilities—and you have high overall self-worth. If you have high self-esteem, you also feel good about your relationships with other people. You feel loved, appreciated, and accepted by your friends and family members.

In contrast, people who have *low self-esteem* doubt their own self-worth and may feel negatively about their traits, skills, and abilities (Figure 15.6). People with low self-esteem may wish they could change their looks, intelligence, or athletic skills. They may feel left out of social groups and disconnected from other people. They may also question whether other people like or respect them, in part, because they do not really like or respect themselves.

Some people think that having high self-esteem means bragging about yourself or being conceited. In reality, however, people with low self-esteem are more likely to show off because they are trying to convince other people of their worth. People with high self-esteem feel good about themselves, so they are not worried about acting in a particular way to get other people to like them.

Most teenagers suffer bouts of low self-esteem from time to time. This is a normal part of adolescence. As teenagers struggle to figure out who

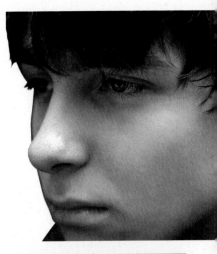

Figure 15.6

Lack of self-worth, doubt about abilities and relationships, and a desire to change one's self can all be signs of low self-esteem. *Based on what you've read in this lesson, how would you describe your own self-esteem?*

they are, they feel uncertain about themselves at times. This uncertainty can cause people to feel lost, or to feel that they do not measure up to others.

Why Self-Esteem Matters

Your self-esteem has a major impact on many different aspects of your life. It affects how well you do in school, how easily you make friends, and how you manage disappointments and frustrations.

This does not mean that people with high self-esteem only experience good situations and never encounter problems. They are, however, better able to cope with mistakes and disappointments than others. People with high self-esteem view negative events and their failures as learning experiences, not as proof of their weakness. Moreover, when they run into obstacles, people with high self-esteem can accept reality and make a new plan. They are also more comfortable asking other people for help and support when needed.

People who have high self-esteem have great decision-making skills. They feel good about themselves, trust their own judgment, and follow their own values. They are confident that they can make the right decision, even in difficult situations. When they are pressured to go along with the crowd, people with high self-esteem have the courage to make the choice they believe is right or take responsibility for a bad choice.

People with low self-esteem, however, often worry about what other people think of them. Being concerned about the opinions of others makes people with low self-esteem vulnerable to peer pressure. They can feel unable to resist pressure to engage in unhealthy behaviors. Unfortunately, these behaviors can have long-term health consequences.

Building self-esteem is not easy, but it can happen as people learn to work through issues and accept who they are. Through experience, people can begin to see how they can take charge and have a positive outcome, thereby improving self-esteem.

Factors That Affect Self-Esteem

Feeling good about yourself is harder for some people than it is for others. Factors that can affect self-esteem include

- social interactions with family members, friends, and others;
- home, school, community, and cultural environments;
- life events;
- media, such as television, movies, and social networking sites;
- body image; and
- personal perceptions.

Many factors can affect self-esteem, but other people have a major impact on how people see themselves. This is especially true during early childhood. Children with parents and guardians who treat them lovingly, which can mean praising them often, generally develop a sense of pride in who they are. On the other hand, children who grow up receiving constant criticism and rejection from their parents and guardians may develop low self-esteem. Social interactions, whether positive or negative, can have a lasting effect on how people feel about themselves.

Personal perceptions also greatly affect how people feel about themselves. Teenagers with low self-esteem may criticize their own appearance and friendships. Some people constantly criticize and find fault with themselves. People who constantly belittle themselves create a negative mindset that erodes their psychological well-being over time. They often do not even notice this negativity, which, unfortunately, can cause others to distance themselves from the person. This further compounds the person's low self-esteem.

Another factor that influences people's self-esteem is how they think about their intelligence, meaning how smart they believe they are (or are not). When most people think about intelligence, they focus on a very narrow view of intelligence, meaning academic knowledge. This is the kind of intelligence that is assessed by standardized tests, such as the SAT or ACT, and often by high school grades.

Intellectual health is much broader than simply knowing facts, figures, and calculations. People who have high intellectual health are curious and enjoy learning new information, whether in an academic setting or on their own.

CASE STUDY   Recognizing the Signs of Poor Mental and Emotional Health

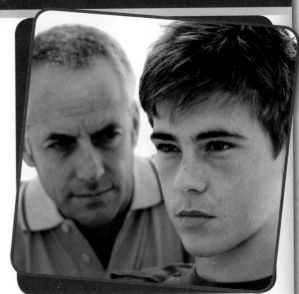

Matt is a 14-year-old high school freshman. For as long as he can remember, his father has criticized his performance in school and in other areas. If Matt has even a single *B* on his report card, his father yells at him for not doing well. When Matt's father watches his basketball games, he criticizes Matt's performance.

Matt is worried about how he will do in high school. He feels he is not as smart as other students, even though he got mostly *A*s in eighth grade. Matt also worries that other people view him negatively, just like his father does. When other students sit with him in the cafeteria, Matt believes they do so because they feel sorry for him and not because they like him. Matt decided not to try out for the basketball team this year because he assumed he would never make it.

Thinking Critically

1. What factors contribute to Matt's low self-esteem?

2. What are some strategies Matt could try to develop a more positive self-image?

3. What advice would you give Matt and other teenagers like him to help them improve their mental and emotional health?

They can think in a clear and organized fashion, and can also think creatively and critically. They enjoy being stimulated by other people's thoughts and ideas, and sharing their own ideas with others.

Self-Actualization

In addition to having high self-esteem, another important part of feeling good about yourself is believing that you are living up to your full potential. Psychologist Abraham Maslow described this feeling as *self-actualization*, meaning you are striving to be the best person you can be.

Maslow's Hierarchy of Human Needs

How do you reach your full potential? According to Maslow, achieving self-actualization occurs only after you meet your basic needs. As shown in Figure 15.7, people strive to meet different types of needs after their basic needs are met.

At the most basic level, people must be able to meet their physical needs for survival. These needs include having food to eat, water to drink, and shelter from extreme cold and extreme heat. Once the basic physical needs are met, people work on meeting the needs listed in the next level. People need to feel secure or safe in their surroundings, including home, school, and work environments.

The next level of Maslow's hierarchy focuses on the need for love and acceptance. This need includes feeling connected with friends and family members and having emotional support from those around you.

Figure 15.7

Where would you place yourself on Maslow's hierarchy of needs? Which needs in your life are being met? Which needs are not being met?

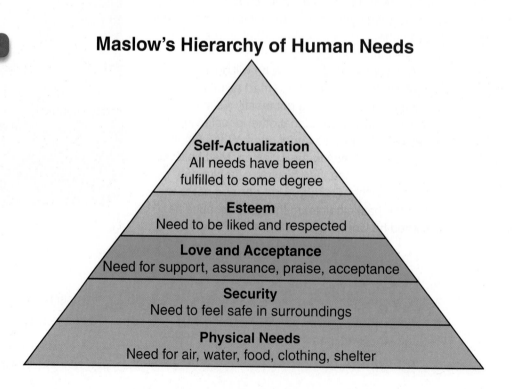

Maslow's Hierarchy of Human Needs

Self-Actualization
All needs have been fulfilled to some degree

Esteem
Need to be liked and respected

Love and Acceptance
Need for support, assurance, praise, acceptance

Security
Need to feel safe in surroundings

Physical Needs
Need for air, water, food, clothing, shelter

The fourth level of Maslow's hierarchy focuses on the individual, and particularly on a person's need to feel good about him- or herself. People also have a need for respect from those around them and a need to feel good about themselves.

Finally, the highest level of needs is the need for self-actualization—the need to reach your full potential. People who are self-actualized continually strive to do everything they are capable of doing. They are focused on continuing to grow, learn, and develop throughout their lives to be the best they can be.

Achieving Self-Actualization

People who are achieving self-actualization and reaching their full potential share certain characteristics. These include

- accepting themselves and others for who they are;
- feeling self-motivated instead of relying on other people to provide motivation;
- working actively to solve problems in the world and in their community, including taking responsibility for finding solutions and helping other people to resolve problems;
- viewing the world with a sense of appreciation, inspiration, and pleasure;
- enjoying spending time with other people, but also feeling a need for independence and time alone; and
- feeling at peace with themselves and the world.

People who are self-actualized also experience moments of intense positive feelings, including joy, wonder, and awe. These experiences lead people to feel inspired, strengthened, and even transformed.

Lesson 15.3 Review

Know and Understand Assess

1. List three factors that can affect self-esteem.
2. Define the term *self-actualization*.
3. According to Maslow, when does self-actualization occur?
4. List each level of Maslow's hierarchy of human needs.
5. List three characteristics of people who are achieving self-actualization.

Analyze and Apply

6. Distinguish between self-image and self-esteem.

7. Compare and contrast people who have high self-esteem with people who have low self-esteem.

Real World Health

Research historical figures or famous people and identify someone you would consider to be a "self-actualized" person. Then write a paper about the person and why you believe he or she has reached this level. After writing the paper, give an oral presentation about it in class. Explain the person you chose and what he or she has done to be considered a self-actualized person.

Improving Your Mental and Emotional Health

Key Terms 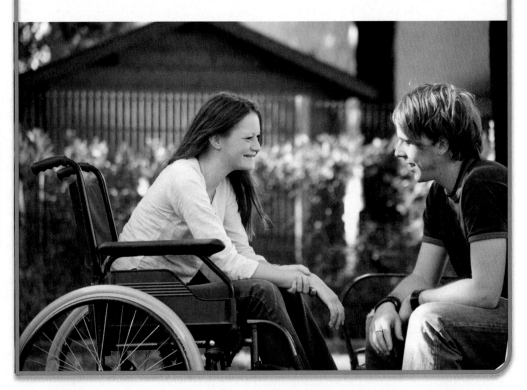 E-Flash Cards

In this lesson, you will learn the meanings of the following key terms.

citizenship
philanthropists
rumination

Lesson Objectives

After studying this lesson, you will be able to

- identify characteristics of people with good mental and emotional health;
- describe strategies for improving mental and emotional health;
- give examples of strategies for improving physical health;
- recognize strategies for improving intellectual health; and
- explain when professional help is needed to improve mental and emotional health.

Before You Read

Tip Chart
Create a chart similar to the one shown below and label the columns physical health, emotional health, *and* intellectual health. *As you read the lesson, fill in the chart with tips given for how teenagers can improve their health in these areas.*

Physical Health	Emotional Health	Intellectual Health

Warm-Up Activity

Your Healthful Activities
Identify actions you take that help you maintain your mental and emotional health, such as discussing problems with a friend. On a separate piece of paper, list these activities and explain the importance of being mentally and emotionally healthy.

You know the importance of taking care of your physical health by eating the right foods, getting plenty of physical activity, and avoiding illnesses and injuries. Did you know that taking care of your mental and emotional health is just as important as taking care of your physical health?

If you feel that your self-esteem could use a boost, there are ways you can improve it with some time and effort. In this lesson, you will learn some strategies for improving your mental and emotional health.

Characteristics of Good Mental and Emotional Health

People with good mental and emotional health share certain traits and characteristics, including the following:

- *having a zest for life*—People who have a zest for life enjoy living and are able to laugh and have fun. They strive to live life to the fullest and see the positive side of situations.

- *being responsible*—Responsible people plan ahead and think before they act. They follow through on what they say they will do and accept the consequences of their decisions.

- *maintaining a sense of balance*—People who maintain a sense of balance in their lives enjoy spending time with other people, but also feel comfortable spending time alone (Figure 15.8).

- *being trustworthy*—People who are trustworthy are honest and fair in their interactions with other people. They do not lie, cheat, steal, or take advantage of others. They are loyal to their friends and family members.

- *being respectful*—People who are respectful treat others with the same courtesy and respect they want be treated with themselves. They are tolerant and accepting of other people's beliefs and values, considerate of other people's feelings, and use good manners. They listen carefully and with an open mind when other people are talking. They manage conflicts with others in constructive ways.

- *being compassionate and kind*—People who are compassionate and kind help people who are in need and thank people who help them. **Philanthropists** are people who make charitable donations to help improve other people's well-being.

- *demonstrating good citizenship*—**Citizenship** describes the status of a person who is recognized by the laws of a state or country as having the rights and duties of all members of that community. People who are good citizens are involved in school and community activities, and work with others to improve their schools and communities. They stay informed about relevant issues, obey laws and rules, and respect authority.

philanthropists
individuals who make donations to improve others' lives and well-being

citizenship
the legal status of being entitled to the rights and duties of a community

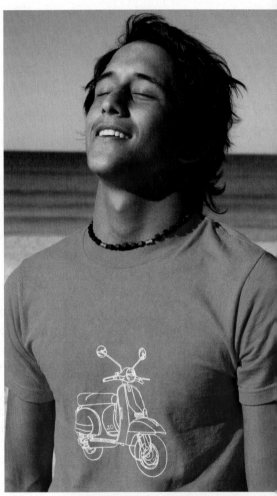

Figure 15.8

Being comfortable spending time alone is a sign of good mental and emotional health. *Why do you think being comfortable with alone time is healthy?*

Strategies for Improving Your Mental and Emotional Health

People who are mentally and emotionally healthy are better able to cope with life's challenges and stresses. They monitor and take care of their own thoughts and feelings and avoid stress and negative emotions whenever possible. They also maintain a balance in their lives between work and responsibilities and play and relaxation.

There are a number of strategies you can use to help improve your mental and emotional health. Trying different approaches will let you determine which of the following strategies help you the most.

Spend Time in Nature

Spending time in nature can boost your mood. Research shows that simply walking through a garden can lower a person's stress and blood pressure. You can improve your own mental and emotional well-being by hiking in the mountains, walking on a beach, or strolling through a park (Figure 15.9).

Develop Strategies for Reducing Stress

Experiencing stress is a part of life. Even the many small stresses of life can sometimes build up and impact a person's mental and emotional health. Strategies for reducing stress may include going for a run or bike ride, writing in a journal, or spending time with friends. Keep in mind the strategies that are most effective and adjust others as necessary to make them work better for you.

Set and Work toward Goals

One of the best strategies for feeling better about yourself is to set realistic goals and work toward accomplishing them. Think about some goals you would like to set for yourself, such as keeping your room clean. Then develop specific strategies for reaching these goals by setting sub-goals, such as organizing your closet.

Achieving the goals you set for yourself feels good, and also builds self-confidence and increases self-esteem. Try to avoid holding yourself to unreasonable standards, however. Each step you take to complete a goal is a positive step. If you miss the goal, reevaluate your progress and then adjust your goals as needed.

Have Fun

Some teenagers feel overwhelmed by the demands of daily life, including homework, chores, extracurricular activities, and after-school jobs. It is important that you also find time in your day, or at least in your week, to spend time doing activities you enjoy. Think about what makes you feel happy and then schedule some time to do those activities.

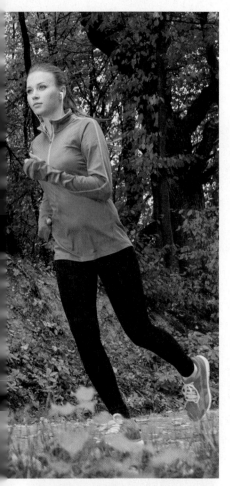

Figure 15.9

Spending time in nature can be a healthy way of calming yourself and caring for your mental and emotional well-being.

Focus on the Good, Not the Bad

Some people spend lots of time each day focusing on what is not going well in their lives. They worry about upcoming exams and tryouts and become absorbed by memories of events that did not go well in the past. They may also obsess about factors they cannot change. This type of negative thinking, which is called *rumination*, can trigger anxiety and depression.

It is much healthier to focus on the events that are good in your life. When negative thoughts enter your mind, shift your focus to something positive and good that has happened. Try to see mistakes or disappointments as opportunities to learn and grow, and not as major crises.

rumination
the act of thinking repeatedly about something for a long period of time

Maintain Close Relationships

Having close and supportive relationships is an essential part of having a healthy life (Figure 15.10). Make sure to develop and maintain close relationships with family members and friends. Join groups in which you can meet people with similar interests, or do volunteer work. Choose to spend time with people who have a positive outlook on life.

Strategies for Improving Your Physical Health

Improving your physical health will lead to improvements in your mental and emotional well-being. Some of the best strategies you can use to improve your physical health include the following:

- getting adequate sleep
- practicing good nutrition
- getting plenty of physical activity
- avoiding risky behaviors

Strategies for Improving Intellectual Health

There are many ways you can work on improving your intellectual health in your daily life. These strategies can be as simple as asking people around you about their jobs, their interests, and places they have lived or visited. You can also read for pleasure, play games, and develop new interests.

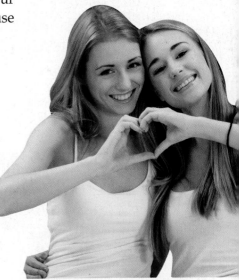

Figure 15.10

Maintaining close, healthy relationships can be challenging, but even one close relationship can greatly improve your life. *What are some qualities of close, healthy relationships? How many of these relationships do you have in your life?*

Make Good Decisions

Some decisions are small and relatively easy to make, such as what to eat for breakfast. Other decisions are much more serious and can be difficult to make, such as choosing a career path. People with good mental and emotional health feel good about the decisions they make.

After you make a decision and act on it, review the outcome. In some cases, you may feel strongly that it was the best choice for you. In other cases, you may realize that the choice you made was wrong. In these situations, you can often learn from the experience. Ask yourself why you made that choice and what you should have done differently. This process of self-reflection will help you make better choices in the future.

Develop New Skills and Interests

Learning new skills and developing new interests gives you a sense of ability and adventure, which boosts your self-esteem and improves your mental and emotional health (Figure 15.11).

You may not even realize some of your talents because you have never tried a particular activity. To find out what talents you might possess, you can join classes and clubs in your school or community. You can also watch online how-to videos to help you develop new skills. Visit places that might help you discover new interests, such as an art museum (many museums provide free or very low-cost admission to students). Attend a poetry reading, dance performance, or musical at your high school or in the community. What other ways can you think of to expand your intellectual health?

Figure 15.11

Discovering and developing new skills and talents can boost your self-esteem and increase your intellectual health.

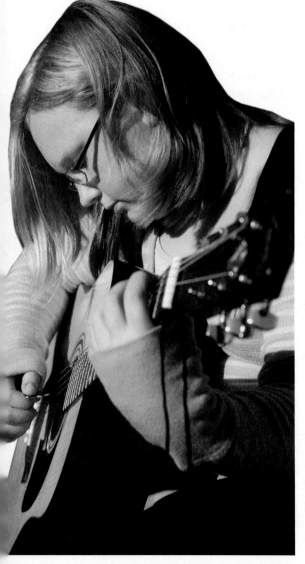

Play Games

One of the best ways of improving your intellectual health is to play games that strengthen your knowledge base, such as trivia games. Games that strengthen creativity, such as charades, can also help improve your intellectual health. You can also work on increasing your intellectual health by taking quizzes on the Internet to test your general knowledge, such as by locating all of the states on a map, remembering important historical dates and figures, and solving math puzzles and logic games.

Read a Book for Pleasure

Some high school students read mostly what they are assigned to read for school. Another great way to improve your intellectual health, however, is to find a book to read during your free time. Reading books helps you learn new words, imagine new places and people, and gain empathy and understanding for other people's perspectives.

Get Help When You Need It

If you make a real effort to improve your mental and emotional health and still do not feel better, consider getting help from a counselor or other mental health professional. These experts are trained to help people who are feeling upset about their lives.

Improving Mental and Emotional Health

The strategies listed below can help you improve your mental and emotional health.

- Take care of your physical health. Get enough sleep, engage in regular physical activity, and eat nutritious foods.

- Make time for relationships to ensure that you stay connected to family members and friends.

- Join a club, group, or volunteer activity to work for a cause you find meaningful. This will help you feel good about yourself and meet people who have common interests.

- Set goals and develop plans to meet them. Chart your progress.

- Determine strategies for reducing stress that work well for you.

- Designate some time each day to have fun and take a break from the demands of daily life.

- Focus on what is positive in your life and stop dwelling on events that are not going well.

- View mistakes as valuable learning opportunities.

If you feel you might benefit from this type of professional help, talk to an adult you trust, such as a parent or guardian, teacher, guidance counselor, or doctor. This adult can put you in touch with a professional who can help you. If the adult you consult does not follow through, then confide in another responsible adult. Remember, asking for help is not a sign of weakness, but rather a sign of strength and courage. You do not need to struggle with mental and emotional health problems alone. Acknowledging your problem is the first step toward feeling better about your life.

Lesson 15.4 Review

Know and Understand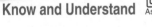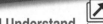

1. List three characteristics of people with good mental and emotional health.

2. What does *citizenship* mean?

3. List four strategies for improving mental and emotional health.

4. List three strategies for improving physical health.

5. List three strategies for improving intellectual health.

Analyze and Apply

6. Research two well-known philanthropists. What characteristics do they have in common? How do they differ?

7. Identify strategies you have used to improve your mental and emotional health. Evaluate the effectiveness of each strategy. How would you modify a strategy to make it more effective?

Real World Health

Many people struggle with improving their mental and emotional health and need to seek professional help. Design a "help sheet" that identifies the names and contact information of health resources available in your community. Organize your list by grouping the different types of professional help into categories, such as hotlines, agencies, and nonprofit organizations. Research each organization to find out as much as you can about its regulations and policies regarding mental, social, and emotional well-being. Distribute the pamphlets in your school and throughout your community.

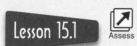
Making Sense of Your Emotions

Key Terms

emotional intelligence   optimism
emotions   resilience
empathy

Key Points

- People experience many different emotions, some of which are unpleasant.
- Learning how to manage emotions can help teenagers as they experience the common emotional ups and downs that occur during adolescence.
- People who have high emotional intelligence are able to express their emotions in healthy, positive ways.

Check Your Understanding

1. Which of the following is a common unpleasant emotion experienced by teenagers?
   A. joy
   B. gratitude
   C. jealousy
   D. pride

2. The first step to managing your emotions is to _____.
   A. acknowledge your feelings
   B. identify your feelings
   C. develop resilience and coping skills
   D. get relief from your feelings

3. *True or false?* Burying emotions deep inside can help them go away more quickly.

4. People who have high emotional intelligence show high levels of _____.
   A. stress
   B. pride
   C. loneliness
   D. empathy

5. **Critical Thinking.** Compare optimism with resilience.

 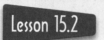
Establishing Your Identity

Key Terms

androgynous   gender roles
ethnicity   gender stereotypes
gender identity   identity

Key Points

- People often focus on different parts of their identities at different ages.
- Gender and ethnicity are factors that influence a person's identity.
- Erik Erikson, a famous figure in psychology, believed that people go through a series of stages in life in which they focus on accomplishing different goals.
- By high school, teenagers have typically formed their own moral code and know which behaviors they believe are right and wrong.

Check Your Understanding

6. Internal thoughts and feelings are a part of a person's _____ identity.
   A. physical
   B. active
   C. social
   D. psychological

7. *True or false?* As children enter adolescence, their focus often shifts from social identity to physical identity.

8. The _____ in a person's life, such as parents, teachers, or older students, can influence identity formation.

9. *True or false?* According to Erikson, forming a distinct identity is necessary before someone can form intimate relationships.

10. *True or false?* By the time they reach high school, teenagers have typically formed their own sense of moral code in terms of what behavior they believe is right and what behavior they believe is wrong.

11. **Critical Thinking.** Give an example of a gender stereotype. How might this gender stereotype lead to unfair treatment of a specific gender?

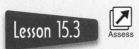

Understanding Self-Esteem

Key Terms

self-actualization   self-image
self-esteem

Key Points

- Self-image and self-esteem are influenced by life experiences and interactions with others.
- People may have high or low self-esteem depending on how they feel about their own self-worth.
- Many factors affect self-esteem, but other people and personal perceptions have a major impact on how people see themselves.
- People who are achieving self-actualization and reaching their full potential share certain characteristics.

Check Your Understanding

12. *True or false?* Self-esteem is closely related to self-image.

13. *True or false?* People with high self-esteem are more likely to show off because they are trying to convince other people of their worth.

14. *True or false?* Media, such as television shows, movies, and social networking sites can affect a person's self-esteem.

15. Children who grow up receiving constant criticism and rejection from their parents may develop _____.

16. According to Maslow, achieving self-actualization occurs only after you meet your _____.

17. When people are living up to their full potential, they are achieving _____.
    A. intellectual health
    B. personal perceptions
    C. self-esteem
    D. self-actualization

18. **Critical Thinking.** Why does self-esteem matter?

Improving Your Mental and Emotional Health

Key Terms

citizenship   rumination
philanthropists

Key Points

- People who are mentally and emotionally healthy are better able to cope with life's challenges and stresses.
- Mental and emotional health is closely linked with physical and intellectual health.
- People can develop effective strategies to help them improve their mental and emotional, physical, and intellectual health.
- People may need to seek professional help from a counselor or mental health professional to improve their mental and emotional health.

Check Your Understanding

19. People who make charitable donations to help improve other people's well-being are called _____.

20. People who focus a lot on what is *not* going well in their lives are engaging in an unhealthy thinking pattern called _____.

21. Which of the following is a good strategy for improving intellectual health?
    A. Read only what you are assigned to read for school.
    B. Make decisions quickly and then do not think about them again.
    C. Ask other people questions.
    D. Spend time in the sun.

22. *True or false?* Asking for professional help to improve mental and emotional health is a sign of strength and courage.

23. **Critical Thinking.** How does improving your physical or intellectual health lead to improvements in your mental and emotional well-being?

Chapter 15 Skill Development

Health and Wellness Skills

24. **Advocate for Health.** Imagine you have noticed a lot of tension within your school during the last couple of weeks and you feel it is important for your peers to verbally express their feelings. Create a telephone hotline at your school for your peers to call anonymously. Research peer hotlines, noting how and why they are created, and then develop a list of questions for peer mediators to use while assisting those who call.

25. **Comprehend Concepts.** Think of a character with low self-esteem from a cartoon, movie, book, or TV show that you enjoy. Be prepared to describe your character in detail when you present to the class. Analyze this character's self-esteem by answering the following questions on a separate piece of paper:
    - How does this character feel about him- or herself?

- What are some examples that demonstrate the character's lack of self-esteem?
- What are some of the character's flaws?
- How would this character be different if he or she had high self-esteem?
- How does this character's family and friends affect his or her self-esteem?
- What is one way this character could boost his or her self-esteem?

26. **Analyze Influences.** Identify a song that changes your mood because of the lyrics or beat. After choosing a song, write a one-page paper explaining how this song affects your mood. Does the song affect your mood positively or negatively? Do you interpret the lyrics the way the artist intended? Do you have a connection to this song because of your past life experiences?

Hands-On Activity
Self-Esteem Project

The term *self-esteem* describes how you feel about yourself. This activity will help you understand what negative remarks can do to a person's self-esteem.

Materials Needed
a container, a water balloon, an empty two-liter bottle, a safety pin, and paper towels

Steps for This Activity
1. For two days, listen to your peers interact with one another. Every time you hear a peer make a negative statement toward someone else, even as a joke, record it on a sheet of paper.

2. After the two days have passed, gather in small groups of about four people. Within your group, compile all the negative comments that your group heard on a new piece of paper. As you discuss these statements, make sure to keep them anonymous.

3. Assign each member of the group a number. Person one will fill the bottle with water. Person two will fill the water balloon from the bottle, tie it, and place it in the container. Person three will be "the reader," and person four will be in charge of the safety pin.

4. After the balloon is full of water, the reader (person three) will begin reading one negative statement at a time. Person four will hold the water balloon over the container. After each statement is read, person four will use the safety pin to carefully poke one hole in the balloon. This will continue until all of the statements have been read.

5. After the statements have been read and the holes have been poked in the balloon, consider the following questions. What does the balloon look like now? Imagine that the balloon resembles the person on the receiving end of those negative comments. Describe that person's self-esteem.

Core Skills

Math Practice

The following graph shows percentages for number of visits of 2.6 million teens who received outpatient mental health services. Study the graph and then answer the following questions.

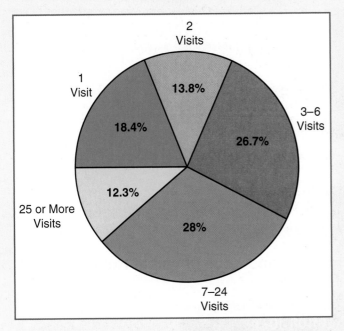

27. How many teens visited outpatient mental health services 7–24 times?
    A. 55,000
    B. 1 million
    C. 728,000
    D. 615,000

28. What percentage of teens visited outpatient mental health services more than 2 times?
    A. 67%
    B. 23%
    C. 100%
    D. 60%

29. How many more teens visited outpatient mental health services 1–6 times than visited 7–25 times?
    A. 500,000
    B. 250,000
    C. 450,000
    D. 483,600

Reading and Writing Practice

Read the passage below and then answer the questions.

Some teenagers feel overwhelmed by the demands of daily life, including homework, chores, extracurricular activities, and after-school jobs. It is important that you also find time in your day, or at least in your week, to spend time doing activities you enjoy. Think about what makes you feel happy and then schedule some time to do those activities. Remember that engaging in activities that make you feel happy is an important part of maintaining good mental and emotional health.

30. What is the main idea of this passage?
    A. Demands of daily life cause some teenagers to feel overwhelmed.
    B. Teenagers have too many responsibilities after school.
    C. Make time to have fun to help maintain good mental and emotional health.
    D. Take an entire week to do fun activities.

31. The word *inundate* is a synonym for which term in the passage?
    A. extracurricular
    B. important
    C. schedule
    D. overwhelmed

32. Which of the following is an antonym for the word *happy*?
    A. dissatisfied
    B. contented
    C. on cloud nine
    D. at peace

33. In a journal, keep track of how you spend your time for one week. Then, write an essay in response to the following questions: How much time did you spend doing activities you enjoy? Do you effectively balance your responsibilities and leisure time? Are there changes you would like to make in your weekly activities to improve your mental and emotional health?

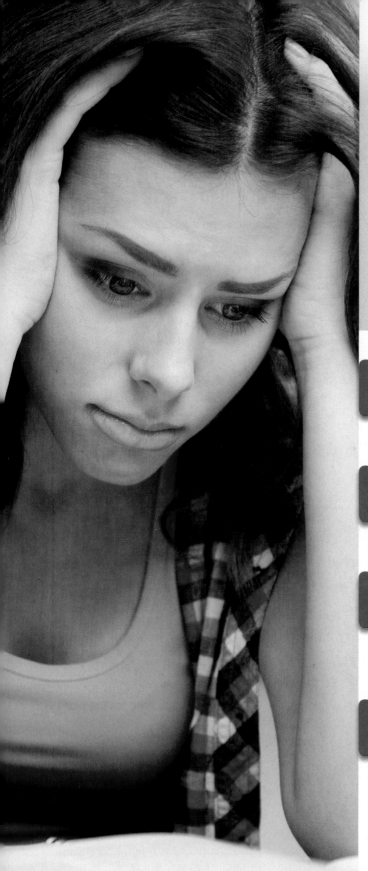

Chapter 16

Managing the Stress in Your Life

Lesson 16.1

What Is Stress?

Lesson 16.2

Stress and Your Physical Health

Lesson 16.3

Stress and Your Intellectual and Emotional Health

Lesson 16.4

Managing Stress

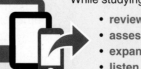

While studying this chapter, look for the activity icon ⬈ to:
- **review** vocabulary with e-flash cards and games;
- **assess** learning with quizzes and online exercises;
- **expand** knowledge with animations and activities; and
- **listen** to pronunciation of key terms in the audio glossary.

G-WLEARNING.com

www.g-wlearning.com/health/

What's Your Health and Wellness IQ?

Take this quiz to see what you do and do not know about stress and managing stress. If you cannot answer a question, pay extra attention to that topic as you study this chapter.

1. *Identify each statement as* True, False, *or* It Depends. *Choose* It Depends *if a statement is true in some cases, but false in others.*
2. *Revise each* False *statement to make it true.*
3. *Explain the circumstances in which each* It Depends *statement is true and when it is false.*

Health and Wellness IQ Assess

1. Only negative events cause stress, not positive events.	True	False	It Depends
2. Your heart rate reacts to stress by slowing down to save energy.	True	False	It Depends
3. Interpersonal relationships can cause stress.	True	False	It Depends
4. Stress can sometimes lead you to perform at your best.	True	False	It Depends
5. Stress disrupts memory.	True	False	It Depends
6. During times of high stress, you should take a break from exercising to give your body a rest.	True	False	It Depends
7. People who experience high levels of stress are more likely to get a cold.	True	False	It Depends
8. Watching a funny movie is a good way to reduce stress.	True	False	It Depends
9. People who write in a journal to reduce stress have lower rates of illness.	True	False	It Depends
10. Social media can cause stress.	True	False	It Depends

Setting the Scene

Imagine that you are about to give an oral report, confront a friend who let you down, or interview for a job. All of these situations might cause you to feel *stress*. Many people find public speaking stressful, and giving an oral report causes them to feel anxious—a psychological reaction. Physical reactions may include trembling, sweaty palms, and an upset stomach.

Stress is unavoidable—everyone experiences it at times. You may even be feeling it as you read this chapter, especially if you will be tested on it tomorrow. Experiencing too much stress at once, or being unable to manage stress, can lead to health problems.

In this chapter, you will learn what causes stress and how stress can impact your health. You will also learn some personal stress management techniques.

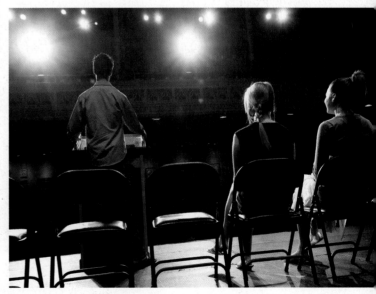

What Is Stress?

Key Terms E-Flash Cards

In this lesson, you will learn the meanings of the following key terms.

conflicts

stress

stressor

Before You Read

Quiz Yourself

Before reading this lesson, read the statements below and consider whether you agree or disagree. After you have read the lesson, consider the statements again and decide whether you agree or disagree. Did your opinion change based on new evidence?

1. *Stress is unavoidable.*
2. *Stress affects you only psychologically.*
3. *People only feel stress from major life events.*
4. *Some stressors can last a few minutes, while others last for hours, days, or even weeks.*
5. *Stress can be positive or negative.*
6. *Your perception of an event does not affect how much stress you will experience from that event.*

Lesson Objectives

After studying this lesson, you will be able to

- differentiate between types of stress;
- understand that stress can be caused by positive or negative events;
- describe how perception influences stress; and
- recognize sources of stress for teenagers.

Warm-Up Activity

Perception Deception

On an index card, describe the most stressful event you have ever experienced. Do not include your name on the card. Shuffle the cards around the class and read the card you end up holding. If you would also experience stress about the event described on the card, draw an X at the bottom of the card. Shuffle the cards several more times, until each person has read 10 cards. Then, find your own card. How many other people were also stressed about your event? Does this surprise you? Why or why not?

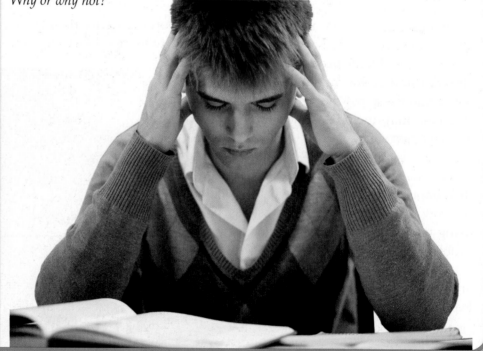

T he physical and psychological reaction of your body to the challenges you face is known as *stress*. A *stressor* is a factor that causes stress.

Types of Stressors

Have you ever taken a test for a driver's license? been asked to the prom? been pressured to do something you don't want to do? These are a few examples of the types of stressors teenagers may experience. Stressors can be categorized and experienced in different ways.

Acute/Short-Term Versus Chronic/Long-Term

Some stressors are sudden and short-lived. This type of *acute stress* comes from the normal demands and pressures of daily life. Acute stressors include experiences like taking a final exam or having a job interview. Your body can manage this type of stress because it doesn't last very long.

People can also experience stressors that continue over long periods of time. This type of *chronic stress* describes ongoing stress that seems to have no clear end in sight. Chronic stressors may include feeling unsafe in your neighborhood or worrying about a loved one who is ill. Chronic stress can lead to depression and hopelessness. It can also produce physiological responses that affect nearly every system in the body.

Major Life Events Versus Daily Hassles

Moving to a new school and losing a loved one are examples of major life event stressors. Researchers have created tables that assign values to the most common major life events. Figure 16.1 lists a sampling of these events in descending order, beginning with the most stressful. The more of these events you experience (especially those at the top of the list), the more stress in your life.

Some stressors are small, but annoying, daily life experiences (Figure 16.2). These can include losing a favorite pair of jeans or arriving late for class. Since these daily hassles occur frequently, they can create more overall stress than major life events.

Negative Versus Positive Events

Sometimes stress feels unpleasant—a knot in the stomach before a big test, for example. Stress can also produce excitement, such as the surge of energy before a championship game.

stress
term for the body's physical and psychological response to traumatic or challenging situations

stressor
any factor that causes stress

Figure 16.1 Major Life Event Stressors for Teens

Death of a parent

Experience parents' divorce

Experience parents' separation

Moving for a parent's job

Death of a close family member

Experience an illness or injury

Experience a parent's remarriage

Parent loses his or her job

Parents reunite after separation

Mother goes back to work

Family member's health changes

Mother becomes pregnant

Experience difficulty in school

New brother or sister in the family

New teacher or class

The family finances change

Break-up with boyfriend or girlfriend

Close friend experiences illness or injury

Fighting more or less with brothers or sisters

Fear of violence at school

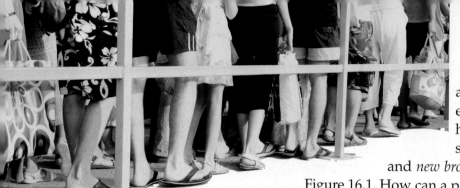

Figure 16.2

Daily experiences such as waiting in long lines or being stuck in traffic may seem like small stressors. As they accumulate, however, these situations can magnify stress in a person's life. *What stressful situations do you experience on a daily basis?*

 Personal Profile

How Much Stress Are You Feeling?

These questions will help you assess how much stress you are experiencing right now.

I feel I have too many activities to do at once. **yes no**

I have lower grades than I would like to have. **yes no**

I feel let down or disappointed by my friends. **yes no**

I have conflicts with my family or friends. **yes no**

I don't have enough time for sleep. **yes no**

I don't have enough time to relax and have fun. **yes no**

I feel lonely. **yes no**

I don't have enough time to exercise. **yes no**

Add up the number of yes answers to assess your level of stress. The more yes answers you have, the greater your level of stress.

conflicts
disagreements or problems that result from opposing actions or views

Although stress is often associated with negative events, positive events can also cause stress. You may have noticed that positive events, such as *parents reunite after separation* and *new brother or sister in the family*, are listed in Figure 16.1. How can a positive event cause stress?

Suppose you are going to the prom. First, your to-do list will grow, which can cause stress, especially if you're already busy. You will have to shop for a dress or tuxedo and arrange transportation. You may have to negotiate a curfew with your parents or ask for time off from your job. You will have to make some decisions, such as what you will wear and how you will pay for it. Although the prom is a positive event, all of these related steps can cause stress.

Same Stress, Different Perception

Your belief about or perception of an event can also influence the stress you experience. If two people experience the exact same event, each person may interpret or think about it in a different way. The meaning a person assigns to an event is a better predictor of how stressful it is than the event itself.

Suppose Joshua and Colleen both fail a math test. Joshua believes failing the test will cause him to be rejected by the college of his choice. For Joshua, this event is very stressful and even life-changing. Colleen views failing the test as unfortunate, but she plans to study harder so she'll do better next time. The event is therefore less stressful for Colleen.

Sources of Stress for Teenagers

The amount of stress a person feels depends on how he or she views the stressor. Most teenagers face similar sources of stress. When facing these stressors, you may benefit from viewing them as a shared experience with your peers.

Relationships

Personal relationships can be major sources of stress when conflicts arise. *Conflicts* are disagreements or problems that occur when individuals have opposing views or interests. The effects of conflict-related stress may become clear after an argument with a friend or parent. The unpleasant exchange may leave you feeling anxious.

Family. Many teenagers experience some conflict at home with a parent or guardian (Figure 16.3). These conflicts often involve differences of opinion about family rules. Some teenagers must cope with the added stress of major family changes, such as their parents' divorce and remarriage. Other teenagers may have a parent with a serious health problem.

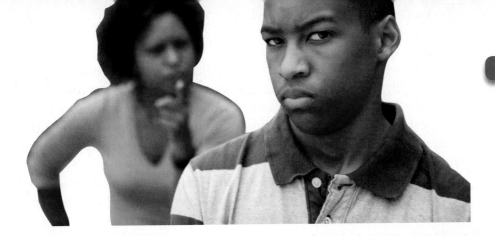

Figure 16.3

Relationships with parents can be a source of stress, especially when these relationships include frequent conflict. *How did you handle the last argument you had with your parents or caregivers?*

Peers. Relationships with friends and peers can also generate stress, at least at times. Stress caused by interpersonal relationships can result from rejection, exclusion, negative peer pressure, or loneliness. Other factors sometimes cause relationships to end, such as having to relocate to a new school. The loss of peer relationships can also cause stress.

School

Many high school students feel pressured to do well in school. They may worry about their grades, upcoming tests and quizzes, and completing homework assignments. Students have to balance the demands and expectations of different teachers, which can be overwhelming at times.

Academic pressure can be especially intense for students who are applying to highly competitive colleges. While staying on top of their academic classes, these students must take standardized tests and complete college applications that can be lengthy. They must balance schoolwork with other activities such as after-school jobs and sports practices. The feeling of having too much to do in too little time can create considerable stress.

Environment

People also experience stress caused by their environment, including the physical aspects of the environment in which they live. Some teenagers live in homes that are crowded and noisy. Coping with noise, a lack of privacy, and clutter can increase stress levels.

Health in the Media

Can Social Media Cause Stress?

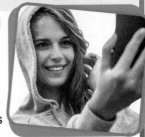

Many teenagers think of social media as a good way to stay connected with friends and family. Being socially connected in this way can reduce stress, but it can also create stress. In one study, researchers asked college students about their use of Facebook and how it made them feel. Some students reported that using Facebook made them anxious. In fact, the more Facebook "friends" they had, the more likely they were to feel stressed by social media.

Having to respond to friend requests created stress for many students—10% of them reported that they disliked receiving the requests. In addition, 63% of the students said they put off replying to a friend request. Rejecting friend requests caused 32% of students to feel guilty and uncomfortable.

People may also feel anxious about what they post on Facebook. For example, if people want to be viewed as cool and mature, they may worry excessively about how others interpret their posts. They may worry about having fewer "friends" than other people and about being left out of the social activities posted by others. People may worry that their own lives are less interesting and less exciting than those of their peers. All of these factors may help explain why Facebook can create stress.

Thinking Critically

1. Do you think social media causes the same level of stress for all teenagers, or are some more bothered by it than others? Explain your answer.

2. What are some strategies that could help you and your friends avoid stress associated with social media?

3. Do you think Facebook has the potential to reduce stress? Consider ways in which Facebook could decrease levels of stress.

Another type of environmental stress is caused by the circumstances in which people live. These circumstances can include concerns about money and safety. Children in families with serious financial problems may worry about getting enough to eat or becoming homeless. They may feel stress about not having money for new clothes or for fees to participate in school events.

Other teenagers may feel stress from living in a neighborhood with relatively high levels of crime. They may worry about being robbed or injured while traveling to and from school.

Have you ever felt stress while waiting in a long line to order food? Being in an environment where you have little or no control, even for brief periods of time, can also make you feel stressed.

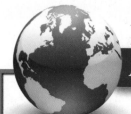

Local and Global Health

Are Some Countries More Stressful Than Others?

According to a large study conducted by an international organization, people in some countries have higher overall life satisfaction than those in other countries. People in these countries may therefore experience lower overall stress. The organization's researchers scored the overall life satisfaction reported by people around the world. They used a scale of 1 to 10 (with 1 meaning *least satisfied* and 10 meaning *most satisfied*) to record people's life satisfaction. Mean, or *average* scores were calculated and the overall life satisfaction scores for selected countries are listed below.

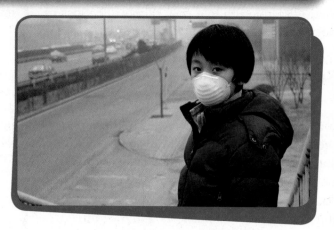

- Norway   7.6
- Australia   7.4
- Canada   7.4
- Korea   6.9
- Mexico   6.9
- United States   6.9
- United Kingdom   6.9
- Chile   6.6
- Spain   6.5
- Japan   6.1
- Russian Federation 5.3
- Turkey   5.3

What factors do you think influence levels of satisfaction? Countries with the highest life satisfaction typically have

- lower rates of unemployment, meaning less fear about failing to meet basic needs;
- lower levels of pollution, including less smog and noise;

- better living conditions, including less crowding and violence; and
- higher rates of affordable healthcare.

These factors are all linked to reduced stress. This may lead to increases in levels of life satisfaction, as well as improved physical health.

Thinking Critically

1. Why do you think levels of life satisfaction in the United States are lower than those in some other countries, including Canada, Australia, and Norway?

2. Do you think the factors predicting life satisfaction are the same in different countries? Explain your answer.

3. This study only examined life satisfaction. Is this the best way to assess levels of stress? Why or why not? What might be a better way to examine differences in stress in different countries?

How Levels of Stress Change across the Life Span

The feeling of having too much to do can cause considerable stress. Researchers have found that this feeling is more common for people during certain times in their lives. People in different age groups were asked if they had enough time to do what they wanted to do each day. The chart to the right shows the percentage of people in each age group who responded negatively to the question.

Analyzing Data

1. These statistics show that a majority of adults from 18 to 64 years of age feel they have too much to do. This feeling is much less common in older adults. What factors do you think contribute to this change?

2. These statistics describe overall stress across the life span for men and women combined. If these statistics were separated by gender, how do you think the percentages for men and women would compare? Explain your answer.

3. This data was collected from individuals 18 years of age and older. What do you think data on people 13 to 17 years of age would show? Why?

Age Range in Years	Percentage of People Reporting Not Enough Time
18 to 29 years of age	54%
30 to 49 years of age	53%
50 to 64 years of age	54%
65 years of age and older	21%

Inner Conflict

Pressure that you exert on yourself can also cause stress. Have you ever felt stressed because you had to make a difficult decision? Having to make choices, especially choices between two desirable options, can cause stress. For example, suppose you had to decide whether or not to take a part-time job. If you took the job, you would have money to buy the things you want, but you would have limited free time for friends. If you didn't take the job, you would have your afternoons free, but you'd have little money. Having to make this type of choice causes stress for many people.

Lesson 16.1 Review

Know and Understand Assess

1. Identify each of the following stressors as either acute or chronic.
   A. interviewing for a job
   B. living in an unsafe neighborhood
   C. planning for prom
   D. taking a final exam

2. Provide one example of a major life event, and one example of a daily hassle.

3. List three possible stressors for teenagers.

4. Describe *inner conflict*.

5. Give three examples of positive stress.

Analyze and Apply

6. Analyze why the same stressor can create a lot of stress for one individual and very little stress for another individual.

7. Evaluate the cause of stress in one of your relationships.

Real World Health

Write a letter to your health teacher and tell him or her about the stressors you are facing in school this year. Include at least 10 stressors. You should also explain how you plan to manage the stress you are experiencing.

Stress and Your Physical Health

Key Terms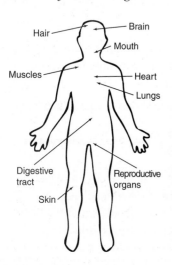

E-Flash Cards

In this lesson, you will learn the meanings of the following key terms.

fight-or-flight response
lymphocytes
stress hormones

Lesson Objectives

After studying this lesson, you will be able to

• understand how the body reacts to stress;

• explain the stages of the body's response to stress;

• summarize how stress affects different body systems; and

• describe the link between stress and illness.

Before You Read

Body Worksheet

On a blank piece of paper, draw a body and label its parts, as shown in the diagram below. Discuss with your classmates the different ways stress affects each part of the body. You should include diseases brought on by stress. After reading this lesson, add the effects you have learned about to your drawing.

Warm-Up Activity

Stress Web

Different types of stress are listed in the chart below. How many of these types of stress do you experience on a regular basis? In a class discussion, give specific examples of stress in your life, how the stress affects you, and how you respond. Do others react to the same or similar stress in the same way you do?

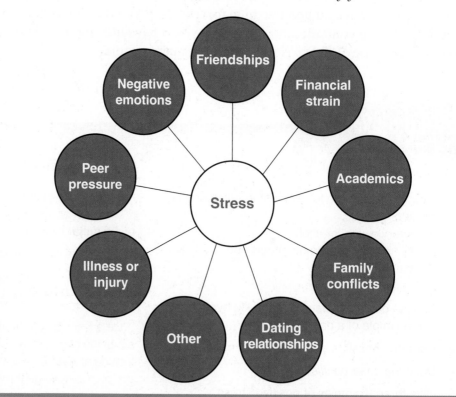

T hink about a time when you were about to do something very stressful, such as take an important standardized test or give an oral presentation. How did your body react in this situation? Did you start breathing rapidly or develop a headache? These are normal reactions your body can have when facing a stressful situation. In this lesson, you'll learn how and why stress can impact your body.

The Body's Response to Stress

Your body reacts in specific ways when you encounter threatening situations, such as a stressful job interview (Figure 16.4). All types of stressors can trigger the same physiological responses.

If you experience a relatively brief threat, your body has plenty of resources stored up to respond. The body's response changes over time, depending on how long the stressor continues. Generally, your body's response to stress can be divided into three stages:

- **Alarm stage**: Your body mobilizes all of its resources to fight off a threat, either by attacking or escaping from the threat. This physiological reaction to a threat is called the *fight-or-flight response*. To prepare for either fighting off or escaping from a predator, your body undergoes several changes, including increases in heart rate, blood flow, and sweat production. The pupils of your eyes widen to improve your vision. In addition, physiological processes unrelated to fighting off a threat, such as digestion and reproduction, are stopped or slowed down. This allows your body to focus its resources where they are most needed.

- **Resistance stage**: Your body continues to devote energy to maintaining its physiological response to the threat. Heart rate, blood pressure, and breathing are still rapid, which helps deliver oxygen and energy quickly to various parts of your body.

- **Exhaustion stage**: If the threat persists, the body may stay in a state of physiological arousal for a long time. In this case, the body's resources will be used up and exhaustion will occur.

fight-or-flight response
the body's physiological impulse to either fight off or flee from threatening situations

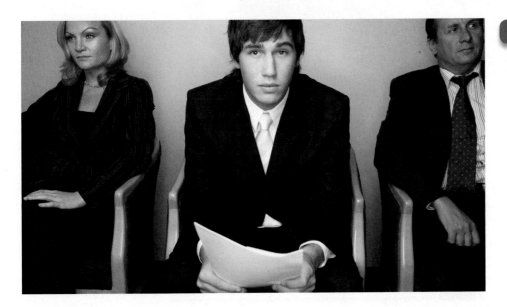

Figure 16.4

Situations that you perceive to be threatening—whether they are actually threatening or not—can trigger your body's response to stress. *What situations trigger your body's response to stress?*

During times of stress, the body devotes large amounts of energy to reacting to that immediate threat. Over time, this energy can run out and the body can become open to infection or disease development. This is why people who experience chronic stress are at a greater risk of developing a number of illnesses and diseases, including the following:

- ulcers
- diabetes
- colds and flu
- asthma
- headaches
- eczema and hives
- back pain
- gastrointestinal disorders
- hernias
- cancer
- cardiovascular disease

Stress may also exacerbate preexisting physical problems or diseases. This is why people with heart disease or high blood pressure are often told to avoid stress whenever possible.

Stress and Body Systems

Stress impacts different body systems, which can then lead to many health problems (Figure 16.5). Body systems particularly affected by stress include the nervous, endocrine, cardiovascular, immune, and reproductive systems.

The Nervous System

The nervous system consists of the brain, the spinal cord, and the neural pathways that bring information to and from the brain. This body system sends messages to the brain that your body is receiving particular sensations—such as touch and pain.

Figure 16.5

In response to a threat or stressful situation, the brain and nervous system send a message to the adrenal glands, which release epinephrine and norepinephrine. These hormones trigger physiological changes that mobilize the body to either fight or flee. Body resources are temporarily diverted away from some areas of the body to areas directly involved in running away or fighting the threat.

Fight-or-Flight Response

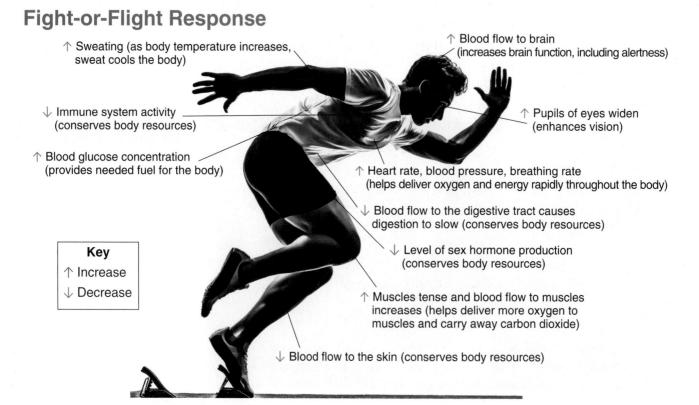

↑ Sweating (as body temperature increases, sweat cools the body)

↑ Blood flow to brain (increases brain function, including alertness)

↓ Immune system activity (conserves body resources)

↑ Pupils of eyes widen (enhances vision)

↑ Blood glucose concentration (provides needed fuel for the body)

↑ Heart rate, blood pressure, breathing rate (helps deliver oxygen and energy rapidly throughout the body)

↓ Blood flow to the digestive tract causes digestion to slow (conserves body resources)

↓ Level of sex hormone production (conserves body resources)

Key
↑ Increase
↓ Decrease

↑ Muscles tense and blood flow to muscles increases (helps deliver more oxygen to muscles and carry away carbon dioxide)

↓ Blood flow to the skin (conserves body resources)

Research in Action

Is Procrastinating Bad for Your Health?

Did you know procrastination could be harmful to your health? Researchers in one study examined how college students managed the stress of their schoolwork. Early in a semester, the students were assigned a paper to complete by the end of the semester. At the beginning and end of the semester, students were asked about their stress levels and any physical symptoms they were experiencing, such as coughs or sore throats.

Early in the semester, students who procrastinated experienced less stress than other students. The procrastinating students, however, experienced greater stress at the end of the semester when postponing the paper was finally catching up with them. The procrastinating students also had more symptoms of illness and were more

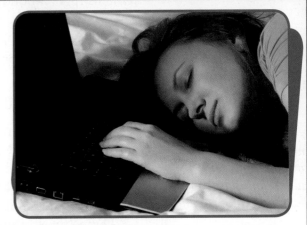

likely to have gone to the health center on campus for treatment. On the other hand, the students who made a plan and kept up with their regular coursework avoided the stress faced by those who ignored their assignments.

Thinking Critically

1. Why do you think there is a link between procrastinating early in the semester and having more symptoms of illness later in the semester?
2. This study only examined college students. Do you think the same results would be found in high school students? Why or why not?
3. How do you think someone who procrastinates could change his or her work habits? Is it possible to stop procrastinating? If so, how?

The nervous system is responsible for mobilizing your body to react to a threatening situation because it regulates many other body systems. In the face of a threat, your nervous system prompts various body systems to act. These systems increase respiration and heart rate, decrease digestion and reproduction, and send blood to the muscles. These physiological changes improve your body's ability to respond to threatening situations.

The Endocrine System

The endocrine system is a set of glands that release hormones into the bloodstream. These hormones then travel through the bloodstream to cause changes in a particular body tissue or organ. During times of stress, the central nervous system stimulates the endocrine glands to secrete *epinephrine* and *norepinephrine*, which are known as the **stress hormones**. These hormones trigger the physiological effects that help the body respond quickly to a threat.

stress hormones
hormones that trigger the body's physiological response to stress; epinephrine and norepinephrine

The Cardiovascular System

The primary function of the cardiovascular system is to pump blood throughout the body. The blood carries oxygen to all the body's cells and organs, and removes carbon dioxide from the body.

People who are stressed show increased cardiovascular activity, including a faster heart rate and higher blood pressure. When blood pressure remains high, a buildup of fatty acids and glucose on blood vessel walls can occur over time. The vessels narrow and the heart must work harder to pump blood through them. This chronic wear and tear that results from stress can cause considerable damage to the heart and the arteries.

The Immune System

lymphocytes
white blood cells that eliminate or disable foreign and possibly infected cells

The body's immune system, which defends against infection and disease, produces blood cells called **lymphocytes**. When foreign cells carrying infection or disease enter your body, they are killed or disabled by lymphocytes. Lymphocytes are classified as either *T cells* or *B cells* depending on their role in the immune response.

During times of stress, your body is focused on escaping from or fighting off a specific threat. The immune system receives fewer of the body's resources as long as the threat continues. As a result, people who experience stress over long periods of time have fewer immune cells in their bodies. These people are more likely to develop infectious diseases than those who are not stressed.

The Reproductive System

The reproductive system consists of a group of organs that work together to allow for the creation of new life. During times of stress, amounts of particular hormones, such as *cortisol*, increase in the body. These hormones affect the body's sex hormones by causing their levels to decrease. The result is lower levels of sperm in the body (for boys and men) and the restriction of ovulation (for girls and women). Lower levels of sex hormones in the body also decrease people's feelings of sexual arousal and can reduce fertility.

Lesson 16.2 Review

Know and Understand Assess

1. Which stage of the body's response to stress is also known as the *fight-or-flight response*?

2. Why are chronically stressed people at greater risk of developing a number of illnesses and diseases?

3. Explain the nervous system's role in response to stress.

4. Which body system secretes epinephrine and norepinephrine?

Analyze and Apply

5. Analyze the effect of stress on heart health.

6. Evaluate why the reproductive and immune systems' functions decrease rather than increase during times of stress.

Real World Health

Imagine that today is your first day at your new job as a physician. You have spent years studying at and attending medical school to prepare for this day. Your first patient comes in with high blood pressure, anxiety, digestion and sleep problems, and diabetes. Write a dialogue between you and the patient in which you explain how stress leads to these health problems. Then create a stress management plan that your new patient can follow.

Stress and Your Intellectual and Emotional Health

Lesson Objectives

After studying this lesson, you will be able to

- summarize how stress affects cognitive ability;
- recognize how stress contributes to emotional problems; and
- understand behavioral problems caused by stress.

Warm-Up Activity

Reacting to Words

As a class, place seven posters labeled Stress, Time Management, Organization, Exercise, Fun, Frustrating, *and* School *around the classroom. Then split into seven groups and take turns discussing each poster's topic. When your group stands in front of a poster, discuss what you associate with that poster's label. Have one group member write everything your group says on the poster. After one minute of discussion, rotate to the next poster and repeat. Once every group has written on every poster, return to your seats. Discuss what has been written on each of the seven posters.*

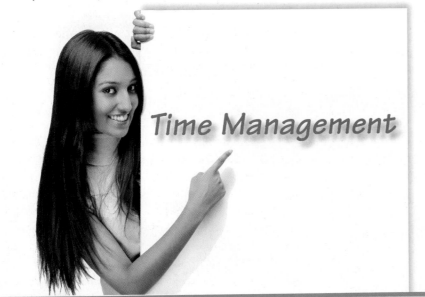

Key Terms E-Flash Cards

In this lesson, you will learn the meanings of the following key terms.

cognitive ability

depression

hippocampus

post-traumatic stress disorder (PTSD)

Before You Read

KWL Chart: The Effect of Stress

Create a KWL chart like the one shown below to organize what you know, what you want to know, and what you have learned from this lesson about how stress affects your intellectual and emotional health.

K What you **K**now	W What you **W**ant to know	L What you have **L**earned

S tress can influence thoughts, feelings, and behaviors. This lesson focuses on how stress impacts your intellectual and emotional health.

Cognitive Problems

cognitive ability
the capacity to think and reason

One of the major ways in which stress impacts intellectual health is by affecting your **cognitive abilities**, or how you think and reason. Stress impacts your ability to think clearly and remember information.

Stress and Thinking

Researchers have studied people who were facing or had faced a threatening event—a test, for example. In many cases, these people had trouble concentrating or focusing on a task, partly because they were distracted by their thoughts about the threatening event.

People experiencing high levels of stress are also at greater risk of being physically injured. For example, a person who is jogging while feeling stressed may be too distracted to pay full attention to the road. This lack of concentration could lead the jogger to trip and become injured (Figure 16.6).

People experiencing stress are also more likely to think negative thoughts. Not surprisingly, these types of thoughts increase stress levels and make it harder to focus on performing tasks well.

Stress increases physiological arousal, which can lead to poor decision-making. When people feel stressed, they are more likely to make impulsive, or quick, decisions. They may forget to consider all the options or the advantages and disadvantages of each choice.

Stress and Memory

hippocampus
the part of the brain involved in the formation and storage of memory

Stress can also cause memory problems. The hormones that are released when stress is experienced disrupt the functioning of the **hippocampus**— the part of the brain involved in memory. By disrupting the hippocampus'

Figure 16.6

High levels of stress can interrupt concentration and lead to physical injuries or accidents. *How does stress affect your concentration? What can you do to improve your concentration when you are highly stressed?*

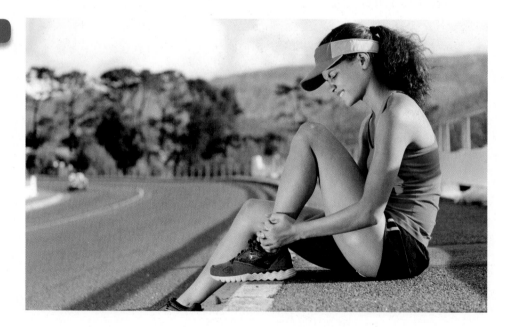

function, these hormones impair a person's ability to create new memories or recall old memories.

Emotional Problems

People facing stressful events often experience strong negative emotions. These emotions can include nervousness, fear, anxiety, helplessness, frustration, irritability, hostility, and anger. Negative emotions caused by a stressful event can trigger hostile behavior toward others.

People's emotional reactions to stressful events vary depending on the type of stressor involved. People who have experienced a major loss may feel disbelief, shock, and numbness. They may also feel a sense of loss and sadness, loneliness, and isolation. Although these emotions can feel overwhelming at times, they are normal reactions to experiencing a major loss.

Certain types of stress can cause some people to develop emotional problems. If someone already has an emotional problem that makes coping with normal daily life challenging, stress can make the problem worse.

Depression

People who experience chronic stress have a greater risk of developing depression. *Depression* is a mood or emotional state characterized by feelings of low self-worth and a complete lack of interest in daily life activities. Researchers have found that the brains of people experiencing chronic stress have lower levels of hormones and other chemicals that make people feel good. Lower levels of particular hormones also cause changes in the body, which can contribute to depression. These changes include a lower level of energy, reduced appetite, and difficulty sleeping.

depression
an emotional state characterized by a feeling of worthlessness and a lack of interest in daily life

Post-Traumatic Stress Disorder

Post-traumatic stress disorder (PTSD) may occur after a person experiences an extremely frightening and upsetting event. These events include natural disasters, war, terrorist events, and sexual assault (Figure 16.7).

Symptoms of PTSD include

- nightmares and recurring thoughts about the event;
- feeling detached, numb, and uncaring;
- an inability to remember parts of the upsetting event;
- lack of interest in normal activities;
- avoidance of people and situations that are reminders of the event;
- difficulty concentrating;
- being easily startled;
- feeling irritable and angry;
- difficulty falling or staying asleep; and
- feelings of guilt.

post-traumatic stress disorder (PTSD)
a mental disorder that results from an extremely stressful event, and which is characterized by flashbacks to the event, feelings of numbness and guilt, and difficulty sleeping

Figure 16.7

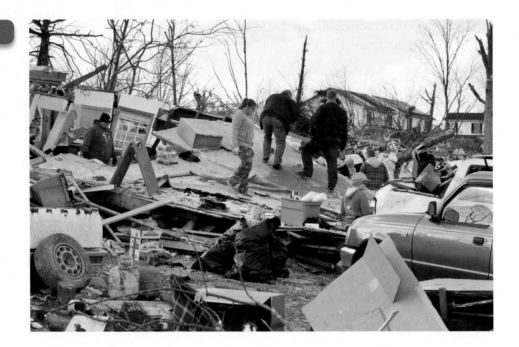

Some people recover rather quickly from traumatic experiences. Others have a strong and lingering reaction. In some cases, these reactions may last for many years.

Behavioral Problems

Can you recall a time when you were stressed out? Perhaps you had several important assignments due at once, or your family was moving to a new town. How did stress influence your behavior? People who experience stressful events can have any or all of the following behavioral problems:

- difficulty falling or staying asleep
- a tendency to cry easily
- loss of appetite
- loss of interest in normal activities

Unfortunately, the behavior of people during times of stress can make effective coping even more difficult. When people are experiencing stress and don't get enough sleep or proper nutrition, their bodies can become run down. A body that is run down has fewer resources to cope with stress, which makes coping particularly difficult.

Interpersonal Conflict

Can you recall a time when you were stressed and you lashed out at someone you cared about, such as a friend or family member?

Stress can cause people to feel frustrated and angry, which can lead to conflict with others (Figure 16.8). People who are experiencing stress often don't treat others as nicely as they should because they are feeling distracted and overwhelmed. In some cases, stress can have very negative consequences, including violence, in relationships. For example, major financial stress is associated with increases in domestic violence. Agencies that assist victims of domestic violence receive more calls during times of high unemployment, when many families are experiencing major financial stress. Couples who report experiencing financial stress are also more likely to get divorced than those who don't experience this type of stress.

Unhealthy Lifestyle Choices

Considerable research reveals that people experiencing high levels of stress are more likely to engage in behaviors that are harmful to their health than those who aren't under stress. High levels of stress are associated with the following unhealthy lifestyle choices:

- smoking cigarettes
- using alcohol or drugs
- eating more foods that are high in fat and sugar
- eating fewer vegetables
- exercising infrequently

Research also shows that people experiencing high levels of stress are less likely to engage in health-promoting behaviors, or take care of themselves. They tend to get less sleep, for example, which is associated with negative health outcomes.

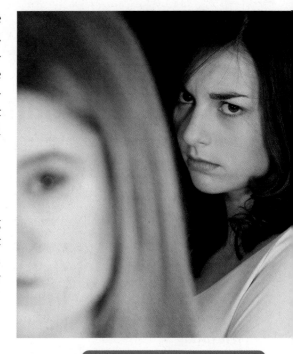

Figure 16.8

Stress can lead to feelings of anger and frustration, which may cause conflict between stressed individuals and the people around them. *How do your interactions with your friends change when you are stressed?*

Lesson 16.3 Review

Know and Understand Assess

1. Explain how stress influences decision making.
2. How do hormones affect memory?
3. Define the term *depression*.
4. List two behavioral problems associated with stress.

Analyze and Apply

5. Depression is often accompanied by a sense of hopelessness. Using what you have learned in this lesson, explain why you think this link exists.
6. Compare and contrast depression and post-traumatic stress disorder (PTSD).

Real World Health

Read the "Dear Abby" letter below and then write a short paragraph identifying the kinds of cognitive, emotional, and behavioral problems Karl is likely to experience as a result of his stress. How might his performance in school suffer?

Dear Abby,
Hi. The lawn hasn't been mowed in weeks, and my room looks like WWII. I fell down the steps because my brother left his skateboard on the stairs. My mom is complaining that I don't spend enough time with the family, and I have a seven-page paper due on Wednesday. I feel like I am going to explode.

Sincerely,
Karl

Managing Stress

Key Terms 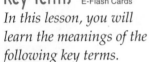 E-Flash Cards

In this lesson, you will learn the meanings of the following key terms.

meditation

positive reappraisal

progressive muscle relaxation

visualization

Lesson Objectives

After studying this lesson, you will be able to

- recall strategies for reducing or avoiding stress;
- describe how to create a time management plan;
- understand when you should seek professional help for stress; and
- summarize the benefits of stress.

Before You Read

Word Cloud

On a separate piece of paper, make predictions about what you will learn in this lesson based on the "word cloud" below. Then, gather into groups of three or four and share your predictions. Finally, choose your group's five best predictions and share them with the class.

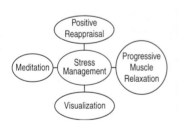

Warm-Up Activity

The Perfect Day

Imagine that you entered a contest and won a "perfect day." As the winner, you choose what you will do and where you will go on your perfect day. Describe your perfect day in detail through the morning, afternoon, and evening. You only have $50 to spend and either a car with a tank of gas or free public transportation for the day. You must be home by 11 p.m.

After you have outlined your perfect day, share your description with the class. Discuss the importance of free time as it relates to stress management. Also discuss how good time management might lead to more free time and more opportunities to have your "perfect day."

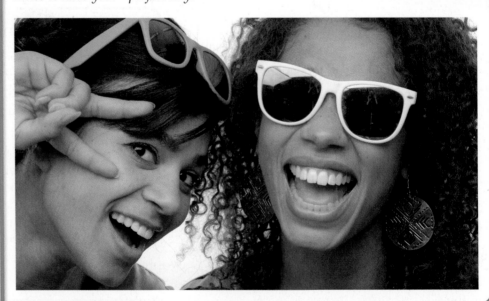

L earning how to manage stress is an important part of staying healthy. People who effectively manage the challenges they face and minimize the negative consequences of stress are called *resilient*. The term *resilience* describes a person's ability to cope with stressful situations, and to return to relatively normal functioning. Not all stress is bad, and when managed properly, may even provide benefits.

Using Stress Management Techniques

You can use many strategies to better cope with stress and become more resilient. Some techniques work better in certain situations than in others.

Manage Your Time

One of the best ways to decrease stress is to manage your time well. Many stressors—such as the feeling of having too much to do at once—can be avoided with careful planning, or *time management*. Planning can be very important when attempting to reduce stress.

To create a time management plan, you should first make a list of everything you need to do. Then break down the big tasks on your list into smaller ones. Create a schedule that describes when you need to accomplish each task and stick to that schedule. This technique is a simple way to keep track of what you have to do and to make sure you get everything done.

Set Limits

People often take on commitments they don't have time or energy for because they have a hard time saying *no*. Being helpful to others is admirable, but committing to many events can create stress when your calendar is already full. Learning to set limits can help you manage stress.

Maintain a Positive Attitude

You can reduce stress by thinking about certain situations in a new and positive way. For example, being stuck in a traffic jam may make you frustrated and anxious. You could come up with productive ways of using that downtime, however, such as making a mental list of what you'd like to do later.

You could also change your perspective on a problem. A strategy called ***positive reappraisal*** suggests that you look for positive aspects of stress-causing events—even negative events. Suppose you tried out for a role in a play or for a spot on the basketball team and you weren't chosen. Not being chosen means you will have more time for homework, which should improve your grades.

positive reappraisal
the strategy of focusing on the positive aspects of a stressful event

Distract Yourself

Many situations that cause stress are either overwhelming or beyond a person's control. These situations may include family financial problems or a debilitating illness. Intense focus on these types of problems can increase stress.

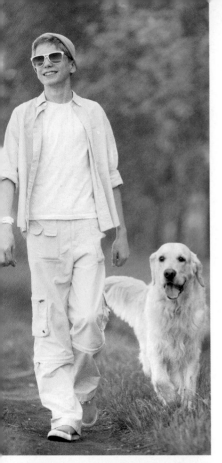

Figure 16.9

When you are overwhelmed by a stressful situation, distract yourself by participating in an activity such as walking. *What activities help you manage stress?*

visualization
the strategy of imagining a pleasant environment when faced with stress

progressive muscle relaxation
the strategy of tensing and then relaxing each part of your body and breathing deeply to relieve stress

meditation
the strategy of clearing negative thoughts from your mind and relaxing your body to relieve stress

Finding distractions can be a good way of managing stress that is consuming your thoughts. Some distraction strategies include

- going for a walk (Figure 16.9);
- volunteering in the community; and
- reading a good book.

These distraction strategies can also help manage stress caused by everyday problems that are beyond your control, such as bad weather. This strategy does not work for all problems, however. For example, if you are anxious about an upcoming science test, developing a study plan is a better way of reducing stress than finding distractions.

Laugh

Another effective way of managing stress is laughter. Humor may help people cope with stressors by distracting them from their problems. If you are feeling stressed, watch a funny movie or TV show, or talk to someone who makes you laugh.

Use Relaxation Techniques

Another useful way to manage stress is to change how your body responds to potentially threatening situations. Instead of becoming tense, you can teach your body to relax using several different techniques.

Deep Breathing. Taking slow, deep breaths helps your brain and body calm down and relax. In turn, deep breathing can have a number of physical benefits, including lowering your heart rate and decreasing your blood pressure.

Visualization. Some people have success using *visualization* to reduce stress. This technique involves thinking about or imagining being in a pleasant environment. For example, if you enjoy the beach, you might imagine the sound of waves crashing and the warmth of the sun on your skin.

Progressive Muscle Relaxation. *Progressive muscle relaxation* is a technique in which you tense and then relax each part of your body until your entire body is relaxed. Practicing deep breathing as you relax each part of your body increases the effectiveness of this technique.

Meditation. The goal of *meditation* is to reduce negative or stressful thoughts that can lead your body to become tense. During meditation, you clear your mind of all negative and stressful thoughts and concentrate on relaxing your body.

Yoga. Yoga involves performing a series of postures and breathing exercises (Figure 16.10). Performing yoga poses involves balance, flexibility, and intense concentration, which requires both physical and mental discipline.

Take Care of Yourself

During times of stress, many people neglect their physical needs. Failing to take care of yourself increases your risk for illness, which can further contribute to stress. During these times, it's important to eat well to provide your body with the energy and nutrients it needs. You also need regular exercise and adequate sleep.

Avoid Tobacco, Alcohol, and Drugs. People who are experiencing stress sometimes use tobacco, alcohol, or drugs to feel better. This approach to managing stress can lead to even more serious problems, which only serve to increase stress. Using substances to deal with stress can contribute to

- social problems with friends who aren't comfortable with substance use;
- academic problems that result from substance use; and
- legal problems due to trouble with law enforcement.

Physical Activity. Engaging in physical activity is a great way to reduce stress. People who engage in regular physical activity experience fewer negative physiological effects of stress. Physical activity reduces the effect of stress on cardiovascular responses, including heart rate and blood pressure. Exercising the muscles also helps them relax.

Express Your Feelings

Simply expressing your feelings—verbally or in writing—can be a good strategy for reducing stress.

Talk to a Friend or Family Member. One of the best strategies for managing stress is to talk to the people who you trust most. The people you confide in may have useful advice for how to handle your problem. They might have been in a similar situation before and can provide helpful insight and suggestions. They might also help you think about the problem in a new way.

Even if a solution is not found, simply talking about your problems can be effective for reducing stress. Sharing your thoughts and feelings—instead of keeping them bottled up inside you—can reduce the amount of stress you feel.

Write in a Journal. Reflecting on problems can also help release and manage stress (Figure 16.11). You can do this by keeping a journal to write about your problems and how you feel about them.

Seek Professional Help When Needed

Recovery from major stressors—such as the death of a loved one or a major natural disaster—can be especially difficult. People experiencing such stressors can become frustrated and discouraged. It is helpful to remember that recovery takes time.

People who experience symptoms of stress for more than a couple of weeks should talk to a mental health professional. These professionals are trained to diagnose mental health problems and to help people cope with the emotional problems caused by stress. Professionals who can help include psychologists, social workers, therapists, and guidance counselors.

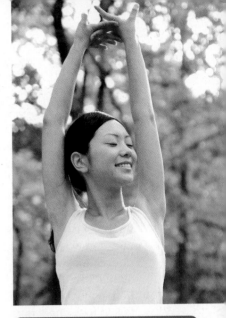

Figure 16.10

Yoga is a relaxation technique that requires intense concentration and discipline. *Why do you think yoga is considered a relaxation technique?*

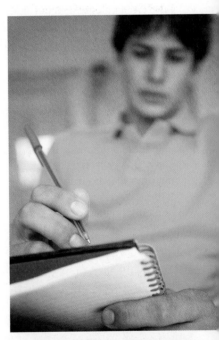

Figure 16.11

Writing about your feelings and thoughts can be a helpful technique for managing stress.

Why Managing Stress Feels Good and Helps You Stay Healthy

Liliana is a 14-year-old freshman. When she started high school, Liliana didn't know many other kids because her family had just moved to town. At the beginning of the year, Liliana's grades were low and she felt less prepared for high school than the other students in her classes. Liliana felt very stressed when she had a test or an assignment due. She began having persistent headaches and stomachaches, which sometimes kept her home from school. Liliana's English teacher suggested she talk to the school nurse about her health problems.

According to the nurse, Liliana's symptoms were the result of stress. The nurse suggested several strategies to reduce Liliana's level of stress and help her perform better in her classes. First, Liliana decided to spend 10 to 15 minutes each Sunday night looking over upcoming assignments for the week and planning when she would do each assignment. Second, she signed up for a yoga class to help her relax her mind and body. Third, Liliana planned to take a bike ride after school each day to relax and clear her mind before starting on her homework.

Liliana is confident these stress-management strategies will lead to greater success in her classes and fewer stress-related health problems.

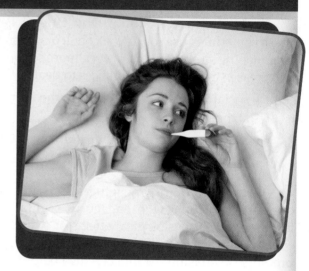

Thinking Critically

1. What do you think are the primary factors that led Liliana to develop health problems?

2. What are some other strategies that might help Liliana feel better?

3. What advice would you give to other teenagers to prevent them from feeling overwhelmed and becoming sick like Liliana?

Figure 16.12

In moderate amounts, stress can cause psychological and physiological arousal, leading to increased levels of energy and performance.

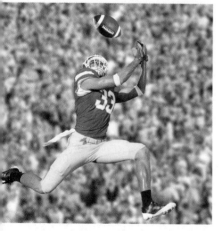

It is especially important to seek help from a professional if the symptoms of stress last for more than a couple of weeks, and if they interfere with your ability to function in daily life. For example, people who are experiencing severe stress may have trouble getting out of bed in the morning. They may lose their desire to eat and experience severe weight loss. You can talk to an adult you trust—a parent, doctor, or guidance counselor for example—for information on a mental health professional in your area.

Benefiting from Stress

A certain amount of stress is unavoidable. When stress is managed properly, however, it can be used to your benefit (Figure 16.12). For example, experiencing threatening or stressful events can help you develop important skills for managing future stress. People who experience stressful situations are able to learn valuable skills by coping with and adapting to such challenges. These skills can be useful later when faced with a new stressful situation.

There are also physiological benefits from experiencing stress. Moderate levels of stress can increase physiological arousal, which is a state of feeling

Reducing Stress

The strategies listed below can help you reduce the stress you feel, and improve your psychological and physical health. Remember that different strategies work for different people, so try a few to see what works best for you!

- Develop a plan for managing assignments and obligations. Having a plan can reduce stress by giving you a sense of control.

- Distract yourself from problems, at least for a little while. Take a bike ride, watch a movie, or read a good book.

- Talk to a friend, sibling, parent, or someone else you trust about your problems. You might get some useful advice on managing your stress. Simply sharing your feelings will help reduce the stress you feel.

- Take care of yourself. During times of stress, eat healthy foods, exercise regularly, and get enough sleep.

- Watch a funny television show or movie. Laughter is a great way to reduce stress.

- Maintain a positive attitude. Try to see the good aspects of challenging situations whenever possible.

- Find ways to relax. Take a yoga class, go for a run, or try meditating to relax your body and clear your mind.

---

especially physically and psychologically excited. In this state, people have extra energy that can help them perform at their best.

Physiological arousal can improve performance in high-level athletes because this state of excitation increases energy and concentration. Increased levels of arousal can also improve performance on other types of tasks, including delivering a speech, performing on stage, interviewing for a job, and taking a test.

Next time you are feeling stressed, try viewing it as a learning experience from which you can benefit in the future. Harness your response to stress to improve your performance on a test, the stage, or the field.

Lesson 16.4 Review

Know and Understand

1. Define *resilience*.
2. List six strategies to reduce or avoid stress.
3. What are the indications that someone may need professional help to deal with stress?
4. Name five relaxation techniques.
5. Why is writing in a journal therapeutic?

Analyze and Apply

6. Select an upcoming project or assignment and create a time management plan to organize your work.

7. Generate a list of ways you could express your feelings in addition to those mentioned in this chapter.

Real World Health

Stress Buster Calendar Draw a calendar of the next 30 days, including the month, dates, and any official holidays. Then, in the boxes for each day, write one thing you can do to decrease your stress level. Do not repeat any activities; each day should be different. Display your calendar somewhere in your room and try to do all of the activities on your calendar.

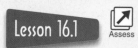
What Is Stress?

Key Terms

conflicts   stressor

stress

Key Points

- Types of stress vary based on duration, source, or the individual's perception. Some types of stress can be positive.
- Stress can be caused by both positive events, such as the prom, and negative events, such as a big test.
- Sources of teen stress can be relationships, school demands, the teen's environment, or of the teen's own making.
- The stress you experience can be influenced by your perception of an event.

Check Your Understanding

1. The body's reaction to stress is both psychological and _____.
   - A. emotional
   - B. short-lived
   - C. physical
   - D. None of the above

2. Identify each of the following stressors as either acute or chronic.
   - A. invitation to prom
   - B. living in unsafe neighborhood
   - C. final exam in chemistry
   - D. immediate family member diagnosed with cancer

3. *True or false?* Daily hassles do not cause stress.

4. Which of the following statements about stress is true?
   - A. A person's perception of an event has no effect on how stressful the event is.
   - B. Although stress is often associated with negative events, positive events can also cause stress.
   - C. Daily life events do not contribute to stress.
   - D. Both A and B

5. List four sources of stress for teenagers.

6. **Critical Thinking.** Analyze the two ways environment can cause stress.

 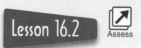
Stress and Your Physical Health

Key Terms

fight-or-flight response   stress hormones

lymphocytes

Key Points

- Different types of stressors lead to the same physiological responses in the body.
- The body goes through three stages when responding to stress—alarm, resistance, and exhaustion.
- Stress affects many of the body's systems, which can lead to health issues.

Check Your Understanding

7. The changes in heart rate, blood flow, sweating, and vision that the body undergoes in reaction to a threat is called _____.
   - A. fear
   - B. adrenaline
   - C. fight-or-flight
   - D. alarm reaction

8. Which stage of stress response is characterized by the body's resources being depleted?
   - A. exhaustion
   - B. alarm
   - C. resistance
   - D. fight-or-flight

9. Which of the following is a hormone secreted by the endocrine system during the stress response?
   - A. epinephrine
   - B. norepinephrine
   - C. estrogen
   - D. Both A and B

10. *True or false?* Lymphocytes are receptors in the nervous system that receive particular sensations such as touch, pressure, temperature, and pain.

11. Which body system is responsible for mobilizing the body to react to a threatening situation?
    - A. cardiovascular system
    - B. reproductive system
    - C. nervous system
    - D. immune system

12. During times of stress, _____ increases in the body, causing the body's sex hormones to decrease.
    A. cortisol
    B. lymphocyte
    C. epinephrine
    D. None of the above

13. **Critical Thinking.** Compare how the various body systems respond during stress.

Stress and Your Intellectual and Emotional Health

Key Terms

cognitive ability   post-traumatic stress
depression   disorder (PTSD)
hippocampus

Key Points

- Stress affects the ability to think clearly and remember information.
- Chronic stress or extremely frightening events can trigger emotional problems.
- Behavioral problems such as interpersonal conflict can arise as a result of stress.

Check Your Understanding

14. *True or false?* Stress impacts intellectual health by affecting your cognitive abilities.

15. *True or false?* Stress-induced physiological arousal improves decision-making skills.

16. The _____ is the part of the brain involved in memory.
    A. epinephrine
    B. hippocampus
    C. cortisol
    D. lymphocyte

17. Which of the following statements about depression is true?
    A. People who experience chronic stress have a greater risk of developing depression.
    B. Low levels of particular hormones can contribute to depression.
    C. Depression is characterized by feelings of low self-worth and a complete lack of interest in daily life activities.
    D. All of the above

18. *True or false?* Post-traumatic stress disorder (PTSD) occurs after experiencing an extremely frightening and upsetting event.

19. **Critical Thinking.** Analyze why behavior problems make coping with stress even more difficult.

Managing Stress

Key Terms

meditation   progressive muscle
positive reappraisal   relaxation
                                 visualization

Key Points

- Many strategies exist to help you reduce the stress you experience.
- Creating a time management plan can help you stay on track and avoid stress.
- When stress interferes with your daily life, you should seek professional help.
- Stress can be beneficial when managed properly.

Check Your Understanding

20. Which of the following phrases best describes a resilient person?
    A. purposefully avoids challenges and stressful situations at any cost
    B. actively seeks out challenges and stressful situations
    C. effectively manages stressful situations and challenges as they arise
    D. None of the above

21. *True or false?* Distraction would be an effective strategy for dealing with stress related to an upcoming final exam.

22. Which of the following is *not* a relaxation technique for relieving stress?
    A. deep breathing
    B. synchronization
    C. meditation
    D. visualization

23. *True or false?* Journaling can be an effective way to manage stress.

24. **Critical Thinking.** Analyze how you can benefit from stress.

Health and Wellness Skills

25. **Analyze Influences.** Tear one piece of paper into 16 squares and arrange the squares in rows of four on your desk. Write the names of four people who mean the most to you on four of the squares. Write your four most important roles, now or in the future, on four more squares. On the next four squares, write your four most treasured material possessions. On the last four squares, write four activities you enjoy. Next, everyone in your class should get up and walk around the room, throwing away one or two squares from other students' desks. Consider which squares are left. How would you feel about losing the squares that were thrown away? Consider how all of your squares affect your ability to manage stress in your life.

26. **Practice Healthy Behaviors.** In a small group, discuss your dream car. How much time and money would you spend taking care of it? Now, consider: How does the amount you'd be willing to spend taking care of your car compare to the amount you'd spend managing your health and stress levels? Write a short paragraph describing what you *should* be doing to manage your stress and care for yourself.

27. **Comprehend Concepts.** Bring two balloons to class and find a partner. One partner should brainstorm all of the stressors a teen might face in any given day. The other student should brainstorm stress-management techniques. After brainstorming, take turns listing stressors and stress-management techniques. Every time a stressor is listed, blow a small amount of air into the balloon. Every time a stress-management technique is given, let a little bit of air out of the balloon. Write a short paragraph about what you learned.

28. **Make Decisions.** Chris is a junior in high school and is trying to get accepted into a competitive college next year. Math has always been a problem for Chris, and his math grade is at an all-time low. Every weekend is crucial study time to help Chris earn his desired grades. His youth group is having a big retreat this weekend, and all of his friends are going. Chris has not spent any time with his friends lately because of his stressful academic situation. Using the DECIDE model, help Chris make a decision about the trip.

Hands-On Activity
Goalball

Explaining your stressful situations to someone you trust is a good stress-management technique. This activity will give you a chance to confide in your classmates and get their feedback on some stressful situations.

Steps for this Activity

1. Write your name on a blank sheet of paper and then describe a task you need to complete by the end of the month. The task could be a set of chores, a homework assignment, or an extracurricular activity.

2. Crumple up the piece of paper and throw it across the room.

3. Walk around the room and retrieve a random piece of paper. Read the task and create a smaller, more manageable goal the person can use to get closer to the large goal. Make sure the goal you write is *SMART* (specific, measurable, action oriented, realistic, and timely) and is something the person could accomplish this week.

4. Return the sheet of paper to the person whose name is written at the top.

5. When you get your paper back, consider the goal the other person created for you. Then write a short paragraph reflecting on how the smaller, more achievable goal alters your perception of the larger task, if at all. Why do you think setting small goals is helpful for managing stress?

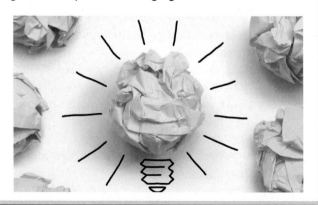

Core Skills

Math Practice

School can be a source of stress for high school students. Answer the following questions using information about the percentage of 15-year-olds from different countries who agreed with the statement "My teachers expect too much of me at school."

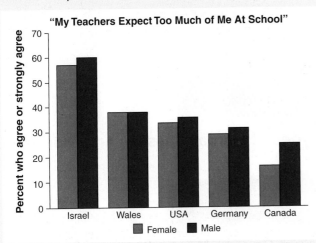

"My Teachers Expect Too Much of Me At School"

29. The boys agree or strongly agree with the "teachers expect too much" statement more than the girls agree in every country *except* _____.
    A. the United States
    B. Germany
    C. Wales
    D. Canada

30. In which country is the ratio of boys who agree with the statement to girls who agree closest to a 2 to 1 ratio?
    A. the United States
    B. Canada
    C. Israel
    D. Germany

31. Which of the following statements best describes the comparison between the number of female Israeli students and female Canadian students who agree or strongly agree with the statement?
    A. More than 3 times as many Israeli students agree or strongly agree.
    B. More than 4 times as many Canadian students agree or strongly agree.
    C. 31 percent more Israeli students agree or strongly agree.
    D. Insufficient information is provided to answer the question.

Reading and Writing Practice

Read the passage below and then answer the questions.

When stress is managed properly it can be used to your benefit. Experiencing threatening or stressful events can help you develop important skills for managing future stress. People who experience stressful situations are able to learn valuable skills by coping with and adapting to such challenges.

Moderate levels of stress can also increase physiological arousal, which is a state of feeling especially physically and psychologically excited. In this state, people have extra energy that can help them perform at their best.

Next time you are feeling stressed, try viewing it as a learning experience from which you can benefit in the future. Harness your response to stress to improve performance on a test, the stage, or the field.

32. What is the author's main idea in this passage?
    A. People often have a difficult time adapting to stressful situations.
    B. Stress can contribute to a state of physiological arousal.
    C. Stress can be beneficial when managed properly.
    D. People perform better under stress due to fear.

33. Which of the following best describes a physiological benefit of stress?
    A. learning valuable skills by coping with a challenge
    B. extra energy contributing to optimal performance
    C. a moderate level of stress
    D. All of the above

34. In this passage, which of the following definitions best applies to the author's use of the word *harness*?
    A. to place a yoke on
    B. to tie together
    C. to utilize
    D. None of the above

35. Write a paragraph describing a time when you used stress to your benefit.

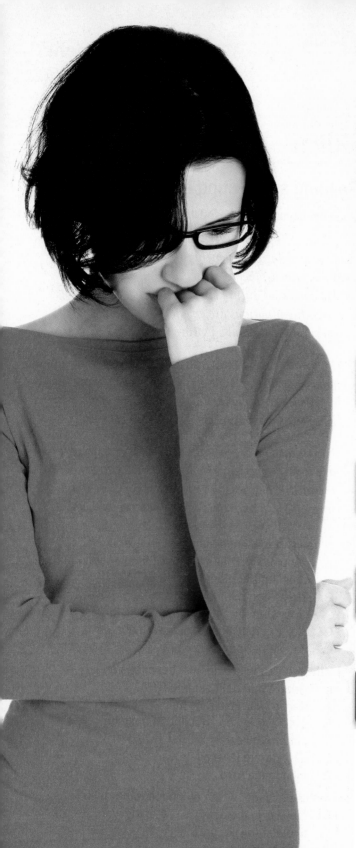

Chapter 17

Mental Illnesses and Disorders

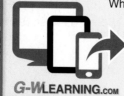

While studying this chapter, look for the activity icon ⬀ to:
- **review** vocabulary with e-flash cards and games;
- **assess** learning with quizzes and online exercises;
- **expand** knowledge with animations and activities; and
- **listen** to pronunciation of key terms in the audio glossary.

G-WLEARNING.com

www.g-wlearning.com/health/

Take this quiz to see what you do *and* do not *know about mental illness and its impact on health. If you cannot answer a question, pay extra attention to that topic as you study this chapter.*

1. *Identify each statement as* True, False, *or* It Depends. *Choose* It Depends *if a statement is true in some cases, but false in others.*

2. *Revise each* False *statement to make it true.*

3. *Explain the circumstances in which each* It Depends *statement is true and when it is false.*

Health and Wellness IQ Assess

1. Anxiety and depression are two of the most common types of mental illnesses and disorders.	True	False	It Depends
2. Phobias are a mental disorder.	True	False	It Depends
3. Untreated depression can have serious consequences.	True	False	It Depends
4. People with autism have trouble interacting with other people.	True	False	It Depends
5. Most people with a mental disorder could get over it if they just tried hard enough.	True	False	It Depends
6. Someone who talks about suicide or writes about it on social media is probably just joking.	True	False	It Depends
7. Suicide is a leading cause of death among teenagers in the United States.	True	False	It Depends
8. Medications can be useful in treating mental disorders.	True	False	It Depends
9. Being physically active can be an effective strategy for coping with negative feelings and stress.	True	False	It Depends
10. If you're a good enough friend, you can cure your friend's mental disorder.	True	False	It Depends

Setting the Scene

What do Abraham Lincoln, Ludwig van Beethoven, Vincent van Gogh, Ernest Hemingway, and Charles Dickens have in common? Are you surprised to learn that all of these successful people suffered from serious mental health conditions? Mental health conditions are surprisingly common and treatable. In fact, many people who are affected by mental health conditions have active, productive, and fulfilling lives.

In this chapter you will learn about different types of serious mental health conditions, what is thought to cause these conditions, and how they can be successfully treated. You will also read about how some mental health conditions may contribute to the risk for suicide. You will learn to recognize some characteristics of those who are considering suicide, and what you and others can do to help prevent people from committing suicide.

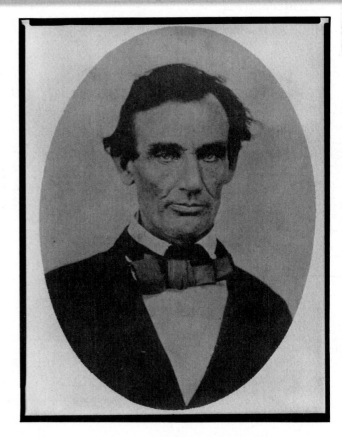

Types of Mental Illnesses and Disorders

Key Terms E-Flash Cards

In this lesson, you will learn the meanings of the following key terms.

antisocial personality disorder

anxiety disorder

bipolar disorder

borderline personality disorder

major depression

mental illness

panic attacks

schizophrenia

Before You Read

KWL Chart: Mental Disorders

Create a KWL chart like the one shown below. Write what you know and what you want to know about mental disorders in the appropriate columns. In the third column, list what you learn as you read this lesson.

K What you Know	W What you Want to know	L What you have Learned

Lesson Objectives

After studying this lesson, you will be able to

- define the terms *mental illness* and *mental disorder*;
- describe types of anxiety disorders;
- differentiate between depression and major depression;
- identify other types of mental illnesses and disorders; and
- recognize symptoms for different types of mental illnesses and disorders.

Warm-Up Activity

Empathy Exercise
Mental illnesses and disorders impair people's ability to function in daily life. On a separate sheet of paper, make a list of what you do every day. The list can include what you must do as well as what you choose to do. Next to each item on the list, write your answer to this question: How would being unable to do this affect my physical, emotional, intellectual, and social health?

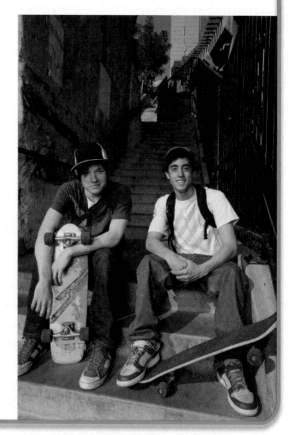

A lmost everyone struggles with feelings of anxiety, sadness, and the occasional irrational fear. Sometimes, however, mental and emotional problems are so severe that people are unable to function in daily life. This lesson describes some of the more serious types of mental health conditions people experience.

Defining Mental Illnesses and Disorders

A *mental illness* is a medical condition that is characterized by a mental or emotional problem so severe that it interferes with daily functioning. For example, a fear of being in public places could lead a person to avoid going to school, work, or even to visit with family and friends.

The terms *mental illness* and *mental disorder* are often used interchangeably because they both refer to serious mental health conditions involving thoughts, feelings, or behaviors. Anxiety and depression are two of the most common types of mental disorders.

mental illness
a medical condition in which a person experiences mental or emotional problems severe or persistent enough to interfere with daily functioning; also known as mental disorder

Anxiety

Almost everyone experiences anxiety in some situations. Common signs and symptoms of anxiety may include an increased heart rate, rapid breathing, sweaty palms, and an upset stomach.

People who experience extreme anxiety in particular situations have an **anxiety disorder**. These people have extreme and unrealistic worries about daily life events, experiences, or objects (Figure 17.1). Different types of anxiety disorders include the following:

- *Panic disorder.* People with panic disorder experience **panic attacks**, or episodes of intense fear that something bad is going to happen. Panic attacks are accompanied by severe physical symptoms, such as heart palpitations and nausea.

anxiety disorder
a mental illness characterized by extreme or unrealistic worries about daily events, experiences, or objects

panic attacks
episodes of intense fear that are often accompanied by serious physical symptoms

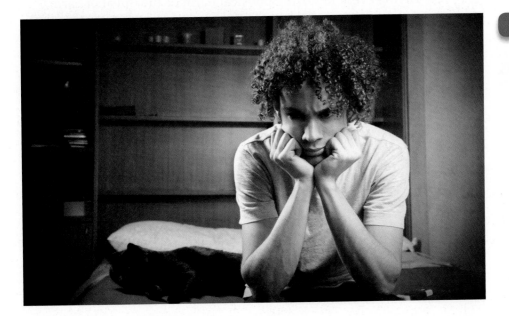

Figure 17.1

Anxiety disorder is characterized by intense, unrealistic worrying about everyday events, experiences, and objects. *At what point do you think worrying becomes unrealistic? Give an example of realistic worrying and an example of unrealistic worrying.*

Bryce is a 15-year-old sophomore in high school. He has always enjoyed doing outdoor activities with his family. Last summer, Bryce was camping with his uncle when they came across a copperhead snake. The snake struck at Bryce's uncle, but fortunately only bit into his jeans and not into his skin.

Although Bryce's uncle was fine, Bryce is now very afraid of having another encounter with a snake. His fear has led him to stop doing outdoor activities. He even avoids his backyard because he is worried about seeing a snake. Bryce also feels anxious if he sees a photo of a snake.

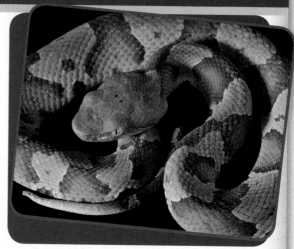

Thinking Critically

1. What do you think are the primary factors that led Bryce to develop these symptoms?

2. What are some strategies Bryce could use to manage his anxiety about snakes?

---

major depression
a mental illness characterized by intense and ongoing negative feelings such as hopelessness, sadness, or loneliness; also known as clinical depression

- *Generalized anxiety disorder.* People with generalized anxiety disorder have a pattern of constantly worrying about many different activities and events, even though these worries are not based in reality.

- *Phobias.* People with phobias have extreme anxiety caused by specific objects or situations. People with *social phobia*, also called *social anxiety disorder*, have a strong fear of being judged by other people and of feeling embarrassed.

- *Obsessive-compulsive disorder (OCD).* People with OCD have persistent and obsessive thoughts or feelings that they manage by engaging in ritualized behavior.

- *Post-traumatic stress disorder (PTSD).* People who live through a terrifying event involving physical harm or the threat of harm, such as a war or natural disaster, may develop PTSD. People with PTSD experience extreme stress or fright, even when they are not in danger. They may also experience recurring flashbacks of the event.

Depression

Everyone feels sad and depressed at times. These feelings are normal (Figure 17.2). For most people, these feelings of sadness and depression improve and go away over time.

For other people, feelings of depression are very intense, do not go away, and negatively affect their daily lives. People who experience these ongoing

Figure 17.2

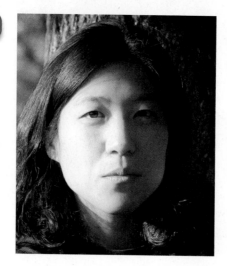

Major life events, such as the loss of a loved one, can cause short-term, often intense, feelings of loss and sadness. These feelings are normal if they eventually go away. *Think of a time when you experienced intense, short-term sadness. How did you manage those feelings? What helped alleviate them?*

negative feelings have *major depression*, or *clinical depression*, which is a serious mental disorder. People with major depression also experience changes in their patterns of thinking and behavior. Professional treatment provided by a mental health specialist is often needed to overcome major depression.

Some of the following symptoms are characteristic of people with major depression:

- a decreased interest in previously enjoyed activities
- feeling worthless
- extreme tiredness and loss of energy
- weight loss or gain
- difficulty sleeping
- trouble concentrating
- irritability, anger, and hostility
- recurrent thoughts of death

Untreated depression can have serious consequences. People who have major depression are more likely to engage in behaviors that are harmful to their health. People who are clinically depressed are also at greater risk of developing various health problems.

Other Types of Mental Disorders

In addition to anxiety and depression, other mental disorders can also affect a person's ability to function in daily life.

Bipolar Disorder

People who have *bipolar disorder* experience periods of intense depression that alternate with periods of *manic*, or mentally and physically hyperactive, moods. During the periods of depression, any of the symptoms of major depression may occur. Symptoms of the manic mood may include poor judgment, little need for sleep, and hyperactive behavior. Another symptom is a lack of self-control, which may include binge drinking, binge eating, drug use, sexual behavior, or out-of-control spending.

Schizophrenia

People who have *schizophrenia* typically experience symptoms such as irregular thoughts, delusions or false beliefs, and hallucinations. People diagnosed with schizophrenia may believe that people are threatening or plotting against them. They may also show inappropriate emotional reactions, such as laughing when they hear someone has died.

Personality Disorders

People with personality disorders show consistent patterns of inappropriate behavior. A common personality disorder is *antisocial personality disorder*. People with this disorder show a disregard for social rules, a

Personal Profile

How Much Anxiety Are You Feeling?

These questions will help you assess how much anxiety you may be feeling from day to day. I become afraid for no reason at all. **yes no** I easily become upset or feel panicky. **yes no** I feel like I am falling apart and unable to control my feelings. **yes no** I feel more nervous and anxious than usual. **yes no** I can feel my heart beating fast, although I am not exercising. **yes no** I am bothered by stomachaches or indigestion. **yes no** I have *fainting spells*, or periods of time when I feel faint. **yes no** I am bothered by headaches and neck and back pains. **yes no** *Add up the number of yes answers to assess how anxious you are feeling. The more yes answers you have, the more anxiety you are experiencing. Take this test at different times to see how your level of anxiety changes based on various experiences.*

bipolar disorder
a mental illness characterized by intense periods of depression closely followed by extreme positive, or manic, feelings

schizophrenia
a mental illness characterized by delusions, hallucinations, and irregular thought patterns

antisocial personality disorder
a common mental illness characterized by disregard for social rules, a tendency for impulsive behavior, and indifference toward other people

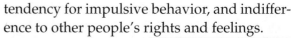

Does Too Much TV Make You Depressed?

Researchers surveyed over 4,000 healthy high school students to determine if media usage is linked to depression. The average amounts of daily media usage for the teenagers in the study were:

- 2.3 hours watching TV with an additional 37 minutes watching movies or videos
- 2.3 hours listening to music
- 25 minutes playing computer games

Seven years later, researchers revisited the study subjects and tested them for depression. Researchers omitted data from people who reported feeling depressed as teenagers to eliminate the possibility that depressed teens tend to use media more often. The researchers found that the people who were depressed in their 20s had watched more television as teenagers—an average of 22 more minutes per day—than those who were not depressed. Other forms of media, including computer games and videos, were not linked with depression.

Researchers suggest that the time people spend watching TV leaves less time for physical activity and sleep, which help prevent depression. Exposure to television may also make people feel anxious or lead them to develop low self-esteem, which can contribute to depression. This is because television programs often present an unrealistic view of the world. Images of people who are wealthier, more physically attractive, and happier than themselves can cause people to become dissatisfied with their own lives.

Thinking Critically

1. You just read a few different explanations for the link between watching too much TV and feeling depressed. Which of these explanations do you find most convincing and why? Use evidence to support your answer.
2. Given this study's finding, what advice would you give to other teenagers, or younger siblings, about watching television? Should this research influence how much television or what types of shows someone watches? Why or why not?

borderline personality disorder
a mental illness characterized by a person showing extreme instability in his or her self-concept and relationships

tendency for impulsive behavior, and indifference to other people's rights and feelings.

People who have **borderline personality disorder** show instability in their own self-concept and interpersonal relationships. They may get very angry at someone for cancelling plans because they fear abandonment. They may also show extreme shifts in their attitudes about other people, such as idealizing a dating partner and then believing that person does not truly care about them.

Autism Spectrum Disorder (ASD)

Autism spectrum disorders are complex mental disorders usually diagnosed in childhood. People with ASD typically have problems with normal interpersonal interactions. They can have difficulty communicating with other people and understanding other people's points of view.

Although symptoms of ASD can vary, people often

- have difficulty making eye contact;
- fail to respond to verbal attempts to gain their attention;
- engage in repetitive motions or unusual behaviors;
- have a strong preference for a familiar routine;
- fail to appropriately use gestures; and
- have delayed language development.

ADD/ADHD

Attention deficit disorder (ADD) and *attention deficit hyperactivity disorder (ADHD)* are the most commonly diagnosed mental disorders in children and adolescents. People with ADD typically have difficulty paying attention, whereas those with ADHD also tend to act impulsively and behave hyperactively. These disorders often occur at different degrees of severity.

People who have ADD or ADHD may show many different types of symptoms. Generally, these symptoms include

- having difficulty focusing or sitting still;
- being quickly bored with tasks and activities (Figure 17.3);
- having difficulty organizing and completing a task;
- having difficulty listening to and following instructions;

- talking nonstop or being in constant motion;
- having difficulty waiting; and
- blurting out inappropriate comments without awareness of the impact of this behavior on others.

Eating Disorders

As you learned in chapter 5, eating disorders are illnesses characterized by serious changes in eating behavior. These disorders can include *anorexia nervosa*, *bulimia nervosa*, and *binge-eating disorder*. People with eating disorders may have symptoms that include eating extremely small amounts of food or severely overeating, engaging in unhealthy weight loss strategies, and having a substantial concern about and focus on body weight or shape.

Addictions

Sometimes people are addicted to a particular substance, such as alcohol, nicotine, or drugs. People can also be addicted to a behavior, such as gambling or using social media. Alcohol and drug addiction also increases the risk of developing certain types of mental disorders, particularly depression, anxiety, and paranoia.

Self-Injury

Self-injury occurs when people intentionally harm themselves. *Self-mutilation*, or *cutting*, is the most common form of self-injury, in which a person makes small cuts on his or her body. Other forms of self-injury may include burning, drinking harmful products such as bleach, or punching. Although self-injury is not technically a mental disorder, this behavior is often addictive. Self-injury is also linked with some mental disorders, including depression and borderline personality disorder. Self-injury typically occurs because people are unable to effectively manage or control their emotions.

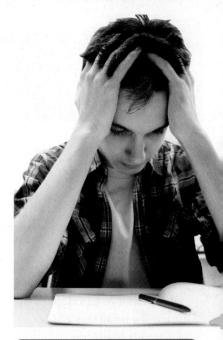

Figure 17.3

People with ADD or ADHD often have difficulty concentrating for long periods of time, which can result in frustration and poor school performance.

Lesson 17.1 Review

Know and Understand Assess

1. Why are the terms *mental illness* and *mental disorder* often used interchangeably?
2. List five types of anxiety disorders.
3. Which mental disorder involves periods of intense depression that alternate with periods of manic moods?
4. Which two mental disorders are most commonly diagnosed in children and adolescents?
5. List three symptoms of eating disorders.

Analyze and Apply

6. Compare antisocial personality disorder and borderline personality disorder.
7. Why do some people intentionally harm themselves?

Real World Health

Use the Internet to find an interview with a person who has a mental illness. Examine the characteristics of this person's mental health condition, and the effect of the disorder on his or her life. Write a short paragraph about your findings.

What Causes Mental Illnesses?

Key Terms E-Flash Cards

In this lesson, you will learn the meanings of the following key terms.

cognitive distortions
concussion
genetic predisposition
traumatic brain injury
  (TBI)

Before You Read

Mindmap

In a mindmap like the one shown below list some factors that cause mental illness. Categorize these as Environmental Factors, Biological Factors, *or* Psychological Factors. *As you read the lesson, list the new factors you learn about under these same categories.*

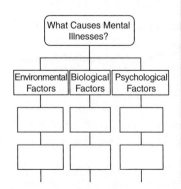

Lesson Objectives

After studying this lesson, you will be able to

- describe biological factors that may cause mental illnesses and disorders;
- identify traumatic life experiences that may trigger a mental illness or disorder; and
- describe psychological factors that may cause mental illnesses and disorders.

Warm-Up Activity

Changing Your Inner Dialogue

How often do you have negative thoughts about yourself that can erode your mental health? For one day, keep track of the negative thoughts, put downs, and critical comments about yourself that run through your mind. If you feel like sharing, compare your final list with a friend or classmate. The next day, when you notice a negative thought, write or type it into the first column of a chart, such as the one shown below. When you finish reading this lesson, fill in the second and third columns of the chart.

Thought	Cognitive Distortions (see Figure 17.6)	Talking Back to the Thought
Example: *I didn't do well on that test. I'll never get into college now.*	Example: *catastrophizing*	Example: *My score on one exam will not keep me out of college.*

T he cause or causes of most mental illnesses and disorders are unknown. Most research suggests, however, that many mental illnesses and disorders are caused by a combination of biological, environmental, and psychological factors.

Biological Factors

Biological factors influence a person's physical makeup. These factors include the person's genes, injuries, and even events that occurred before he or she was born.

Genetics

The genes people inherit from their biological parents can determine their risk for developing mental illnesses and disorders (Figure 17.4). People who have a family member with depression or schizophrenia are at a greater risk of having these disorders themselves. This suggests that people with certain genes are more likely than others to develop a particular mental illness or disorder. These people have a *genetic predisposition*, or vulnerability, to that illness.

Genes may influence the levels of particular chemicals in the brain. People with certain mental disorders have abnormal levels of these chemicals. In some cases, the levels of particular chemicals are too low. People with major depression may have lower levels of the chemical *serotonin* in their brains. Serotonin helps regulate mood. In other cases, the level of a chemical may be too high. People with schizophrenia have higher-than-normal levels of another chemical, *dopamine*, in their brains.

Having a genetic predisposition to developing a particular mental illness does not mean that a person will develop that illness. Most experts believe that a person's life situation or circumstances play a major role in whether the illness actually develops.

Brain Injury

People who experience a serious brain injury are at greater risk of developing some mental illnesses and disorders. *Traumatic brain injury (TBI)* occurs when a severe blow or jolt to the head damages the brain. A *concussion* is a type of brain injury that results from a blow to the head or the body. Contact sports injuries and motor vehicle accidents are common causes of TBIs and concussions. Concussions result in disorientation, confusion, nausea, and weakness, and may cause memory loss or unconsciousness. Although usually temporary, concussions can lead to serious complications and should be treated by a doctor.

Brain injuries may cause temporary or permanent changes to brain function. Irreversible brain changes can result in depression, anxiety, personality changes, and aggression. People with brain injuries are also at greater risk of developing a substance abuse problem. In these situations, alcohol and drugs may be used in an attempt to regulate negative mood or pain.

genetic predisposition
a hereditary vulnerability to various diseases and illnesses

traumatic brain injury (TBI)
damage caused by a severe blow or jolt to the head, which may alter mental functioning

concussion
a brain injury resulting from a severe blow to the head, characterized by nausea, confusion, weakness, memory loss, and unconsciousness

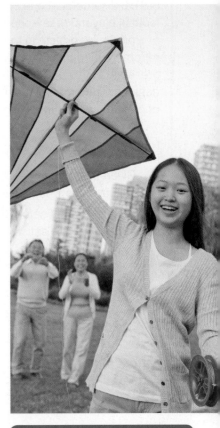

Figure 17.4

Having a genetic predisposition does not mean a person will develop the illness.

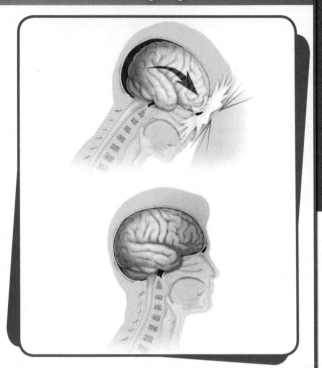

One of the most common injuries to occur during football and other contact sports is concussion. Wearing proper equipment and following rules and safety guidelines when playing sports can help reduce the risk of concussion. Despite safety precautions, however, the CDC reports that there are still millions of people who experience a concussion each year.

For some people—especially those who have repeated concussions—brain changes can pose greater risks for developing certain mental disorders. In one study of 67 college football players, researchers found higher levels of a particular protein in the blood of players who reported being hit in the head several times. The presence of this protein in the blood indicates brain damage. The protein is linked to the development of brain disorders, including epilepsy and dementia.

Thinking Critically

1. Given these findings, do you think there should be rules to limit body contact that can cause concussions when playing certain sports? Provide details to support your response.

2. What rules and safety guidelines are in place at your school to protect student athletes? Do you think these rules are satisfactory? Why or why not? Provide details to support your response.

Environment during Pregnancy

A pregnant woman who experiences certain events or engages in unhealthy behaviors may increase the risk that her baby will someday develop a mental illness or disorder. These events and behaviors include

- consuming alcohol or drugs;
- eating poorly or not getting proper nutrition;
- experiencing a major stress or trauma;
- being exposed to a virus, toxins, or certain chemicals; and
- experiencing medical complications during birth, such as a disruption in the flow of oxygen to the baby's brain.

Environmental Factors

Environmental factors are events and stressors that occur in a person's life and may contribute to the development of a mental disorder. Some

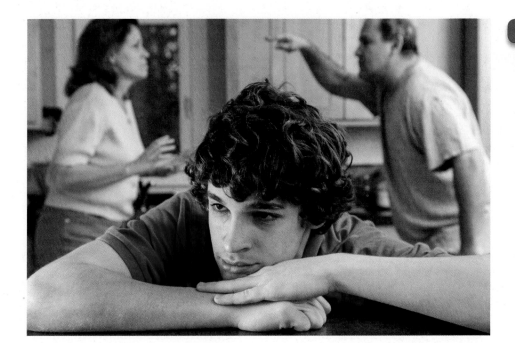

Figure 17.5

Traumatic life experiences, such as a significant family conflict, can increase a person's risk for developing a mental illness or disorder.

experts believe that traumatic life events and stressors can trigger the development of a mental disorder in people who are genetically vulnerable to it.

Traumatic life experiences that can trigger a mental disorder include the following:

- the death of a loved one
- divorce
- significant family conflict (Figure 17.5)
- financial pressures
- moving or changing jobs or schools
- abuse or neglect
- substance abuse

Recovery from traumatic experiences may take a few weeks or months, but the effects may also last longer.

Psychological Factors

Psychological risk factors include feelings of inadequacy, low self-esteem, anxiety, and anger. People who have unhealthy patterns of thinking, or *cognitive distortions*, about the world around them are also at greater risk of developing a mental disorder. Feelings of loneliness and difficulties relating to other people are often common among these individuals. These people may believe the negative feelings they experience will never go away. Some of the common cognitive distortions are described in Figure 17.6.

In some cases, negative feelings are caused by biology, such as the levels of particular chemicals in a person's body or how his or her brain functions. Traumatic life experiences can also lead to these feelings and thought patterns. Fortunately, people can learn to correct these distortions, leading to improved mental health.

cognitive distortions
unhealthy thinking patterns that people have about the world around them

Figure 17.6 Cognitive Distortions

Thinking Pattern	Description and Examples	To challenge this type of thinking, ask yourself...
Black-and-White Thinking	People categorize everything as either all good or all bad. They do not view situations in more complex and nuanced ways. They either think, "I am perfect," or "I am a failure."	What is positive about this situation?
Jumping to Conclusions	People assume they know what other people are thinking and why they behave as they do. For instance, if they encounter people who are unfriendly, they jump to the conclusion that the people do not like them. In reality, the people may just be shy.	What evidence do I have for my conclusion? Is there another explanation I am not considering?
Catastrophizing	People believe that every event—even a relatively inconsequential event—has a huge and negative possible consequence. For example, if they do poorly on one exam, they believe they will never get into college.	Will this event necessarily lead to the conclusion I am dreading, and will that be so bad?
Control Fallacies	People believe they are victims of circumstances; they do not see their role in creating situations. If they get a low grade on an English paper because they procrastinated, they blame their teacher for not providing enough time.	What was my role in creating this situation? What could I have done differently to achieve a different outcome? How can I prevent this in the future?
Emotional Reasoning	People believe that whatever they feel at the moment is a permanent condition. If they spend a weekend feeling lazy and bored, they believe they are and will always be lazy and bored.	Have I always felt this way in the past? If not, why do I believe I will always feel this way in the future?
Fallacy of Change	People believe they can pressure or persuade other people to change. In reality, a person cannot change anyone except him- or herself.	Have my efforts to change this person been successful in the past? Can I accept that this person will never change and if not, do I want to stay in this relationship?
Always Being Right	People constantly try to prove that their attitudes and behaviors are correct. In an argument with another person, they focus more on winning an argument than on issues and feelings.	How would I feel if I were in the other person's shoes? Is this really a right or wrong issue? What is more valuable: being right or maintaining this relationship?

Lesson 17.2 Review

Know and Understand

1. List three biological factors that can contribute to the development of a mental illness or disorder.
2. What does it mean when a person has a *genetic predisposition* to develop a mental illness or disorder?
3. List three symptoms of a concussion.
4. List five traumatic life experiences that can trigger a mental illness or disorder.

Analyze and Apply

5. Describe how the environment during pregnancy may increase the risk of a person someday developing a mental illness or disorder.
6. Compare two common cognitive distortions.

Real World Health

Choose one category of factors that cause mental illness—biological, environmental, or psychological. Then, select three mental illnesses that you read about in the chapter and that you think would be heavily impacted by the type of cause in your chosen category. For each mental illness, research answers to the following questions:

- What causes this mental illness?
- Which age groups are directly impacted?
- What are the major symptoms of this particular mental illness?
- What are some treatment options for this mental illness?

Understanding and Preventing Suicide

Lesson Objectives

After studying this lesson, you will be able to

- identify risk factors associated with suicide;
- describe how suicide impacts other people in the victim's life;
- recognize signs that someone may be at risk of attempting suicide; and
- describe suicide prevention strategies.

Key Terms E-Flash Cards

In this lesson, you will learn the meanings of the following key terms.

suicide clusters

suicide contagion

survivors

Warm-Up Activity

Myths and Facts about Suicide

List everything you have heard about suicide. Then categorize each item as a myth or a fact, as shown in the chart below. Compare your chart with a partner. Do you and your partner have any of the same statements on your lists? If so, did you agree on which items are myths and which items are facts?

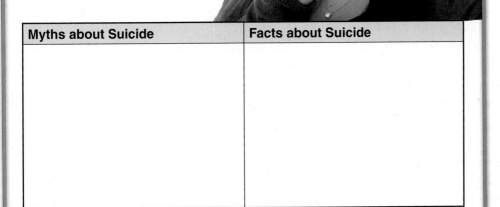

Myths about Suicide	Facts about Suicide

Before You Read

Self-Assessment

As you are reading this chapter, complete four of the following six outcome sentences on a separate sheet of paper.

I feel…

I learned…

I'm beginning to wonder…

I rediscovered…

I'm still not sure of…

I was surprised that…

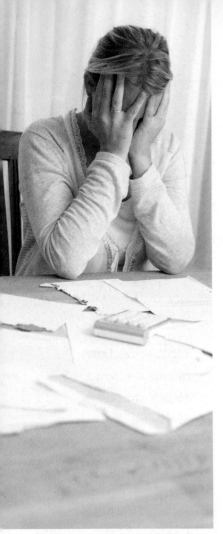

Financial crisis can be a risk factor for suicide.

W hen people are thinking about committing suicide, they feel like their lives are never going to get better—but they are wrong. Eventually, many of these people recover and later realize that illness contributed to their feelings of hopelessness and despair. This is why it is important for people who are thinking about suicide to get help.

Risk Factors Associated with Suicide

Suicide is one of the leading causes of death among teenagers and young adults in the United States. Trying to predict who is at risk of committing suicide is difficult. Many personal, social, and environmental factors may contribute to this behavior. One major risk factor is a previous suicide attempt. A person who has attempted suicide before is more likely to make a future attempt. Other potential risk factors may include a history of mental disorders and a history of alcohol and substance abuse.

It is important to remember, however, that many people with mental illnesses, including teenagers, never try to commit suicide.

Family Factors

People from certain types of family backgrounds may be at greater risk of attempting suicide. People whose biological parents experience depression may be at greater risk of developing depression themselves, so they may also be at greater risk of committing suicide.

Difficult relationships among family members may also increase the risk for suicide attempts. Crises such as financial hardships, issues of abuse or neglect, or substance abuse and addiction problems, may further strain family relationships and increase risk factors (Figure 17.7).

Environmental Factors

Serious stressors in a person's environment can lead someone who is already depressed to consider suicide. People who experience long-term stress in their environments, such as abuse or neglect, are also at greater risk of attempting suicide. Teenagers who are bullied by their peers are at greater risk of thinking about and attempting suicide (Figure 17.8).

Hearing about the suicide of someone else, even a stranger, may increase the risk for certain people to attempt suicide themselves. This copying of suicide attempts is called *suicide contagion*. Some communities or groups experience a series of suicides among members in a relatively short period of time. These are called *suicide clusters*, when one person in a community or group commits suicide and then other people within the same community or group copy this behavior.

The Impact of Suicide on Others

Survivors, or people who lose a loved one to suicide, often feel anger, guilt, and sadness. Survivors may suffer with guilt because they were unable

suicide contagion
term for the copying of suicide attempts after exposure to another person's suicide

suicide clusters
a series of suicides in a community over a relatively short period of time

survivors
people who lose a loved one to suicide

to prevent the death. They may feel rejected and abandoned by the victim. Also, because suicide deaths are sudden, survivors are unable to prepare themselves for this loss.

Survivors may feel embarrassed or ashamed by the suicide. In addition, many people are uncomfortable with the topic of suicide, and may blame the victim instead of supporting the survivors. Unfortunately, this means survivors may not get the support they need following their loss.

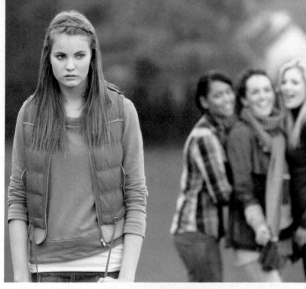

Preventing Suicides

Most people who make a suicide attempt show some warning signs about their intentions. They often tell someone about their plans beforehand or hint at such plans in other ways. Some people may say they feel like they have no reason to live, or they may seem obsessed with death. It is very important to take any mention of suicide seriously, even if the person seems to be joking.

Warning signs that can indicate a person is at risk of attempting suicide include changes in eating and sleeping habits and withdrawal from friends, family, and regular activities. Disregard for personal appearance, changes in personality, giving away valued possessions, and loss of interest in activities previously enjoyed are also signs.

If you ever find yourself thinking about hurting yourself, or if you know someone who may be thinking about suicide, there are steps you can take to get help. First, always take thoughts or mention of suicide very seriously. Talk to an adult you trust immediately. This person can put you in touch with a mental health professional who can help.

If a person confides in you about having suicidal thoughts, you cannot keep this secret. Talk to someone who can help immediately, or call 911 or a suicide hotline number to reach a trained counselor. If you are getting help for someone, it does not mean you are breaking confidentiality.

Figure 17.8

Being bullied or experiencing other forms of abuse can make someone more likely to attempt suicide. *What should a person do if he or she is contemplating suicide because of bullying or other forms of abuse?*

Lesson 17.3 Review

Know and Understand
Assess

1. List three risk factors associated with suicide.
2. Define the term *survivors* as it relates to a possible suicide.
3. List five warning signs that can indicate a person is at risk of attempting suicide.
4. What should you do if you know someone who may be thinking about attempting suicide?
5. Do most people who attempt suicide keep their intentions private or secret?

Analyze and Apply

6. Explain the difference between *suicide contagion* and *suicide clusters*.

Real World **Health**

Research strategies for suicide prevention and design a pamphlet containing useful strategies that can be handed out to students at your school. Include information listing available community and national resources for assisting those at risk of attempting suicide.

Getting Help for Mental Illnesses and Disorders

Key Terms
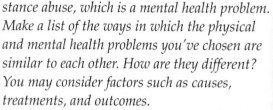
E-Flash Cards

In this lesson, you will learn the meanings of the following key terms.

antidepressants
antipsychotics
family therapy
stigma

Lesson Objectives

After studying this section, you will be able to

- summarize barriers to seeking treatment for mental illnesses and disorders;

- describe treatments for mental health illnesses and disorders;

- identify how medications are used to help treat mental illnesses and disorders; and

- recognize how to help a loved one who has a mental illness or disorder.

Before You Read

Identifying Resources
Using a chart like the one shown below, identify resources for people suffering from mental illnesses and disorders. Write Resources for People with Mental Illnesses *in the middle oval, and list any resources you can think of in the surrounding circles.*

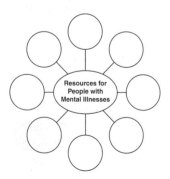

Warm-Up Activity

Mental and Physical Illnesses
How are mental and physical illnesses and disorders similar? On a separate sheet of paper, list a physical health problem and a mental health problem. For example, the images here show a broken leg, which is a physical health problem, and substance abuse, which is a mental health problem. Make a list of the ways in which the physical and mental health problems you've chosen are similar to each other. How are they different? You may consider factors such as causes, treatments, and outcomes.

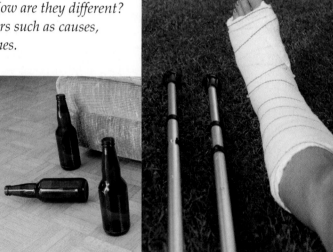

Generally, people are able to manage negative feelings. At times, however, these feelings can be very intense or overwhelming, and may linger for a week or longer. Under these circumstances, negative feelings may suggest a mental illness or disorder.

Although everyone can benefit from getting help when they are struggling with negative feelings, people with mental illnesses and disorders need specific types of help. All mental illnesses and disorders are treatable, so people can effectively manage these conditions with some help.

Barriers to Seeking Help

Unfortunately, people with mental health concerns sometimes do not get the help they need. These people may assume their negative feelings will go away on their own. Most mental illnesses and disorders, however, do not improve without treatment. Untreated mental illnesses and disorders may even get worse and lead to larger problems. These people may also be dealing with external barriers to getting help for their condition.

Social Stigma

The social *stigma*, or negative and often unfair beliefs, about mental illnesses and disorders can cause people with these conditions to not seek help (Figure 17.9). Social stigma may also cause people to

- deny they have a problem;
- feel shame and embarrassment about their illness or disorder; and
- fear that they will lose an opportunity—a job, a scholarship, or a leadership position—because of their condition.

People who experience a mental illness or disorder may mistakenly believe that they should be able to fix their illness or disorder on their own. These people need to realize that their condition requires a doctor's treatment just like a physical problem.

Cost of Treatment

People may be reluctant to seek help because of a cost they may be unable to afford. Although mental health professionals do charge for their services, a person's health insurance may cover a portion of the expenses. Some mental health clinics may also provide therapy services at no cost or a reduced rate.

Treatments for Mental Health Concerns

Researchers are trying to find ways of identifying people who are vulnerable to mental illnesses and disorders. As researchers better understand how the human brain works, they are also creating new treatments so people with mental illnesses and disorders can live healthy and productive lives.

stigma
a negative or unfair belief circulated within society

Figure 17.9

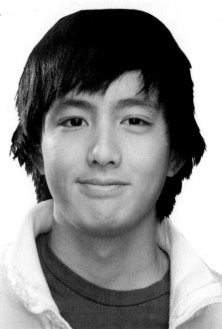

The stigma surrounding mental illnesses and disorders can prevent people from getting the help they need, putting them at greater risk for suicide. *What are some practical ways you can battle the stigma attached to mental illnesses and disorders?*

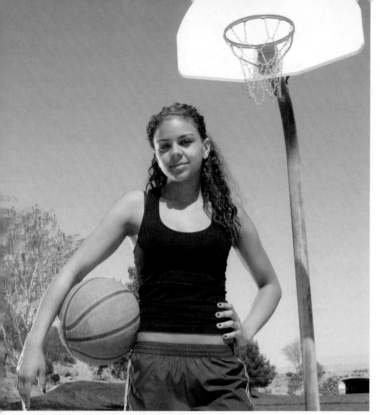

Figure 17.10

During treatment, people learn to cope with negative feelings or stress in positive ways, such as exercise, journaling, and other healthy activities.

family therapy
a method of treatment in which members of a family meet together with a therapist

antidepressants
type of medications that make certain chemicals in the brain more available to combat depression

Individual Therapy

A therapist is a professional who is trained to diagnose and treat people with mental illnesses and disorders. Therapists include professionals such as psychologists, psychiatrists, social workers, and counselors.

The information people share with therapists is completely confidential in most cases. If a therapist believes their patient may hurt him- or herself, or someone else, the therapist may share that information with a parent or guardian. Therapists can help people understand their feelings and behaviors in an accepting and nonjudgmental way. Therapists may also have specific suggestions for how people can understand their thought processes and help themselves feel better. Therapists can help people learn to cope with their problems in healthy, positive ways (Figure 17.10).

Family Therapy

Family therapy, in which all family members meet together with a therapist, helps families build positive, functional relationships and strengthen interactions. Family therapy can also help members of a family support one member with a mental illness or disorder through treatment and recovery.

Support Groups

In *support groups*, a therapist meets with a group of people who share a common problem. Strategies for managing this problem are shared and discussed with all group members at the same time. People can feel a great deal of support from the group because members truly understand the problems they are facing. Members of support groups also gain information about what strategies were helpful for others.

Medication

Medications, which are prescribed by doctors—usually psychiatrists—often work by changing a person's biology. People who have the following mental illnesses or disorders are often treated through the use of medications in conjunction with therapy:

- **Depression.** *Antidepressants* are used to make certain chemicals in the brain, such as serotonin, more available, which can reduce or eliminate symptoms.

- **ADHD.** Stimulants are used to increase the levels of norepineph-rine and dopamine in the brain, which helps improve memory and attention span.

- **Anxiety disorders.** Medications used to treat people with anxiety disorders often slow down the central nervous system, which makes people feel calmer and more relaxed.

- **Schizophrenia.** *Antipsychotics* can be used to manage the symptoms of schizophrenia, which may include hallucinations.

- **Bipolar disorder.** *Lithium* is commonly used to help control the extreme highs and lows experienced by people with bipolar disorder.

- **Substance abuse.** In addition to therapy, treatment for addictions and substance abuse may include taking certain medications long enough to help people manage withdrawal symptoms.

Managing Medication Side Effects. Most medications have some side effects, which can include tiredness and weight gain or loss. In some cases, medications can have very serious side effects. Some types of medication can cause damage to major organs. Some teenagers who take certain types of antidepressants can experience *increases* in suicidal thoughts and behaviors. Due to side effects, people who take these medications are regularly monitored by a doctor or mental health professional. Blood tests are often ordered to check for correct levels of effectiveness or dangerous side effects.

Using Medication with Therapy. Many researchers believe that medications are most effective when used along with some type of therapy. People with depression may take medication, but could also benefit from therapy to help correct their negative, unhealthy thought patterns.

antipsychotics
type of medication used to manage the symptoms of schizophrenia

SKILLS FOR HEALTH AND WELLNESS

Coping with a Loved One's Mental Illness or Disorder

If you know someone who is mentally ill, the following strategies created by the National Alliance on Mental Illness (NAMI) may be helpful:

- Remember that you cannot cure a mental disorder any more than you can cure someone's broken leg or high blood pressure. You are not a trained medical professional.

- Remember that it's not your fault this person developed the disorder.

- Try to separate your feelings about the disorder and its symptoms from the feelings you have toward your family member or friend.

- Remember that it is often difficult for a person to accept that they have a mental illness or disorder.

- Recognize that other people may not understand or accept your friend or family member's disorder.

- Understand that the symptoms shown by your family member or friend may change over time.

- Make sure to take care of your own needs—do not neglect your health.

- Talk to a therapist or join a support group for people whose loved ones have a mental disorder. Remember, you are not alone in your experience.

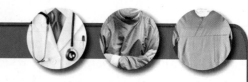

Mental Health Careers

Many different types of careers involve helping people improve their mental and emotional health in various ways.

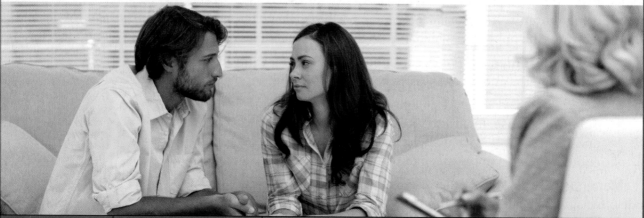

Career	Typical Education and Training	Typical Job Duties and Demands	Career Resources
Psychiatrist	bachelor's degree, followed by a medical degree (MD), and a certification exam	diagnoses and treats mental illnesses and disorders; should have an interest in science and in working directly with patients	American Psychiatric Association
Psychologist	doctoral degree (PhD or PsyD) and a licensing exam	studies mental processes and behaviors, and provides psychotherapy to treat mental disorders; should be able to work well with people who are experiencing mental and emotional problems	Society of Clinical Psychology, American Psychological Association
Clinical Social Worker	master's degree and supervised clinical therapy	diagnoses and treats mental, behavioral, and emotional issues; may work in mental health clinics, schools, hospitals, or private practice; should have good listening and communicating skills	National Association of Social Workers
Psychiatric Nurse	nursing degree (RN) followed by specialized training in psychiatry and psychotherapy, and direct clinical training	interviews and tests patients to learn symptoms and patterns of illness; develops plans to provide treatment and care; should be able to provide counseling to patients and their families	American Psychiatric Nurses Association
Marriage and Family Therapist	bachelor's degree (a master's degree is required in some states) followed by direct clinical training	assess, diagnose, and treat mental illness and psychological disorders that occur within marriages and families; should work well with people individually, in couples, and in families	American Association for Marriage and Family Therapy

Exploring Careers

1. Think about your interests, strengths, and weaknesses. With these in mind, which career described above appeals most to you? Which career does not interest you? Explain your answers.

2. Do you know a person who works in one of these careers? If so, ask why the person chose this career and what he or she likes most and least about the work.

Inpatient Treatment

In some cases, a person's mental illness or disorder causes such serious problems that he or she needs care in an *inpatient* clinic or hospital. This type of treatment is used only when people are at serious risk of harming themselves or others. People who are very depressed and suicidal may need to be hospitalized for a period of time to make sure they do not attempt suicide. In the hospital, people receive around-the-clock supervision, medication, and therapy.

Helping a Loved One

If you are concerned that someone you care about has a mental illness or disorder, share your concerns with that person in an open and honest way. Simply saying that you are worried and would like to help lets that person know you are available. You could also offer to find a mental health professional who can help and accompany your loved one to talk to the professional.

Sometimes a person who is experiencing a mental disorder is not interested in seeking help. You need to intervene when you suspect someone is suicidal, but otherwise, you need to accept that it is not your responsibility to solve that person's problem. It is also important to remember that you should not try to protect people from the consequences of their disorder. This type of protection simply enables people to continue having the disorder without treatment. For example, if your friend is too depressed to complete his homework, doing the assignment for your friend just helps him hide the seriousness of his condition from people who could offer help.

Remember that sometimes people just need more time before they are ready to get the help they need. Take immediate action, however, if you suspect someone is contemplating suicide, or has taken steps toward suicide. Call 911 or take the person to the hospital right away.

Lesson 17.4 Review

Know and Understand 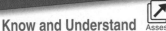 Assess

1. List three reasons people do not seek help for mental health conditions.

2. Define the term *therapist* and give an example.

3. List four treatments for mental health concerns.

4. Which treatment option would be best for someone who is very depressed and suicidal?

Analyze and Apply

5. Compare antidepressants and antipsychotics.

6. How can you help a loved one who has a mental illness or disorder?

Real World Health

Research the resources available in your community to help people with mental health conditions. Make a list of the organizations and then select one to contact. Find out how the organization determines what help and treatments a person needs. What are the availability and cost of these services?

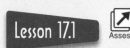

Lesson 17.1

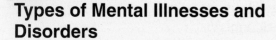

Types of Mental Illnesses and Disorders

Key Terms

antisocial personality
  disorder
anxiety disorder
bipolar disorder
borderline personality
  disorder

major depression
mental illness
panic attacks
schizophrenia

Key Points

- Mental illnesses and disorders are so severe that people are unable to function in daily life.
- Two of the most common types of mental illnesses are anxiety and depression.
- Other mental disorders that can impair the ability of people to function in daily life include bipolar disorder, schizophrenia, personality disorders, ASD, ADD/ADHD, eating disorders, addictions, and self-injury.

Check Your Understanding

1. People who experience extreme anxiety in particular situations have a(n) _____.

2. People who live through a terrifying event involving physical harm or the threat of harm may develop _____.
   A. ADHD
   B. ASD
   C. OCD
   D. PTSD

3. People who have _____ typically experience symptoms such as irregular thoughts, delusions or false beliefs, and hallucinations.
   A. bipolar disorder
   B. schizophrenia
   C. antisocial personality disorder
   D. autism spectrum disorder

4. *True or false?* Alcohol and drug use increases a person's risk of developing certain types of mental disorders.

5. **Critical Thinking.** Explain the difference between depression and major depression.

Lesson 17.2

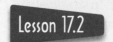

What Causes Mental Illnesses?

Key Terms

cognitive distortions
concussion

genetic predisposition
traumatic brain injury (TBI)

Key Points

- Most research suggests that mental illnesses and disorders are caused by a combination of biological, environmental, and psychological factors.
- A biological factor is something that influences a person's physical makeup, such as his or her genes, injuries, and even what occurred before he or she was born.
- Traumatic life events or stressors can contribute to the development of a mental illness or disorder.
- Identifying and challenging unhealthy patterns of thinking can lead to improved mental health.

Check Your Understanding

6. *True or false?* The cause or causes of most mental illnesses and disorders are known.

7. *True or false?* People with major depression have higher-than-normal levels of dopamine in their brains.

8. Divorce, financial pressures, the death of a loved one, and abuse and neglect are all examples of _____ factors that can contribute to the development of a mental disorder in people who are genetically vulnerable to it.

9. Feelings of low self-esteem, anxiety, and anger are all examples of _____ that can increase a person's likelihood of developing a mental illness or disorder.
   A. biological factors
   B. environmental factors
   C. psychological factors
   D. traumatic life events

10. **Critical Thinking.** What cognitive distortions do you recognize in your own thinking? What questions could you ask yourself to challenge these distortions?

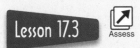

Understanding and Preventing Suicide

Key Terms

suicide clusters   survivors
suicide contagion

Key Points

- People who are thinking about suicide need to get help to eliminate their negative feelings.
- Many personal, social, and environmental factors may contribute to suicide attempts.
- Suicide has a major impact on other people in the victim's life.
- Most people who attempt suicide exhibit some warning signs about their intentions.

Check Your Understanding

11. The copying of suicide attempts is called _____.

12. *True or false?* It is important to take any mention of suicide seriously.

13. Which of the following is a warning sign that a person is at risk of committing suicide?
    A. seeing a therapist to talk about personal problems
    B. joining a support group
    C. giving away valued personal possessions
    D. None of the above

14. **Critical Thinking.** Describe the impact suicide can have on other people in the victim's life.

Getting Help for Mental Illnesses and Disorders

Key Terms

antidepressants   family therapy
antipsychotics   stigma

Key Points

- Most mental illnesses and disorders do not improve without treatment.
- Individual and family therapy and support groups help people learn to cope with their problems in healthy, positive ways.
- Medications are used to treat many mental illnesses and disorders by helping people manage their symptoms.
- Treating mental illnesses and disorders is very challenging, and people with specific professional training are needed to help with such problems.

Check Your Understanding

15. Social stigma may cause people to _____.
    A. admit they have a problem
    B. feel happy and positive about their mental illness or disorder
    C. recognize they need help to fix their illness or disorder
    D. feel ashamed or embarrassed about their illness or disorder

16. *True or false?* The information shared with a therapist is, in most cases, confidential.

17. People often take _____ to manage the symptoms of schizophrenia.
    A. antidepressants
    B. antipsychotics
    C. stimulants
    D. lithium

18. _____ is a medication commonly used to help control the extreme highs and lows experienced by people with bipolar disorder.

19. *True or false?* People who are very depressed and suicidal may need to receive inpatient treatment at a clinic or hospital for a period of time to make sure they do not attempt suicide.

20. *True or false?* People who have a mental illness or disorder need to be protected from the consequences of their disorder.

21. **Critical Thinking.** Compare family therapy and support groups.

Health and Wellness Skills

22. Communicate with Others. This chapter identified several strategies for preventing suicide. Find a partner and film a one- or two-minute commercial promoting one of these strategies. Once it is finished, play the commercial for your class.

23. Practice Healthy Behaviors and Reduce Health Risks. On a separate piece of paper, list some of the factors that might contribute to mental illness in your life. Then, consider how you might manage each factor to lower your risk for mental illness. For each factor, identify three different actions you can take this week that will help you control that factor.

24. Access Information. Many resources exist for those struggling with mental illness or contemplating suicide. Using the Internet, research the contact information of all the mental health resources available in your community. Then, design a poster organizing your information and present that poster to the class.

25. Advocate for Health. Imagine that your principal has asked you to lead a program to educate your peers on the topic of suicide. Design two or three school events that you think will give your peers the most important facts about suicide and encourage them to seek help if they need it.

Hands-On Activity
Mental Illness Insight

Go back and read the "Setting the Scene" feature at the beginning of this chapter. Pay particular attention to the first paragraph and reflect on what you read.

A lot of extremely successful people struggle with mental illness. This activity will help you gain more insight into what those people's lives are like.

Steps for This Activity

1. Choose a famous person with a mental illness who is intriguing to you and then research his or her life. During your research, seek to answer the following questions:

   - What are the signs and symptoms of mental illness in this person's life?

   - What social stigma has mental illness caused in this person's life?

   - Does mental illness affect this person physically? If so, how?

   - How does mental illness affect this person's thoughts and emotions?

   - How is this person being treated for his or her mental illness? What treatment options are available in your community for the person's given situation?

   - Has mental illness affected this person's accomplishment? If so, how?

2. Make a poster or collage that illustrates the information you found.

3. Present your poster to the class. Be prepared to discuss the ideas that you found most interesting in your research.

4. If you can, display your poster in the school hallway where others can learn about your findings.

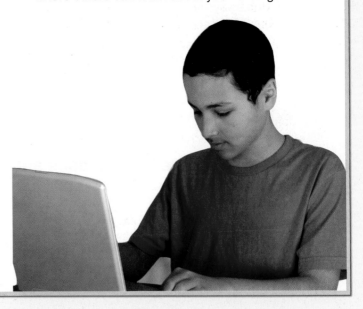

Core Skills

Math Practice

The following graph shows the percentage of adolescents 12 to 17 years of age who have experienced a *major depressive episode* (MDE) in the past year. Study the graph and then answer the questions below.

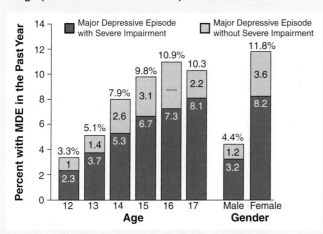

26. What percentage of 15-year-olds experienced an MDE *with* severe impairment?
    A. 5.6
    B. 6.7
    C. 4.5
    D. 7.6

27. How does the percentage of 16-year-olds who experienced MDEs differ from the percentage of 13-year-olds who experienced MDEs?
    A. The percentages are the same.
    B. More 13-year-olds experienced MDEs than 16-year-olds.
    C. There is not enough information to answer this question.
    D. Approximately twice as many 16-year-olds experienced MDEs than 13-year-olds.

28. Approximately how much larger is the percentage of females with MDEs as compared to males?
    A. 4 times more
    B. 6.5 times more
    C. 2.5 times more
    D. 10 times more

29. What percentage of 16-year-olds experienced an MDE *without* severe impairment?
    A. 2.5
    B. 3.6
    C. 4.1
    D. 1.8

Reading and Writing Practice

Read the passage below and then answer the questions.

Environmental factors are events and stressors that occur in a person's life and may contribute to the development of a mental disorder. Some experts believe that traumatic life events and stressors can trigger the development of a mental disorder in people who are genetically vulnerable to it.

Traumatic life experiences that can trigger a mental disorder include the following:

- *the death of a loved one*
- *divorce*
- *significant family conflict*
- *financial pressures*
- *moving or changing jobs or schools*
- *abuse or neglect*
- *substance abuse*

Recovery from traumatic experiences may take a few weeks or months, but the effects may also last longer.

30. What main point is the author conveying in this paragraph?
    A. Traumatic events cause mental illnesses and disorders.
    B. A genetic vulnerability must be present for a person to develop a mental illness or disorder.
    C. Environmental factors in a person's life may help contribute to a person developing a mental illness or disorder.
    D. Everyday stressors do not contribute to mental illness.

31. The word *defenseless* is a(n) _____ for *vulnerable*.
    A. antonym
    B. metaphor
    C. simile
    D. synonym

32. Find an article to read about a traumatic life event that contributed to a person's development of a mental illness or disorder. Write a one-page summary of the article to share with the class.

Unit 7 Social Health and Wellness

Chapter 18   **Healthy Family and Peer Relationships**

Chapter 19   **Dealing with Conflict, Violence, and Abuse**

Big Ideas

- The quality of your relationships with others is an important part of your health and wellness.

- By employing communication, conflict resolution, and other strategies, you can create healthy relationships.

- Violence and abuse, which take many forms, often leave a lasting impact on victims.

- It is never acceptable to use violence or abuse to resolve conflicts.

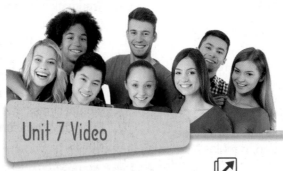

Unit 7 Video

Can Bullies Be Stopped? Videos

A student becomes the target of physical abuse, ridicule, and cyberbullying in school and out. Although the student is tormented by only a few people, many bystanders participate in the bullying. How can the student's friends help him?

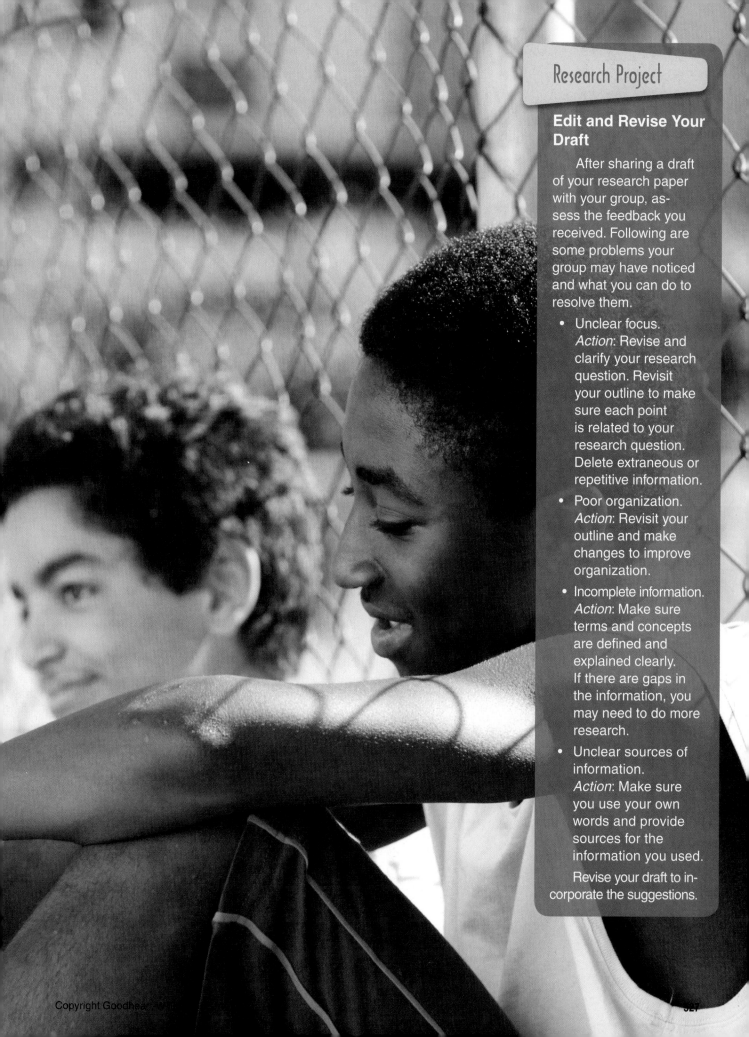

Edit and Revise Your Draft

After sharing a draft of your research paper with your group, assess the feedback you received. Following are some problems your group may have noticed and what you can do to resolve them.

- Unclear focus. *Action*: Revise and clarify your research question. Revisit your outline to make sure each point is related to your research question. Delete extraneous or repetitive information.

- Poor organization. *Action*: Revisit your outline and make changes to improve organization.

- Incomplete information. *Action*: Make sure terms and concepts are defined and explained clearly. If there are gaps in the information, you may need to do more research.

- Unclear sources of information. *Action*: Make sure you use your own words and provide sources for the information you used.

Revise your draft to incorporate the suggestions.

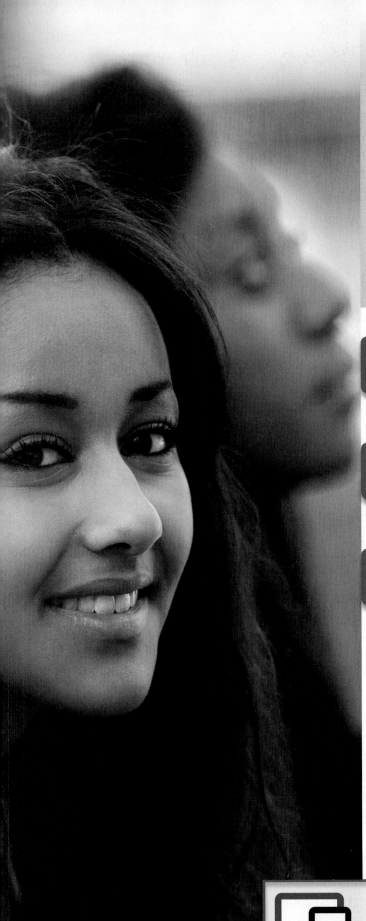

Lesson 18.1

Healthy Family Relationships

Lesson 18.2

Healthy Friendships

Lesson 18.3

Healthy Dating Relationships

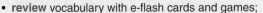

While studying this chapter, look for the activity icon ↗ to:
- **review** vocabulary with e-flash cards and games;
- **assess** learning with quizzes and online exercises;
- **expand** knowledge with animations and activities; and
- **listen** to pronunciation of key terms in the audio glossary.

G-WLEARNING.com   www.g-wlearning.com/health/

Take this quiz to see what you do *and* do not *know about healthy relationships and their impact on health. If you cannot answer a question, pay extra attention to that topic as you study this chapter.*

1. *Identify each statement as* True, False, *or* It Depends. *Choose* It Depends *if a statement is true in some cases, but false in others.*

2. *Revise each* False *statement to make it true.*

3. *Explain the circumstances in which each* It Depends *statement is true and when it is false.*

Health and Wellness IQ Assess

1. Culture and language are passed down through families.	True	False	It Depends
2. Nonverbal communication is just as important as verbal communication.	True	False	It Depends
3. Active listening is part of the communication process.	True	False	It Depends
4. It is important to follow the rules your parents and guardians set, even if you don't agree with them.	True	False	It Depends
5. Jealousy is a normal part of friendship.	True	False	It Depends
6. Infatuation is another word for love.	True	False	It Depends
7. Peer pressure can have positive as well as negative effects.	True	False	It Depends
8. Sibling rivalry is healthy and leads to positive feelings.	True	False	It Depends
9. The best way to get over a breakup is to quickly begin a new dating relationship.	True	False	It Depends
10. In healthy dating relationships, the two people's separate identities become blended into a single identity.	True	False	It Depends

Setting the Scene

Relationships are the bonds and connections you have with other people. Think about the many ways you are connected to other people and how they are connected to you. Your social network includes family members, friends, classmates, and people in your community. Consider how you and the people in your life affect each other.

In this chapter, you will learn how to identify healthy relationships. You will learn communication skills and other skills that can help you build healthier relationships with the various people in your life. Common problems in relationships are discussed, as well as strategies for managing issues with family members, friends, and romantic partners.

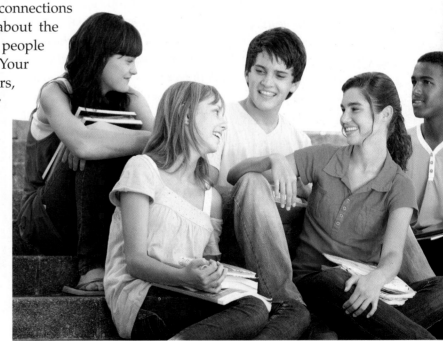

Healthy Family Relationships

Key Terms E-Flash Cards

In this lesson, you will learn the meanings of the following key terms.

active listening

communication process

feedback

nonverbal communication

sibling rivalry

verbal communication

Before You Read

Give One, Get One

Create a chart like the one shown below with as many rows as you need. In the "Give One" column, list information that you already know about healthy family relationships. In the "Get One" column, list the new information you learn as you read the lesson.

Give One (what you already know)	Get One (new information)

Lesson Objectives

After studying this lesson, you will be able to

- analyze the functions of the family;
- differentiate between verbal and nonverbal communication;
- identify three strategies for effectively communicating with others;
- utilize strategies to promote healthy relationships with parents and siblings; and
- recognize various changes that occur within families.

Warm-Up Activity

Verbal and Nonverbal Communication

Communication between people can be either verbal or nonverbal. For example, the teenagers in the photo shown here are engaged in different types of communication. The girl is writing, which is a form of verbal communication. Both teenagers' facial expressions, posture, and eye contact are forms of nonverbal communications. List other examples of verbal communication and nonverbal communication. Search for images—online and in magazines and newspapers—that illustrate each example you listed. Share the images with your class and describe the type of communication that is being shown in each image.

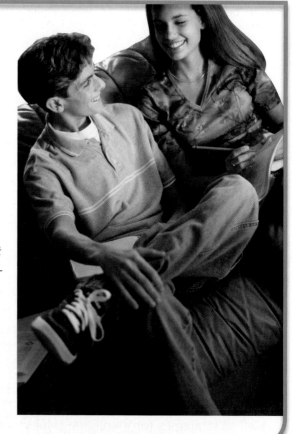

The very first relationships you had were probably with your family members. Most people spend lots of time with members of their *immediate family*, meaning their parents and siblings. People may consider these family relationships to be among their closest. Family relationships are unique because functions of the family and interactions among family members differ from functions and interactions in other types of relationships.

Functions of Family Relationships

Family relationships have several unique functions that make them different from other relationships. Unlike other types of relationships, families have the responsibility of providing for members' physical needs, fulfilling mental and emotional needs, and educating and socializing their children.

Provide for Physical Needs

Families typically provide for the physical needs of their members, including food, clothing, and a place to live. Family members also ensure that you are healthy and safe. Your parents or guardians may take you to the doctor and dentist on a regular basis. They set rules—even rules you don't like—with the goal of keeping you safe and healthy.

Meet Mental and Emotional Needs

Families also help meet mental and emotional needs of their members, such as the need for love, self-esteem, and emotional comfort. For example, your parents or guardians may attend your school performances and sporting events. They may celebrate your birthday and your achievements. The support and love you receive from your family members make you feel secure and good about yourself. Many people rely on their families for advice about how to solve problems or handle challenges they are facing.

Educate and Socialize Children

People learn about culture, values, and traditions through their families (Figure 18.1). People learn language from their families as well as information about culture and religion. All families have unique traditions, which may include celebrating special occasions, holding particular values and beliefs, and participating in certain religious rituals.

People also learn important social skills from their families. Relationships with family members, such as siblings and cousins,

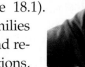

help people learn about cooperation, sharing, and compromise. Families also help teach their children communication skills, which are important in every relationship.

Types of Communication

Effective communication is perhaps the most important part of a healthy relationship. The *communication process* involves sending a message, such as thoughts, ideas, feelings, and information, to a receiver, such as a family member. Effective communication happens when the receiver understands the message and sends *feedback*—a constructive response—to communicate that the message was received and understood. The communication process continues with further exchange of messages. Two types of communication are used to send messages—verbal and nonverbal communication.

Verbal Communication

Verbal communication involves the use of words to send an oral (spoken) or written message. You use verbal communication all the time—through everyday conversation, text messages, phone calls, e-mails, social media posts, letters, and notes. For example, telling a parent you will be home at a certain time is a form of verbal communication.

Nonverbal Communication

Communication involves more than just words. You also communicate with your face and body. *Nonverbal communication* involves communicating through facial expressions, body language, gestures, tone and volume of voice, and other signals that do not involve the use of words. Your nonverbal communication shows people whether or not you are paying attention and are interested in the conversation. These signals are an especially important part of showing respect for the person communicating with you.

Nonverbal communication includes

- eye contact or lack of eye contact (Figure 18.2A);
- facial expressions, such as smiling, frowning, or eye rolling (Figure 18.2B);
- gestures, such as nodding, shaking the head, or moving the hands (Figure 18.2C);
- posture, such as leaning forward, facing away, or slumping in a chair (Figure 18.2D);
- tone of voice, such as friendliness, doubt, or sarcasm;
- volume of voice, such as loud or soft; and
- *intonation*, or pitch of voice, such as high-pitched or low-pitched.

communication process
the process by which ideas, thoughts, feelings, and information are exchanged

feedback
a response that signals a message has been received and understood

verbal communication
the use of spoken or written words to send messages

nonverbal communication
the use of body language, tone, volume, and other methods to send messages

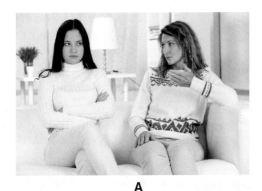

A

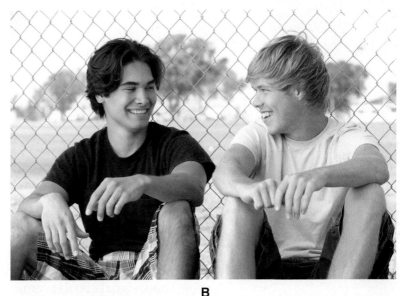

B

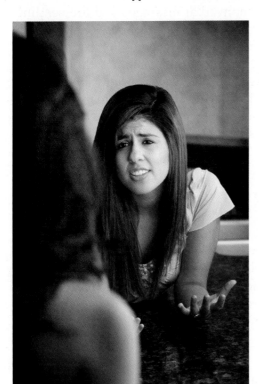

C

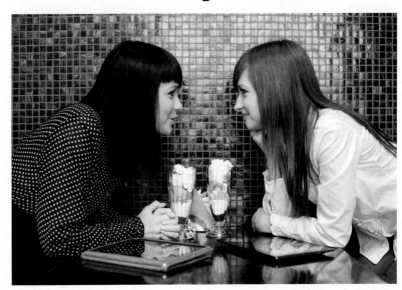

D

Effective Communication Strategies

In healthy relationships, people communicate their thoughts, values, and feelings. They know they will be listened to and supported by the other person in the relationship. Many communication techniques encourage effective, open communication. You can use these techniques to communicate care, consideration, and respect for yourself and others.

Use Active Listening. Good communication requires good listening skills. By focusing on what the other person is saying, you make sure you understand his or her point of view, and convey respect for him or her.

Active listening involves two key steps. First, focus your full attention on the person who is talking. Don't think about your response or something else while he or she is speaking. Second, acknowledge and repeat what you heard in your own words to make sure you heard correctly. Active listening is a great way to avoid misunderstandings. Also, if you carefully listen to what others say to you, they are more likely to do the same for you (Figure 18.3).

Figure 18.2

Nonverbal messages can be communicated through a variety of body movements, such as lack of eye contact (A), facial expressions (B), hand gestures (C), and posture (D). *Analyze the photos shown here and describe what message each nonverbal cue is communicating.*

active listening
the practice of concentrating on what a person is saying

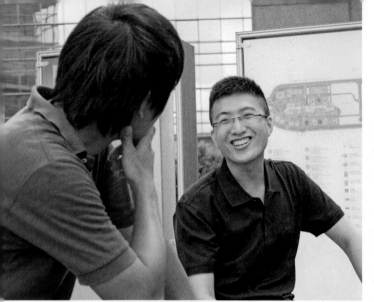

Figure 18.3

When you use active listening, you show respect for the speaker and avoid many misunderstandings, creating an environment in which both individuals can speak and be heard. *Examine your listening skills. What aspects of active listening do you already use?*

Clearly Express Your Needs and Preferences. To communicate effectively, people need to clearly state their wants, needs, opinions, and feelings. A sign of bad communication in a relationship is when one person expects the other person to be a mind reader. Some people assume that others should be able to pick up on their subtle hints and know how they are feeling. This is a poor communication strategy.

Watch Your Nonverbal Communication. Be aware of the nonverbal messages you are sending. What messages do your facial expressions and body language communicate to others? For example, suppose you are having a conversation with your sister and, as she speaks, you look down at your phone and periodically roll your eyes. These signals do not communicate active listening or respect for your sister. Eye contact, nodding your head, and leaning forward would communicate that you value what she is saying.

Strategies for Resolving Common Conflicts in Family Relationships

Family relationships are some of the most important relationships you will have in your life. These relationships, however, can be difficult at times. It is particularly important to develop strategies for resolving conflicts that arise within family relationships.

Parents

Many teenagers experience some conflict in their relationships with parents or guardians. Conflicts between parents and teenagers can get worse during adolescence. Identifying common problems in these relationships and using certain strategies can help strengthen the relationship between parents and teens.

Common Problems in Parent-Teen Relationships. Many problems between parents and children are the result of conflicting goals. One major goal teenagers have is to figure out who they are as unique individuals apart from their family. Adolescence is a time of self-exploration. During this time, teenagers naturally push for more freedom, independence, and responsibility.

On the other hand, parents' goals include keeping their teens safe and healthy and teaching them how to function well in society. To do so, parents set rules and limits that teens might find restrictive. This is one reason why conflicts between parents and children often escalate during adolescence.

Strategies for Maintaining Healthy Parent and Caregiver Relationships. Some effective strategies for preventing conflicts with family members include the following:

- Share your plans with your parents or caregivers ahead of time. Make sure to get their approval before you make a commitment. Revise the plan, if needed, and answer any questions parents may have.

- Discuss family rules with your parents or guardians. If you disagree with a rule, calmly explain why you think it should be changed. Your parents may agree to reconsider the rule.

- Follow your family's rules, even if you disagree with them. Remember, these rules may be relaxed or disappear completely if you show responsible behavior and a willingness to obey the limits set for you.

- Remain calm. When you have a disagreement, do not resort to yelling and do not walk away. Show your parents or guardians that you are capable of having a mature discussion and that you can be responsible.

- Spend time doing enjoyable activities with your family. You might suggest having a special family dinner one night a week or planning a trip. These types of activities can bring families together.

Siblings

Sibling relationships are often the earliest friendships people have. Many siblings also have a reputation, however, for fighting and arguing.

Common Problems in Sibling Relationships. Even when siblings are biologically related, or are raised in the same household, they may not share interests. Siblings may have different personalities, find different activities interesting, or have different ways of handling major life events. These differences can create conflict, especially when people spend a lot of time together (Figure 18.4 on the next page).

Another source of problems common among siblings is competition. Competing with a sibling for various material and nonmaterial items is called *sibling rivalry*. Examples of sibling rivalry include competing for a parent's attention or fighting over use of the family car. When teasing is involved, feelings of competition may increase. Sibling rivalry may encourage negative feelings, such as resentment, anger, or jealousy.

Strategies for Maintaining Healthy Relationships with Siblings. Some effective strategies for managing sibling relationships include the following:

- Get away from tense situations and cool down. By taking a break from a heated situation, you will avoid making the argument worse.

- Express how you feel to your sibling. Communication is the first step in resolving conflict. Try to work with your sibling to find solutions to your disagreement, and show respect for his or her ideas (Figure 18.5 on the next page).

- Talk to your parents about the conflict and see if they have advice for how you could find a good solution.

Personal Profile

How Well Do You Communicate?

These questions will help you assess how well you communicate in your close relationships. Imagine a conversation with someone you are close to, and answer the following questions.

I can calmly express how I feel when we disagree. **yes no**

I listen carefully to what he or she says. **yes no**

I repeat what he or she says in my own words to make sure I understand **yes no**

I maintain eye contact when we are talking. **yes no**

I nod when listening to show that I am paying attention. **yes no**

I calmly and clearly express my needs and preferences when we disagree. **yes no**

I avoid using sarcasm and ridicule when we disagree. **yes no**

I do not assume that he or she understands what I mean without clearly explaining something. **yes no**

Add up the number of yes answers to assess your use of good communication strategies. More yes answers means you are more likely to use effective communication strategies, and more no answers means you tend to use less effective communication strategies.

sibling rivalry
competitive feelings and behaviors that exist between siblings; may include competing for attention, praise, or material objects

Differences in personalities and interests can cause conflict between siblings, especially because siblings typically spend so much time together. *What kinds of sibling conflicts have you witnessed or experienced?*

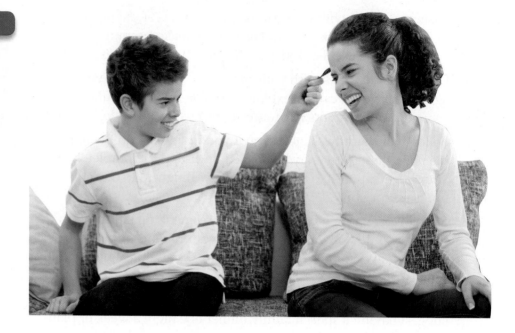

By using constructive communication to solve conflicts, siblings can strengthen their relationships and enjoy each others' company. When conflicts are resolved, sibling relationships can be some of the closest relationships in a person's life.

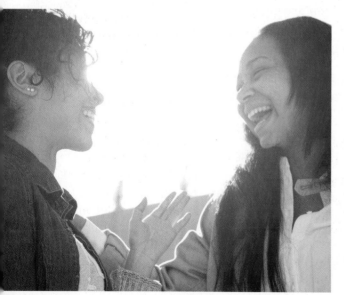

- Compromise when you experience recurring issues. Try to work out a solution that both you and your sibling think is fair. Together, you can develop specific rules for handling ongoing sources of conflict.

- Designate personal space for each person. For example, if you share a bedroom with a sibling, talk to him or her about designating areas for each of you.

- Respect your sibling's space and privacy. Do not enter a sibling's room without knocking. If you share a room, respect your sibling's private space within that room.

Maintaining good sibling relationships is important today and for the rest of your life. Try to find enjoyable ways of spending time with your siblings. This could include going for a bike ride or having a family game night.

Changes in Family Relationships

All families encounter changes over time, such as a physical or mental illness, loss of a job, or relocation to a new community. Change can create stress in a family and disrupt family relationships. These changes are a normal, although difficult, part of family life.

Earlier you read that even positive changes—such as a job promotion, graduation from high school, or having a new baby in the house—can create stress. This is because new events can lead to changes in how family members interact in daily life. For example, suppose a parent gets a big promotion at work. This may mean that the parent must work longer hours or travel more. Other family members may need to take on additional

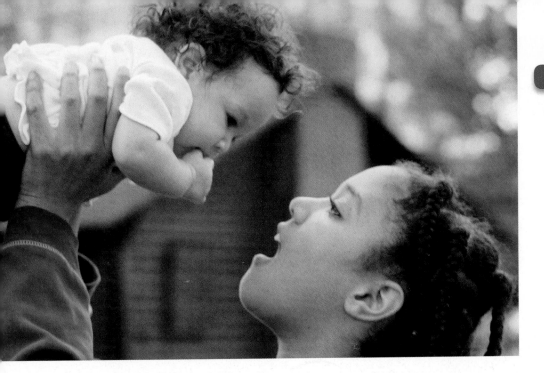

Figure 18.6

Changes in a family's structure—whether they are painful (a death in the family) or joyous (the birth of a new baby)—can pose new challenges for existing family members. *What changes to your family's structure have occurred over the past five years?*

chores at home. Similarly, the arrival of a new baby is a positive event, even exciting, but it can lead to various stresses. Just a few of these stresses include concern about paying for day care and disrupting sleep for other family members.

Some of the most challenging changes families experience are changes in family structure—the addition or loss of a family member. These changes include the birth or adoption of a new family member, separation or divorce, remarriage, serious illness, and death (Figure 18.6). Although these events can be difficult, healthy families can work through them together. Sometimes families even grow closer when dealing with changes such as these.

Lesson 18.1 Review

Know and Understand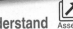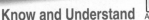

1. Name three functions of family relationships.
2. List three social skills that people usually learn from their families.
3. Describe *active listening*.
4. Name at least three effective communication strategies.
5. Explain *sibling rivalry*.

Analyze and Apply

6. What is the difference between verbal and nonverbal communication? List one example of each type of communication.
7. Select one issue that typically causes you to argue with your parents. Which strategy would you select to help prevent a conflict about this issue?

8. Why are changes in the family structure (a loss or addition of a family member) often stressful for the family? What strategies could a family use to adjust to a new family structure?

Real World   Health

Conflict will exist to some degree in almost all families, whether that conflict is with a parent, caregiver, or a sibling. Within your own family, discuss and create a plan to work through recurring conflicts or other conflicts that might arise among family members. Review the communication skills that you learned in this lesson, and implement these skills and strategies in your family plan.

Healthy Friendships

Key Terms E-Flash Cards

In this lesson, you will learn the meanings of the following key terms.

acquaintances

clique

diversity

Before You Read

Interpreting Headings

Before reading this lesson, your teacher will list this chapter's main lesson headings on chalkboards or dry-erase boards around the room. Without talking, move around the room and write one or two sentences describing what you already know about each lesson heading. You may also write comments or questions responding to other students' ideas. Your teacher may ask that you do this activity using an online editing application instead of physical boards. After reading the lesson, go back around the room and add the new information you learned under each lesson heading.

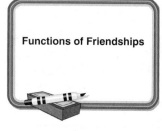

Functions of Friendships

Lesson Objectives

After studying this lesson, you will be able to

- determine the functions of friendships;

- distinguish between different types of friendships, including *acquaintances*, *best friends*, and *virtual friends*;

- evaluate common issues in friendships, such as cliques, jealousy, and changes over time, and the impact each issue has on a friendship;

- differentiate between positive and negative types of peer pressure; and

- devise a plan to use strategies for maintaining healthy friendships.

Warm-Up Activity

My Best Friend

Who is your best friend? Find a picture of you and your best friend. On a separate sheet of paper, write a short paragraph explaining why you consider this person your best friend. Then write a second paragraph to answer the following questions: Is this a healthy relationship? Why or why not?

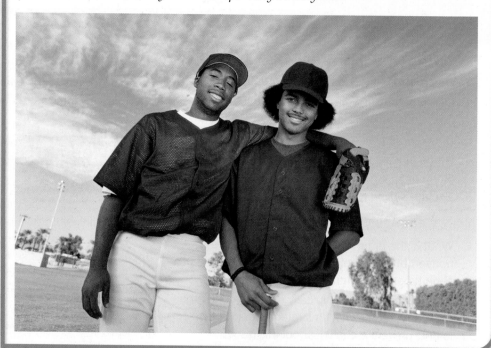

F riendships are some of the most important relationships in your life. Your friendships develop because of mutual respect, care, trust, and affection. Friendships are especially important during adolescence when relationships with peers can become the center of your world.

Functions of Friendships

Healthy relationships fulfill some basic human needs, including the need to belong to a group and feel connected with and loved by other people (Figure 18.7). Your relationships impact you emotionally. An argument with a friend can make you feel angry or sad. A smile or a compliment from a friend or a classmate can lift your spirits.

Relationships also play a crucial role in your physical health. Researchers have found that people with good social support are less likely to get sick than people who lack social support. People with good social support also tend to recover from illnesses faster and even live longer. Relationships filled with tension and conflict, however, can have the opposite effects on health.

Friendships allow you to learn more about yourself, receive and provide emotional support, and gain skills for communicating and resolving conflicts. Different friendships satisfy different needs.

Types of Friendships

The term *friendship* is used to describe many different types of relationships. For example, you probably know the difference between your very closest friends and your more casual friends. Perhaps you have a single friend who you consider your best friend. You may also have many *acquaintances*—people you know and interact with, but may not consider friends.

In a diverse culture, you are likely to meet people who see the world differently than you do. *Diversity* is present in a group of people with various backgrounds, including different ages, genders, ethnicities, and cultures. In healthy relationships, each person respects the other person for who they are. They celebrate differences, and avoid making assumptions based on stereotypes or prejudices. Diversity in a culture can broaden people's knowledge. Ideally, each person challenges and learns from the other person, while respecting the other person's values.

In the past, most people had friends who lived in their neighborhood or city. Today, however, many people have friends who live farther away. You may have *virtual friends*, or people you met through social networks, chat rooms, or gaming. Although true friendships can some-

acquaintances
individuals with whom you interact regularly but may not consider friends

diversity
the wide range of backgrounds, ages, ethnicities, and genders represented in a group of people

Figure 18.7

Healthy relationships—and the feelings of love and belonging they create—greatly improve a person's quality of life and mood. These relationships also provide a strong support network. *What are the healthy relationships in your life? How do those relationships make you feel?*

times develop between virtual friends, particularly if you share some real-life friends, be careful about sharing information with people you have only met online. You can learn more tips about staying safe when meeting people online in Chapter 19, and in the Background Lessons at the end of your textbook.

Most people also have relationships within their communities. These relationships may be with people in your neighborhood, town, or religious organization. Many people also have professional relationships within their school, workplace, or volunteer job. These include relationships with nonfamily adults, such as teachers, employers, and doctors. It is important to have healthy relationships within your community. You can build healthy relationships in your community by treating other people with respect, being open and honest about what you think and feel, and being reliable and trustworthy.

Common Problems in Friendships

clique
a small group of friends who intentionally turn away people who may want to interact with or befriend them

Although friendships enrich your life in many ways, they can also be a source of problems. Cliques, jealousy, changes over time, and peer pressure are common types of problems in friendships.

Cliques

Many high school students enjoy spending time with groups of friends. Sometimes groups of friends exclude other people, which can lead to hurt feelings. A *clique* is a small group of friends who deliberately exclude other people from joining or being a part of their group (Figure 18.8).

People who are part of a clique can feel pressured to act a certain way to fit in, or adopt the attitudes and behaviors of group members. Cliques can also pressure group members to act in ways that endanger their health and wellness. For example, a group may encourage cigarette smoking. In this way, cliques can reduce each person's individuality and compromise well-being, which is unhealthy.

SKILLS FOR HEALTH AND WELLNESS

Developing New Friendships

If you feel shy or anxious about meeting and getting to know new people, the following strategies can help:

- Before you start a conversation, pick a topic or common interest to discuss.
- Compliment people on something you notice about them, such as a piece of clothing, jewelry, or their skill in a certain activity or class.

- Get involved in activities such as sports, music, school clubs, or volunteer opportunities to meet people your age who share common interests.
- Be friendly when you meet new people to discover whether you share anything that could be the basis for developing a friendship.

Jealousy

Jealousy may sometimes occur in a friendship. You may feel jealous of your friend's achievement in a particular area, such as schoolwork, athletics, or music. You may also feel jealous of other aspects of a friend's life, such as his or her home, dating relationship, or family life. Feelings of jealousy are normal if they occur once in a while, but continuous jealous feelings can harm a relationship over time.

Honestly expressing your emotions, including jealousy, can prevent negative thoughts from building up over time and eroding your friendship. If you value your friendship and want to maintain it, try to move beyond feelings of jealousy.

Changes over Time

Friendships evolve as people change over time. Experiencing physical, emotional, and social changes can lead to changes in your friendships. This is particularly true if you and a friend change in different ways. You may no longer share the same interests with your childhood friends. You may need to stop spending time with a friend, or take a break from the friendship.

Sometimes old friendships are maintained, but they change in some way. For example, you might see an old friend less frequently as your interests and peer groups change. You might find that you prefer spending time with different people if you feel less close with your old friends.

If you feel as though you and a friend are drifting apart, tell your friend how you feel. If both of you are interested in maintaining the friendship, you can work together to find ways of remaining close.

Peer Pressure

Peer pressure is a common element present in friendships. Two different types of peer pressure exist—positive and negative.

Positive Peer Pressure

Although people often associate peer pressure with negative activities, peer pressure can also have a positive influence. For example, you might feel pressured to participate in community service projects with a school group or athletic team (Figure 18.9). A friend may encourage you to study harder and improve your grade in a class. In these cases, pressure from peers can help you broaden your perspective on the world, contribute to your community, or succeed in a certain class.

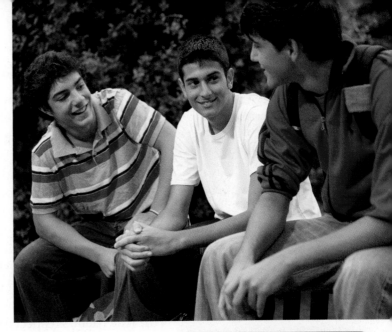

Figure 18.8

Although having a group of close friends is healthy, *cliques* can sometimes form and exclude others. *Why do you think some groups of friends exclude other people? How does it feel to be excluded?*

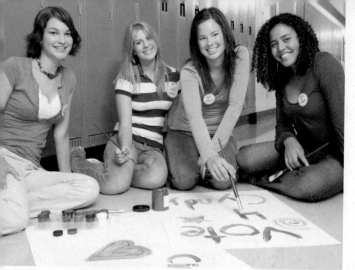

Figure 18.9

Positive peer pressure encourages you to do things that are healthy for you and your community. *When have you experienced positive peer pressure?*

Negative Peer Pressure

In some friendships, however, one person pressures another to do something he or she is not comfortable doing. A teenager may be pressured to drink alcohol, cut class, or tease a classmate to fit in with a group of friends. Most people want to be liked and to fit in with a group. They may decide to go along with certain behavior even if they are uncomfortable with it. They may worry about being ridiculed if they do not join in with the group activity. Sometimes teenagers worry that standing up for what they believe could cause them to lose a friendship.

In healthy friendships, this type of negative peer pressure does not occur. True friends respect each other's choices. If you are experiencing negative peer pressure, you have the right to stand up for what you believe, and to walk away from situations that make you uncomfortable. If a friend ends a relationship with you over this choice, he or she does not respect you and your friendship. Standing up to peer pressure is especially important when friends are doing something that could hurt you or someone else.

What can you do to stand up to peer pressure? Strategies you can use to respond to negative peer pressure include the following:

- Focus on your own thoughts, feelings, and values, and make sure your actions reflect your core beliefs.
- Have the strength and self-confidence to walk away from a situation, or from people who make you uncomfortable.
- Choose friends who have values similar to yours so you are less likely to experience this type of pressure. People who share your values, goals, and beliefs will probably support your decisions.
- Support other people when they resist peer pressure. Sometimes having just one other person say, "I agree, this is a bad idea," is all it takes to change a group's behavior.
- If peer pressure continues over time, talk to someone you trust—a parent, teacher, or guidance counselor.

Strategies for Healthy Friendships

Arguing with friends is not unusual. Determining whether someone shares your core values and beliefs can take time, especially if you are still trying to figure out what you believe. Even when arguments arise, however, there are ways to maintain healthy friendships over time.

Make Time for Relationships

It takes time and energy to maintain close relationships with friends and family members. Even when you are busy with homework, sports, or a job, you should try to find time to connect and spend time with the important people in your life.

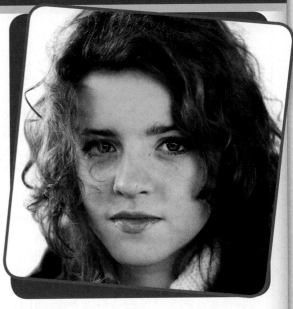

After Kim, a freshman in high school, moved to a new town, she was eager to make new friends. After a few lonely weeks of school, she started hanging out with a group of juniors and seniors she met in an after-school club. At first, Kim enjoyed spending time with her new friends; they were funny, mature, and had a good time together. When her new friends talked about their weekend plans, however, Kim started to feel less comfortable. Weekend plans for these students often involved drinking alcohol, and Kim does not drink. One of Kim's friends offered her an alcoholic drink and seemed surprised when Kim said *no*. Kim is worried that if she doesn't start drinking with them, her new friends won't want to hang out with her anymore.

Thinking Critically

1. What are some strategies Kim could use to resist the pressure she feels to drink?

2. Do you think Kim's friendship with the group can survive if she refuses to drink alcohol or smoke? Why or why not?

3. What advice would you give other teenagers who find themselves pressured by peers to engage in unhealthy behaviors?

Step away from the Screen

The best relationships are formed, and maintained, through face-to-face interactions instead of screen-to-screen interactions. Direct communication is an important part of having a close relationship. Make sure not to rely too much on virtual interaction. One of the best ways to keep a relationship strong is to step away from screens—including your phone, TV, video games, and computer—and make time to be physically present with someone.

Be a Good Friend

The best relationships are *reciprocal*, meaning each person contributes equally to the relationship. Make sure you are being a good friend, meaning you listen carefully to what your friends are saying, and do not interrupt, judge, or criticize them when they are talking. Some additional strategies that can keep your friendships strong include the following:

- Support and encourage your friends, and celebrate their successes.

- Avoid teasing or criticizing your friends.

- Work with your friends to solve disagreements and problems, and collaborate to reach an agreement when necessary.

- Express your feelings openly during conflicts, and listen carefully to your friend's perspective.

- Apologize if you hurt your friend and try to find ways to make amends.

Research in Action

The Hazards of Driving with a Friend

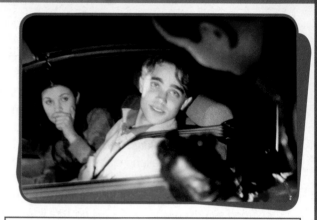

Most states have laws that prohibit new teenage drivers from driving with their peers as passengers. These laws were created after numerous studies found that teenagers who drive with friends are much more likely to speed and have a car accident.

Researchers in one study examined data from 677 drivers—all between 16 and 18 years of age—who were involved in serious car crashes to determine factors that may have contributed to these crashes. The researchers' findings revealed that both male and female drivers who had passengers in the car were more distracted than those without passengers. In fact, 20% of female drivers and 25% of male drivers reported being distracted by something inside the car just before the car accident.

The crashes were caused by different factors for each gender. Male drivers with distracting passengers were more likely to crash as a result of speeding or reckless driving. In contrast, female drivers were more likely to crash due to other distractions, such as texting, talking to friends, using a cell phone, or eating.

Thinking Critically

1. Using reliable online sources, research and compare the rate of car accidents among teen drivers to accidents among older adults. Are teen drivers more distracted by the presence of peers? Why or why not?

2. Create a hypothesis to explain the differences in gender as they relate to car accidents. Why do male and female teen drivers show different patterns of distraction?

3. Given the findings of this study, what do you think high schools, parents, and driving schools should do to prevent such accidents? How would you implement these changes?

Lesson 18.2 Review

Know and Understand Assess

1. Identify three functions of friendships.

2. Define *acquaintance*.

3. Describe *diversity*.

4. Identify three common sources of problems in friendships.

5. Explain the difference between negative and positive peer pressure.

Analyze and Apply

6. Ideally, how does diversity impact friendships?

7. Explain how physical, emotional, and social changes can lead to changes in a friendship over time.

8. How might prolonged jealousy damage a friendship?

Real World Health

Suppose that a social network posts ads for people seeking new friends. Write a personal ad for the website describing the new friendship that you hope to create. What type of person would you want as a friend? What kinds of characteristics would you prefer in a friend? What will you bring to the friendship? Be honest about what you want and would give to this friendship, and be original with your ad.

Healthy Dating Relationships

Lesson Objectives

After studying this lesson, you will be able to

- differentiate between attraction, closeness, and commitment in a relationship;
- assess the importance of maintaining individuality, balance, open communication, support, and safety in a dating relationship;
- recognize characteristics and signs of an unhealthy dating relationship;
- develop strategies for forming a healthy dating relationship; and
- identify feelings that result from a breakup.

Key Terms E-Flash Cards

In this lesson, you will learn the meanings of the following key terms.

exclusive

infatuation

sexual assault

Warm-Up Activity

Similarities and Differences

In this chapter, you have learned about many types of healthy relationships. What are some qualities healthy dating relationships have in common with healthy friendships and family relationships? What are some qualities unique to each type of relationship? In a diagram like the one shown here, map these similarities and differences.

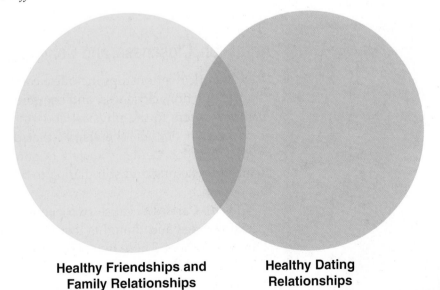

Healthy Friendships and Family Relationships

Healthy Dating Relationships

Before You Read

Think-Ink-Pair-Share

Before reading this lesson, read the lesson objectives and list the main topics you think will be presented in this lesson. List the information you already know about these topics. Then pair up with a classmate and share and record your knowledge in a table similar to the one below.

What I know	What my partner knows

D ating relationships are a new type of relationship for many teenagers. The decision to begin dating is personal, and different people feel ready to begin dating at different times. Some teenagers are interested in and ready for dating earlier than their peers. These teens may feel attracted to a person in a romantic way and decide to act on those feelings. Other teenagers may not feel this type of attraction for someone else just yet. Additionally, some families may have rules that limit or forbid dating until a certain age.

Identifying when a relationship is healthy is important. Perhaps you have already seen examples of healthy and unhealthy relationships. This lesson will discuss differences between healthy and unhealthy dating relationships, strategies for forming healthy relationships, and strategies for coping with the end of a relationship.

Characteristics of Healthy Dating Relationships

How do you know if you are in a healthy romantic relationship? All types of healthy relationships—family, friendship, and dating—share similar qualities, such as honesty and trust, mutual respect, and care and commitment (Figure 18.10). Healthy dating relationships have other qualities in addition to these. The following are important qualities of healthy dating relationships:

- attraction, closeness, and commitment
- maintained individuality
- maintained balance
- open communication
- support
- love
- physical intimacy
- safety

Figure 18.10

Healthy dating relationships are characterized by honesty, trust, mutual respect, care, and commitment; teens should be wary of dating relationships that are characterized by anything less. *How do you think you could measure these healthy characteristics in a dating relationship?*

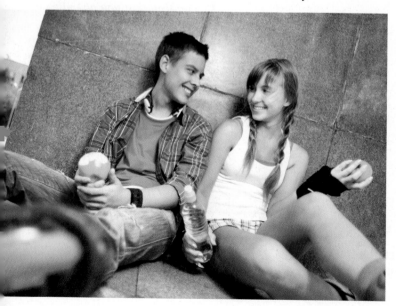

Attraction, Closeness, and Commitment

Romantic relationships include a combination of attraction, closeness, and commitment. *Attraction* refers to the physical and emotional connection or the "chemistry" that draws people together. Being attracted to someone means it is exciting and stimulating to be with that person.

Closeness arises because two people share special feelings and thoughts that they do not share with others. These two people develop a bond. Closeness is seen between friends, but friends may not share attraction for each other. Attraction without closeness is called a *crush*.

Finally, healthy dating relationships include commitment. Commitment means promising to be *exclusive*, or romantically involved only with your dating partner. Commitment also means that you agree to try to maintain the relationship over time and work through problems when they occur instead of just ending the relationship at the first sign of trouble.

Individuality

Some people think that when a person is in a dating relationship, his or her life should revolve around the relationship. They may think that being part of a couple is more important than being an individual. In healthy dating relationships, however, each person maintains his or her own unique identity. The relationship does not redefine a person. Each person's core values, beliefs, and sense of self remain the same.

When you enter a dating relationship, stay true to yourself and assert your individuality. Each person in the relationship should respect the other's separate identity. Remember that your personality and individuality attracted you to each other. Continue meeting your own responsibilities and doing activities you enjoy as an individual.

Balance

People in a dating relationship often want to see their boyfriend or girlfriend regularly. Making time for friends and family members, however, is also important. In a healthy dating relationship, people balance the different relationships in their life and do not prioritize one relationship over all others (Figure 18.11).

People in a dating relationship should also trust each other to spend time with friends and be alone. Your boyfriend or girlfriend should not get angry with you for talking to other people or for spending time with family and friends. You each have the right to enjoy time with other people and spend time on your own.

Balance in a healthy relationship also refers to a balance of power. The relationship is unbalanced if one person makes all the decisions without consulting the other person. In a healthy dating relationship, time and activities are shared equally and fairly. Each person gets the chance to choose activities and decide how to spend time together. You each need to share your thoughts and feelings and permit each other to do so. This requires open, honest communication.

Open Communication, Honesty, and Respect

Healthy dating relationships are characterized by good communication, honesty, and respect. Both people in a relationship should feel comfortable expressing their likes, dislikes, goals, values,

Figure 18.11

While teens may be tempted to devote all their time and energy to a dating relationship, they should maintain balance and nurture all the relationships in their lives. *What do you think would be a healthy ratio of time spent on a dating relationship to time spent on other relationships?*

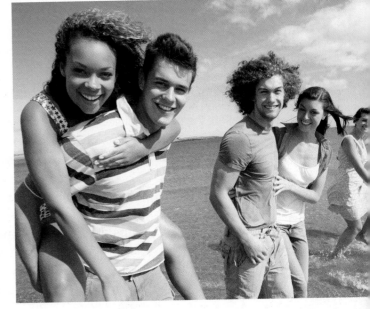

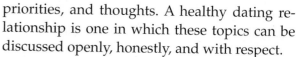

Health in the Media

No, Everyone Else Is *Not* in a Dating Relationship

You've probably seen movies or TV shows about teenagers who never seem to study for class or take out the garbage. These teens and all of their friends are too busy trying to find the boy or girl of their dreams.

Teenage dating relationships in movies and television programs are often unrealistic portrayals of what these relationships are actually like in real life. Media images often emphasize the fun and exciting aspects of dating relationships. The media also shows teens engaging in risky behavior, often without any consequences.

Although relationships may seem easygoing in the media, romantic relationships can be confusing and complicated in reality. Teens sometimes feel rejected by the boy or girl they want to date. They can also have conflicts with their dating partner, such as feeling pressured to engage in behaviors they do not feel comfortable doing.

Versions of teenage life shown by the media may make some people feel pressured to start dating before they are ready. Others may begin dating before they feel genuine affection for someone. Although it may seem like most teenagers in the media are dating, many teens in real life are not in romantic relationships.

Thinking Critically

1. Do you agree that television shows and movies provide unrealistic versions of teenage dating relationships? Explain your answer.

2. How might inaccurate portrayals of teenage dating in the media influence high school students? middle school students? What are the negative effects of these images? Are there any positive effects, and if so, what are they?

infatuation
term for intense romantic feelings based largely on physical attraction

priorities, and thoughts. A healthy dating relationship is one in which these topics can be discussed openly, honestly, and with respect.

In contrast, dishonesty can undermine any relationship. For example, if you say you need to study but your boyfriend or girlfriend finds out you went shopping with friends instead, he or she may have trouble trusting you again. In these situations, hurt feelings should be discussed openly and honestly. Usually, two close and loving people can talk about an issue and work together to resolve a problem.

Support

One of the most important aspects of a healthy relationship is that each person supports the other person in good times and in bad. Both people should support each other's successes, happiness, talents, interests, and goals. If your boyfriend or girlfriend does well in an audition for the school play, you can be supportive by celebrating with and being happy for him or her. You should also support your partner when he or she is sad, hurt, or struggling. Helping each other through tough times can bring you closer together and strengthen your relationship.

Love

Over time, love may develop in a dating relationship. Feelings of love describe an intense affection for and attachment to another person. Love develops gradually as people get to know each other on a more intimate level.

Feelings of love are often confused with infatuation. **Infatuation** describes intense romantic feelings for another person that develop suddenly and are usually based on physical attraction. These feelings are often not returned by the other person. The person experiencing infatuation may not know the other person very well or at all.

Love may also be confused with feelings of passion. Dating relationships often begin because two people feel attracted to each other. Passion can be very powerful and exciting, especially when it is a new emotion for teenagers. Passion is typically short-lived, however, partly because it is based in physical attraction rather than a deeper, longer-lasting emotional connection.

Physical Intimacy

Unlike other types of relationships, dating relationships often include some type of physical intimacy, such as holding hands and kissing. These are ways for people in close dating relationships to express affection for one another. Physical intimacy does not necessarily mean sexual activity. People can express affection for each other in many other ways besides sexual activity.

Before you start dating, you should know how you feel about being physically intimate with another person. It is better to know your limits before you are in a situation that requires a quick decision. You should also feel comfortable communicating your limits to your dating partner. In healthy dating relationships, each person is open about his or her limits regarding different types of intimacy, and the other person accepts and respects these limits. Your partner may even feel relieved that you are clear and honest about your limits.

Many factors, including your values, religion, and judgment, will influence decisions you make about physical intimacy. You may also wish to abstain from sexual activity to decrease your risk of developing sexually transmitted infections, HIV/AIDS, and pregnancy. It is possible to maintain a rewarding, fun, healthy romantic relationship without engaging in sexual activity.

Some teenagers feel pressured by their dating partners to engage in physically intimate or sexual behavior that does not feel comfortable. It is important to remember that this type of pressure does not exist in healthy dating relationships. Your partner should never tease you when you refuse to do something that makes you uncomfortable.

Safety

In healthy dating relationships, each person feels safe with the other person. Your dating partner should never make you feel unsafe (Figure 18.12). Each person respects the other's personal boundaries and cares for his or her well-being. Part of maintaining a safe relationship is informing your parents or guardians about the relationship. Be honest with them. Your parents will need to know the person you are dating, where you are going with him or her, and when you will be home.

Signs of an Unhealthy Relationship

While you are in a romantic relationship, or even a friendship, you may have trouble seeing the signs of an unhealthy relationship. This is especially true for people who were raised in an environment where a lack of respect, kindness, and trust was considered normal, and where anger and verbal or physical abuse was present.

In an unhealthy relationship, one or both people in the relationship may feel used, ignored, or unappreciated. One person may feel that he or she is more

Figure 18.12

If you ever feel unsafe in your dating relationship, then your relationship is unhealthy. Feeling unsafe can be caused by someone crossing your personal boundaries, choosing harmful words, or being physically forceful.

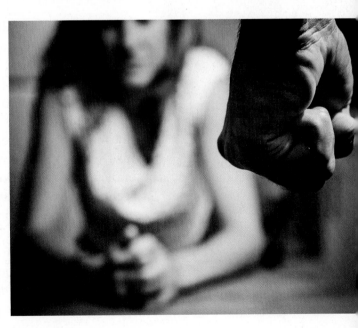

interested in maintaining the relationship than the other person. People in unhealthy relationships may feel angry, sad, or anxious. In some cases, they may even feel unsafe.

Your partner should never physically force you to do something you do not want to do. Forcing someone to engage in any type of sexual activity against his or her will is **sexual assault**. Sexual assault and *rape*, or nonconsensual sexual intercourse, are serious crimes that have serious consequences. If you are sexually assaulted, you should report the act to an adult you trust right away. Seek medical help and get out of the abusive relationship. This type of pressure and mistreatment is *never* part of a healthy dating relationship. You will learn more about sexual assault and unsafe dating relationships in a later chapter.

Your relationship is also unhealthy if any of the following scenarios have occurred:

- you endure angry outbursts
- you feel you cannot say anything right
- you feel you are constantly fighting
- you are made fun of or threatened
- your partner is *possessive*, or extremely jealous
- your partner tells you to stay away from your friends or family
- your boyfriend or girlfriend has raised a hand as if to hit you
- you have been slapped, choked, kicked, or otherwise physically assaulted
- you have been pressured or coerced into having sex

All of these are signs that you need to get out of the relationship. If you have been hit or threatened with violence, you should tell someone you trust and get out of that relationship as soon as possible. Some teenagers make excuses for their boyfriend's or girlfriend's abusive behavior. Making excuses for this behavior is a sure sign that something is wrong.

The End of a Dating Relationship

The reality is that many high school dating relationships eventually end (Figure 18.13). These relationships often do not last long, partly because teenagers' goals and beliefs are still forming and changing during these years as they try to figure out their own identities. This means it can be hard to maintain a dating relationship during high school.

Breakups can be emotionally painful, especially for the person who does not want to end the relationship. It is important, however, to recognize when a relationship is not working. No matter how a relationship ends, both people involved will probably find it difficult to cope. Common feelings following the end of a relationship include sadness, anger, physical illness, and loneliness (Figure 18.14). These feelings are a normal reaction to the end of a relationship and will heal over time.

Some people try to cope with the loss of a dating relationship by quickly beginning a new relationship. By doing this, however, they do not allow themselves time to process their feelings about the end of their previous relationship.

sexual assault
the act of forcing someone into sexual activity that he or she does not want

While a breakup can be emotionally painful for one or both members of the relationship, breakups are a normal part of teen dating. *Have you experienced a breakup? If so, have you learned anything about handling breakups that you would pass on to others as advice?*

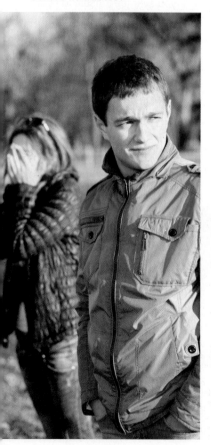

Some of these feelings can spill over into the new relationship, which is unfair to new dating partners. They deserve to be with someone who is focusing on the new relationship rather than continuing to cope with the loss of a past relationship.

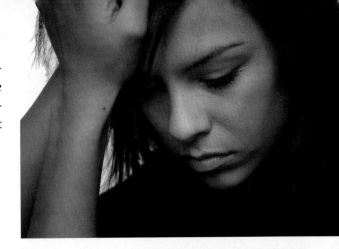

Strategies for Forming Healthy Dating Relationships

If you are like many teenagers, you have either already had or are interested in having a romantic relationship. Strategies you can use for forming a healthy relationship include the following:

- Get to know the person you might want to date. Talk to this person at school, during an activity, or on the phone before going out with him or her. This will help you figure out if you share common interests.

- Go out with a group that includes the person you are interested in. This is called *group dating*, and it is a good way to get to know a potential dating partner. Being with a group reduces the pressure of having to keep a conversation going with someone you are just getting to know. Group dating is also a good way to stay safe, especially if you do not know the person very well.

- Find ways to cope with your nerves. You may feel nervous about talking to or meeting with the person you may want to date. These feelings are normal and the other person will probably be nervous, too. If talking makes you nervous, plan activities that do not require much conversation, such as seeing a movie, playing miniature golf or bowling, or going to a school dance.

Figure 18.14

Breaking up with a dating partner can cause feelings of sadness, anger, and loneliness. These feelings are normal, and it is important to express and cope with them in healthy ways.

Lesson 18.3 Review

Know and Understand Assess

1. Identify at least six characteristics of a healthy dating relationship.

2. Define *exclusive*.

3. Explain the difference between love and infatuation.

4. Define *sexual assault*.

5. List at least eight signs of an unhealthy relationship.

Analyze and Apply

6. Why is maintaining individuality important in a dating relationship?

7. Someone once said, "Love does not consist in gazing at each other but in looking together in the same direction." Explain how this quote reflects the ideas presented in this lesson.

8. Why are attraction, closeness, and commitment important in a dating relationship? How is a dating relationship impacted if one of these characteristics is missing?

Real World Health

Create your own "Dating Bill of Rights." Include your own rights and responsibilities, as well as the rights and responsibilities of your dating partner.

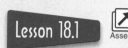

Lesson 18.1

Assess

Healthy Family Relationships

Key Terms

active listening
communication process
feedback

nonverbal communication
sibling rivalry
verbal communication

Key Points

- The family fulfills three main functions: providing for physical needs, fulfilling mental and emotional needs, and educating and socializing their children.
- Verbal communication involves the use of words to send a message.
- Nonverbal communication involves communicating through body language, facial expressions, eye contact, and tone and volume of voice, but not words.
- Relationships with parents and siblings can be improved by using various strategies.
- When family relationships or structures change, the family experiences stress and a period of readjustment.

Check Your Understanding

1. *True or false?* The family's only function is to help family members meet their basic physical needs.

2. Which of the following is an example of parents meeting the emotional needs of their children?
   A. attending their child's school performance
   B. teaching their child the importance of following rules and respecting adults
   C. providing their child with clothing
   D. teaching their child about family traditions

3. When a listener responds to the speaker to communicate that the message was received and understood, the listener is sending _____.

4. Which of the following is an example of verbal communication?
   A. rolling your eyes
   B. sending a text message
   C. nodding your head
   D. raising the volume of your voice

5. Leaning forward to show interest when someone is speaking to you is an example of _____.

6. Why is active listening important in the communication process?

7. **Critical Thinking.** Why might nonverbal messages be misunderstood? Are the meanings of nonverbal messages the same everywhere? Explain how relying on nonverbal communication may result in a misunderstanding between two people.

8. **Critical Thinking.** How does sibling rivalry affect the relationship between siblings?

Lesson 18.2

Assess

Healthy Friendships

Key Terms

acquaintances
clique

diversity

Key Points

- Friendships allow you to learn more about yourself, receive and provide emotional support, and gain communication and conflict management skills.
- Common sources of problems in friendships include cliques, jealousy, and changes over time.
- Peer pressure can be positive or negative.
- Various strategies can be used to help keep your friendships strong and remedy common conflicts.

Check Your Understanding

9. Which of the following is an example of how friendships affect your physical health?
   A. Friendships allow you to learn more about yourself.
   B. A smile or a compliment from a friend or a classmate can lift your spirits.
   C. People with good social support tend to recover from illnesses faster.
   D. Friendships allow you to receive and provide emotional support.

10. *True or false?* An acquaintance is someone you know, but is not a close friend.

11. A group of people with various backgrounds, including various ages, genders, ethnicities, and cultures describes _____.
    A. cliques
    B. diversity
    C. stereotypes
    D. prejudice

12. A small group of friends that deliberately excludes other people from joining or being a part of their group is called a _____.
    A. clique
    B. club
    C. stereotype
    D. prejudice

13. *True or false?* Experiencing physical, emotional, and social changes can lead to changes in your friendships.

14. *True or false?* Peer pressure is always negative.

15. Which of the following is an example of positive peer pressure?
    A. Your best friend hands you a cigarette.
    B. Your boyfriend or girlfriend encourages you to stay out past your curfew.
    C. A friend in your study group encourages you to study harder for the next exam.
    D. Your teacher recommends that you try out for the debate team.

16. Which of the following is *not* a strategy for maintaining a healthy relationship?
    A. Support and encourage your friends, and celebrate their successes.
    B. Avoid teasing your friends.
    C. When in a disagreement, give your friend "the silent treatment."
    D. Apologize if you hurt your friend and try to find ways to make amends.

17. **Critical Thinking.** How might prolonged jealousy damage a friendship?

 Lesson 18.3   Assess

Healthy Dating Relationships

Key Terms

exclusive   sexual assault
infatuation

Key Points

- Healthy dating relationships include attraction, closeness, commitment, individuality, balance, open communication, support, love, and safety.

- Couples do not have to be sexually active to have a healthy dating relationship.
- Signs of an unhealthy dating relationship include angry outbursts, constant fighting, threatening or belittling, possessiveness, jealousy, isolation from friends and family, physical abuse, and sexual assault or forced physical intimacy.
- Breakups can be stressful and emotionally challenging, but hurt feelings eventually heal.
- Group dating and getting to know a person are two strategies for forming healthy dating relationships.

Check Your Understanding

18. The physical and emotional connection that draws people together is called _____.
    A. infatuation
    B. love
    C. exclusivity
    D. attraction

19. *True or false?* Being *exclusive* in a relationship means you promise to be romantically involved with only your dating partner.

20. *True or false?* Maintaining your individuality in a relationship means that your core values, beliefs, and goals should change to match your dating partner's values, beliefs, and goals.

21. Which of the following is *not* an example of balance in a dating relationship?
    A. making time for family, friends, and a dating partner
    B. openly discussing decisions together
    C. sharing responsibilities
    D. spending free time only with a dating partner

22. Intense romantic feelings for another person that develop suddenly and are usually based on physical attraction are known as _____.

23. *True or false?* You can express affection for a dating partner in ways other than sexual activity.

24. Forcing someone to engage in any type of sexual activity against his or her will is called _____.

25. *True or false?* The best way to cope with the end of a dating relationship is to quickly begin a new relationship.

26. **Critical Thinking.** If your friend was going through a breakup, what healthy strategies could you suggest for coping with the end of the relationship?

Health and Wellness Skills

27. **Access Information.** In each community, city, or state, different resources exist to help victims of sexual assault or domestic violence. Research these types of resources within your own community or area. After gathering your information, create a brochure with information that might help one of these victims.

28. **Communicate with Others.** Eventually you will encounter people who disagree with you about certain health topics. When responding to a person you don't agree with, you may find it difficult to effectively communicate your knowledge and opinions while remaining respectful. With a partner, select one controversial health-related topic of your choice. Hold a discussion in which each of you argues different sides of an issue. Practice using strategies for overcoming communication barriers and disagreements.

29. **Advocate for Health.** Effective communication includes using audio and visual methods to present a message. Work together in small groups to create a public service announcement (PSA) that discusses signs of an unhealthy dating relationship. Include visual messages in your PSA, such as pictures, graphics, or clips, as well as audio.

30. **Practice Healthy Behaviors.** Suppose you are out on a date with your new girlfriend or boyfriend. He or she suggests that you go to a party where there is a large group of teenagers and no adults or parents are home. Drugs and alcohol are present at the party, and as the night progresses, couples begin going in and out of bedrooms. Your date begins pressuring you to drink and do drugs, and starts being very physical. What would be your personal plan of action in this type of situation? Write a short paragraph or script about what you would do.

Hands-On Activity
Healthy Relationships Tool Kit

Healthy relationships can sometimes be difficult to maintain. At times you may wish that you had a tool kit to help you out when relationships become difficult. This activity will allow you to create that kit, with items that symbolize what has been discussed in this chapter.

Materials Needed

- brown paper bag
- colored markers or pencils
- pictures from magazines or the Internet
- items to include in your kit

Steps for this Activity

1. Collect three to five items that remind you of the characteristics of a healthy relationship. These items can be related to any type of relationship mentioned in this chapter and can be related to characteristics like honesty, communication, or your relationship goals.

2. Decorate the outside of your paper bag with drawings or pictures that reflect the characteristics most important to you in a healthy relationship.

3. Place your collected items into your bag.

4. Share the meaning behind some or all of your items or pictures with the class. Use evidence that you learned in this chapter to explain why you chose these items and pictures for your Healthy Relationships Tool Kit.

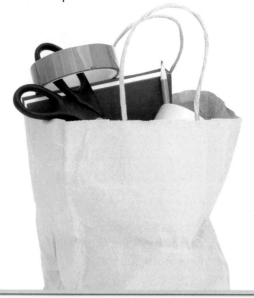

Core Skills

Math Practice Assess

The following table lists the number of households in the United States with related children younger than 18 years of age. Analyze the table and answer the questions that follow. Round your answers to the nearest whole number.

Number of Households with Related Children	
Number of Children	**Number of Households**
1 child	15,902,634
2 children	13,414,048
3 children	5,430,075
4 or more children	2,400,746

31. What is the total number of households surveyed in this study?
    A. 38,000,518
    B. 37,147,503
    C. 15,902,634
    D. 2,400,746

32. What percentage of households has only one child younger than 18 years of age as a resident?
    A. 15%
    B. 28%
    C. 37%
    D. 43%

33. What percentage of households has three related children younger than 18 years of age as residents?
    A. 15%
    B. 28%
    C. 37%
    D. 43%

34. What percentage of households has three or more related children living in one household?
    A. 6%
    B. 15%
    C. 21%
    D. 50%

Reading and Writing Practice Assess

Read the passage below and then answer the following questions.

In the past, most people had friends who lived in close proximity. Today, however, many people have friends who live farther away. You may have virtual friends, or people you met through social networks, chat rooms, or gaming. Although true friendships can sometimes develop between virtual friends, particularly if you share some real-life friends, you should be careful about sharing information with people you have met only online.

35. Based on the context, what is the meaning of the word *proximity*?
    A. nearness
    B. farness
    C. diversity
    D. ethnicity

36. Based on the content, what is the meaning of the word *mutual*?
    A. possessive
    B. unique
    C. virtual
    D. shared

37. According to the passage, how is the development of friendships different today when compared to the past?
    A. In the past, most people developed friendships with people who lived farther away, but today people develop friendships according to proximity.
    B. Today, many people have friends who live farther away. In the past, most people developed friendships according to proximity.
    C. True friendships developed in the past, but are less likely to develop today.
    D. There is no difference between how people develop friendships today when compared with the past.

38. Write a brief paragraph describing how technology has made an impact on the development of friendships and how people communicate.

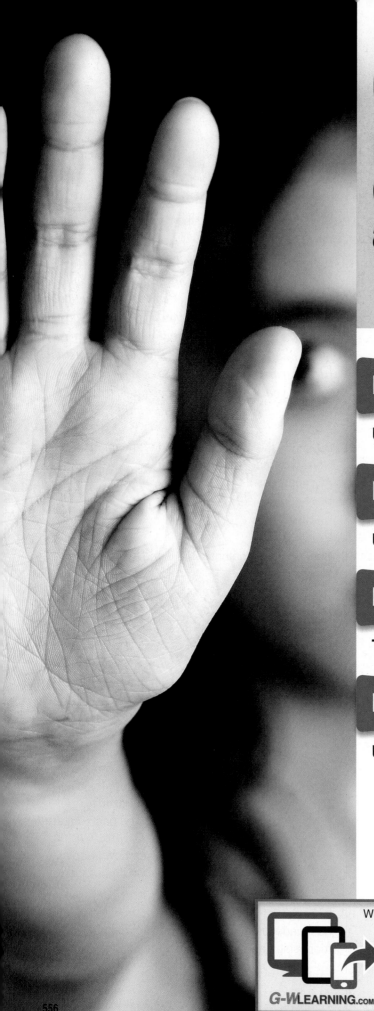

Chapter 19

Dealing with Conflict, Violence, and Abuse

Lesson 19.1

Understanding Conflict

Lesson 19.2

Understanding Violent Behavior

Lesson 19.3

The Reality of Family Violence

Lesson 19.4

Unwanted Sexual Activity

While studying this chapter, look for the activity icon to:
- **review** vocabulary with e-flash cards and games;
- **assess** learning with quizzes and online exercises;
- **expand** knowledge with animations and activities; and
- **listen** to pronunciation of key terms in the audio glossary.

G-WLEARNING.com

www.g-wlearning.com/health/

What's Your Health and Wellness IQ?

Take this quiz to see what you do *and* do not *know about conflict, violence, and abuse. If you cannot answer a question, pay extra attention to that topic as you study this chapter.*

1. *Identify each statement as* True, False, *or* It Depends. *Choose* It Depends *if a statement is true in some cases, but false in others.*

2. *Revise each* False *statement to make it true.*

3. *Explain the circumstances in which each* It Depends *statement is true and when it is false.*

Health and Wellness IQ Assess

	True	False	It Depends
1. If they are not resolved, conflicts can escalate; a minor conflict can become a major conflict.	True	False	It Depends
2. Using aggressive behavior is a good strategy for resolving conflicts.	True	False	It Depends
3. Mediators solve conflicts for other people.	True	False	It Depends
4. A person who sees violence in the media is at an increased risk of acting violently.	True	False	It Depends
5. Alcohol use tends to reduce violent behavior.	True	False	It Depends
6. Hazing is a harmless activity that brings a group of people closer together.	True	False	It Depends
7. Most rapes and sexual assaults are committed by strangers.	True	False	It Depends
8. Most abuse of older adults is committed by strangers.	True	False	It Depends
9. If you see someone engaging in a violent behavior, such as hazing, bullying, or sexual assault, you should mind your own business and not get involved.	True	False	It Depends
10. People who commit violence and abuse have often been victims of violence and abuse.	True	False	It Depends

Setting the Scene

You might think you don't have to worry about violence, especially if you live in a community with a low crime rate. Violence affects virtually all teenagers at some point in their lives, however, no matter where they live or how safe they feel.

Violence often has devastating effects on teenagers' health. This chapter will try to help you understand why violence occurs. Since violence is a social problem as well as a personal problem, you will also learn what the government, schools, and communities are doing to combat it. Most importantly, you will learn about strategies that can help you prevent and resolve conflicts that may lead to violence.

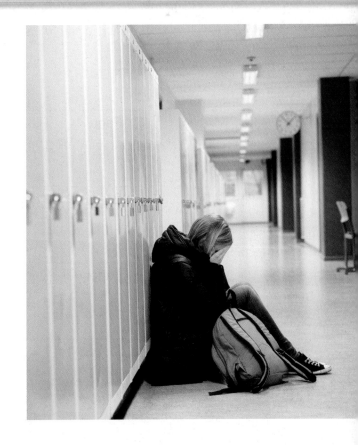

Understanding Conflict

Key Terms E-Flash Cards

In this lesson, you will learn the meanings of the following key terms.

aggressive
assertive
compromise
mediation
mediator
peer mediation

Before You Read

SQ3R Reading Method
*Use the SQ3R reading method to study this lesson. First, **S**urvey the lesson by glancing through it. Then, rewrite the headings and subheadings as **Q**uestions that might be answered within the text. **R**ead the lesson to find answers to your questions. **R**ecite the information and record it in your notes. Finally, **R**eview the lesson to make sure you didn't miss anything.*

Survey
Question
Read
Recite
Review

Lesson Objectives

After studying this lesson, you will be able to

- describe factors that cause conflict;
- describe consequences of conflict; and
- summarize strategies for resolving conflict.

Warm-Up Activity

Conflict Comic Strip
What is the most recent conflict you've had with someone? Illustrate this conflict in a short, six-panel comic strip formatted like the one shown here. Describe what was said, and try to show any nonverbal elements of communication such as body language and movement. Then write a paragraph to explain whether this conflict was handled in a healthy or unhealthy way. You will consider your answer again in the Real World Health activity at the end of this lesson.

Panel 1	Panel 2
Panel 3	Panel 4
Panel 5	Panel 6

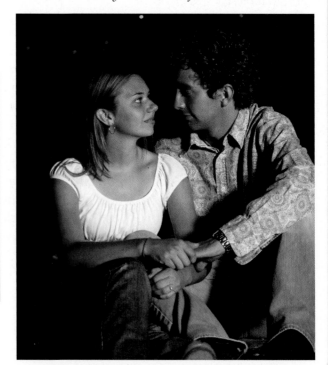

C onflict is a normal part of everyday life, and it is not always bad. Engaging in conflict can have positive outcomes for yourself and your relationships. Understanding conflict—including what causes conflict and how to best prevent and resolve conflict—is important.

Factors That Cause Conflict

Many different factors can lead to *interpersonal conflicts*, which are conflicts between people or groups of people (Figure 19.1). Conflicts occur when different people have different priorities, values, and needs. Conflicts also occur when people or groups have misunderstandings.

Consequences of Conflict

In some cases, people try but are unable to resolve a conflict, which can lead to serious and lasting consequences. Conflicts that last a while often *escalate*—meaning relatively minor conflicts become major problems. Unresolved conflicts can have negative effects on a person's psychological and emotional well-being. Interpersonal conflict can even impact a person's physical health. Conflict is a particular type of stress, and people who experience long-term stressors in the form of conflict can develop serious health problems.

Many people worry that discussing their conflicts with other people can destroy a relationship or make the conflict worse. In reality, working through a conflict can actually strengthen a relationship. When people decide to work together to resolve a conflict, they show their commitment to the relationship.

Strategies for Resolving Conflict

Your interpersonal interactions may be pleasant most of the time, but conflicts are sure to arise. Learning strategies for resolving conflict in productive and positive ways is important because conflict is an inevitable part of life.

Embrace Differences

Remember that people have different personalities and different perspectives on the world. You do not need, or even want, everyone in your life to be identical copies of you. In some cases, you simply need to accept the differences between yourself and the important people in your life to avoid unnecessary conflict.

Figure 19.1

Interpersonal conflicts can be caused by any number of factors, including differences of opinion and preexisting conditions, such as stress. *Think of the interpersonal conflicts you've had in the last month. Why did they occur? What factors contributed to these conflicts?*

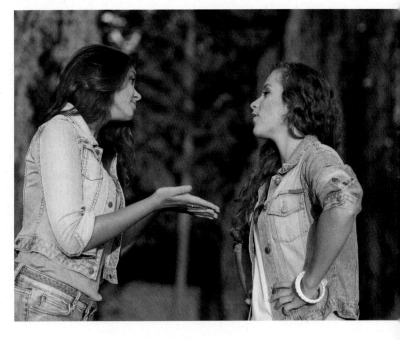

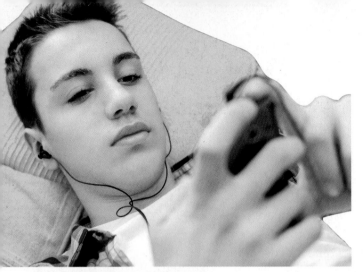

Figure 19.2

When you are in the middle of a heated conflict, you should take time to manage and control your feelings. Keep calm by withdrawing to cool down, if necessary.

Talking with friends or family members who have different interests, experiences, and views of the world can be invigorating and exciting. These people can introduce you to ideas, foods, music, places, and activities that you might not otherwise experience.

Keep Calm

Sometimes feelings get heated when people are in the middle of a conflict. In some cases, intense feelings, such as disappointment and frustration, can make a conflict worse. After all, it is hard to communicate effectively when you are feeling very emotional.

A good strategy for resolving conflict is to learn to manage and control your anger. Although everyone gets angry at times, you need to be able to share your feelings without becoming violent or abusive.

Some types of conflict are easier to resolve after time has passed. If you feel too angry or upset to have a productive conversation about a conflict, walk away and give yourself and the other person a chance to calm down (Figure 19.2).

Share Your Feelings

Sometimes conflicts continue, or grow worse, because the people involved do not share their feelings. Instead of trying to pretend you are not upset, talk about the conflict with someone. Ignoring the conflict does not give you or the other person involved a chance to resolve the problem and work out a solution.

You might also find it helpful to talk to someone you trust about your feelings. Explaining the situation to someone else can help you work out how you feel and offer you a new perspective.

Listen

Sometimes people are so focused on seeing a conflict from their own perspective that they have difficulty imagining any other perspective. This makes conflicts harder to resolve. The next time you have a conflict with someone, listen carefully to what that person is saying and try to understand his or her perspective.

compromise
an arrangement in which each side of a disagreement gives in a little to the other

assertive
a style of behavior in which you speak honestly about and act appropriately on your needs, feelings, and goals

aggressive
a style of behavior in which you speak or act toward others in a demanding and insulting way

Compromise

Some conflicts can be resolved relatively easily if both sides agree to give in a little, or **compromise**. Through compromise, each side can reach a solution that is acceptable for all people involved. For example, if you and your friends disagree about which movie to see, you could agree to see one movie this weekend and the other movie next weekend. Effective compromise is only possible, however, if both sides are willing to be flexible.

Be Assertive (Not Aggressive)

When you are **assertive**, you speak honestly about your feelings, needs, and goals. This is different from **aggressive** behavior, which is demanding and insulting. Behaving aggressively often makes it harder to effectively resolve conflicts, and can even cause conflicts to escalate.

To be more assertive, use *I-statements*, such as "I am hurt when you..." instead of *you-statements*, such as "You are never there for me when...". Telling other people how you feel helps them understand your perspective without making them feel attacked.

Suppose your friend has been spending more time with his or her new dating partner instead of with you, and you confront him or her about this. You could use an aggressive approach by saying, "You are really a lousy friend." Or you could use an assertive approach instead and say, "I feel hurt about not getting to spend much time with you anymore." The assertive approach lets the other person understand how you are feeling without insulting them, which can just escalate conflict further.

Seek Outside Help

In some cases, a conflict is too serious or too difficult for the people directly involved to manage by themselves. In this situation, an outside individual with a neutral perspective can help the people or groups find a good solution.

Mediation is a strategy for resolving difficult conflicts by involving a neutral third party, or *mediator*. During mediation, both parties in the conflict separately share their perspective of the conflict with the mediator. The mediator then brings the two parties together to share their views and tries to help them reach an agreement. Conflict resolution programs in many high schools provide *peer mediation*, in which specially-trained students work with other students to resolve conflicts (Figure 19.3).

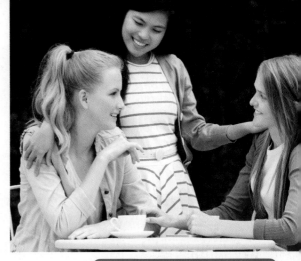

mediation
a method of resolving conflict that involves a third, neutral party

mediator
a neutral third party who helps resolve conflicts by listening carefully to each perspective

peer mediation
a method of resolving conflict in which a neutral peer listens to both parties in the disagreement and helps them reach a solution

Lesson 19.1 Review

Know and Understand
Assess

1. List at least two reasons why a conflict might occur.

2. List five strategies for resolving conflict.

3. Explain how assertive behavior differs from aggressive behavior.

4. What is the role of a mediator?

Analyze and Apply

5. Why can ignoring a conflict actually make the conflict worse? Create a scenario that provides support for your reason(s).

6. Compare effective and ineffective compromises.

Real World **Health**

Now that you have learned some strategies for resolving conflict, analyze the comic strip you created for the Warm-Up Activity at the beginning of this lesson. What strategies did you use to resolve that conflict? How healthy were those strategies? What strategies could you have used instead? Choose one or two strategies you think would have resolved the conflict in a better way and then draw a new comic showing how that conflict may have ended differently.

Understanding Violent Behavior

Key Terms E-Flash Cards

In this lesson, you will learn the meanings of the following key terms.

assault
bullying
hazing
homicide
human trafficking
identity theft
school violence

Before You Read

3-2-1 Chart

Before you read this lesson, make a chart like the one shown below. List three facts you discover while reading, two facts you find interesting, and one fact you still question.

3 Facts I Discovered	1. 2. 3.
2 Facts I Find Interesting	1. 2.
1 Fact I Still Question	1.

Lesson Objectives

After studying this lesson, you will be able to

- list risk factors for violent behavior;
- describe different types of violence; and
- practice methods of violence prevention.

Warm-Up Activity

Your School

Think about any instances of school violence that have occurred in your community. How safe and comfortable do you feel at your school? How did these instances affect your feelings of safety and comfort? In a chart like the one shown here, outline some factors that make you feel safe at school and some factors that make you feel unsafe.

Factors that Make Me Feel Safe at School	Factors that Make Me Feel Unsafe at School

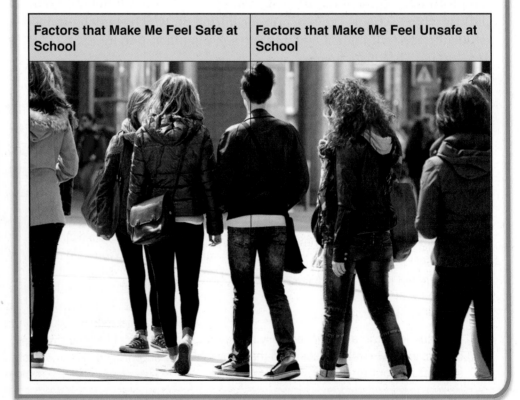

W hen conflicts cannot be effectively resolved, they can escalate to interpersonal violence. *Violence* is the intentional use of physical force, or the threat of physical force, to injure another person. A physical attack is referred to as an **assault**. **Homicide**, or *murder*, is the third leading cause of death for teenagers and young adults. Violence can also refer to behavior that results in psychological injury, as in the case of someone who spreads gossip or rumors that are harmful to someone else (Figure 19.4).

assault
the threat or use of physical force to injure another person

homicide
the killing of one human by another; murder

Violence Risk Factors

Even highly trained experts have trouble predicting what might lead one person to engage in a terrible act of violence. Factors about the person and factors about the person's environment or situation can have an impact and lead to violence.

Mental or Emotional State

Feeling frustrated is one factor that can lead a person to behave violently. Sometimes aggression may seem like the easiest way to release pent-up anger, especially for people who feel like they don't have other good ways of expressing those emotions. Hurting someone else is never an acceptable way of releasing aggression.

Personal Gain

Some people use violence, or the threat of violence, to get what they want. Some people use violence to retaliate against someone else. People who engage in violent behavior may receive punishment for their behavior from parents, their school, or even the police. They may also get injured as a result of their aggressive actions.

Exposure to Violence

Children whose parents behave violently toward one another are more likely than others to behave violently toward other children. These children are also more likely than others to behave violently toward their own romantic partners later in life. Similarly, people who have been bullied may repeat this type of aggression toward others, leading to a cycle of violence. Exposure to violence in the neighborhood or the media can also lead to aggression and violent behavior.

Alcohol and Drug Use

Alcohol and drug use impairs people's ability to use good judgment and consider the

Figure 19.4

Whether it causes physical injury or psychological injury, violence has lasting effects on its victims, and should be taken seriously. *What physical and psychological injuries are being inflicted on this teen?*

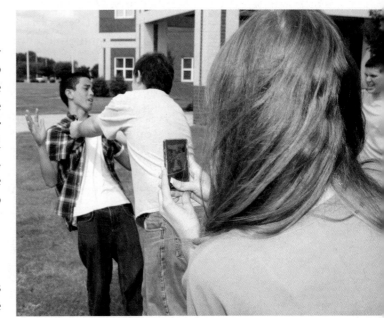

Do you think playing violent video games increases the likelihood that a person will behave aggressively? Researchers have used video games to examine how exposure to violence in the media contributes to aggression. In one study, men and women were randomly assigned to play either a violent video game or a nonviolent game.

After playing one of these two games for 10 minutes, study participants were given a task to perform with another student. The task gave participants the ability to punish their partners by blasting their ears with loud levels of noise through headphones. Receiving these blasts was very unpleasant. The researchers wanted to know which group of people would give their partners a louder blast of noise—those who played the violent game, or those who played the nonviolent game.

People who played the violent game chose to send higher levels of noise to their partners than those who played the nonviolent game. Gender also played a role in participants' behavior. Men who played the violent game blasted their partners with higher levels of noise than women who had also played the violent game. This study leads to the conclusion that being exposed to violence in video games can cause people to behave more aggressively in their daily lives.

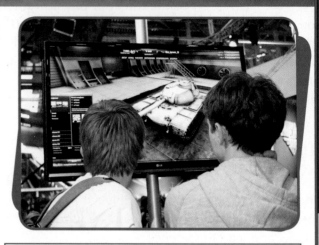

Thinking Critically

1. What do you think explains the findings of the study? How exactly does playing a violent video game lead to aggression in the real world?

2. This study found that playing a violent video game had a stronger impact on levels of noise blasts for men than for women. Were you surprised by this gender difference? Why or why not?

3. Given the results of this study, do you believe there should be new laws or regulations about violent video games? If so, what should these be? If not, why not?

consequences of their actions. Many victims of violence report that their attackers were under the influence of alcohol. Alcohol use is also associated with most cases of family violence, including violence between romantic partners and child abuse.

Availability of a Weapon

Research clearly shows that having access to a weapon increases a person's risk of behaving violently. If your parents or guardians own a gun, ask them to keep it unloaded in a locked cabinet. If you know someone who carries a gun or brings any weapon to school, tell an adult you trust, such as a teacher, parent or guardian, or school nurse.

Types of Violence

Many different types of violence exist, and violence occurs in many places—even places where people should feel safe, such as homes and schools. Schools can be especially unsafe for students who are assaulted or experience bullying and hazing. *School violence* is any violent behavior that occurs on school property, on school buses, and at school-sponsored events.

Bullying

Bullying is a type of aggressive behavior in which someone intentionally and repeatedly causes another person injury or discomfort (Figure 19.5). This can refer to physical or psychological injuries. Indirect and verbal bullying involves excluding someone from a group of friends, spreading rumors, and making fun of other people. Typically, the person who is being bullied has done nothing to cause the bullying and has trouble effectively defending him- or herself.

Cyberbullying. *Cyberbullying* is a form of bullying that takes place electronically. Cyberbullies may embarrass, harass, or threaten their peers by

- sending people mean or threatening e-mails or text messages;
- blocking people's e-mail addresses or "unfriending" them on social media sites for no reason;
- spreading personal or embarrassing information about people;
- hacking into people's e-mail accounts or social media pages and impersonating them to others; and
- creating websites to ridicule or embarrass other people.

In some ways, cyberbullying is similar to traditional bullying. Both can have a severe negative impact on people who are targeted. The victims can become depressed, have lower self-esteem, and experience problems at school.

In some ways, however, the impact of cyberbullying can be worse than traditional bullying. Information can be spread rapidly and widely as people forward e-mails and texts, and post messages on websites and social media pages. People can hide behind fake screen names online, allowing them to make comments they would never make in person. This can increase the harshness of a cyberbullying attack and cause additional anxiety to the victim. Victims of cyberbullying do not feel safe from attacks anywhere, even in their own homes.

Figure 19.5

Bullying doesn't have to involve physical violence. *How is the teen in this photo being harmed? How is this bullying?*

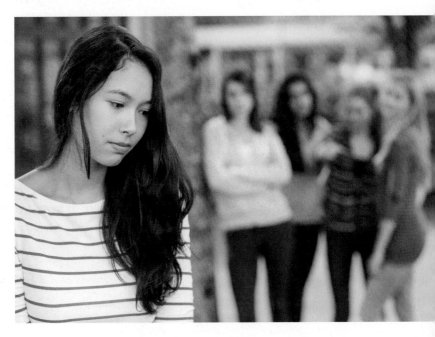

What Victims Can Do. Many teenage victims of bullying find it helpful to

- tell a trusted adult about what is happening;
- avoid the person who is bullying them whenever possible;

- calmly tell the bully to stop it;

- avoid reacting to the bully;

- do not respond to any taunts or name calling as your response may cause the bully to increase the behavior;

- stay near friends or adults when fearful of running into the bully;

- if you cannot avoid a cyberbully, stay off the Internet as much as possible; and

- print or save threatening or abusive messages and postings as proof of the bullying.

Internet Violence

identity theft
fraudulent act of stealing and using a person's personal information; often for financial gain

In addition to cyberbullying, other forms of violence can take place on the Internet. *Identity theft* happens when someone uses information about you without your permission. A person who gains access to personal information about you, such as your birthdate, address, or social security number, can open a credit card or buy a phone in your name. You could then be legally required to pay those bills.

Child sexual abuse can also begin or take place on the Internet. Online predators meet children and teenagers in chat rooms, on social networking sites, and through instant messages. They try to develop trust and form relationships with potential victims, and later on suggest meeting in person. You will learn more about child sexual abuse in the next lesson of this chapter.

To protect yourself from Internet violence, follow these steps:

- Keep your passwords secret, even from friends.

- Use privacy settings on social media accounts so strangers cannot see what you are posting.

- Let your parents or guardians know what you are doing online and with whom you are interacting.

- If anything happens online that makes you uncomfortable, talk to a trusted adult.

Hazing

hazing
a humiliating or dangerous activity that someone is required to perform to become part of a group

Hazing is any humiliating or dangerous activity that someone is required to perform, often as part of being accepted by a group. Hazing practices include excessive alcohol consumption, sleep deprivation, and physical punishment. Newcomers often submit to hazing because they want to fit in. Hazing can occur in any group setting and can be dangerous, which is why most states have laws against hazing.

Gang Violence

Gangs are groups of adolescents and young adults who engage in violent and illegal activities. These activities can include drug dealing; robbery; assault, especially of rival gang members; and vandalism.

Some teenagers join a gang to feel like part of a group and gain a sense of identity. Other people join gangs as a result of peer pressure, to make money, or to provide protection for themselves and their families.

Teenagers who join gangs almost always become involved in committing acts of violence. These teens may be pressured to commit a violent crime as an initiation into the gang. Because of the strong link between gangs and violence, teenagers in gangs often go to prison or become victims of violence.

People who join gangs are likely to have

- grown up in an area with widespread gang activity;

- family members or friends who are in gangs;

- lived in a home with violence or a lack of adult supervision; and

- negative feelings about themselves or feel hopelessness about the future.

Human Trafficking

Human trafficking is a form of modern slavery in which people are forced to perform some type of job or service against their will. In some cases, people are forced to work long hours for very little money. Their employers use threats of violence or other types of pressure to force them to continue working. For example, if a person is not a United States citizen, an employer could threaten to call immigration authorities to have the person put in jail.

Sex trafficking is a particular type of human trafficking in which people are forced to engage in sexual activity against their will. Sometimes people are forced to engage in sexual activity with another person for money. This type of sex trafficking is prostitution. Sex trafficking also includes forcing someone to pose for sexually explicit photographs. These types of sex trafficking are often advertised on websites, and the United States government is taking steps to combat avenues for human trafficking.

If you or someone you know is a victim of human trafficking, it is important that you talk to a trusted adult, such as a teacher, coach, doctor, or nurse. You can also call the National Human Trafficking Hotline (1-888-373-7888) or text HELP to BeFree (233733).

Hate Crimes

Victims of hate crimes are targeted because of their race, ethnic origin, disability, sexual orientation, or religion. Hate crimes include vandalism, offensive graffiti, and verbal threats as well as violent assaults and physical attacks.

Personal Profile

Are You Participating in Hazing?

Suppose you belong to a group that subjects new recruits to "tests" before they become full-fledged members of the group. These questions will help you assess whether your group is engaging in hazing.

Would I get in trouble for participating in this activity if my parents were watching? **yes no**

Would I get in trouble for participating in this activity if a teacher or coach were watching? **yes no**

Am I being asked to keep these activities secret? **yes no**

Am I doing something illegal? **yes no**

Am I being asked to do something that goes against my values? **yes no**

Am I being asked to do something that causes emotional distress or stress of any kind to myself or others? **yes no**

Am I being asked to do something that could physically harm myself or someone else? **yes no**

Do I feel pressured to do this activity to be accepted by the group? **yes no**

Add the number of yes answers to assess whether your group is engaged in hazing. The more yes answers, the more likely it is that the group is hazing others.

human trafficking
form of modern-day slavery involving the use of force or coercion to make a person perform some type of job or service against his or her will

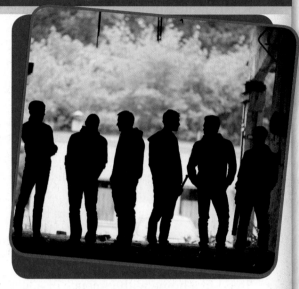

Robert is a 15-year-old sophomore in high school. He always had good grades, but recently, his grades have slipped. Since his parents separated, Robert's brother has lived with his mother and Robert has lived with his father. Robert goes home alone every day after school and doesn't feel like doing homework.

In the last month, Robert has started spending time with a new group of friends after school. These friends don't care about school and many of them are in a gang. Robert knows some gangs are involved in activities that could get him in trouble, or even result in serious injury. He also enjoys feeling like he's a part of a group. He doesn't know what to do.

Thinking Critically

1. What factors are leading Robert to consider joining a gang? How might Robert change those factors?

2. What are some strategies that could help Robert get back on track with his schoolwork and avoid getting involved in gang activities?

3. What kinds of trouble might Robert experience if he does join a gang?

4. What advice would you give other teenagers in the same situation as Robert?

Hate crimes tend to have a lasting impact on the victim as well as on his or her community. This is because people who commit hate crimes target not just a single person, but rather a larger group of people who share an identity.

In most cases, people who commit hate crimes are driven by stereotypes, prejudice, and misinformation. These attackers tend to have low self-esteem, which they try to improve by putting other people down. Some people who commit hate crimes have been victims of violence and aggression at the hands of family members.

Most states have laws against hate crimes. These laws increase the punishment for crimes such as vandalism or assault that were committed against someone as a hate crime.

Sexual Violence

Sexual violence describes any form of sexual activity that is attempted without the other person's consent. You will read more about sexual violence in the last lesson of this chapter.

What Schools Are Doing about Violence

People who study violence prevention say that individuals can only do so much. Schools and communities must get involved to create a culture that has zero tolerance for violent behaviors.

School violence prevention programs teach students the skills to identify situations that could lead to violence, solve problems without violence, communicate effectively, and manage conflict. Schools that have implemented violence prevention programs often experience a decrease in the rate of violent acts committed by students. In fact, school violence prevention programs are associated with improvements in positive behaviors among students, including better attitudes toward school and homework, better social relationships, and more order and discipline in classrooms.

Schools can use the following strategies to prevent violent behaviors, such as bullying and hazing:

- Select strong, positive, responsible student leaders who display appropriate behavior and will not be afraid to speak out against violence.
- Develop positive team-building activities, such as community service opportunities.
- Make sure all students know that violence of any form will not be tolerated and that there will be serious consequences for those who violate this rule.
- Provide specific examples of violent acts that had serious consequences to make the point that potential outcomes of violence can be severe.
- Install a buddy system in which older students have a responsibility to look out for younger students.
- Encourage all students to immediately report any violent behaviors they observe.

Lesson 19.2 Review

Know and Understand

1. List four risk factors for violence.
2. Where does school violence occur other than on school property?
3. List three forms of cyberbullying.
4. What is *hazing*?

Analyze and Apply

5. What feelings or experiences might make someone more likely to join a gang?

6. Which violence prevention strategy discussed in this lesson do you think would be most effective at your school? Why?

Real World Health

Homicide is the third leading cause of death for teenagers and young adults. Why do you think this is? Using your local library or the Internet, research this statistic and the most common reasons for these homicides. Then write a short newspaper editorial describing your findings and suggesting one or two strategies to lower the rate of teen homicide.

The Reality of Family Violence

Key Terms E-Flash Cards

In this lesson, you will learn the meanings of the following key terms.

child abuse

child sexual abuse

domestic violence

elder abuse

neglect

voyeurism

Before You Read

Deciphering Meaning in Context

Before you read this lesson, create a three-column chart like the one shown below. While you are reading the lesson, list facts that interest you in the left column and then list what you think those facts mean in the middle column. After reading the entire lesson, revisit this chart. If your understanding of a fact has changed based on the context of the entire lesson, write your new interpretation in the third column.

The text says...	I think the text means...	Now I think the text means...

Lesson Objectives

After studying this lesson, you will be able to

• describe domestic violence;

• list forms of elder abuse;

• identify types of child abuse; and

• summarize the consequences of child abuse.

Warm-Up Activity

How Can You Help?

Read the following scenario and reflect on how you might be able to help in this situation. Pair and share with another classmate to discuss different alternative actions.

You find one of your friends crying outside of the school cafeteria. When you finally get her to talk, she tells you that she was hit by her boyfriend, and that he screamed at her repeatedly. She has a bruise on her cheek and is obviously shaken up. You want her to tell your school counselor or her parents, but she doesn't want to tell anyone. What, if anything, do you do?

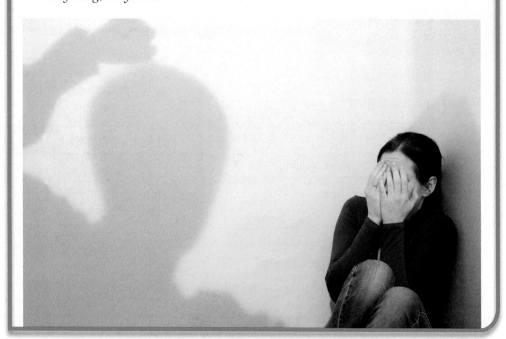

S ome families have serious problems that prevent them from meeting the needs of their members. In these families, physical, mental, and emotional abuse, or sexual mistreatment occurs.

Any member of a family can be the victim of family violence or abuse. All types of abuse are wrong, no matter who is committing the abuse and who is being abused.

Domestic Violence

Domestic violence is abuse that involves couples who are married, dating, or in a romantic relationship. This type of abuse occurs when one person in a relationship uses physical violence or mental or emotional abuse to try to control or dominate the other person. It can also include the threat of physical violence. Domestic violence is sometimes referred to as *spousal violence, intimate partner violence*, or *dating violence* (Figure 19.6).

Domestic violence often starts when one person threatens and verbally abuses the other. This behavior then escalates to violent physical attacks. Domestic violence can occur in person or electronically, and may occur between current or former partners.

Victims of domestic violence may suffer physical injuries, such as bruises or broken bones. They also suffer emotionally and experience depression, anxiety, fear, and shame. Victims of domestic violence may feel socially isolated and alone, in part because they do not want to tell anyone about the abuse.

Dating violence is common, even among high school and college students. In some cases, violence in an adolescent dating relationship can lead to problems with violence in future adult relationships. This is why it is essential to get out of a relationship the very first time that violence occurs. Abuse and violence should not occur in healthy relationships.

Elder Abuse

Older adults who are victims of *elder abuse* are abused in their homes, nursing homes, or other living situations. Elder abuse is typically committed by family members or paid caregivers. This abuse can take the following forms:

- physical abuse, including inappropriate use of medications or restraints
- verbal, emotional, or psychological abuse, including ignoring calls for help
- sexual abuse
- financial abuse, including the theft of money or real estate
- neglect, including failure to provide food, water, medications, and basic hygiene

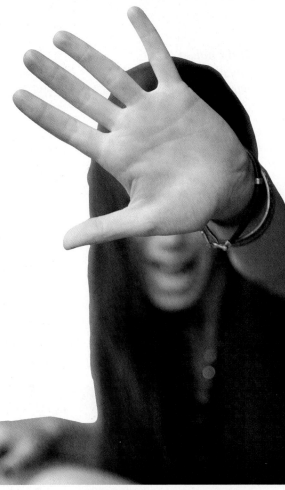

Figure 19.6

Domestic violence occurs within a romantic relationship and can be physical or verbal abuse. *What are some examples of physical and verbal domestic abuse?*

domestic violence
physically, mentally, or emotionally abusive behavior that occurs within a romantic relationship

elder abuse
any abuse or neglect that harms or seeks to harm an older adult

child abuse
any abuse or neglect that
harms or seeks to harm a
child

child abuse
any abuse or neglect that harms or seeks to harm a child

child sexual abuse
a type of abuse that involves using a child for sexual stimulation

voyeurism
looking at someone for sexual pleasure

neglect
a type of abuse that involves caregivers not meeting a dependent person's basic needs

---

Figure 19.7

While neglected children are not intentionally harmed, their basic physical and emotional needs are not being met. These children are likely to experience long-lasting physical and psychological effects due to being neglected. *What are the basic needs of a child? What are some examples of neglect?*

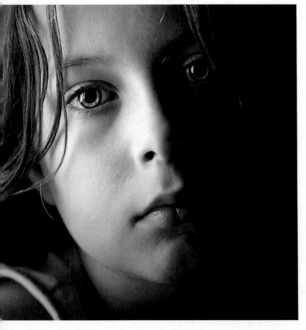

Many cases of elder abuse go unreported. Older adults who are abused and neglected feel helpless, lonely, and distressed. They also tend to die earlier than older adults who have not been abused.

Child Abuse

Each year in the United States, over 700,000 children between the ages of 2 and 17 experience some form of abuse or neglect. *Child abuse* includes physical, emotional or psychological, and sexual abuse committed by parents or caregivers. People who abuse children may have been abused themselves. They may feel depressed or have unhealthy thoughts about children. Teenagers sometimes abuse younger children.

Sometimes children and teenagers who are abused blame themselves. It is important to remember that the victim is *never* responsible for the abuse—abuse is caused by the abuser's problems.

Child Sexual Abuse

Child sexual abuse is a specific type of abuse in which an adult uses a child for sexual stimulation. The adult uses pressure, force, or deception to make the child engage in sexual activity, which can include

- intimate kissing;
- sexual touching;
- using the child to create pornography or forcing the child to view images of sexual activity;
- exposure or "flashing" of body parts to the child; and
- *voyeurism* (looking at, or *ogling*, for sexual pleasure).

Many people believe that only strangers commit sexual abuse. In about 90% of cases, however, children are abused by someone they know well, such as a family member, neighbor, or other trusted adult. Most sexual abusers of children are male.

It is hard to know how many children are sexually abused since many cases are not reported to the police. Research estimates indicate, however, that one in four girls and one in six boys will be sexually abused before they reach 18 years of age.

Neglect

Child abuse is often viewed as something that is intentionally done to a child, such as an act of violence. However, child abuse also includes neglect.

Children who are abused through *neglect* are not intentionally harmed, but their basic physical, emotional, medical, or educational needs are not met by their parents or guardians (Figure 19.7). Neglect also includes the failure to protect a child from harm, which can occur when a child is inadequately supervised or exposed to a dangerous living situation.

Consequences of Child Abuse

Your sense of well-being comes from knowing that you have the love, support, and respect of your family members and caregivers. When people are abused or neglected, their sense of well-being is shattered. Not surprisingly, that can have serious consequences. People who experience abuse may also suffer physical injuries (Figure 19.8).

A child who is abused may experience short- and long-term physical and psychological problems. Some children will even die from the abuse. In fact, over 1,500 children in the Unites States die from abuse or neglect each year. Unfortunately, some children who are abused and neglected will continue the cycle of violence when they have children.

Physical consequences of abuse may include brain damage, blindness, motor impairments, and cognitive impairments. Abused children are also more likely than others to develop health problems and diseases as adults, including heart disease, cancer, liver disease, and obesity.

Children who are abused are also more likely than others to behave in ways that can harm their health. Abused children have an increased risk of

- smoking;
- becoming alcoholics;
- abusing drugs;
- engaging in high-risk sexual behaviors;
- being delinquent;
- doing poorly in school and failing to graduate from high school; and
- being arrested as juveniles and adults.

Not surprisingly, children who are abused or neglected are also at greater risk of experiencing psychological problems. The psychological problems experienced by abused or neglected children include depression,

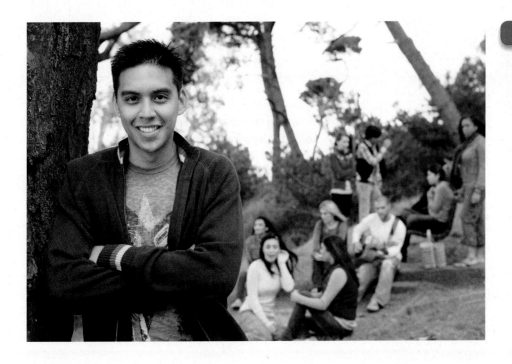

Figure 19.8

Although they can face great obstacles, abused children can grow up to live fulfilling and productive lives, especially if they seek help in managing their feelings and thoughts about the abuse.

anxiety, eating disorders, and post-traumatic stress disorder. The stress of ongoing, or *chronic*, abuse may also cause children to develop learning, attention, and memory problems. These problems increase the likelihood that abused children will struggle in school.

Finally, child abuse can impair a person's ability to establish and maintain healthy intimate relationships in adulthood. People who do not experience love, trust, and support in their early relationships may have trouble building healthy relationships with others later.

Fortunately, children who have been abused are not doomed to an unhappy and unhealthy life. They can get help to feel better about themselves and others, and live fulfilling lives.

Treating Abusers

People who commit abuse or neglect have serious problems. Many of them were victims of this type of behavior themselves. Others have problems such as

- substance abuse or addiction;
- mental disorders, including depression; or
- low self-esteem.

People who commit abusive or violent acts may benefit from specific types of treatment. In the case of parents or guardians who abuse their children, treatment could include education on appropriate parenting techniques.

For people who commit sexual violence, treatment may include training to increase empathy for victims. The abuser's misconceptions about abuse, such as a belief that victims asked for or enjoyed the attack, can be corrected through this treatment method. Treatment also includes training that helps abusers stop acting on their preference for sexual behavior that hurts others.

Lesson 19.3 Review

Know and Understand Assess

1. List three types of abuse.
2. List five forms of elder abuse.
3. What is child neglect?
4. List three physical consequences of child abuse.

Analyze and Apply

5. Why might children and teens who are abused blame themselves for the abuse?

6. How can being abused as a child affect a person's relationships in adulthood?

Real World | Health

Mandated reporters are people who are required by law to report any suspected cases of child abuse and neglect. Examples of mandated reporters may include police officers, human services workers, teachers, and doctors. Conduct research to find out about the laws for reporting child abuse in your state. Create a colorful fact page of your findings.

Unwanted Sexual Activity

Lesson Objectives

After studying this lesson, you will be able to

- describe types of sexual violence;
- identify consequences of sexual violence;
- define *rape*;
- describe steps for treatment after a sexual assault; and
- recognize behaviors that are types of sexual harassment.

Key Terms E-Flash Cards

In this lesson, you will learn the meanings of the following key terms.

acquaintance rape

consent

rape

sexual harassment

sexual violence

statutory rape

Warm-Up Activity

What is Sexual Consent?

Saying "yes" in a strong, clear manner would be an obvious verbal agreement for sexual consent, just as saying "no" strongly and firmly proclaims an obvious lack of consent. Working with a partner, brainstorm some other examples of consent and lack of consent and list them in the appropriate columns on a sheet of paper formatted like the chart below. Include both verbal and nonverbal messages.

Ways to Convey Consent	Ways to Not Consent
Saying "Yes"	Saying "No"

Before You Read

Three Questions

Based on its title, key terms, and objectives, what are three questions you'd expect to be answered in this lesson? List your questions in a chart like the one below. After reading the lesson, revisit your questions and write answers to them. If a question was not addressed, research an answer and write it in the answer column in a different color.

Questions	Answers
1.	
2.	
3.	

sexual violence

any sexual activity to which one party did not consent

T he term used to describe sexual activity involving someone who did not give consent for the activity to occur is ***sexual violence***. Although sexual violence can happen to anyone at any age, teenagers are especially vulnerable. This is partly because teenagers' physical, emotional, and sexual development are all at different levels, and their sex drives are particularly strong. People who are more sexually experienced may take advantage of teenagers. Some teens may have poor judgment or decision-making skills, and others may just act impulsively.

This lesson examines sexual violence, which includes rape and sexual harassment. You will learn skills that will help you refuse unwanted sexual activity and avoid becoming a victim of sexual violence.

What Is Sexual Violence?

rape

sexual intercourse to which one party did not consent

Threatening or forcing someone into sexual activity is wrong and illegal. Sexual violence includes *rape*, or nonconsensual sexual intercourse. The following behaviors are also sexual violence if consent is not given:

- kissing
- sexual touching, including the touching or fondling of body parts through a person's clothing
- exposure of a person's genitals to another person
- sexual harassment
- photographing a person who is nude
- attempted sexual intercourse, even if penetration does not occur
- exposing someone to pornography

Sexual violence includes the sexual abuse of children by family members, domestic abuse of one spouse by another, and both stranger rape and *date rape*. Although more males than females carry out acts of sexual violence, both males and females can be victims of sexual attacks.

Lack of Consent

consent

a direct, verbal, non-coerced agreement from someone who is capable of making an informed decision

Lack of consent is an important part of the definition of sexual violence. **Consent** is direct, verbal agreement that occurs when someone clearly says *yes*. Consent does *not* occur if someone says *no* or nothing at all. People cannot assume a person is agreeing to engage in a particular behavior unless the person specifically, verbally expresses a willingness to do so. Without *mutual consent*, or consent by both people, unwanted sexual activity is sexual abuse or rape. Some states are considering laws requiring people to have this type of *affirmed consent* before engaging in any type of sexual activity.

Some people are not legally capable of giving consent to sexual activity. Consent can only be given by someone who is informed, or who fully understands what he or she is agreeing to do. People do not consent to engage in sexual behavior under the following conditions:

- they are pressured or coerced by someone else

- they are under the influence of drugs or alcohol (Figure 19.9)
- they have certain types of disabilities or disorders, such as a cognitive disability
- they are asleep or unconscious
- they are younger than a particular age—16, 17, or 18 years of age, depending on the state

The person who commits the sexual violence act is entirely to blame if sexual activity occurs under any of these circumstances. In these cases, the victim is *never* to blame.

Laws prohibit sexual activity between adults and adolescents because adolescents are considered incapable of giving consent. The crime of **statutory rape** occurs when an adolescent engages in sex with an adult. An adult can be charged with statutory rape even if the adolescent consented to having sex.

Some people believe that if two people are in a dating or an intimate relationship, any kind of sexual activity must be consensual. This is false—no one, not even a dating partner, has the right to pressure or coerce someone else to engage in sexual activity. More than half of sexual-violence victims know their attackers.

Consequences of Sexual Violence

Sexual violence can impact the health and well-being of victims in lasting and destructive ways. Sexual violence can also have lasting and harmful effects on the victim's family, friends, and his or her community.

Impact on Physical Health

Many people who experience sexual violence develop physical health problems. Many are also physically injured as a result of the rape. Physical side effects of sexual violence can include

- bruises, burns, and broken bones;
- pelvic pain;
- gastrointestinal disorders;
- migraines and other frequent headaches; and
- back pain.

Victims of sexual violence are also sometimes left with an unwanted pregnancy or a sexually transmitted infection.

Impact on Emotional Health

Victims of sexual violence experience both short- and long-term psychological injuries. Common psychological symptoms following a sexual attack include shock, denial, fear, anxiety, shame, guilt, and confusion.

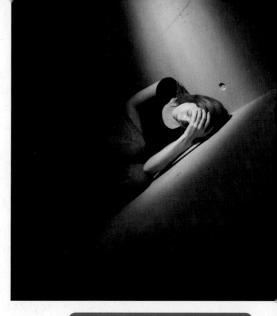

Figure 19.9

If someone is unconscious or under the influence of drugs or alcohol, he or she is unable to give consent. Having sexual intercourse with such a person is, therefore, considered rape. *How can you tell if someone is able or unable to give consent?*

statutory rape
sexual activity that occurs between an adult and an adolescent

These symptoms may disappear or lessen with time. Some people who have experienced sexual violence may develop post-traumatic stress disorder or become depressed.

In some cases, people who have experienced sexual violence attempt to cope with this trauma by engaging in risky health-related behaviors. As a result, the person may experience further health problems.

Impact on Social Health

Sexual violence can also impact a person's social health and well-being, especially if the person inflicting the violence is a trusted person. People can become hesitant to trust others as a result of sexual violence, which can cause problems in intimate relationships. Some victims of sexual assault feel alienated from their family members and friends.

Victims are sometimes scolded for dressing a certain way or having too much to drink. Victims are never to blame for sexual violence, but they may feel shame and guilt if they blame themselves. Their self-esteem can suffer and they may withdraw from their friends and family. Many victims of sexual crimes fear blame, so they do not report the crimes to law enforcement officials or their friends and family members.

Rape

Although rape involves sexual violence, experts say that it is not an act of sex, but an act of power and aggression. Rapists use force, violence, weapons, or alcohol and drugs to make other people submit to sexual acts.

Rapists can be strangers or acquaintances. People are more likely to be raped by someone they know and trust than by a stranger. Some people use the term *acquaintance rape* to refer to rape committed by someone the victim knows. In incidents of acquaintance rape, a rapist takes advantage of being trusted, and may use alcohol or drugs to reduce the victim's ability to resist sex (Figure 19.10).

acquaintance rape
unwanted sexual intercourse that is committed by someone the victim knows

Figure 19.10

Most victims of sexual assault are attacked by acquaintances, and alcohol and drugs are often involved. *What precautions can you and your friends take to guard against sexual violence?*

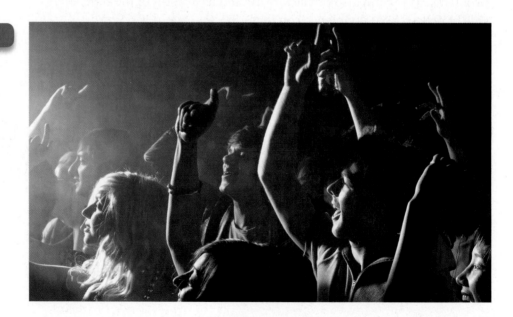

Preventing Assault

You can reduce your risk of becoming a victim of unwanted sexual activity or sexual abuse, including date rape. The following strategies can help you prevent assault:

- Be aware of your surroundings. People talking on their cell phones or wearing headphones are easier targets.

- Avoid walking alone, especially at night. If you must walk alone at night, stay in well-lighted areas and avoid alleys and bushes where someone might hide.

- Never accept a ride from or give a ride to a stranger, no matter how nice that person may appear.

- If you are walking alone, have your keys out before you get to your car. Examine the inside of your car *before* you get in. Lock your doors immediately after you get inside.

- If you are attacked, yell *stop* or *stay back* to attract attention from other people.

- The first few times you go out with someone, make sure you are with friends in a group setting or in a public place.

- Avoid using alcohol or other drugs, which can impair your ability to sense danger, resist sexual activity, and make good decisions.

- When you are attending a party or going out with friends, let adults know where you will be and who will be there. Don't go to parties that are unsupervised by adults, such as parties that occur when someone's parent is out of town.

- Do not leave a drink unattended or accept a drink from someone you don't know or trust. Certain drugs, called *date rape drugs*, are sometimes slipped into an unsuspecting person's drink. People in a drowsy, disoriented, or unconscious state are easy prey for attackers.

- Don't leave a party with someone you don't know well. Never go alone to unfamiliar, isolated places with people you do not know very well.

- Don't stay in a situation with someone who makes you nervous or uncomfortable, or who pressures you to do something you don't want to do. Leave the situation and call a friend, parent, or guardian immediately.

- Make your intentions and refusal known with a clearly and firmly stated *No, get away!* if the person does not respect your refusal.

Getting Treatment

When people are sexually assaulted or threatened with sexual assault, they should try to stay calm. If possible, they should stall the attacker so they have time to get help. They may be able to scare off their attacker by saying they have a sexually transmitted infection. In some cases, they may need to passively submit to the attack to avoid getting hurt. Their top priority is to stay alive (Figure 19.11 on the next page).

After a rape, the victim should immediately call 911 to get help. It is important to get medical attention right away at a hospital or clinic. The person will be examined and treated for physical injuries and tested for sexually transmitted infections. He or she can receive medications to decrease the chances of developing a sexually transmitted infection. If the rape victim is a female, she may also receive medications to decrease her chance of becoming pregnant.

Rape is a crime—even if the victim knows the person who committed the rape—and it should be reported to the police. The police can only arrest the attacker if they know what occurred and can collect evidence. A person who is raped should not change clothes or take a shower before going to the police station or hospital, since evidence can be gathered from clothes and hair.

Figure 19.11 What a Rape Victim Should Do

Was it rape? It was rape if consent was not given for sexual intercourse to occur. Consent can never be legally given by minors or by an intoxicated or unconscious person. After a rape has occurred, the next steps are important for the victim's safety and health.

1.	Get to a safe place away from the rapist or rapists.
2.	Get medical care to treat injuries and prevent sexually transmitted infections.
3.	Talk to doctors about preventing pregnancy.
4.	Contact police to report the rape. This can prevent another rape.
5.	Save evidence such as clothing with blood or semen on it in case police need this to investigate the rape.
6.	Remember details about the rapist, the location, and the time.
7.	Share your experience and feelings with at least one trusted adult.
8.	Get psychological counseling to help cope with your feelings.
9.	Know that rape is *only* the rapist's fault.

Figure 19.12

Victims of sexual assault can get help dealing with their traumatic experiences by confiding in a counselor, trusted adult, or religious leader. Sometimes talking about these feelings can help victims move forward.

Many people who have been sexually assaulted find it helpful to talk to specially-trained counselors. Some people who have been victims find support by talking to others who have been through this type of trauma.

A school nurse, doctor, or local rape crisis center can provide information about specially trained counsellors and local support groups. Victims might also find it useful to talk to other adults they trust. Parents, the family physician, religious leaders, and guidance counselors are examples (Figure 19.12).

Supporting Survivors of Sexual Assault

If you know someone who has been sexually assaulted, he or she may or may not want to talk about the attack. Follow the victim's lead and do not ask too many questions. Try to be a good listener, and do not judge or blame the victim for what happened. Here are some helpful messages to convey to a person who has experienced an assault:

- "I'm glad you're alive."
- "It's not your fault."
- "I'm sorry it happened."
- "You did the best you could.

Remember, the victim is *never* to blame for an attack.

School-Based Programs

Many high schools and colleges have programs that educate students about

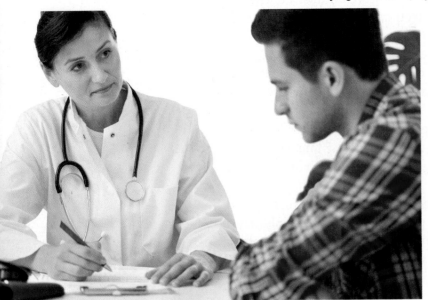

intimate partner violence. These programs also help teach students about the importance of stepping in if you believe an assault might occur. For example, Safe Dates is a program designed to prevent emotional, physical, and sexual abuse in high school dating relationships. The goals of this program are to

- change norms about dating violence;
- improve skills for resolving conflicts;
- promote awareness of the importance of getting help if abuse occurs; and
- decrease rates of abuse in dating relationships.

Research shows that teenagers who participate in such a program report fewer incidents of physical and sexual dating violence.

Sexual Harassment

Sexual harassment is unwanted sexual attention. Unfortunately, it is fairly common among adolescents. Most victims are female, and most perpetrators are male. However, both males and females can commit sexual harassment and be the victims of such harassment.

Like other types of sexual violence, sexual harassment can be devastating for victims. Sexually harassed teens can become depressed and anxious, lose sleep, withdraw from normal activities, and hate going to school. Changes in behavior, such as avoiding usual activities and missing school, could be signs of depression or anxiety caused by sexual harassment.

sexual harassment
any unwanted sexual attention

Sexual harassment, whether verbal or nonverbal, involves giving unwanted sexual attention to a person through gestures, words, or other methods. *What is an example of sexual harassment?*

What Is Sexual Harassment?

Sexual harassment can be either verbal or nonverbal (Figure 19.13). Verbal sexual harassment includes the use of words, gossip, and threats. People who tell sexual jokes and make inappropriate or intimidating sexual comments to others are guilty of sexual harassment.

Sexual harassment can also occur when sexual comments are not directed at someone, but just spoken in the presence of a person who is made uncomfortable by the comments. Spreading rumors of a sexual nature, either through word of mouth or technology, is also sexual harassment.

Nonverbal sexual harassment includes instances when sexual gestures are directed at someone or are made in reference to someone. Nonverbal sexual harassment includes pinching, rubbing, or brushing up against someone in an inappropriate way.

If you are unsure whether someone's behavior counts as sexual harassment, ask yourself these questions: How does it makes you feel? Do you want the behavior to stop? If the behavior makes you feel bad and you want the person to stop, you are experiencing sexual harassment.

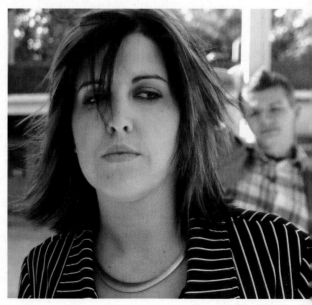

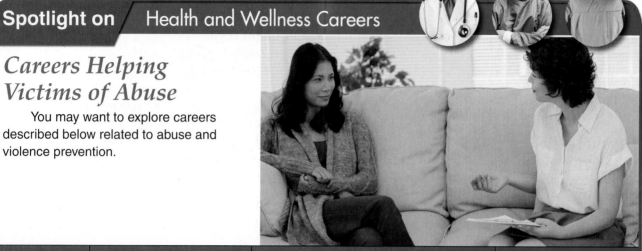

Careers Helping Victims of Abuse

You may want to explore careers described below related to abuse and violence prevention.

Career	Typical Education and Training	Typical Job Duties and Demands	Career Resources
Police Officer and Detective	ranges from high school diploma to college degree, plus graduation from an agency's training program; must meet rigorous physical and personal qualifications	Police officers protect people's lives and property. Detectives collect evidence and investigate possible crimes.	National Sheriffs' Association; International Association of Chiefs of Police; US Marshals Service
School Psychologist	four-year college degree, plus a three-year master's degree; must pass a certification exam	School psychologists work with students individually and in groups to manage behavioral, academic, and social problems. They may also work with teachers and parents to develop strategies for managing students' behavior, and provide training to students, parents and teachers about managing crisis situations and substance abuse problems.	National Association of School Psychology (NASP)
Child Protection Social Worker	Bachelor of Social Work (BSW) or Bachelor of Science (BS) degree, and potentially a Master's of Social Work (MSW) degree, plus state licensure	Child Protection Social Workers investigate potential cases of child abuse and neglect. They interview people and gather information, and intervene if necessary.	Children's Bureau, Administration for Children and Families; National Association of Social Workers
School Social Worker/ School Adjustment Counselor	four-year college degree followed by a master's degree, and state licensure	School Social Workers or Adjustment Counselors work with individuals and groups to provide interventions that promote the social and emotional well-being of students. They may provide individual and group counseling, consult with teachers and administrators, and deliver classroom and school-wide interventions.	American School Counselor Association; National Association of Social Workers

Exploring Careers

1. Think about your interests, strengths, and weaknesses. With these in mind, which career described above appeals most to you? Which career does not interest you?

2. Do you know someone who works in one of these careers? If so, ask this person why he or she chose this career and what she or he likes most and least about the work.

What You Can Do

Victims of sexual harassment often feel powerless to stop the behavior. They may even be accused of causing the harassment. Certain steps can be taken, however, to make the behavior stop. First, victims should know that sexual harassment is not their fault. They did nothing to deserve to be treated in this way.

Victims also need to document their experiences by writing down details of events, dates, locations, and possible witnesses to the harassment. They should print or save e-mails, pictures, videos, texts, social media posts, and other evidence of the harassment that can be used to report the activity and stop it.

In some cases, people can talk directly to the person harassing them and ask them to stop. In many cases, however, this can be intimidating. Most schools and workplaces have a sexual harassment policy. If the harassment occurs at work, people can report it to their supervisor or to someone in human resources. At school, people can speak with their teachers, counselors, or principal to ask for help. If you are ever sexually harassed and you are not sure what to do, talk to a trusted adult.

How Bystanders Can Help

If you observe someone else being sexually harassed, do not speak to the harasser; this can cause worse behavior. Try to get the person being harassed away from the situation by coaxing him or her to leave with you.

If you feel unsafe or uncomfortable getting involved when you observe sexual harassment, tell a teacher, guidance counselor, or principal. Remember that harassment is wrong, painful, and criminal. Notifying someone who can stop it is the right thing to do.

Lesson 19.4 Review

Know and Understand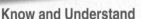

1. List three examples of cases in which people are incapable of giving consent.
2. Why should a victim not change clothes or shower after a rape occurs?
3. Give one example of verbal sexual harassment and one example of nonverbal sexual harassment.
4. List two ways a bystander can help someone who is being sexually harassed.

Analyze and Apply

5. Why does consent not occur if a person says nothing at all?

6. Why do experts call rape an act of power and aggression more so than an act of sex? Develop an argument either supporting or disagreeing with this view.

Real World Health

Think about situations in which you might be vulnerable to violence. For each of these situations, create a personal safety plan by outlining three to five actions you could take to help keep yourself safe. What steps could you take to prevent danger? If you found yourself in an emergency situation, what steps could you take to seek help?

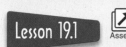

Chapter 19 Review and Assessment

Understanding Conflict

Key Terms

aggressive   mediation
assertive   mediator
compromise   peer mediation

Key Points

- Conflict may occur between people or groups for a variety of reasons.
- Unresolved conflicts may have serious consequences.
- Learning strategies for dealing with conflict can help people resolve conflict in positive ways.

Check Your Understanding

1. *True or false?* Conflict is a part of everyday life.

2. *True or false?* Working through a conflict can strengthen a relationship.

3. A productive method for solving conflict is to _____.
   A. use *I-statements*
   B. use *you-statements*
   C. be aggressive
   D. avoid sharing feelings

4 _____ is a program in which specially-trained students work with other students to resolve conflicts.

5. **Critical Thinking.** Explain why controlling anger is important to resolving a conflict.

Key Points

- Violence results in physical or psychological damage.
- Some risk factors increase the likelihood of a person exhibiting violent behavior.
- Types of violence include school violence, bullying, Internet violence, hazing, gang violence, human trafficking, hate crimes, and sexual violence.
- Many schools have taken steps to help prevent violence.

Check Your Understanding

6. A physical attack is referred to as a(n) _____.

7. _____ is a type of aggressive behavior in which someone intentionally and repeatedly causes another person injury or discomfort.
   A. Hazing
   B. Bullying
   C. Homicide
   D. Assault

8. *True or false?* Newcomers often submit to hazing because they want to fit in.

9. In _____, victims are targeted because of their race, ethnicity, sexual orientation, or religion.

10. **Critical Thinking.** Explain why people who have used alcohol or drugs are more likely to engage in violent behavior.

11. **Critical Thinking.** Explain why a person who engages in hate crimes is likely to have low self-esteem.

Understanding Violent Behavior

Key Terms

assault   human trafficking
bullying   identity theft
hazing   school violence
homicide

The Reality of Family Violence

Key Terms

child abuse   elder abuse
child sexual abuse   neglect
domestic violence   voyeurism

Key Points

- Domestic violence occurs within couples who are married, dating, or in a romantic relationship.
- Types of elder abuse include physical abuse, financial abuse, and neglect.
- Child abuse may include emotional or sexual abuse.
- Children who are abused may experience short-term and long-term physical and psychological effects.
- People who commit abusive or violent acts may benefit from specific types of treatment.

Check Your Understanding

12. _____ is a type of abuse that involves couples who are married, dating, or in a romantic relationship.

13. *True or false?* Victims of elder abuse are abused only in nursing homes.

14. _____ is the ogling of someone's body for sexual pleasure.

15. *True or false?* Children who are abused are more likely than others to behave in ways that can harm their health.

16. *True or false?* Children who are neglected are not intentionally harmed.

17. **Critical Thinking.** Why can victims of domestic violence feel lonely and isolated from other people?

18. **Critical Thinking.** Why might violence in adolescent relationships lead to problems with violence in future adult relationships?

 Lesson 19.4   Assess

Unwanted Sexual Activity

Key Terms

acquaintance rape	sexual harassment
consent	sexual violence
rape	statutory rape

Key Points

- Sexual violence may include various behaviors, such as sexual touching, sexual harassment, and exposure to pornography.
- Without mutual consent, sexual activity is categorized as abuse or rape.
- Sexual violence can have consequences that affect the victim's physical, emotional, and social health.
- Rape victims should report the crime and receive medical treatment immediately.
- Many schools have programs that help educate students about intimate partner violence.
- Sexual harassment may be verbal or nonverbal.
- Most schools and workplaces have a sexual harassment policy.

Check Your Understanding

19. Nonconsensual sexual intercourse is _____.

20. A person cannot give consent to engage in sexual behavior if he or she is _____.
    - A. over the age of 18
    - B. awake and alert
    - C. pressured or coerced
    - D. able-bodied

21. _____ occurs when an adolescent engages in sex with an adult.

22. *True or false?* An adult can be charged with a crime even when an adolescent consents to have sex.

23. *True or false?* Victims of sexual violence may experience post-traumatic stress disorder.

24. _____ refers to rape committed by someone the victim knows.

25. *True or false?* A person who is raped should shower before going to the hospital.

26. *True or false?* People can be sexually harassed through social media.

27. **Critical Thinking.** What type of treatment is recommended for people who have been sexually assaulted?

28. **Critical Thinking.** Why might victims feel powerless to stop sexual harassment?

Health and Wellness Skills

29. **Access Information.** Look through the local news and find a current event that involves one of the types of conflict, violence, or abuse discussed in this chapter. Consider the strategies and prevention methods you learned in this chapter and apply them to the news story you found. Rewrite the article so that those involved in the situation implement your strategies and reach a different outcome.

30. **Advocate for Health.** Design a pamphlet about what someone should do if he or she is in an abusive situation. Include the signs of abuse, some basic steps to take in an abusive situation, and where to go for help. If you can, include the names and contact information of local resources for victims of abuse. Distribute your pamphlet in your school or community.

31. **Be an Advocate.** In small groups, learn more about human trafficking in schools by visiting the website of the National Center on Safe Supportive Learning Environments. With guidance from your instructor, choose one aspect of human trafficking and find out about its definition, risks, ways to identify trafficking, and how to prevent and protect one's self from dangerous situations. Create a poster of your findings to display in school.

32. **Practice Healthy Behaviors and Reduce Health Risks.** An important way of sharing your feelings without the other person feeling attacked and becoming defensive is to use an *I-statement* instead of a *You-statement*. For example, saying "I feel hurt when you share my private information with other people," instead of saying "You violated my trust and you're a terrible person." Convert the following *You-statements* into *I-statements*.
    You-statement: "You always remind me to do my homework. Why can't you let me try to do it on my own?"
    You-statement: "You didn't tell me you were going to Joe's party. Didn't you know I would find out?"
    You-statement: "You always make me clean my room when you know I am trying to get to work on time."
    You-statement: "You always make me babysit my little brother, and you never offer to pay me or thank me."
    Write two to three more *I-statements* that may help you start a conversation to help resolve a conflict.

Hands-On Activity
Program against Violence

Now that you understand more about the different types of violence, why violence occurs, and strategies to prevent and resolve conflicts, design a school-based or community-based program that will raise awareness about one type of violence.

Steps for this Activity

1. Study your school or your community, and identify existing programs that target violence. Organize these programs according to the types of violence discussed in this chapter. This list will show you which types of violence may be insufficiently targeted in your community.

2. As a class, choose a type of violence you want to target. Is there a program that already exists for this type of violence, but is not very successful? Do you, as a student, see a specific need that school or community leaders may not see?

3. Decide what type of program you want to create. If you are changing an existing program, decide how you will give it new life. Use as many resources as possible, including adults who work in these areas, as you create your program.

4. Once you create your program, obtain any school or community permissions you may need.

5. Assign necessary roles and responsibilities within your program, and complete any necessary training. For example, if your program is based on peer mediation, select students who are suited for this task and have them trained in peer mediation.

6. Develop a media campaign to advertise your program. Write a creative slogan that highlights your area of focus and communicates information about what services your program will offer. This campaign could include advertisements in the local or school paper, brochures or pamphlets, and social media announcements.

7. Put your program into action as a class and observe the results.

Core Skills

Math Practice

The following table shows percentages of rape and sexual assault committed against females by number of offenders and victim-offender relationship for three periods of five years each. Study the graph and then answer the following questions.

Offender characteristic	Period 1	Period 2	Period 3
Number of offenders			
One	93%	91%	90%
Two or more	7%	9%	10%
Victim-offender relationship			
Stranger	21%	25%	22%
Nonstranger	79%	75%	78%
Intimate partner	28%	30%	34%
Relative	9%	3%	6%
Well-known/casual acquaintance	42%	42%	38%

33. In period 2, what percentage of victims were attacked by nonstrangers?
    A. 25%
    B. 75%
    C. 78%
    D. 79%

34. In period 3, what percentage of victims were assaulted by more than one offender?
    A. 7%
    B. 9%
    C. 10%
    D. 90%

35. In period 3, how much higher a percentage of victims was assaulted by well-known/casual acquaintances than by strangers?
    A. 16%
    B. 22%
    C. 38%
    D. 78%

36. Including all three periods, which ratio best reflects attacks by nonstrangers as compared to attacks by strangers?
    A. 2 to 1
    B. 1 to 1
    C. 3 to 1
    D. 6 to 1

Reading and Writing Practice

Read the passage below and then answer the questions.

In some ways, cyberbullying is similar to traditional bullying. Both can have a severe negative impact on people who are targeted. The victims can become depressed, have lower self-esteem, and experience problems at school.

In some ways, however, the impact of cyberbullying can be worse than traditional bullying. Information can be spread rapidly and widely as people forward e-mails and texts, and post messages on websites and social media pages. People can hide behind fake screen names online, allowing them to make comments online that they would never make in person. This can increase the harshness of a cyberbullying attack and cause additional anxiety to the victim. Victims of cyberbullying do not feel safe from attacks anywhere, even in their own homes.

37. What is the main idea of this passage?
    A. Many teens are bullies.
    B. Social media makes it easy to bully others.
    C. Cyberbullying can be worse than traditional bullying.
    D. Victims of cyberbullying are never safe.

38. Why can fake screen names increase the harshness of cyberbullying attacks?
    A. Anonymity allows people to have higher self-esteem.
    B. Bullies can spread information more rapidly.
    C. Photographs can be used easily in cyberbullying.
    D. People will make comments online that they would never make in person.

39. Which of the following statements is false?
    A. Victims of bullying can become depressed.
    B. Information spreads slowly through social media.
    C. Harsher attacks increase the victim's anxiety.
    D. Cyberbullying victims are not even safe in their homes.

40. Write a paragraph about steps you can take to prevent cyberbullying. Share your paragraphs in class.

Unit 8 The Human Life Cycle

- Sexual reproduction involves the combination of genetic material from a male and a female.

- During pregnancy, a woman needs medical care to ensure the health of her newborn.

- Every stage of the human life cycle—from infancy to older adulthood— is associated with physical, emotional, intellectual, and social changes.

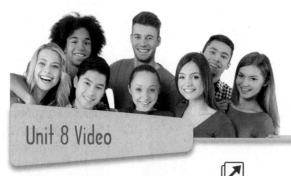

Unit 8 Video

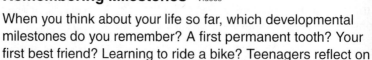

Remembering Milestones Videos

When you think about your life so far, which developmental milestones do you remember? A first permanent tooth? Your first best friend? Learning to ride a bike? Teenagers reflect on their past and the milestones they remember.

Rewrite the Paper

You've incorporated feedback from group members into your outline and draft. You're now ready to write the final version of your research paper. As you write your paper, be sure to list footnotes and use the format (font, font size, paper type, line spacing, and so forth) specified by your teacher.

If you aren't sure about spelling or grammar, check it using a dictionary or an online source. When you are done, make sure to proofread your work and correct any errors. The pages should be numbered.

As you worked on your research project, you may have found interesting photographs, drawings, charts, or graphs that relate to the subject. You may incorporate these visual elements into your paper, making sure to cite the source of each.

Congratulations! You've answered your research question, hopefully learned something new and interesting about an aspect of health and wellness, and, as an added bonus, sharpened your writing skills.

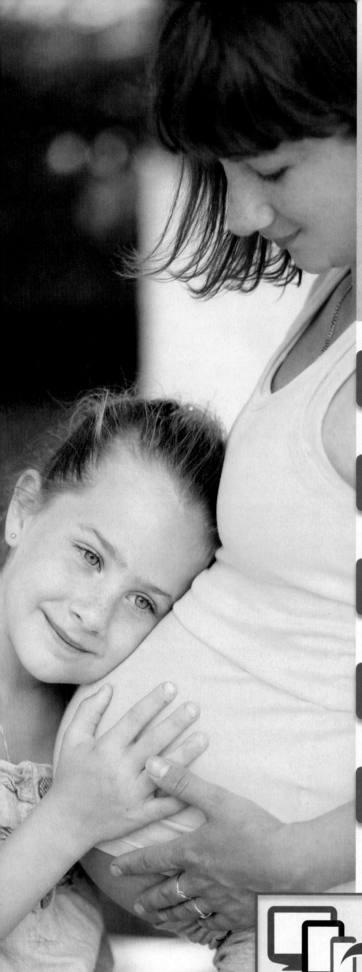

Chapter 20
Reproduction and Pregnancy

Lesson 20.1

Sexual Reproduction

Lesson 20.2

The Human Reproductive System

Lesson 20.3

Pregnancy

Lesson 20.4

Prenatal Care and Pregnancy Problems

Lesson 20.5

Reproductive System Diseases and Disorders

While studying this chapter, look for the activity icon to:

- **review** vocabulary with e-flash cards and games;
- **assess** learning with quizzes and online exercises;
- **expand** knowledge with animations and activities; and
- **listen** to pronunciation of key terms in the audio glossary.

G-WLEARNING.com

www.g-wlearning.com/health/

Take this quiz to see what you do *and* do not *know* about sexual reproduction and pregnancy. If you cannot answer a question, pay extra attention to that topic as you study this chapter.

1. Identify each statement as True, False, *or* It Depends. *Choose* It Depends *if a statement is true in some cases, but false in others.*

2. Revise each False *statement to make it true.*

3. Explain the circumstances in which each It Depends *statement is true and when it is false.*

Health and Wellness IQ Assess

1. The sperm cell determines the gender of the baby.	True	False	It Depends
2. Ova are fertilized inside the vagina.	True	False	It Depends
3. The uterus makes the female hormones estrogen and progesterone.	True	False	It Depends
4. One ovum is released during each menstrual cycle.	True	False	It Depends
5. Alcohol has no effect on a developing fetus.	True	False	It Depends
6. Bleeding is a normal part of the menstrual cycle.	True	False	It Depends
7. Most fibroid tumors are cancerous.	True	False	It Depends
8. Cancer of the prostate affects mainly older men.	True	False	It Depends
9. Sperm can remain alive in the female reproductive tract up to 72 hours after ejaculation.	True	False	It Depends
10. Testes produce the male hormone testosterone.	True	False	It Depends

Setting the Scene

Right now, as you read this textbook, you are an extremely complex organism consisting of trillions of cells. You began your life, however, as a single cell, which was a link in the chain of life reaching back to your most distant ancestors. This single cell was created from the merging of two cells, one from each of your biological parents. The resulting genetic combination produced you—a unique human being who is unlike any that has ever been or will ever exist.

Reproduction, pregnancy, and birth continually renew life. The continuity of human life begins with sexual reproduction. In this chapter, you will learn how this amazing process works, from fertilization to the birth of a child. You will also learn about the key aspects of pregnancy and some of the important diseases and disorders of the reproductive system.

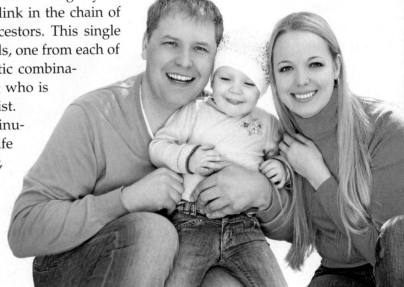

Lesson 20.1

Sexual Reproduction

Key Terms E-Flash Cards

In this lesson, you will learn the meanings of the following key terms.

asexual reproduction

cell division

dominant

fertilization

gamete

inheritance

meiosis

mitosis

ovum

recessive

sexual reproduction

sperm

zygote

Before You Read

Alphabet Brainstorm

List all the letters of the alphabet on a sheet of paper. For each letter, brainstorm a word or short phrase that you associate with the topic of sexual reproduction and inheritance. Then write a summary paragraph using as many of the words and phrases as possible.

A	
B	
C	
D	
E	

Lesson Objectives

After studying this lesson, you will be able to

- distinguish between asexual reproduction and sexual reproduction;

- describe two types of cell division;

- summarize the process of fertilization;

- explain how children inherit their parents' traits; and

- explain the role of chromosomes in gender determination.

Warm-Up Activity

A Unique Cell

Working with a partner, create a picture of a single cell that has resulted from the combination of two original cells. Be creative. The single cell should be unique, but should demonstrate some characteristics of both of the two original cells. You can create your drawing on paper using colored pencils or paint, or you could use a computer software program. Share your drawing with the class, pointing out the ways in which the unique new cell combines features of its "mother" and "father" cells.

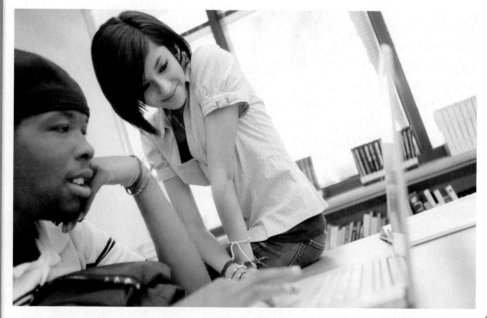

Reproduction is the process by which animals and plants create offspring. Many living things reproduce asexually, which does not require two parents. *Asexual reproduction* produces offspring that are identical to each other and identical to the parent. For example, to reproduce, a yeast cell simply duplicates its genetic material, grows, and divides its contents and genes, producing two new cells.

Humans, other animals, and most plants reproduce sexually. *Sexual reproduction* involves the combination of genetic material from two individuals, a male and a female. In sexual reproduction, each parent contributes a sex cell, called a *gamete*. The male gamete is called a *sperm*. The female gamete is called the *ovum* (plural—*ova*).

Human Sexual Reproduction

Humans reproduce through sexual intercourse. During intercourse, sperm must be deposited within the vagina to cause pregnancy. The sperm are capable of swimming from the vagina to the fallopian tube, where the ovum is located. There, the sperm and ovum combine in a process called *fertilization*.

Human cells have 46 chromosomes occurring in 23 pairs (Figure 20.1). Of these, 22 pairs possess similar structure and genetic material. One pair of chromosomes differs considerably. These are called the *sex chromosomes* because they determine the sex of an individual. A female has two X chromosomes in each cell, and a male has one Y chromosome and one X chromosome in each cell.

Unlike the trillions of other cells in your body, the gametes do not have 46 chromosomes. Instead, each gamete has 23 chromosomes, one half of each of the chromosome pairs. This means that each gamete carries only one sex chromosome. A sperm carries either a Y chromosome or an X chromosome. Each ovum carries one X chromosome.

Cell Division

One cell was created from merging the genetic material from each of your biological parents. How did that single cell become the trillions of cells that make up your body? Cells increase in number through a process called *cell division*. Mitosis and meiosis are the two types of cell division (Figure 20.2).

Mitosis. In *mitosis*, cells copy their genetic material and split into two identical cells, each receiving a complete and identical copy of the genetic material. Mitosis allows organs and body parts to grow in size during development inside the mother. Mitosis also allows growth to continue after birth. The production of new cells by mitosis also repairs worn or injured body parts.

Meiosis. In humans, the sperm and ova are produced by a special type of cell division called *meiosis*.

asexual reproduction
a process that requires only one cell and which produces offspring identical to that cell

sexual reproduction
the process by which the genetic material of two organisms—one male and one female—combine to create offspring

gamete
a sex cell that contains an individual's genetic material

sperm
the male sex cell, which combines with the ovum to create a zygote

ovum
the female sex cell, which combines with the sperm to create a zygote

fertilization
the process by which the sperm and ovum combine to create a zygote

cell division
the process by which cells multiply

mitosis
a type of cell division in which a cell copies its own genetic material and then divides into two identical cells

Figure 20.1

Human cells contain 23 pairs of chromosomes, including sex chromosomes, which determine the sex of an individual. *If an ovum is fertilized by a sperm containing an X chromosome, what sex will the baby be?*

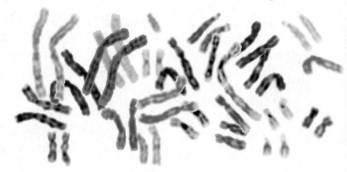

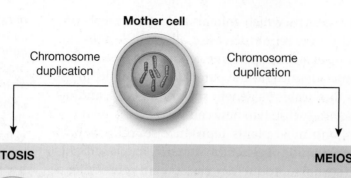

Mother cell

Chromosome duplication

Chromosome duplication

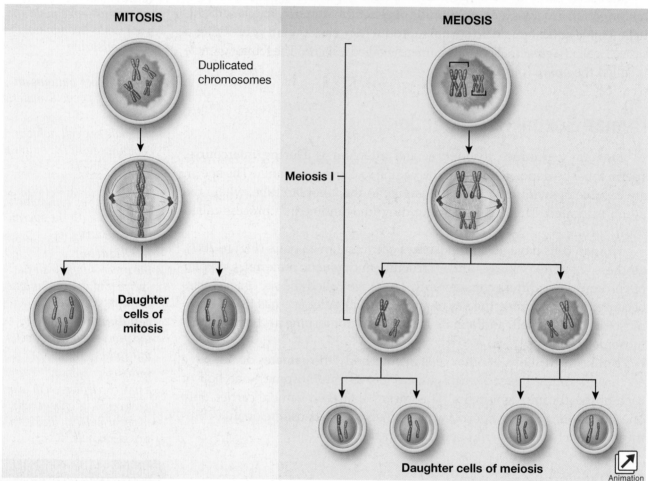

MITOSIS

MEIOSIS

Duplicated chromosomes

Meiosis I

Daughter cells of mitosis

Daughter cells of meiosis

Animation

Figure 20.2

Mitosis (on the left) involves a cell duplicating its genetic material and splitting into two identical cells. Meiosis (on the right) involves a cell splitting its genetic material between two different cells. *Why do sex cells need to split through meiosis? What would happen if they split through mitosis?*

meiosis
a type of cell division in which a cell splits its own genetic material and then divides into two different cells

In meiosis, body cells divide by halving their genetic material, resulting in sperm and ova with just half of the chromosomes found in other body cells.

Fertilization

Fertilization restores the full set of chromosomes to a gamete. During fertilization, a sperm penetrates an ovum and the genetic material merges. The tip of each sperm can break through the outer layers of an ovum. When the first sperm connects with the ovum's cell membrane, a chemical reaction sweeps over the surface of the ovum, forming a barrier to additional sperm. This ensures that just a single sperm fertilizes the ovum.

The nucleus of the sperm, which contains its genes, then meets the ovum's nucleus. On contact, the nuclei fuse and combine their chromosomes, forming a nucleus with half of the mother's genes and half of the father's genes. The fertilized ovum is called a *zygote*. The new combination of genes from two parents produces offspring genetically different from each other and distinct from their two parents.

Fertilization usually involves the union of a single sperm with a single ovum. In rare cases, however, a woman produces two ova that are each fertilized by a different sperm. If each fertilized ovum develops, the result is a pair of *fraternal twins*. Fraternal twins are not genetically identical—they are genetically unique like most brothers and sisters. Even rarer are *identical twins*, which develop when a single fertilized ovum develops, splits in two, and produces genetically identical babies. Although extremely uncommon, these processes can also result in more than two babies.

Inheritance

Inheritance is the process by which characteristics are transmitted from parents to their children. Children resemble their mothers in some ways and their fathers in other ways. A child may inherit his or her mother's straight hair but not her brown eyes. That child could inherit his or her father's green eyes but not his curly hair. Why does this happen?

The first explanation for the child's eye color is simple. Eye color is determined by a number of different genes, not just one gene. A child may not inherit the mother's eye color because he or she did not inherit all the genes necessary to produce brown eyes. Recall that the ovum has only half of the mother's genes, so the ovum may not have all the genes for brown eyes.

The second explanation is that some genes always cause their characteristics in offspring. These genes are called **dominant**. Inherited genes that do not always express their characteristics in the offspring are called *recessive*. You need to inherit just the right genes to get a certain eye color. In contrast, the inheritance of a person's gender is straightforward.

zygote
an ovum that has been fertilized by a sperm and which contains half of a mother's genes and half of a father's genes

inheritance
the transmission of parents' characteristics to their children

dominant
term used to describe genes that are always expressed in offspring

recessive
term used to describe genes that are not always expressed in offspring

---

CASE STUDY   The Mystery of Twins

Marilyn and Carolyn are twins, who were born minutes apart on the same day. They are both girls, and they have the same hair color, eye color, skin color, eye shape, height, build, and facial features. In fact, most people cannot easily tell these sisters apart. Marilyn and Carolyn are identical twins.

Thinking Critically

1. If a pregnancy is supposed to arise from one ovum fertilized by one sperm, what happened to produce two babies—identical twins?

2. Fraternal twins, another type of twin, are not identical. How do fraternal twins develop?

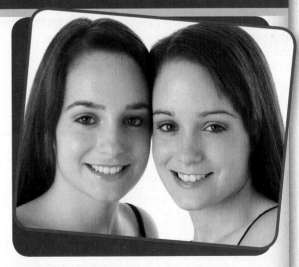

Figure 20.3

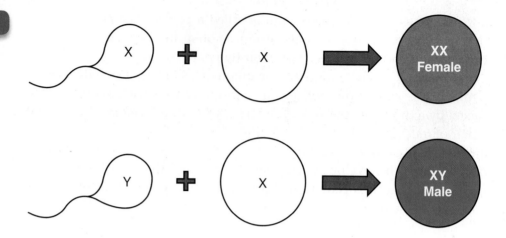

If a sperm containing an X chromosome fertilizes an egg, the developing zygote will have two X chromosomes and will become female. If an egg is fertilized by a sperm containing a Y chromosome, the zygote will have one X and one Y chromosome and will become male.

Gender Determination

A person's gender is determined by the sex chromosome contributed by the sperm cell (Figure 20.3). If a sperm with a Y chromosome fertilizes an ovum, the zygote gets one X and one Y chromosome and is male. An egg fertilized by a sperm with an X chromosome will produce a female.

The X chromosome contains several genes used by both males and females. The Y chromosome, which only males possess, has very few genes. These few critical genes determine a person's gender. During the first few weeks after an egg is fertilized, it produces a small mass of cells called an *embryo*. The embryo contains cells that will develop into ovaries.

If the embryo's cells have the Y chromosome, however, its genes cause these embryonic cells to develop into testes. The testes then produce the male hormone testosterone. Testosterone causes the embryo's cells to turn into the various male organs. The baby then develops with male characteristics.

If the embryo's cells do not have a Y chromosome, the embryo simply continues to develop ovaries. Ovaries then produce the female hormone estrogen, which causes the baby to develop female characteristics.

Lesson 20.1 Review

Know and Understand Assess

1. What type of reproduction requires two individuals?

2. Identify the male gamete and the female gamete.

3. Describe the process of fertilization.

4. How do fraternal twins develop?

5. What is the difference between dominant and recessive genes?

Analyze and Apply

6. Compare and contrast the two types of cell division.

7. How does gender determination occur? Develop a clear, thorough explanation of this process in your own words.

Real World **Health**

Write a paragraph or two explaining why a pair of identical twins who had been separated at birth, raised in different environments, and reunited as adults could be suitable subjects for a study of the effects of heredity versus environment on personality development.

Lesson 20.2

The Human Reproductive System

Lesson Objectives

After studying this lesson, you will be able to

- list the female organs of reproduction;
- explain the functions of female reproductive organs;
- list the male organs of reproduction; and
- explain the functions of male reproductive organs.

Warm-Up Activity

Same/Different Diagram

The female and male reproductive systems are alike in some ways and different in others. Draw a Venn diagram like the one shown below. List characteristics that are specific to the female reproductive system in one circle, and characteristics that are specific to the male reproductive system in the other circle. In the area where the circles overlap, list characteristics that the male and female reproductive systems have in common.

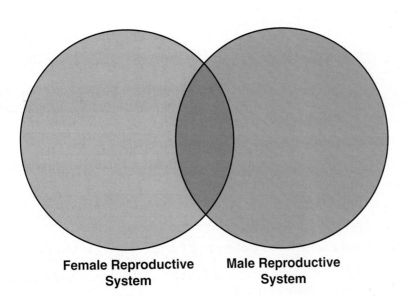

Female Reproductive System   **Male Reproductive System**

Key Terms E-Flash Cards

In this lesson, you will learn the meanings of the following key terms.

clitoris
ejaculation
erectile tissue
fallopian tube
flagellum
menarche
menopause
ovary
ovulation
prostate
semen
testes
uterus
vagina
vas deferens

Before You Read

Choose and Share

Form groups of three or four students. Each group will receive four note cards. After reading an assigned passage from this lesson, each group will find four favorite sentences. Write each sentence on one side of a card, and the reason it was chosen on the other side. Share your cards with the class.

R eproduction is a fundamental characteristic of all living things. Each type of animal and plant possesses specialized organs for the complex process of reproduction. The human reproductive system includes organs that produce the sperm and ova. In addition, the body has organs for sexual intercourse, which permits fertilization. Finally, female reproductive organs protect and nurture the developing baby until birth.

The Female Reproductive System

The female reproductive organs have several functions (Figure 20.4). Some organs make hormones. Other organs produce ova and nurture the fertilized egg as it develops into a baby. In addition, females have organs for sexual intercourse.

Ovaries

ovary
a female reproductive organ that contains ova and produces the hormones estrogen and progesterone

The two **ovaries** are small, almond-shaped organs in the lower abdomen (Figure 20.5 on the next page). Each ovary contains thousands of immature eggs (*ova*). A single layer of nurturing cells, a *follicle*, surrounds each ovum. Each month, a single ovum and its follicle grow toward maturity and are released into the nearby opening of the fallopian tube. Ovaries also make *progesterone* and *estrogen*, the female hormones that control sexual characteristics, the menstrual cycle, and pregnancy.

Fallopian Tubes

fallopian tube
a structure that connects the ovaries to the uterus and guides ova out of the ovaries; uterine tube

One **fallopian tube** (also called a *uterine tube*) leads from each ovary to each side of the uterus. The open ends of the fallopian tubes take in an ovum as it is released from the ovary. If sperm are in the fallopian tube, fertilization may occur here. The fertilized ovum then travels through the fallopian tubes to the uterus.

Figure 20.4 The Female Reproductive System Structure and Function	
Female organ	**Function**
ovary	produces ova and the female hormone estrogen
fallopian tube	carries ovum from ovary to uterus; sperm fertilizes ovum here
uterus	embryo implants in inner lining; encloses and protects fetus; forms part of placenta
cervix	closes the opening to the uterus at the vagina
vagina	sexual intercourse; the birth canal
labia majora	outer, hair-covered folds that cover the opening to the vagina
labia minora	inner, moist membrane-covered folds that enclose the opening of the vagina
clitoris	erectile tissue that is sensitive to sexual stimulation
breasts	produce milk for newborn baby

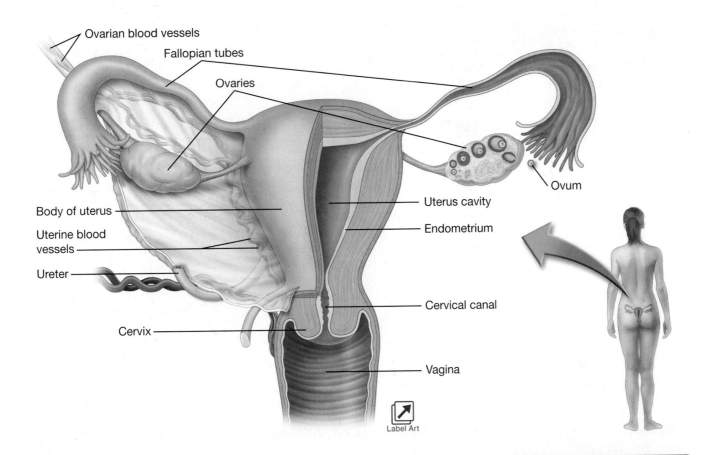

Ovarian blood vessels
Fallopian tubes
Ovaries
Ovum
Body of uterus
Uterine blood vessels
Ureter
Cervix
Uterus cavity
Endometrium
Cervical canal
Vagina

Label Art

Figure 20.5

The female reproductive organs, from a posterior view. Ova are produced in the ovaries and are then swept into the fallopian tubes. If sperm are deposited in the vagina and swim up to the fallopian tubes, then an ovum can be fertilized.

Uterus

The **uterus** is a hollow organ lined with a tissue called *endometrium*. The walls of the uterus contain strong muscles and many blood vessels. A fertilized ovum develops into an embryo and completes fetal development in the uterus.

Vagina and Cervix

The **vagina** is a tube-like structure lined with a moist membrane. Its external opening lies between the legs and leads inward and upward to the uterus. The vagina serves as the *birth canal*, or the passage through which a baby is delivered. The vagina connects with the uterus through the *cervix*, a narrow passage lined with mucus.

External Genitalia

The external sex organs are known as *genitals* or *genitalia* (Figure 20.6 on the next page). During puberty, these organs grow and develop into their adult form. A female's external genitalia include the *mons pubis*, a pad of fat tissue above the labia and vaginal opening. From the mons pubis, the labia extend downward on each side of the vaginal opening. The outer, larger folds are called *labia majora* and the inner, smaller folds are the *labia minora*.

uterus
a hollow organ of the female reproductive system that is lined with endometrial tissue and which houses and nurtures a developing fetus

vagina
a tube-like structure that extends from the external vaginal opening to the cervix, which leads into the uterus

Figure 20.6

The female's external sex organs, also called *genitalia*, include the mons pubis, labia majora, labia minora, and clitoris. *Why are external genitalia important to the reproductive system?*

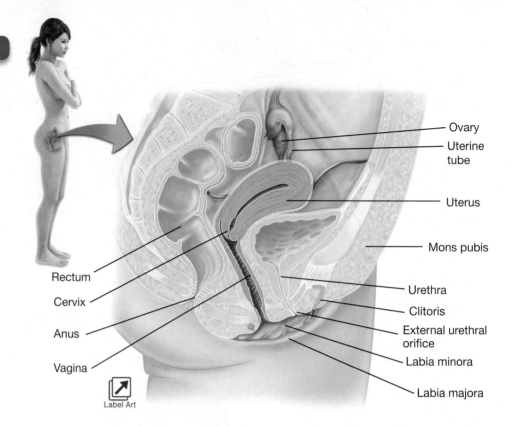

Ovary
Uterine tube
Uterus
Mons pubis
Rectum
Cervix
Anus
Vagina
Urethra
Clitoris
External urethral orifice
Labia minora
Labia majora

Label Art

clitoris
an organ filled with erectile tissue and located above the vaginal opening; swells during sexual excitement

The **clitoris** is located above the vaginal opening and contains sensitive tissue known as *erectile tissue*. Erectile tissue is spongy and filled with many small spaces. During sexual arousal, blood flows into these spaces, causing the organ to swell and enlarge.

The urinary tract is not part of the female reproductive system. In contrast, the urinary tract *is* a part of the male reproductive system as well as the male urinary system.

The breasts contain glands that produce milk. Ducts of the milk glands converge and open at the nipple, which is surrounded by a darkly pigmented area known as the *areola*. Breasts are supported by connective tissue covered with fatty tissue and skin.

Ovulation and Menstruation

After puberty, females experience a menstrual cycle each month. The menstrual cycle includes changes in the body in preparation for a possible pregnancy. A girl's first menstrual cycle, or **menarche**, generally occurs when she is between 10 and 15 years of age. During a monthly menstrual cycle, female hormones cause an ovum to be released from an ovary. Hormones also prepare the uterus for a possible pregnancy. If no pregnancy occurs, menstruation begins (Figure 20.7 on the next page).

Menstruation is the sloughing off of the endometrial lining of the uterus. Blood and some tissues from the uterus are released and pass through the vagina during this time. Menstruation continues throughout a woman's life span, except during pregnancy, and usually ends when a woman is in her late 40s or early 50s. The reproductive years end with **menopause**, when the ovaries stop releasing ova.

menarche
a girl's first menstrual cycle, which typically occurs between 10 and 15 years of age

menopause
the end of a woman's reproductive years, when her ovaries stop releasing ova

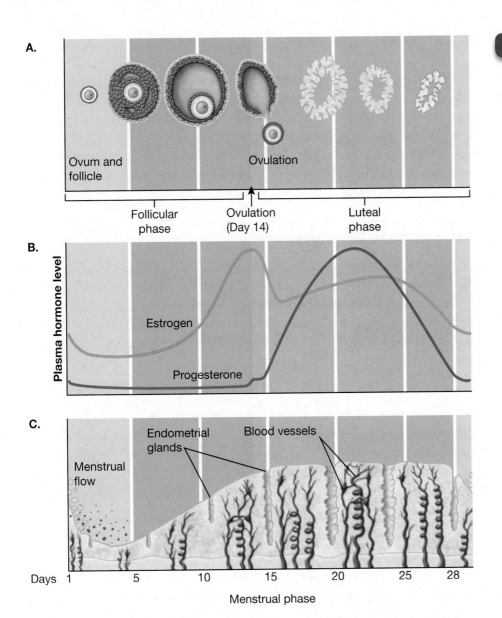

A.

Ovum and follicle

Ovulation

Follicular phase

Ovulation (Day 14)

Luteal phase

B.

Plasma hormone level

Estrogen

Progesterone

C.

Endometrial glands

Blood vessels

Menstrual flow

Days 1   5   10   15   20   25   28

Menstrual phase

Figure 20.7

During the female menstrual cycle, hormones trigger the release of an ovum from the ovaries. The hormone estrogen stimulates the uterus to build endometrial tissue in case of a pregnancy. If no pregnancy occurs, this endometrial tissue is shed.

The menstrual cycle includes a sequence of changes coordinated by sex hormones. During the first half of the cycle, the ovaries secrete the hormone *estrogen*, which is carried by the blood to the uterus. Estrogen stimulates the endometrium of the uterus to thicken and develop more blood vessels. These changes help the uterus deliver nutrients to the developing baby if a pregnancy occurs.

At the beginning of each menstrual cycle, ovarian follicles begin developing within the ovaries. As the menstrual cycle proceeds, the follicles grow and develop with their ova. At the midpoint of the menstrual cycle, ovulation occurs. *Ovulation* is the release of an ovum from one of the follicles.

After ovulation, the empty follicle begins to secrete the hormone progesterone, which stimulates endometrial growth. If no fertilization occurs, progesterone secretion stops and less estrogen is produced. Declining progesterone and estrogen mark the end of the menstrual cycle. At this point, the low hormone levels cause menstruation.

If pregnancy occurs, the empty follicle continues to make high levels of progesterone. This hormone is necessary for maintaining the pregnancy.

ovulation

the release of an ovum from one of the follicles in the ovaries

The Male Reproductive System

The male organs of reproduction produce hormones and sperm. These organs include the testes and penis, seminal vesicles, prostate, and vas deferens (Figures 20.8 and 20.9 on the next page). Male sex organs grow and mature as boys enter puberty in their early teens. An early sign of puberty is growth of the **testes**, organs that produce sperm and the hormone testosterone. Males begin making sperm at puberty and continue to produce sperm throughout their lives.

Testes and Vas Deferens

Two testes are suspended in the *scrotum*, a skin-covered, saclike structure. The testes contain tiny tubes called the *seminiferous tubules*, where sperm develop. When the sperm mature, they enter the *epididymis*, a coiled tube that lies along the outer wall of the testis. The epididymis leads into a tube called the **vas deferens**, which carries sperm to the penis.

Seminal Vesicles and Prostate

Located near the base of the urinary bladder, the *seminal vesicles* and **prostate** secrete fluid that mixes with sperm to form **semen**. Semen contains fluid that protects and nurtures sperm. The semen leaves the vas deferens and enters the urethra in the penis. The *urethra* is a tube that carries urine out of the body through the penis. Semen also passes through the urethra.

Figure 20.8

Side view of the male reproductive organs. Sperm form in the testes (one *testis* shown) and are carried to the penis by the vas deferens. The seminal vesicles and prostate secrete fluid to mix with the sperm and form semen.

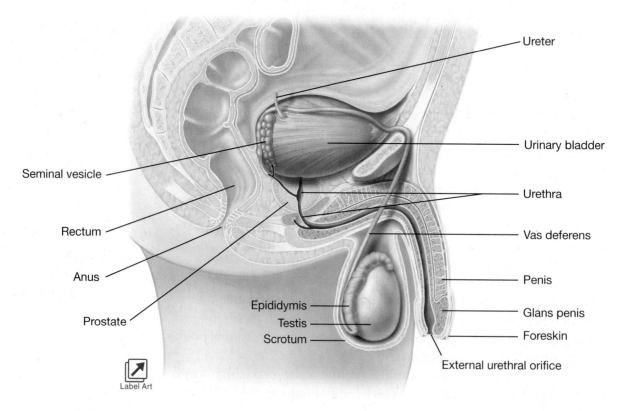

Figure 20.9 Male Reproductive System Structure and Function

Male organ	Function
testes	produce male hormone testosterone and sperm
seminiferous tubules	site of sperm development
epididymis	site of sperm maturation and storage
vas deferens	conducts semen to the penis
seminal vesicles	produce seminal fluid
prostate	produces most of the semen
bulbourethral glands	produce mucus that lubricates the urethra
penis	sexual intercourse
foreskin	flap of skin that covers the tip of the penis
erectile tissue	fills with blood; causes erection

Penis

The penis is the organ used for sexual intercourse and is also part of the urinary system. The penis contains **erectile tissue**, or spongy tissue that fills with blood during sexual excitement. The expanded end of the penis is called the *glans penis*, which is very sensitive to sexual stimulation. A flap of loosely attached skin, called the *foreskin*, covers the glans penis. The foreskin is sometimes removed shortly after birth in a procedure called *circumcision*.

In the male, sexual stimulation causes blood to flow into the erectile tissue of the penis, and results in an erection. The erect penis is capable of being inserted into the vagina for sexual intercourse. Intense sexual stimulation causes waves of contractions in the epididymis and vas deferens, propelling sperm into the urethra. Secretions of the seminal vesicles and prostate gland mix with the sperm, forming semen.

Ejaculation of the semen occurs when muscular contractions forcefully eject the semen out the urethral opening. Ejaculation is usually accompanied by orgasm in males.

erectile tissue
spongy tissue contained in the penis and clitoris that fills with blood during sexual excitement

ejaculation
a process by which muscular contractions expel semen through the urethral opening in the penis

---

SKILLS FOR HEALTH AND WELLNESS

Managing Your Reproductive Health

Reproductive health in adolescence and adulthood is built on a solid foundation of knowledge and skills. These tips for reproductive health will help you make informed decisions about your own health, sex, and pregnancy.

- Understand the process of sexual intercourse and how pregnancy begins.
- Understand how the male reproductive system fertilizes an ovum.

- Learn how to identify certain reproductive disorders so you can get treatment early.
- Research what steps you can take to prevent infertility.
- Understand the normal female reproductive cycle and when pregnancy is possible during that cycle.
- Take precautions to prevent reproductive system cancers and sexually transmitted infections.
- Recognize the signs of pregnancy to begin good prenatal care.

Figure 20.10

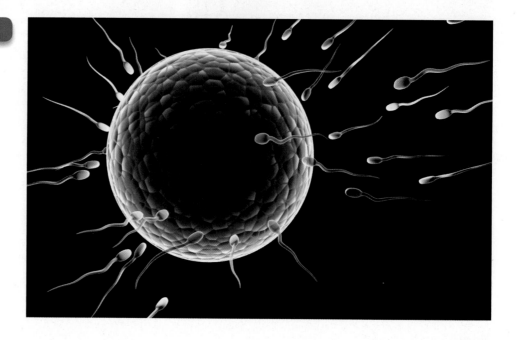

Sperm swim through the cervix into the uterus and then into the fallopian tubes where they may find an ovum. If sperm find and fertilize an ovum, a zygote is formed.

flagellum
a long, whip-like structure on the sperm that propels the sperm through liquid

Semen contains nutrients for the sperm and buffers that protect the sperm from the acidic environment of the vagina. The sperm cells are very small, made up of nothing more than a *flagellum* and a nucleus that contains half of the father's chromosomes. After ejaculation, sperm remain alive and capable of fertilization for 24 to 72 hours in the female reproductive tract.

In the vagina, sperm swim within the seminal fluid using the long, whip-like flagellum and make their way through the cervix, into the uterus, and then up the fallopian tubes. The sperm usually meet the ovum in the upper third of the fallopian tube (Figure 20.10).

Lesson 20.2 Review

Know and Understand

1. Explain the path an ovum takes during ovulation.
2. What is menarche?
3. What role does the hormone progesterone play in menstruation and pregnancy?
4. Which male organs produce sperm?
5. What is the role of the vas deferens?
6. What function does a flagellum fulfill for sperm?

Analyze and Apply

7. What triggers the endometrial lining to release from the uterus when no pregnancy occurs after ovulation?

8. Why is it important that semen contains fluids from the seminal vesicles and prostate?

Real World Health

Your class will be divided into two groups—the female reproductive system group and the male reproductive system group. In your group, brainstorm the various parts of your system, including hormones, organs, and other anatomical structures. Assign each part to a student. Once you have received your assignment, make a sign that describes the function of your part. Then, as a group, write a one-page explanation of the functioning of your assigned system. Exchange your description with the other group.

Lesson Objectives

After studying this lesson, you will be able to

- describe the process of cleavage;
- describe the process of implantation of a zygote;
- explain the functions of the placenta and umbilical cord;
- describe the stages of embryonic development;
- discuss the stages of fetal development; and
- explain how pregnancy is confirmed and measured.

Warm-Up Activity

Cell Division

When a sperm fertilizes an egg, the result is a single cell. As shown in the illustration below, that cell divides repeatedly—a process that ultimately creates the trillions of cells that make up the adult human body. You read about this type of cell division, called mitosis, earlier in this chapter. Search online for a video animation that depicts the process of mitosis in human cells. Then write a description of what you saw. Include any questions you had as you watched the video. Answer your questions as you read the lesson, or consult additional online and printed resources.

    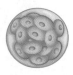 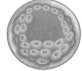

Key Terms
E-Flash Cards

In this lesson, you will learn the meanings of the following key terms.

amnion
blastocyst
chorion
chorionic gonadotropin
cleavage
differentiation
embryo
germ layers
gestation
implantation
obstetrician/gynecologist (OB/GYN)
organogenesis
placenta
umbilical cord

Before You Read

Identifying VIPs

As you read, use sticky notes to indicate Very Important Points in the text—the VIPs. These can consist of points of interest, confusion, or a place where you remembered a connection to other information. When you have finished reading the lesson, meet with a group and discuss the VIPs you selected. List the points that group members agree should be VIPs.

cleavage
the process through which a single-celled zygote divides into many cells

blastocyst
a ball of cells formed by the cleaving zygote as it travels into the uterus

Figure 20.11

During the process of cleavage, a zygote divides until it is a ball of cells known as a *blastocyst*. A blastocyst may then implant in the endometrial tissue of the uterus and become an embryo. *Why is it important for a blastocyst to implant in the uterus, and not in the fallopian tubes?*

T o become an infant in nine months, a zygote has to change dramatically and rapidly. The changes that take place during pregnancy are dramatic for the developing baby and mother alike.

Cleavage and Implantation

The single-celled zygote undergoes cell division through a process called *cleavage*, which is a type of mitosis. The roughly spherical zygote develops a furrow, which deepens and appears to cleave, or split the zygote into two new cells. These two cells then cleave, producing four cells, and so on (Figure 20.11).

Cleavage produces smaller and smaller cells, so the resulting mass of cells remains small enough to get to the uterus through the tiny passageway of a fallopian tube. Five days after fertilization, the zygote has cleaved seven times, forming a ball of 128 cells. This ball of cells, called a *blastocyst*, has traveled to the uterus. After eight to ten days, the blastocyst implants in the endometrium. This implanted mass of cells is now called an *embryo*.

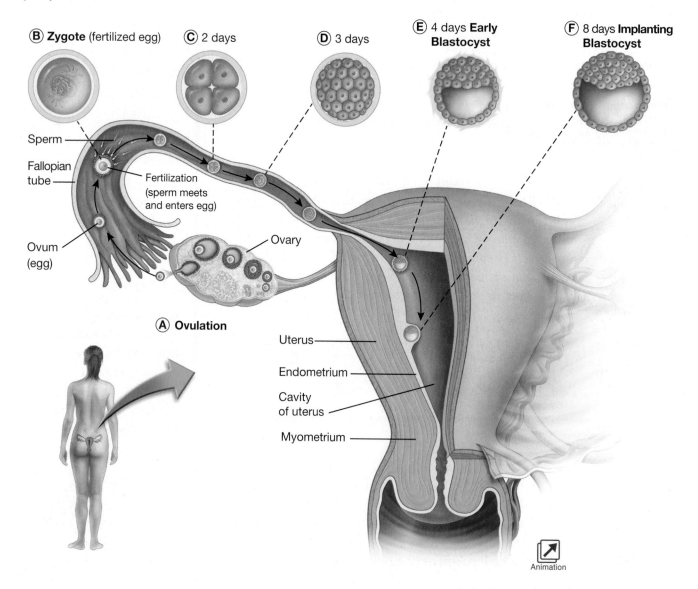

B **Zygote** (fertilized egg) C 2 days D 3 days E 4 days **Early Blastocyst** F 8 days **Implanting Blastocyst**

Sperm

Fallopian tube

Fertilization (sperm meets and enters egg)

Ovum (egg)

Ovary

A **Ovulation**

Uterus

Endometrium

Cavity of uterus

Myometrium

Animation

During *implantation*, the embryo burrows into the endometrium, embedding itself within the lining of the uterus. At the site of implantation in the uterus, the endometrium thickens and develops large, blood-filled spaces called *sinuses*. The implanted embryo soon develops an embryonic membrane called the **chorion**. Fingerlike projections called *villi* extend from the chorion into the sinuses of the endometrium. This merging of embryonic chorion and endometrial tissue creates the **placenta**. An **umbilical cord** made of blood vessels connects the placenta to the developing baby at its abdomen. The umbilical cord and placenta work together to nurture the developing baby.

The placenta secretes the hormone progesterone, which maintains the endometrium in its blood- and nutrient-rich state. The placenta blocks some—but not all—harmful substances from reaching the developing baby. It also prevents many types of microorganisms, such as bacteria, from coming into contact with the embryo or fetus.

Chemicals such as alcohol, nicotine, and many drugs can pass from the mother to the developing baby through the placenta. If a fetus is exposed to alcohol in the womb, the baby can develop *fetal alcohol syndrome*. Babies with fetal alcohol syndrome are underdeveloped and may have some degree of brain damage that affects their ability to learn and communicate.

The placenta obtains oxygen and nutrients from the mother and passes these through vessels of the umbilical cord to the developing baby. Waste products are carried by the umbilical cord from the developing baby to the placenta and the mother.

Embryonic Development

The embryo begins to form the various tissues and organs of a new individual, a process called **differentiation**. During differentiation, embryonic cells adopt a variety of specialized structures and functions. One of the first and most important steps of differentiation is the formation of three types of embryonic tissues called **germ layers**. These layers will eventually make up the three main types of tissues in the body.

Embryonic development proceeds as specialized structures are generated. During a process called **organogenesis**, the organs take their familiar forms and locations. Organogenesis continues for several weeks, completing the basic organization of the organs after eight weeks. The embryo is then considered a *fetus* (Figure 20.12 on the next page).

Fetal Development

Fetal development occurs within an embryonic membrane called the **amnion**, which forms a fluid-filled sac that encloses the fetus, cushioning and stabilizing it. The fetus grows considerably in the remaining months of pregnancy. After nine months, most organs, bones, and muscles have completed their development. The lungs and liver are the last organs to complete development, which happens just before birth.

embryo
a ball of cells formed by the cleaving zygote, and which implants in the uterus

implantation
the process by which an embryo burrows into the endometrial lining of the uterus

chorion
a membrane that develops around the implanted embryo

placenta
the merged chorion and endometrial tissue that surrounds, protects, and nurtures a developing fetus

umbilical cord
a structure that connects the developing fetus to the placenta to provide the fetus with nutrients required for growth

differentiation
the process by which embryonic cells develop into cells with specific structures and functions

germ layers
types of embryonic tissues that will eventually constitute the three main types of tissues in the body

organogenesis
the process by which organs belonging to the developing fetus take their familiar locations in the body

amnion
a membrane that forms a fluid-filled sac, which cushions and protects a developing fetus

Figure 20.12

After organogenesis has occurred and the organs take their familiar places in an embryo, the embryo becomes a fetus. A fetus is about ten centimeters long.

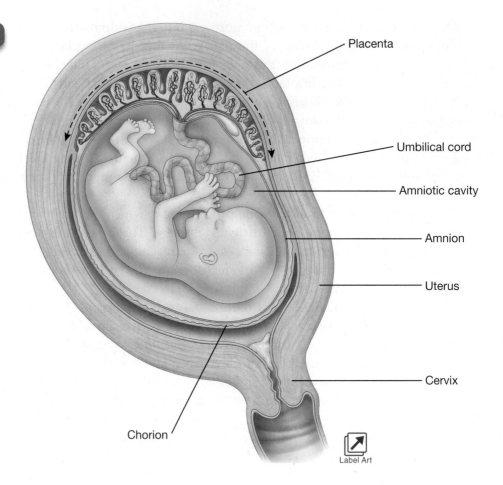

Placenta

Umbilical cord

Amniotic cavity

Amnion

Uterus

Cervix

Chorion

Label Art

The Pregnancy Calendar

During pregnancy, hormones stop ovulation and menstruation from occurring. Therefore, the first sign that a woman is pregnant is often a missed menstrual period. A woman can confirm whether or not she is pregnant by getting a pregnancy test. Urine is tested for *chorionic gonadotropin*, a hormone produced by the chorion of the embryo.

Human gestation is about nine months long. *Gestation* is the period of time from fertilization through birth. Doctors measure pregnancies in weeks. Most babies are born 36–40 weeks after fertilization.

During pregnancy, a mother should make regular visits to an *obstetrician/gynecologist (OB/GYN)*, which is a doctor who specializes in pregnancy, labor, and delivery. On a first visit, the doctor will ask a woman for the date of her last menstrual period to estimate the expected birth date, or *due date*. Very few women deliver their babies on the expected date, but this estimate allows the doctor to monitor fetal development. Doctors generally divide a pregnancy into three stages called *trimesters*:

- The first trimester is from fertilization through week 13 of gestation.
- The second trimester is week 14 through week 26.
- The third trimester is from week 27 through the end of the pregnancy.

chorionic gonadotropin
a hormone that is produced by the chorion; signals pregnancy

gestation
the period of time between fertilization of an ovum and the birth of a baby

obstetrician/ gynecologist (OB/GYN)
a type of doctor who specializes in the female reproductive system, especially pregnancy, labor, and delivery

Figure 20.13 Pregnancy and the Changing Body

Bodily change	Explanation
Breast growth	• Early in pregnancy, the breasts grow and may continue to grow as the milk glands prepare to feed the baby.
Skin changes	• Hormones trigger skin glands to make more oil, which can cause acne. Blood volume increases during pregnancy, so blood vessels in the skin cause a blush or "glow" on the skin. • Brown or yellow patches can appear on the face and a darkly pigmented line might appear running down the middle of the abdomen. • Bluish-purple stretch marks may develop on the abdomen. • Moles and freckles may become more pronounced. • The areola, the pigmented area around the nipples, becomes darker.
Emotional changes	• Mood swings, depression, and anxiety are common.
Unpleasant side effects	• **Nausea and vomiting.** Known as *morning sickness*, this occurs early in the pregnancy. Women may become sensitive to smells, tastes, or thoughts of certain foods. • **Leg swelling.** Pressure of the fetus builds in the abdomen, slowing blood return from the legs. • **Varicose veins.** These enlarged, swollen veins develop in the legs and the area around the vaginal opening due to the buildup of pressure in the abdomen. • **Hemorrhoids.** These varicose veins develop around the anus because of the buildup of pressure in the abdomen. • **Indigestion and constipation.** These side effects are caused by pressure of the growing fetus on the digestive system. • **Frequent urination.** Pressure on the bladder causes it to fill sooner, making it necessary to urinate more frequently. • **Backache, fatigue, and difficulty sleeping.** These are all common side effects.

The Woman's Changing Body

A woman's body changes dramatically during pregnancy as it prepares to nurture and deliver a baby. Women enjoy some aspects of pregnancy, while other changes cause discomfort. Emotional changes, such as mood swings or sudden tearful outbursts, are also normal. If a woman knows what to expect, she will be able to note anything out of the ordinary. For example, bleeding or pain are not expected during pregnancy and require a doctor's attention. Normal changes that accompany pregnancy are listed in Figure 20.13 above.

Lesson 20.3 Review

Know and Understand Assess

1. When does a blastocyst become an embryo?
2. List three functions of the placenta.
3. What is organogenesis?
4. Which organs are the last to complete development?
5. How long is the human gestation period?

Analyze and Apply

6. How can a doctor calculate a baby's due date?

Real World Health

In small groups, create a timeline from the moment that a sperm fertilizes an ovum to moments after birth. Include descriptions of the physical changes that occur during each step of fetal development along the timeline. Present your group's timeline to your class as a poster, video, slide show, comic book, or any other creative format.

Prenatal Care and Pregnancy Problems

Key Terms 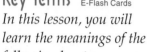 E-Flash Cards

In this lesson, you will learn the meanings of the following key terms.

eclampsia
ectopic pregnancy
gestational diabetes
  mellitus
miscarriage
preeclampsia
prenatal care
stillbirth

Lesson Objectives

After studying this lesson, you will be able to

• describe a pregnant woman's typical doctor visit;

• identify special dietary concerns of pregnant women;

• describe substances that may harm the developing fetus;

• discuss types of complications that can affect a pregnancy; and

• identify health risks for pregnant teens and their babies.

Before You Read

Double Journal Entry

Fold a piece of paper in half to create two columns. In the header for the first column, write Ideas about text. *In the header for the second column, write* Reaction/ connection to text. *As you read this lesson, fill in ideas that you have about information presented in the text, as well as your reactions or connections to the text.*

Ideas about text	Reaction/ connection to text

Warm-Up Activity

Top 10 List

Suppose you are an obstetrician/ gynecologist (OB/GYN). Create a list of the top 10 steps your patients can take to increase their chances of having a healthy pregnancy. This list can include activities and behaviors pregnant women should and should not *do. Share and compare your list with your classmates' lists.*

Receiving good medical care during and after pregnancy is vital for both the mother and baby. A woman should avoid harmful substances and receive good prenatal care as soon as she knows she is pregnant. *Prenatal care* is medical care provided for the mother and the fetus before birth.

prenatal care
medical care provided to the mother and fetus before birth

A Typical Doctor Visit

A pregnant woman typically sees her doctor monthly through the eighth month and weekly during the last month of pregnancy. If a woman has pregnancy complications or a health condition, she will probably see her doctor more frequently throughout her pregnancy (Figure 20.14).

The first doctor visit might include lab tests for diabetes and sexually transmitted infections. At follow-up visits, the doctor performs a routine physical exam to measure a woman's weight and blood pressure. The doctor monitors the fetus's growth by measuring the growth of the woman's abdomen. Around 20 days into a pregnancy, the fetal heartbeat can be detected with a certain type of ultrasound. The doctor might prescribe vitamins that are especially needed during pregnancy, such as folic acid to help build the nervous system of the fetus.

Food and Nutrition

Eating well is the most important thing a mother can do to promote her health and the baby's health. Most expectant mothers should add about 300 calories to their daily diets. Gaining about 25–35 pounds is normal during pregnancy. Pregnant women also need to drink plenty of water.

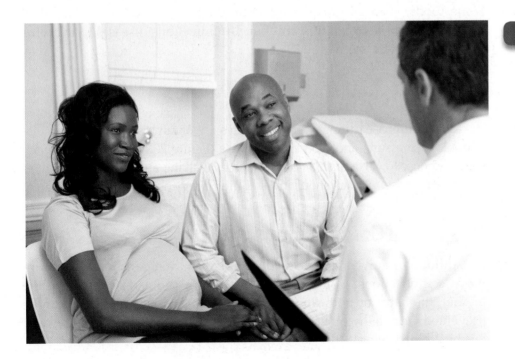

Figure 20.14

A pregnant woman will typically see her doctor monthly until her last month of pregnancy. It is common for doctors to examine their patients more frequently during the last month of the pregnancy.

Foods and Substances to Avoid

Expectant mothers should avoid certain foods and substances. Women should never smoke, drink alcohol, or take illegal drugs during pregnancy. It is well known that heavy alcohol consumption damages the fetus's brain and causes birth defects. Because no one knows what amount of alcohol is safe, most women are advised to avoid it completely.

Researchers have found that pregnant women who smoke risk having their baby too early, which is called *premature birth*. Premature babies have a low birth weight, and some of their organs may be underdeveloped. Babies with a low birth weight have difficulty getting enough oxygen during birth, which can cause brain damage. These babies also often have more respiratory and digestive diseases than others. They have difficulty feeding, gaining weight, and maintaining their body temperature.

Smoking can also cause **stillbirth**, or the death of a fetus, and sudden infant death. The death of an otherwise healthy infant during sleep is called *sudden infant death syndrome (SIDS)*, or *crib death*. The causes of SIDS remain unknown. However, children whose mother smoked during pregnancy have a higher risk of dying from SIDS.

The use of illegal drugs, such as cocaine or marijuana, can cause miscarriage, premature birth, and serious medical problems, including addiction in the baby. Expectant mothers should ask their doctors before taking any medications, herbal medicines, or vitamins. These may be harmful to the fetus.

Pregnant women should also avoid certain foods (Figure 20.15). Foods that contain mercury, such as canned tuna, can damage the fetal brain. Some foods, such as unpasteurized products and raw or undercooked meat, eggs, and fish, can transmit harmful infectious diseases to the fetus and should not be eaten.

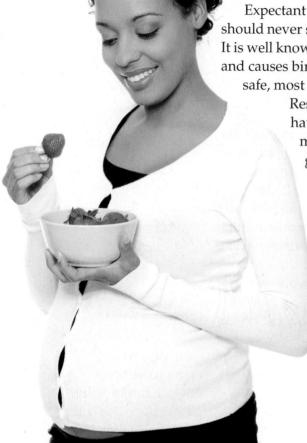

Figure 20.15

Pregnant women should avoid foods and drinks that may be harmful to their babies. *What are some foods and drinks a pregnant woman should avoid?*

stillbirth
the birth of a dead fetus

Physical Activity

Regular exercise during pregnancy helps a woman maintain good circulation, blood pressure, and blood sugar levels (Figure 20.16). Pregnant women should choose lower-impact activities such as walking and swimming as their source of exercise. Women should avoid lifting heavy objects during pregnancy.

Pregnancy Complications

Although many pregnancies turn out well, a significant number involve complications. Complications are health problems that affect the mother, the baby, or both during pregnancy. Many complications can be prevented, and many others can be treated early before they become serious health problems.

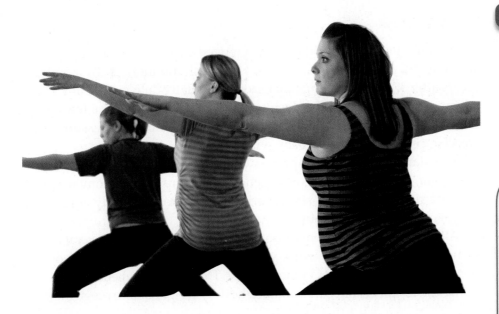

Figure 20.16

Physical activity can help regulate a woman's circulation and blood sugar levels during pregnancy. While a pregnant woman should not engage in high-impact activities, exercise is important to her health and the health of her baby.

Personal Profile

Are you Protecting Your Fertility?

Over ten percent of women in the United States experience infertility. In about one-third of the cases, the problem lies with the man, and about one-third are due to the woman. The following questions will help you assess how well you are protecting your fertility for the future.

Do you drink heavily? **yes no**

Do you use drugs? **yes no**

Do you smoke regularly? **yes no**

Are you exposed to pesticides or other harmful substances? **yes no**

Are you frequently stressed? **yes no**

Do you have a poor diet? **yes no**

Are you overweight or underweight? **yes no**

Have you contracted a sexually transmitted infection? **yes no**

Add up the number of yes answers to assess your chances of having fertility problems in the future. The more yes answers you have, the greater your risk of experiencing fertility disorders.

Ectopic Pregnancy

Occasionally, a narrow or blocked fallopian tube prevents or slows the movement of a fertilized ovum to the uterus. The fertilized ovum may die in the fallopian tube or it might implant there. An ***ectopic pregnancy*** is a serious condition in which the embryo attaches and develops inside the fallopian tube where it cannot complete development.

Most cases of ectopic pregnancy are caused by previous sexually transmitted infections or *pelvic inflammatory disease* (PID) that scar the fallopian tubes and cause them to narrow. An ectopic pregnancy itself damages the fallopian tubes and might prevent future pregnancies.

Endometriosis can also damage or block the fallopian tubes and lead to ectopic pregnancy. *Endometriosis* is a painful condition in which the endometrium grows in abnormal places, such as inside a fallopian tube.

The embryo in an ectopic pregnancy might grow large enough to cause serious problems. Rupture of the fallopian tube can occur suddenly, causing severe abdominal pain, bleeding, fainting, and shock. The placenta is vital for embryonic development, so an ectopic pregnancy cannot survive for long. Treatment for an ectopic pregnancy includes medications that help the body reabsorb the pregnancy and surgery that terminates the pregnancy.

A woman can reduce her risk for ectopic pregnancy by avoiding exposure to sexually transmitted infections. If an infection is suspected, a doctor should be consulted right away.

Miscarriage

Many pregnancies end before a woman even knows she is pregnant. A pregnancy that ends before the 20th week is a *spontaneous abortion*, also called a ***miscarriage***. Miscarriages are fairly common, and many result from a genetic abnormality in the fetus. Miscarriages are also caused by injuries, infections, and other diseases in the mother.

ectopic pregnancy
a condition in which an embryo implants and begins developing in the fallopian tubes

miscarriage
a pregnancy that ends before the 20th week

Preeclampsia

preeclampsia
a condition in which the mother experiences high blood pressure

Preeclampsia is a condition characterized by high blood pressure during pregnancy. Preeclampsia requires medical attention. If this condition occurs after 37 weeks of pregnancy, doctors usually deliver the baby. If preeclampsia occurs earlier, the doctor may treat the mother for a few weeks. She will rest and take medicine that helps control blood pressure. If the preeclampsia is serious, the baby will be delivered.

The danger of preeclampsia is that it can suddenly develop into *eclampsia*, a life-threatening emergency. In eclampsia, the women's blood pressure rises quickly and she experiences seizures. The only cure for eclampsia is to deliver the baby.

eclampsia
a life-threatening emergency in which a pregnant woman's blood pressure rises, causing seizures

Although it has no known cause, preeclampsia is linked to several factors, including pregnancy with twins; young motherhood; and a history of high blood pressure, diabetes, or kidney disease. Doctors recommend that women with a risk for preeclampsia maintain a healthy weight before pregnancy.

Gestational Diabetes Mellitus

gestational diabetes mellitus
a condition in which a woman's body becomes incapable of producing insulin due to the hormones involved in pregnancy

Women who do not have diabetes mellitus can develop it during pregnancy—a condition called **gestational diabetes mellitus**. A person with diabetes mellitus cannot make the hormone insulin, which normally controls the amount of sugar in the blood. During pregnancy, hormones can interfere with the function of insulin. In addition, the placenta causes insulin to become inactive. Therefore, some pregnant women experience low insulin levels and high blood sugar.

Women at risk of developing gestational diabetes have a family history of diabetes mellitus and become pregnant at an older age. A woman has a greater chance of having gestational diabetes if she had it in a previous pregnancy or if she previously had a baby larger than nine pounds. Smoking doubles the risk of developing gestational diabetes.

A pregnant woman can reduce her risk for gestational diabetes by eating a healthful diet, maintaining a healthy weight, not smoking, and exercising regularly. If left untreated, gestational diabetes can cause stillbirth, premature delivery, and high or low birth weight.

Health Risks for Teen Mothers and Their Babies

Most teen pregnancies are not planned. Many teens make the mistake of putting off telling parents about their pregnancy for as long as possible. It is impossible and unsafe to keep the pregnancy secret for long.

Pregnant teens should see a doctor and begin prenatal care as soon as possible. Pregnant teens, especially younger girls, have high-risk pregnancies because their bodies have not finished maturing. Teens are at greater risk than adult women for pregnancy complications, including

- *placenta previa*—a condition in which the placenta blocks the passage of the baby through the birth canal;
- preeclampsia (occurs often in teen pregnancy);

- prolonged labor;
- premature delivery (Figure 20.17); and
- anemia (low levels of red blood cells).

Certain complications and problems occur more often among teen mothers and their babies after birth. These include

- low birth weight—poor growth or early delivery results in smaller and less healthy babies;
- infant death—infants of teen mothers are at greater risk of death within their first year;
- chemical dependence—teens are more likely to abuse drugs and alcohol than adult women, which results in more chemical dependence among the babies born to teenagers;
- poor growth—overall, babies of teen mothers grow poorly compared with babies of adult women; and
- infections—babies of teens are more susceptible to infections than babies of adult women.

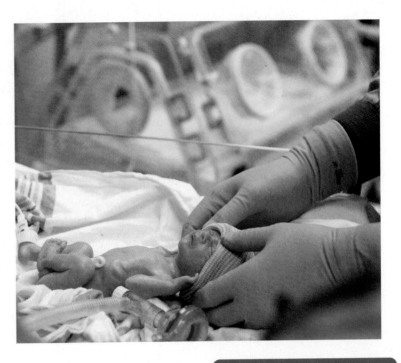

Figure 20.17

Premature babies are very small and are usually kept at the hospital in incubators. Premature babies have a greater risk than full-term babies for many diseases and infections.

For these reasons, pregnant girls must tell a parent, guardian, or other trusted adult about their pregnancy so they can begin prenatal care and start planning for their baby. A girl's priority should be her physical and mental health from pregnancy through parenthood. Pregnant teens should see a doctor as soon as possible.

In addition to a routine examination, the doctor will screen the teenager for STIs, measure her blood sugar, monitor her blood pressure, and begin treatment if anything is out of order. The doctor will also prescribe vitamins that include calcium, iron, and folic acid. Calcium is used to build bones and teeth and for the normal function of most cells in the body. Iron builds hemoglobin, the red pigment that carries oxygen inside every red blood cell, and helps prevent anemia. Folic acid is important for the normal development of the brain and spinal cord.

Nutrition and Diet

Nutrition and rest are key to the mother's and baby's physical and emotional health. Adjusting her diet may be difficult for a girl who has established poor eating habits. Also, pregnant teens face nutritional problems that most adult women do not. The bodies of pregnant teens are still growing. They must obtain enough calories, protein, calcium, water, and vitamins to sustain their own growth, as well as the rapid growth of their developing babies.

Pregnant teenagers should include plenty of fresh vegetables, fruits, whole grains, lean meats, and water in their diets. They should avoid sugars,

Figure 20.18 Teen Health during Pregnancy

Expecting teen mothers should...	Expecting teen mothers should not...
• sleep 6–8 hours each night • eat whole grains • prevent STIs • eat fresh fruits and vegetables • eat lean meats • drink plenty of water • exercise moderately • take prenatal vitamins	• smoke • use drugs • drink alcohol • exercise excessively • diet to lose weight

empty calorie foods, fast food, and soft drinks. Girls should not attempt to lose weight during and after pregnancy. They need calories for the baby's growth, healing and recovery, and making breast milk after birth.

Vital Prenatal Care

Doctors can advise girls on how to care for themselves and their babies. Just like pregnant adult women, pregnant teens must not smoke, drink alcohol, or use drugs during pregnancy (Figure 20.18). Pregnant teens who are using alcohol or tobacco may need assistance from their doctor to stop using these addictive substances.

Moderate, low-impact exercise such as walking and swimming maintains good circulation and a healthy blood sugar level. Pregnant teens do not need extreme exercise during this time, however.

Lesson 20.4 Review

Know and Understand
Assess

1. What vitamin might a doctor prescribe for a pregnant woman and why?

2. What is considered normal weight gain for a pregnant woman?

3. List four problems common to low birth weight babies.

4. List four foods a pregnant woman should avoid.

5. What is an ectopic pregnancy?

6. What steps do doctors recommend to women at risk for preeclampsia?

7. List three complications teen mothers are at risk for during pregnancy.

Analyze and Apply

8. How can a woman reduce her risk for an ectopic pregnancy?

9. Why can a woman who does not have diabetes mellitus develop gestational diabetes mellitus during pregnancy?

Real World Health

Using the top 10 list you created in the opening activity of this lesson, create a colorful brochure or pamphlet for expecting mothers. Elaborate on your list and create a *Pregnancy Wellness* guide that could be given to newly pregnant moms at their first prenatal visit.

Reproductive System Diseases and Disorders

Lesson Objectives

After studying this lesson, you will be able to

- identify disorders of the female reproductive system;
- discuss different types of cancers that affect female reproductive organs;
- identify infections and inflammatory conditions of the male reproductive system; and
- discuss different types of cancers that affect male reproductive organs.

Warm-Up Activity

Myth or Fact?

Take a few moments to consider the following statements about reproductive system diseases and disorders:

1. *Female reproductive system disorders only affect older women.*
2. *During menstruation, girls and women are easily upset.*
3. *Sexually transmitted infections can lead to infertility in both men and women.*
4. *Breast cancer is the second leading cause of cancer deaths in women.*
5. *Prostate cancer and testicular cancer are most common in older men.*

Your teacher will place a piece of paper with the word Myth *on one side of the room and a piece of paper with the word* Fact *on the other side of the room. As your teacher reads a statement aloud, move to the Myth sign if you believe the statement is false, or to the Fact sign if you believe the statement is true. Discuss your choice with the other students who made the same choice. Select a spokesperson to explain your decision to the class.*

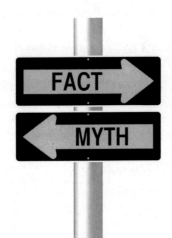

Key Terms E-Flash Cards

In this lesson, you will learn the meanings of the following key terms.

breast cancer
cryptorchidism
endometriosis
epididymitis
fertility
fibroid
orchitis
ovarian cancer
ovarian cysts
premenstrual dysphoric disorder (PMDD)
premenstrual syndrome (PMS)
prostate cancer
prostatitis
testicular cancer
uterine cancer

Before You Read

KWL Chart: Reproductive Diseases and Disorders

*Create a KWL chart to organize what you **K**now, what you **W**ant to know, and what you **L**earned from this lesson about reproductive system diseases and disorders.*

The ability to have biological children is known as *fertility*. In this lesson, you will learn about diseases and disorders that can affect the structure and function of the reproductive system. Some of these conditions can affect fertility in both men and women.

Female Reproductive System

Disorders of the female reproductive system are common. Most of these disorders occur after puberty and affect women of all ages.

Menstrual Disorders

Changes in menstrual periods can be normal. These changes can also arise from pregnancy or underlying diseases (Figure 20.19). If teenage girls notice an abnormality in their periods, they should consult their doctor. Symptoms of menstrual disorders include

- lack of menstruation;
- painful, irregular menstrual periods;
- excessive bleeding; and
- changes in mood, or depression and anxiety.

Premenstrual Syndrome

Premenstrual syndrome (PMS) is a group of symptoms that start one to two weeks before menstruation and stop when menstruation begins. Common symptoms of PMS are

- breast swelling and tenderness;
- acne;
- bloating and weight gain;
- headache;
- joint pain;
- food cravings;
- irritability, anxiety, or depression;

Figure 20.19 Menstrual Disorders		
Disease	**Symptoms**	**Cause**
amenorrhea	lack of menstrual period or menstrual periods stop for several months	pregnancy, breast-feeding, stress, cancer, hormone imbalance, low body weight, excessive exercise, thyroid disorders, anorexia nervosa, athletic training
dysmenorrhea	painful menstruation	PID, endometriosis, fibroids
menorrhagia	excessive menstrual bleeding	hormonal imbalance, fibroids, pregnancy complications, PID, thyroid disorders, endometriosis, and liver or kidney disease; sometimes the cause is unknown
metrorrhagia	bleeding between menstrual periods or irregular periods	fibroids, PID, thyroid disorders, diabetes, and blood-clotting disorders

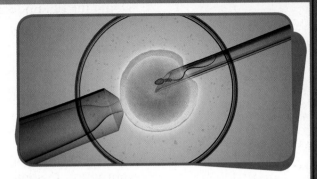

Many couples struggle with infertility. Infertility may be caused by endometriosis, a sexually transmitted infection, or another reproductive system disorder. Luckily, a procedure called *in vitro fertilization* (IVF) has been developed to help such couples. Extensive research on human reproduction led to the development of IVF, which was first used in 1977. In 2010, the prestigious Nobel Prize in Physiology or Medicine was awarded to Robert G. Edwards to recognize his pioneering work on IVF.

In vitro means *in glass* and it once referred to experiments and procedures done in laboratory glassware. This explains why babies conceived through IVF have been called *test tube babies*. However, IVF babies are not born in test tubes. *In vitro* simply refers to procedures done outside of living things—in IVF, fertilization occurs outside the woman's body.

First, doctors obtain ova from the woman. To ensure that this is successful, the woman receives hormone injections that stimulate the ovaries to produce many ova at once. The ova that are obtained are mixed with sperm from the father, which fertilizes several ova. Several healthy embryos are then inserted into the woman's uterus for implantation. Inserting multiple embryos increases the chance that at least one

will successfully implant. More than one embryo may implant, which is why IVF sometime results in twins, triplets, or even more babies.

Since 1978, research has improved the effectiveness and safety of IVF. IVF now makes it possible for thousands of couples to have biological children.

Thinking Critically

1. Do you think people should use IVF when there is an associated risk of multiple births—triplets, quadruplets, or more?

2. The IVF procedure is expensive. Should health insurance companies help infertile couples pay for this procedure?

3. Can this procedure work if the man is infertile? Why or why not?

- mood swings or crying spells; and
- fatigue or trouble sleeping.

The cause of PMS is not known, but hormonal changes trigger the symptoms. Pain relievers may help ease cramps, headaches, backaches, and breast tenderness. Contraceptives may be prescribed by a physician to reduce severe symptoms.

For some women, the physical and emotional symptoms of PMS are severe and interfere with daily living. This condition is known as *premenstrual dysphoric disorder (PMDD)*. In addition to severe PMS symptoms, PMDD includes depression, anxiety, and problems with emotions and mood. Exercise and rest, a well-balanced diet, and stress reduction can relieve symptoms. Antidepressants also help some women with PMDD.

Endometriosis

Endometriosis is a condition in which endometrial tissue grows outside the uterus. In this condition, endometrial tissue can embed and grow on the ovaries, the outer surface of the uterus, the intestines, or other abdominal organs. The cause of endometriosis is unknown, and it cannot be prevented.

premenstrual dysphoric disorder (PMDD)
a condition in which the symptoms of PMS become severe enough to interfere with a woman's day-to-day living

endometriosis
a condition in which endometrial tissue grows in abnormal places, often leading to pelvic pain and infertility

Even outside its normal location inside the uterus, endometrial tissue will respond to the hormones of the menstrual cycle by growing and sloughing off. Endometriosis can cause

- pelvic pain;
- diarrhea or constipation;
- abdominal bloating;
- menorrhagia;
- metrorrhagia; and
- fatigue.

The major complication of endometriosis is *infertility*, or the inability to reproduce. In some cases, a woman's fertility can be restored by treating her endometriosis. Treatment of endometriosis may include pain relievers, hormone therapy, and surgery.

Pelvic Inflammatory Disease

Pelvic inflammatory disease (PID) is a potentially serious but *highly preventable* condition, often caused by sexually transmitted infections. PID causes inflammation and scarring of a woman's pelvic reproductive organs. PID can cause chronic pelvic pain and ectopic pregnancy, and can lead to infertility.

Female Cancers and Tumors

Abnormal cell growth produces benign and malignant tumors. Benign tumors usually remain in the area of the body where they first develop and do not invade nearby tissues. They usually pose few health hazards and may not need treatment. However, *malignant tumors*, or *cancer*, invade nearby normal tissues and can spread to other parts of the body.

Cervical Cancer. *Cervical cancer*, or cancer of the cervix, progresses slowly. If detected early, cervical cancer can be treated effectively. The *Pap test*, or *Pap smear* detects abnormal changes in cervical cells before the cells become cancerous (Figure 20.20). In the Pap test, a doctor swabs the cervix to obtain a sample of cervical cells for study under the microscope. Women should have the Pap test every two to three years beginning at 21 years of age. After they reach 30 years of age, they might test every three to five years. Younger women and girls who are sexually active should also get Pap tests.

Uterine Cancer. *Uterine cancer*, or cancer of the endometrium, is the most common cancer of the female reproductive organs. The cause of this cancer is unknown, but estrogen levels appear to be a factor.

Fibroid Tumors. Fibroid tumors, also called *fibroids*, are benign tumors of uterine muscle. Fibroids are the most common tumor of the female reproductive system. They can cause vaginal bleeding, pelvic and abdominal pain, and an enlarged abdomen. Depending on their size and location, fibroids can make pregnancy difficult or impossible.

Ovarian Cancer. *Ovarian cancer* is difficult to detect in its early stages, which means that the cancer often spreads before a woman experiences symptoms. The symptoms of ovarian cancer can be mistaken for a painful menstrual period except that the sensations do not stop after the period.

uterine cancer
a type of cancer that grows in the endometrium; the most common cancer of the female reproductive organs

fibroid
a benign tumor that grows in the uterine muscle

ovarian cancer
a type of cancer that grows in the ovaries and is often not detected until it has spread elsewhere

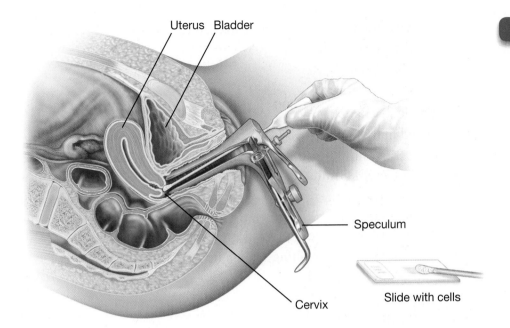

Uterus   Bladder

Speculum

Cervix

Slide with cells

Figure 20.20

During the Pap test, an OB/GYN inserts a *speculum* to hold the vagina open and then swabs a sample of cells from the cervix to detect whether there are any abnormal changes that might signal cancer.

Ovarian Cysts. *Ovarian cysts* are tumors on the ovaries. The cysts can be fluid-filled or they might contain abnormal cells. These cysts are not cancerous, but might need to be surgically removed if they become large and painful.

Breast Cancer and Tumors of the Breast. *Breast cancer* is the second leading cause of cancer-related death in women. Benign tumors of the breast are very common conditions, but they are not as serious as breast cancer. Causes of these benign tumors are not known, but hormones may play a role. Many of these tumors go away without treatment, or they can be removed surgically.

ovarian cysts
noncancerous tumors on the ovaries, which may need to be removed if they cause pain

breast cancer
a type of cancer that grows in the breasts; the second leading cause of death in women

Male Reproductive System

Several disorders affect the male reproductive system. Some of these are preventable while others are not. An understanding of the normal male reproductive system helps men recognize abnormal signs and symptoms if they arise.

Infectious and Inflammatory Conditions

There are several conditions that affect the male reproductive system by causing inflammation. Some of these conditions are the result of a sexually transmitted infection. There are also several cancers that affect the male reproductive organs in particular.

Prostatitis. *Prostatitis* is inflammation or infection of the prostate gland. It is also called *benign prostate hyperplasia*. This condition usually begins when men reach middle age. Most cases of prostatitis have no known cause. The signs and symptoms of prostatitis include lower back or groin pain, difficulty urinating, and blood in the urine. Prostatitis can be treated with pain relievers. If caused by bacteria, it is also treated with antibiotics.

Epididymitis. *Epididymitis* is characterized by inflammation of the epididymis, the organ that stores immature sperm. Signs and symptoms of epididymitis include

prostatitis
inflammation or infection of the prostate gland, leading to pain and blood in the urine

epididymitis
inflammation of the epididymis, which leads to pain, swelling, and possible penile discharge

- testicular swelling, tenderness, and pain;
- scrotal pain;
- painful urination;
- fever;
- penile discharge; and
- blood in the semen.

Urinary tract infections and a number of sexually transmitted infections can cause epididymitis. This condition can be treated with antibiotics.

orchitis
inflammation of the testes, leading to pain, swelling, and possible penile discharge

Orchitis. *Orchitis* is inflammation of the testes. The viral infection *mumps* is the most common cause of orchitis. Other causes include bacterial infections or injury. The signs and symptoms include

- sudden testicular swelling, pain, and tenderness;
- nausea and vomiting;
- fever;
- penile discharge; and
- prostate enlargement and tenderness.

Prevention of orchitis includes receiving a vaccination for mumps and using a protective cup over the genitals during athletic activities.

Local and Global Health

Cervical Cancer Screening and Prevention in the Americas

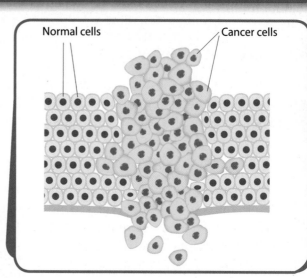

In Central America and South America, the Pap test has had nearly no impact on the number of deaths caused by cervical cancer. Today the death rate from cervical cancer remains seven times higher in Latin America than in North America. To be effective, women need to have a Pap test every two to three years. Many Central and South American women do not get regular Pap smears. Positive tests require follow-up doctor visits, but many of the women with positive tests do not get the required follow-up. If current trends continue, the number of deaths caused by cervical cancer in the Americas is projected to almost double by 2030.

Thinking Critically

1. Why might some women not get Pap tests regularly?
2. How could women's regular use of the Pap test be encouraged?
3. How can follow-up appointments for women with positive Pap tests be encouraged?
4. A newer test called *VIA* allows a doctor to identify cancer while visually examining the cervix. The cancer can be removed right away. How do you think this test and treatment would affect the cervical cancer death rate?

Cryptorchidism. *Cryptorchidism* is a failure of the testes to descend from the abdominal cavity into the scrotum. This condition can easily be detected during an examination when one or both of the testicles cannot be felt in the scrotum. Cryptorchidism can cause infertility and testicular cancer. Treatment includes surgery or hormone therapy.

cryptorchidism
a condition in which the testes fail to descend from the abdominal cavity; a common cause of infertility and testicular cancer

Male Cancers

Adolescent males should be aware of a few cancers that can affect their reproductive organs. The sooner these cancers are detected, the easier they are to treat.

Testicular Cancer. *Testicular cancer* is cancer that is present in one or both testes. Men who experience testicular swelling or feel a painless lump on a testicle should see their physician. Men may also experience aching in the lower abdomen or scrotum as a symptom. A testicular examination should be part of a general physical examination, and young men should conduct regular self-exams.

The cause of testicular cancer is unknown, but known risk factors include cryptorchidism and a family history of testicular cancer. Fortunately, early testicular cancer is treatable.

testicular cancer
a type of cancer that grows in one or both of the testes; treatable if detected early

Prostate Cancer. The signs and symptoms of *prostate cancer* resemble those of prostatitis. A male's age is the single most important risk factor for prostate cancer—most cases occur in men who are 65 years of age or older. Other risk factors include smoking, a high-fat diet, and prostatitis.

Screening tests for prostate cancer exist, but men should consult their doctor about whether they need to have the tests. They are usually given annually after a man reaches 40 years of age. Prostate screening involves the *prostate-specific antigen (PSA)* test, which measures the amount of a substance produced by the prostate that is present in the blood. A doctor also performs a digital rectal exam by inserting fingers (digits) inside the rectum, where the surface of the prostate can be felt.

prostate cancer
a type of cancer that grows in the prostate; the second most common cancer in the world

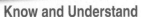

Lesson 20.5 Review

Know and Understand

1. List five common symptoms of premenstrual syndrome.
2. What is the difference between PMS and PMDD?
3. Why does ovarian cancer often spread before a woman experiences symptoms?
4. List three symptoms of prostatitis.
5. What is the most common cause of orchitis?
6. Name two risk factors for testicular cancer.

Analyze and Apply

7. Why might sexual abstinence be the most effective preventive measure for epididymitis?

8. Compare and contrast the male and female reproductive cancers.

Real World Health

Using this lesson as a guide, write a question for an advice columnist to answer. Choose a disorder, describe the symptoms, and ask the columnist what this ailment might be. Be sure not to name the ailment in your question. Use as many facts and descriptors as possible. Trade your paper with a partner.
Now imagine you are the advice columnist. Using the text, find the symptoms your partner describes and discuss the probable cause of the symptoms with him or her.

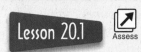

Lesson 20.1

Sexual Reproduction

Key Terms

asexual reproduction	mitosis
cell division	ovum
dominant	recessive
fertilization	sexual reproduction
gamete	sperm
inheritance	zygote
meiosis	

Key Points

- Sexual reproduction involves combining genetic material from the sex cells of each parent.
- Fertilization occurs when the sperm and ovum combine in the fallopian tube.
- Characteristics are transmitted from parents to their children through inheritance.
- A person's gender is determined by the sex chromosome contributed by the sperm cell.

Check Your Understanding

1. *True or false?* Asexual reproduction produces offspring that are identical to each other and to the parent.

2. The type of cell division called _____ allows humans to continue growing after birth.

3. If an embryo's cells carry a Y chromosome, _____.
   A. its genes cause testes to develop
   B. the hormone estrogen is produced
   C. female organs and characteristics develop
   D. its genes cause ovaries to develop

4. **Critical Thinking.** If a man with curly hair and woman with straight hair have a child with curly hair, which gene for hair traits is dominant? How do you know?

Lesson 20.2

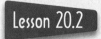

The Human Reproductive System

Key Terms

clitoris	erectile tissue
ejaculation	fallopian tube

flagellum	semen
menarche	testes
menopause	uterus
ovary	vagina
ovulation	vas deferens
prostate	

Key Points

- Females and males have specialized organs for the process of reproduction.
- The menstrual cycle causes changes in the female body to prepare for a possible pregnancy.
- The male organs of reproduction produce sperm.

Check Your Understanding

5. The _____ is the single layer of nurturing cells surrounding each ovum.

6. The female reproductive years end with _____, when the ovaries stop releasing ova.
   A. menarche
   B. menstruation
   C. menopause
   D. ovulation

7. Sperm develop in the _____.

8. **Critical Thinking.** Summarize the sequence of events in the menstrual cycle.

Lesson 20.3

Pregnancy

Key Terms

amnion	gestation
blastocyst	implantation
chorion	obstetrician/gynecologist
chorionic gonadotropin	(OB/GYN)
cleavage	organogenesis
differentiation	placenta
embryo	umbilical cord
germ layers	

Key Points

- The zygote produces new cells quickly.
- The placenta and umbilical cord pass oxygen and nutrients from the mother to the baby.
- Through the process of differentiation, the embryo's tissues and organs begin to form.

Check Your Understanding

9. The _____ secrete(s) the hormone progesterone, which maintains the endometrium.
   A. villi
   B. sinuses
   C. placenta
   D. umbilical cord

10. *True or false?* Chemicals such as alcohol, nicotine, and drugs can pass from the mother to the developing baby through the placenta.

11. **Critical Thinking.** Why is implantation in the endometrium critical for the embryo's survival?

Lesson 20.4 Assess

Prenatal Care and Pregnancy Problems

Key Terms

eclampsia
ectopic pregnancy
gestational diabetes
mellitus

miscarriage
preeclampsia
prenatal care
stillbirth

Key Points

- Good prenatal care is important for a healthy pregnancy.
- Substances such as tobacco and alcohol can harm the fetus.
- Women should be aware of complications that could occur during pregnancy.
- Teen mothers and their babies face significant health risks.

Check Your Understanding

12. *True or false?* Smoking is a major cause of premature birth and low birth weight.

13. *True or false?* Most cases of ectopic pregnancy are caused by prior sexually transmitted infections.

14. _____ is a life-threatening emergency in which the pregnant women's blood pressure rises quickly and she has seizures.

15. **Critical Thinking.** Why do pregnant teens face nutritional problems that adult pregnant women do not?

Lesson 20.5 Assess

Reproductive System Diseases and Disorders

Key Terms

breast cancer
cryptorchidism
endometriosis
epididymitis
fertility
fibroid
orchitis
ovarian cancer
ovarian cysts

premenstrual dysphoric
   disorder (PMDD)
premenstrual syndrome
   (PMS)
prostate cancer
prostatitis
testicular cancer
uterine cancer

Key Points

- Some disorders of the female reproductive system are minor, but others can lead to infertility.
- Various infectious and inflammatory conditions can affect the male reproductive system.
- The earlier that cancers of the reproductive system are detected, the more successful the treatment will be.

Check Your Understanding

16. *True or false?* Disorders of the female reproductive system are common.

17. _____ is a condition in which endometrial tissue grows outside the uterus.
   A. Uterine cancer
   B. Ectopic pregnancy
   C. Endometriosis
   D. Epididymitis

18. _____ is characterized by a failure of the testes to descend from the abdominal cavity.
   A. Prostatitis
   B. Orchitis
   C. Epididymitis
   D. Cryptorchidism

19. *True or false?* A man's age is the single most important risk factor for testicular cancer.

20. **Critical Thinking.** What is the difference between fibroid tumors and ovarian cysts?

Health and Wellness Skills

21. **Comprehend Concepts.** Research shows that a baby costs parents about $850 a month during its first year. Calculate your personal budget for one month including your allowance or work earnings. Subtract your total expenses for a typical month, which might include clothes, food, transportation, hobbies, student activities, and entertainment. Can you remove $850 a month from that budget? If you work 25 hours a week at minimum wage, will this make up the difference? After you have done your budgeting, write a paragraph about how your life would change if you had to support a baby.

22. **Make Decisions.** Lacey and Jeff, who are both 27 years of age, have been married for two years. Recently, they both graduated from law school, and now have entry-level jobs. They are heavily in debt from student loans they took out to attend law school, and they are trying to save money to buy their own home. Should Lacey and Jeff have a baby at this point in their lives? Use the five-step decision-making model given in the first chapter of this textbook to help Lacey and Jeff make the best decision for their family.

23. **Communicate with Others.** Imagine you found out that you have an identical twin. Draw your twin on a piece of poster board. Make sure to consider details such as his or her height, hair color, eye color, and other physical characteristics. On the poster, list at least 10 personality traits you assume your identical twin would share with you. On the back of the poster, list at least 10 personality traits that may be different since your twin was raised in a different environment than you. Share your poster with the class.

Hands-On Activity
Using Genetics to Create a Creature

You have learned that different patterns of inheritance exist because of the dominant and recessive traits you receive from your biological parents. In this activity, you will create a creature that possesses certain physical traits. This activity will help you learn how a combination of genes work together to create a unique organism.

Materials Needed

- water-soluble paint in pink and blue
- small paintbrush
- 1 pink penny (paint a thin pink line around the edge)
- 1 blue penny (paint a thin blue line around the edge)

Steps for this Activity

1. On a separate sheet of paper, create a chart like the one shown here.

2. To determine which trait will be expressed, flip both the pink coin and the blue coin. If a coin lands heads-up, check the appropriate "Heads" column. If it lands tails-up, check the appropriate "Tails" column.

3. In the final column of your chart, circle which trait will be expressed in your creature—the dominant trait or the recessive trait. The dominant trait is expressed if either one or both parents passed it on. A recessive trait is only expressed if both parents passed it on.

4. Repeat steps two and three for each trait in your chart.

5. After you have completed the chart, use the traits in the last column to draw your creature. Compare your creature to your classmates' creatures.

Genetic Trait	Mother (pink)		Father (blue)		Your Creature
	Dominant (heads)	Recessive (tails)	Dominant (heads)	Recessive (tails)	Creature Trait
1. body shape					D= large/round r= small/skinny
2. number of eyes					D= 2 r= 1
3. eye color					D= blue, green, purple r= red, yellow, orange
4. skin color					D= blue, green, purple r= red, yellow, orange
5. skin texture					D= hairy/furry r = smooth
6. skin design					D= solid color r= polka dots
7. tail length					D= short r= long
8. tail color					D= purple, pink, red r= blue, green, black
9. teeth					D=sharp r= round
10. number of arms					D= 2-4 r= 0-1
11. number of fingers					D= 5-10 r= 2-4
12. claw length					D= long r= short
13. number of claws					D= 5-10 r= 2-4
14. number of legs					D= 2-4 r= 0-1
15. ear size					D= large r= small
16. ear shape					D= round r= pointy or square
17. number of horns					D= 2 r= 1
18. horn shape					D= pointy or jagged r= round or curly
19. horn color					D= orange, yellow, green r= red, pink, purple

Core Skills

Math Practice

Study the graph of infertility rates among married women, then answer the questions.

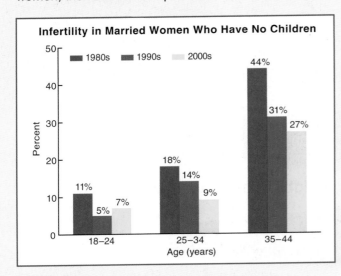

Infertility in Married Women Who Have No Children

24. What percentage of women between 25 and 34 years of age were infertile in the 1980s?
   A. 11%
   B. 18%
   C. 14%
   D. 44%

25. What was the percentage difference of women between 35 and 44 years of age who were infertile in the 1990s as compared to the 2000s?
   A. 4%
   B. 5%
   C. 13%
   D. 31%

26. In the 1980s, what was the ratio of infertile women aged 35–44 to infertile women aged 18–24?
   A. 4 to 1
   B. 2 to 1
   C. 1 to 1
   D. 3 to 1

27. Which grouping of age and year had the least amount of infertility?
   A. age 18–24, 2000s
   B. age 25–34, 2000s
   C. age 18–24, 1980s
   D. age 18–24, 1990s

Reading and Writing Practice

Read the passage below and then answer the questions.

The single-celled zygote undergoes cell division through a process called cleavage, *which is a type of mitosis. The roughly spherical zygote develops a furrow, which deepens and appears to cleave, or split the zygote into two new cells. These two cells then cleave, producing four cells, and so on.*

Cleavage *produces smaller and smaller cells, so the resulting mass of cells remains small enough to get to the uterus through the tiny passageway of a fallopian tube. Five days after fertilization, the zygote has cleaved seven times, forming a ball of 128 cells. This ball of cells, called a blastocyst, has traveled to the uterus. After eight to ten days, the* blastocyst *implants in the endometrium. This implanted mass of cells is now called an* embryo.

28. What is the author's main idea in this passage?
   A. In eight to ten days, a blastocyst becomes an embryo.
   B. A blastocyst is tiny.
   C. A zygote produces many new cells through cleavage.
   D. A blastocyst is made of 128 cells.

29. Five days after fertilization, how many times has a zygote cleaved?
   A. 7
   B. 16
   C. 128
   D. 48

30. Using context, the process of cleavage is to furrow as
   A. reproduction is to mitosis
   B. digging is to a trench
   C. dividing is to multiplication
   D. construction is to cement

31. Analyze how the author uses specific word choices to shape the meaning of this passage. Then rewrite the paragraph using your own word choices. Share your paragraph with the class.

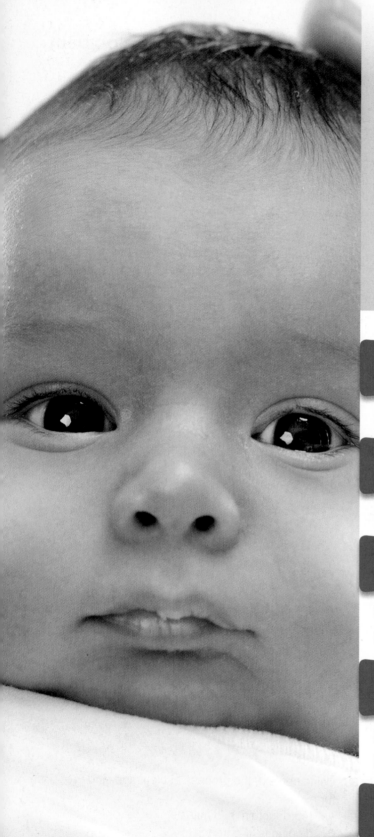

Chapter 21
Childbirth and Parenting Newborns

Lesson 21.1

Childbirth and the First Days

Lesson 21.2

Newborn Care

Lesson 21.3

Newborn Nutrition, Growth, and Development

Lesson 21.4

Bonding, Communication, and Parenting Issues

Lesson 21.5

Teen Parents

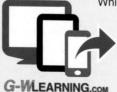

While studying this chapter, look for the activity icon ⬈ to:
- **review** vocabulary with e-flash cards and games;
- **assess** learning with quizzes and online exercises;
- **expand** knowledge with animations and activities; and
- **listen** to pronunciation of key terms in the audio glossary.

G-WLEARNING.com

www.g-wlearning.com/health/

Take this quiz to see what you do and do not *know* about childbirth and parenting. If you cannot answer a question, pay extra attention to that topic as you study this chapter.

1. *Identify each statement as* True, False, *or* It Depends. *Choose* It Depends *if a statement is true in some cases, but false in others.*

2. *Revise each* False *statement to make it true.*

3. *Explain the circumstances in which each* It Depends *statement is true and when it is false.*

Health and Wellness IQ Assess

1. A mother must give birth in a hospital.	True	False	It Depends
2. Only a medical doctor can deliver a baby.	True	False	It Depends
3. A newborn's condition is assessed using the Apgar test.	True	False	It Depends
4. Adopted children cannot have contact with their biological parents.	True	False	It Depends
5. Soon after birth, a baby can recognize the voice of his or her mother or caregiver.	True	False	It Depends
6. Newborns can sleep up to 16 hours each day.	True	False	It Depends
7. Infants need immunizations to protect them from infectious diseases.	True	False	It Depends
8. A baby feeding on breast milk needs no other food or drink.	True	False	It Depends
9. A baby cries because it is sick.	True	False	It Depends
10. Teen mothers have to drop out of high school.	True	False	It Depends

Setting the Scene

A successful parent has the skills of a teacher, nurse, police officer, manager, cook, judge, cheerleader, psychologist, and counselor. Parenting requires maturity; patience; courage; sympathy; toughness; tenderness; and the abilities to plan, organize, lead, and learn. If you think parenting is complicated, you are right. If you choose to become a parent, you will find that parenting is among the most challenging, yet most rewarding, parts of life.

In this chapter, you will learn what happens during childbirth. You'll get a glimpse into the hard work and challenges of parenting during the first months of a baby's life. You will also learn about the responsibilities, challenges, and rewards of parenting. The special challenges and health risks that pregnancy and child rearing pose to teenagers are also addressed.

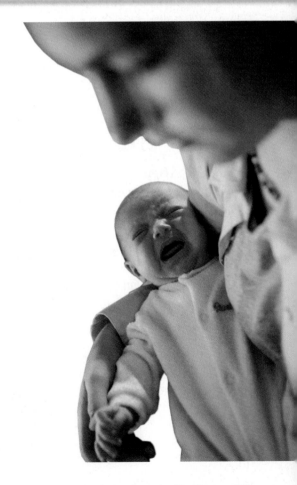

Childbirth and the First Days

Key Terms E-Flash Cards

In this lesson, you will learn the meanings of the following key terms.

adoption
Apgar test
birth plan
birthing center
birthing room
cesarean section (C-section)
dilation
epidural anesthesia
labor
nurse-midwife
oxytocin
reflex
vernix

Before You Read

Before and After
Create a chart like the one below. Before reading, write what you already know and what you want to know about childbirth. After reading, list what you have learned and what you still want to learn.

Before Reading		After Reading	
I know	I want to know	I learned	I want to learn

Lesson Objectives

After studying this lesson, you will be able to

- describe the decisions a couple should make when preparing for childbirth;
- summarize the stages of labor;
- explain the care the baby receives immediately after delivery; and
- discuss reasons people adopt a child and ways to prepare for adoption.

Warm-Up Activity

Baby's New World
Imagine you are a newborn moving from the safety and protection of a dark, serene, fluid-filled space into a bright, busy, air-filled world. Before reading this lesson, write a short children's story that chronicles a newborn traveling from the womb into his or her new surroundings. What sensations does the newborn experience for the first time? How does the newborn feel? Create pictures to accompany your children's story.

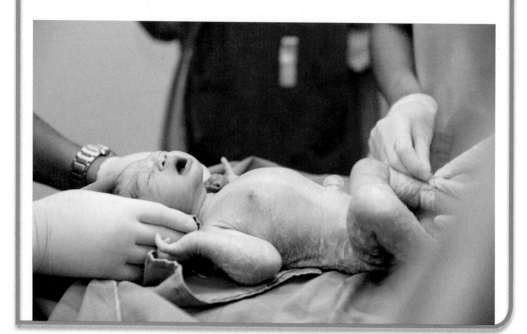

T he birth or adoption of a first child transforms a couple into new parents and changes their lives forever. In this section you will learn about childbirth and rewards and challenges of parenting during the first days of life.

Preparing for Childbirth

Most people have trouble making decisions during the excitement and stress of childbirth. This is why they should prepare early and make important decisions before the big day arrives.

The Birth Setting

As the delivery day approaches, the mother and her doctor often discuss a **birth plan** to address the mother's preferences about the birth process, such as where they will give birth. Many hospitals offer specialized **birthing rooms** with comfortable private facilities in which mothers stay through the whole process of labor and delivery.

Another option is a **birthing center**, which does not have medical facilities and is meant to look and feel like a home. Some mothers may choose to give birth in their own home. While women may feel more comfortable at a birthing center or at home, they should plan how they would get to the nearest hospital in an emergency.

Who Delivers the Baby?

A mother should determine who she would like to help deliver her baby and inform her doctor before the delivery date. Many women choose their OB/GYN (Figure 21.1 on the next page). Other women choose a familiar family doctor who has experience in labor and delivery.

Women can also have the assistance of a certified **nurse-midwife**, a medical professional licensed to help women with routine, medically uncomplicated births. A nurse-midwife often educates women before the birth and later coaches them through the labor and delivery.

Labor and Delivery Issues

The birth process is physically demanding, exhausting, and often painful. The duration and stress of labor vary greatly among women, but it can last many hours. A less stressful birth is beneficial to the new baby.

Pain Management. When preparing for childbirth, a woman should talk with her doctor about pain management during labor and delivery. Many women opt to receive **epidural anesthesia**. In this process, pain medicine is injected into the space surrounding the lower spinal cord, blocking pain from that point down. However, this method cannot be used after labor has progressed beyond a certain point, so it is helpful for women to discuss this option with their doctors before labor begins.

Personal Profile

What Do You Know about Parenthood?

I know whether I want to have children. **yes no**

I understand that adults can adopt children. **yes no**

I know how many children I want to have. **yes no**

I understand the educational and emotional needs of children. **yes no**

I understand the expense of raising children. **yes no**

I know that raising children takes much time and energy. **yes no**

I know how to care for infants and children. **yes no**

I understand that parents remain parents for the life of their children. **yes no**

Add the number of yes answers to assess your understanding of the demands of parenting. The more no answers, the more you need to learn about parenthood.

birth plan
an outline of a mother's preferences for the birth process

birthing room
a private space, often within a hospital, where a mother can give birth surrounded by the familiar comforts of home

birthing center
a nonmedical facility where a mother can give birth in a homelike environment

nurse-midwife
a licensed medical professional who educates women before birth, coaches them through labor and delivery, and aids in routine, uncomplicated births

epidural anesthesia
pain medication used during childbirth

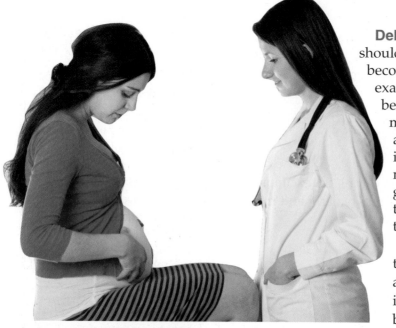

Many women choose an OB/GYN to deliver their baby, although other options are available. *What factors should a woman consider when choosing a doctor to help deliver her baby?*

cesarean section (C-section)
delivery of an infant through an incision made in the mother's abdomen and uterus

labor
the muscle contractions and changes in a woman's body as she gives birth

dilation
the widening and thinning of the cervix

oxytocin
a hormone that triggers strong uterine contractions to push the baby through the cervix and vagina

Delivery Decisions. Women and their doctors should also discuss medical procedures that may become necessary to safely deliver a baby. For example, a ***cesarean section (C-section)*** might be considered if the baby is in distress or the mother's health is in jeopardy. In a C-section, a doctor delivers the baby through an incision in the mother's abdomen and uterus. A doctor may also need to assist a difficult delivery by grasping the baby's head with *forceps*, clamps that allow the doctor to pull the baby through the vagina.

If the baby is having difficulty passing through the birth canal, a doctor might make an incision called an *episiotomy*. This incision is easily stitched closed after birth and heals better than a tear. Before the birth process begins, decisions should be made regarding questions that will arise before and immediately after delivery (Figure 21.2).

Childbirth

As the baby's due date approaches, the woman's hormones prepare her body for childbirth, then trigger and coordinate labor and delivery of the baby. In this section you will learn about childbirth, from the first stages of labor through the delivery of the newborn baby.

Labor

Labor describes the muscle contractions and changes in a woman's body as she delivers her baby. Before labor begins, the mother's body releases hormones that prepare it for labor and birth. Hormones cause ligaments and joints to soften and relax; this permits the baby to pass through the birth canal. Soon after, labor starts with rhythmic uterine muscle contractions. These contractions cause the cervix to thin, stretch, and open, a process called ***dilation***. Finally, the brain releases the hormone ***oxytocin***, which causes

Figure 21.2 Decisions to Make before Childbirth
Who will be present during the birth?
Will the mother use pain medication, and if so, what kind?
Will a doctor or nurse-midwife deliver the baby?
Will the mother have a C-section if recommended?
Will the mother have an episiotomy if recommended?
Will a son be circumcised?
Will the baby be breast-fed or formula-fed?
How will the mother and baby get home?
Will the mother have help caring for the baby at home during the first few weeks?

stronger uterine contractions that push the baby through the cervix and vagina.

The stages of labor occur as follows (Figure 21.3):

- First stage: Regular contractions of the uterus cause the cervix to thin (*efface*) and stretch (*dilate*). This opens the cervix and makes room for the baby to pass from the uterus into the vagina.

- Second stage: The uterine and abdominal muscles push the baby into the vagina and out of the body.

- Third stage: The placenta is delivered.

Some women have difficulty getting labor started even though they are well past their expected due date. In other cases, medical issues require delivery to be sped up through a process called *induction*. A doctor can speed up, or induce, labor contractions by breaking open the membrane that holds the amniotic fluid surrounding the baby. Sometimes doctors give the mother a medication or the hormone oxytocin to induce labor contractions.

After Delivery

Right after birth, mucus and fluids are suctioned from the baby's mouth and nose to allow the baby to take a first breath. The baby's health, responsiveness, and vital signs are evaluated immediately. In the hospital, newborns are screened the first day for a variety of diseases and disorders so treatment can begin promptly, if needed.

Baby's First Medical Exam

After birth, a doctor assesses a newborn's general condition by using the ***Apgar test***. This test is the acronym for the five conditions it assesses:

1. appearance (skin coloration)
2. pulse (heart rate)
3. grimace response (responsiveness to stimulation)
4. activity and muscle tone
5. respiration (breathing rate and effort)

The doctor rates each condition on a scale of 0 to 2, with 2 being the best (Figure 21.4 on the next page). The scores for each condition are added to give the total Apgar score, which ranges from 10 (highest) to 0 (lowest). The Apgar test is usually given to a baby at one minute after birth and again at five minutes after birth. If the score at five minutes is low, the test may be administered for a third time at ten minutes after birth.

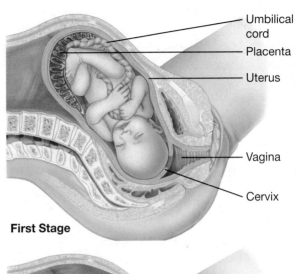

First Stage
— Umbilical cord
— Placenta
— Uterus
— Vagina
— Cervix

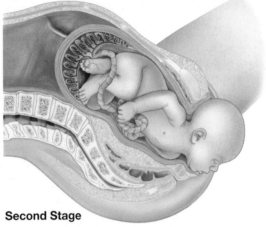

Second Stage

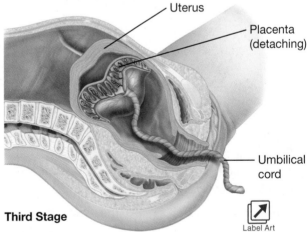

— Uterus
— Placenta (detaching)
— Umbilical cord

Third Stage

Label Art

Figure 21.3

In the first stage of labor, the cervix dilates until it is wide enough for the baby to pass through. In the second stage of labor, *expulsion*, the baby is pushed out through the vagina. Finally, the placenta detaches and is delivered during the third stage of labor.

Figure 21.4 Understanding Apgar Scores

Apgar Condition	2	1	0
appearance (skin coloration)	normal color all over (hands and feet are pink)	normal color (but hands and feet are bluish)	bluish-gray or pale all over
pulse (heart rate)	normal (above 100 beats per minute)	below 100 beats per minute	absent (no pulse)
grimace (responsiveness)	pulls away, sneezes, coughs, or cries with stimulation	facial movement only (grimace) with stimulation	absent (no response to stimulation)
activity (muscle tone)	active, spontaneous movement	arms and legs flexed with little movement	no movement, "floppy" tone
respiration (breathing rate and effort)	normal rate and effort, good cry	slow or irregular breathing, weak cry	absent (no breathing)

Apgar test
the measure of a newborn's health and condition through five basic tests

A score of eight after five minutes means the baby is in good health. Lower scores are common and usually mean the baby needs some attention or more time to adapt. When a very low score persists, something else may be wrong.

In addition to the Apgar test, a doctor does a physical exam and standard blood tests to detect any diseases or abnormalities. A tiny amount of blood is drawn from a heel prick to test for blood sugar abnormalities, thyroid disease, and *phenylketonuria (PKU)*, an inherited metabolic disease. These tests are done right away because these diseases can be controlled if detected early. The baby's first hepatitus B vaccine may be given at the time. Hearing is often tested right away.

The Newborn

There is a great deal of variation at birth, but the average baby weighs 7 pounds, 4 ounces and is 20 inches long. The baby's head may be temporarily misshapen after passing through the birth canal but will return to a normal shape within a few weeks. Newborns may also be temporarily covered with a white protective coating called **vernix**, fine hair, and blood. Their skin may be discolored. The mother's elevated hormone levels may cause the baby's genitals to enlarge, but they return to normal soon.

vernix
a temporary, white protective coating that may cover a newborn at birth

Life in the uterus and passing through the birth canal may also leave the newborn's torso, neck, arms, and legs bent. The newborn's skin may be rough or wrinkled (Figure 21.5). It may have blotches or rashes. All of these conditions are normal and usually disappear as the baby grows.

Premature Infants. Infants who are born at 37 weeks of pregnancy or earlier are considered *premature.* Premature infants may have low birth weights and other physical problems. Their lungs and other organs may not be fully developed and may not function properly. A premature birth may increase the infant's risk of developing infections.

Premature infants may need special care to help them survive and thrive. In the hospital, they are often kept in a *neonatal intensive care unit*, or *NICU.* These units have the equipment needed to diagnose problems and specialized staff to treat them.

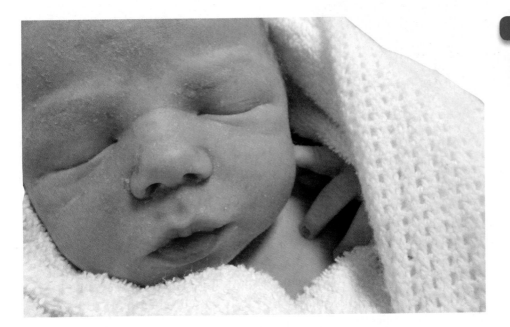

Figure 21.5

Newborns may have bent limbs or wrinkled, blotchy skin from their passage through the birth canal. *Should a mother be concerned if her newborn has some of these conditions?*

Newborns Adapt. Newborns must adapt to a dramatically different world outside of their mother's body. After birth they must breathe, eat, process sights and sounds, and support their bodies against the pull of gravity. Infants make this transition rapidly.

A newborn's brain is born ready to learn. Newborn babies are very alert, often opening their eyes wide, watching faces, and listening to voices. A newborn can recognize his or her mother's voice. Newborn vision starts out blurry, but infants can see objects one foot away—about the distance between the baby and his or her mother's face when she is holding the baby.

Newborn babies do little more than eat and sleep. Their muscles and nerves are not yet coordinated with their brains, and they do not move much. The movements of newborns are reflexes. A *reflex* is an automatic muscle movement in response to a stimulus. For example, if you place an object in the hand of a newborn, the baby will grasp it.

reflex
automatic muscle movement in response to stimulus

SKILLS FOR HEALTH AND WELLNESS

Understanding Parenting

Why do people choose to become parents? Interview an adult to learn about parenting skills and the rewards and challenges of parenting. Beforehand, prepare a list of questions. You can add some of the questions below:

- What are the biggest challenges related to parenting?
- What is a good age to become a parent?
- What do you like the most about parenting?
- Is raising children more or less expensive than you thought?

- How many children do you have, and how did you decide on that number?
- If you work outside your home, how do you provide care for your children while you are at work?
- How do you juggle responsibilities of parenting, work, free time, and household chores?
- What was your biggest surprise when you began parenting?
- How did you learn about being a good parent?

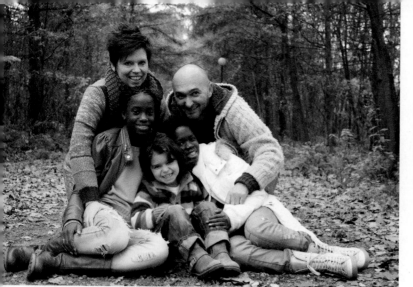

In transcultural adoptions, parents adopt children from different cultures and ethnicities than their own. *What do you think would be a challenge of transcultural adoption? What do you think would be a benefit?*

adoption
the legal placement of a child with someone other than his or her biological parents

Preparing for Adoption

People can also become parents through adoption. *Adoption* is the legal process of permanently placing a child with someone other than the child's biological parents. Sometimes children are placed for adoption after their biological or birth parents have died. In other cases, the biological parents are unable to raise the children for emotional, medical, or financial reasons. Although giving up a child for adoption is often painful and emotionally difficult, these parents realize that another family can better meet the child's needs and provide the child with a safe, loving home. In *open adoptions*, adopted children may have contact with their biological parents. In *closed adoptions*, the birth parents' information is kept private.

States and foreign countries vary in some specific requirements for adoptive parents. In general, parents must be able to pass criminal background and health screenings. They should have the financial and emotional ability to care for a child in a safe and healthful living environment.

Some transitions are challenging and need special attention. For example, adoptive parents may need to prepare for children with special needs, such as illness or disabilities. When an infant or a child is adopted from another country and culture, called a *transcultural adoption*, older children may initially have language problems and some difficulty adapting (Figure 21.6).

Adopting parents need to know as much as possible about the child's history to help the child with any illnesses. The adoptive parents should learn what they can about their child from the birth parents, child welfare agents, or foster families.

Lesson 21.1 Review

Know and Understand Assess

1. Identify the three types of medical professionals a woman might choose to deliver her baby.

2. List two reasons a C-section might be necessary to deliver a baby.

3. What is the role of the hormone oxytocin in labor and delivery?

4. What five conditions of a newborn are assessed by the Apgar test?

5. Describe the difference between an open and a closed adoption.

Analyze and Apply

6. Explain the difference between a birthing room and a birthing center.

7. Compare and contrast childbirth with and without anesthesia.

Real World Health

Research some natural (without drugs) pain management techniques for women in labor. Choose one technique and write a brief description of the technique. Include at least one example of how the technique works.

Lesson 21.2

Newborn Care

Lesson Objectives

After studying this lesson, you will be able to

- describe special concerns related to handling newborns;
- summarize newborns' sleeping habits;
- discuss ways to help prevent sudden infant death syndrome (SIDS);
- explain the importance of properly diapering and bathing an infant; and
- relate information about basic medical care for newborns.

Key Terms E-Flash Cards

In this lesson, you will learn the meanings of the following key terms.

fontanel

pediatrician

sudden infant death syndrome (SIDS)

Warm-Up Activity

The Two Sides of Parenting

New parents are often exhausted due to the constant demands of caring for a newborn baby. With a partner, or in a small group, choose a lullaby and compose new lyrics to its melody. Your new lyrics should describe both the exhaustion and the joy of being a new parent.

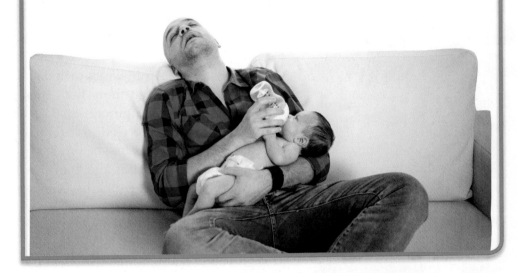

Before You Read

Roundabout Reflections

Your teacher will divide you into groups and assign each group some main headings and subheadings from this lesson. Write your group's assigned headings on a piece of paper and then brainstorm related words and ideas. After 30–45 seconds, pass your papers clockwise to the next group so they can add their ideas. Repeat this process until each group has added their ideas under every heading. After reading the lesson, add what you learned to each paper.

T iny, fragile newborns may frighten new parents. Parents should not be afraid of handling newborns—regular physical contact and interaction with caregivers foster a baby's healthy growth and development. With a few simple precautions, parents can learn to handle newborns safely.

Handling Newborns

Because newborns and young babies have immature immune systems, everyone should wash their hands with soap and water before handling babies. Compared to older children, newborns have weak immune systems.

fontanel
a soft spot on a newborn's skull where the bone has not yet formed

The skull of a newborn has a few soft spots called ***fontanels***, where bone has not yet formed. These soft patches of tissue permit the newborn's skull to pass through the birth canal and allow the baby's brain to grow rapidly after birth. The fontanels convert to bone slowly over the next couple of years. During the first few months, the fontanels should not be touched because they remain soft.

A newborn also has relatively weak neck and shoulder muscles. Therefore, caregivers should support the head and neck when carrying or holding a newborn. Shaking and sudden movements should always be avoided.

By law, infants must travel in a car seat every time they ride in a vehicle. Car seats reduce the chances for serious injury and death among children. A newborn should be placed in a rear-facing car seat in the back seat of the vehicle (Figure 21.7). Children seated in the front seat can be killed or severely injured if an air bag deploys. Parents should always check with their state's laws and guidelines regarding car seats. Parents can visit local fire or police stations with questions—many of them perform car seat inspections to ensure correct installation.

Figure 21.7

Infant car seats should always be placed in the back seat of a vehicle and should face the rear of the car.

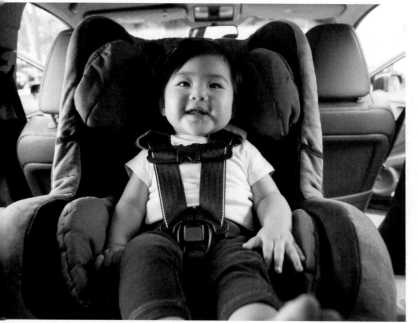

Sleeping Tips

Newborns may sleep 16 hours each day, although they rarely sleep more than two to four hours at a time (Figure 21.8). They waken every few hours to feed. At around three months of age, babies first begin sleeping through the night. At this age, they can typically eat enough during one feeding to sleep for six to eight hours at a time.

Parents and caregivers can help the baby adapt to the day/night cycle by reducing noise, light, and stimulation in the evening. They can also save talking and playing for daytime.

Figure 21.8 Ten Fun Facts about Newborns

1. Newborns sleep 16 hours or more each day.
2. Newborns recognize and respond to the human voice from birth.
3. In the first year of a baby's life, the baby's weight triples, the baby's length increases by 50%, and brain size doubles.
4. Babies have color vision and prefer the primary colors—red, yellow, and blue.
5. Babies prefer looking at curved lines rather than straight lines.
6. Soft background noise often helps babies fall asleep.
7. A mother's breast milk gives her baby immunity to several infections, but not to the germs that cause the common cold.
8. Touching a baby—especially a premature infant—stimulates the baby's growth and weight gain.
9. A baby's stomach is no larger than his or her fist, so a baby needs to eat small meals every two to four hours.
10. Until they are between three and twelve weeks of age, babies do not produce tears when they cry.

Preventing Sudden Infant Death Syndrome

sudden infant death syndrome (SIDS) the death of a healthy baby while sleeping; while the cause is unknown, it may be due to difficulty breathing

The leading cause of death in babies from one month to one year of age is *Sudden Infant Death Syndrome (SIDS)*. The cause of SIDS is unknown, although it may be caused by an infant's inability to breathe properly. It usually occurs while infants are sleeping. Taking the following steps can significantly reduce the risk of SIDS:

- Put babies to sleep on their backs.
- Do not allow anyone to smoke near babies.
- Remove crib padding, fluffy bedding, and pillows from the crib.
- Remove stuffed animals and fluffy toys from the crib.

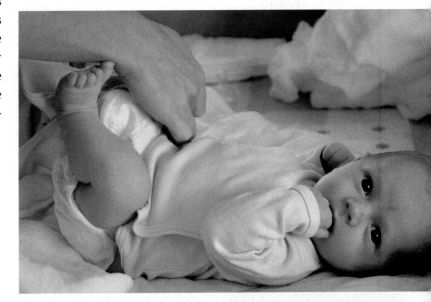

Figure 21.9

Diaper Care and Bathing

Diapers come in either a disposable or cloth form (Figure 21.9). Disposable diapers are more convenient than cloth because they do not need laundering. However, using disposable diapers costs more money in the long run. In addition, disposable diapers, even those labeled "biodegradable," do not break down well in garbage landfills.

Caregivers should have diaper-changing supplies ready and within easy reach. The baby should not be left alone on tables or in cribs with the sides down.

Parents must decide between disposable diapers or cloth diapers. *What are the advantages and disadvantages of disposable and cloth diapers in relation to the environment? in relation to the baby? in relation to the parents?*

Vaccines Do Not Cause SIDS

Parents, doctors, and scientists have been desperate to uncover the cause of sudden infant death syndrome (SIDS), so the syndrome can be prevented. Thanks to research studies, some suspected causes can be ruled out. Childhood vaccines were once prime suspects because infants are vaccinated around the age that SIDS occurs. Scientists at the Institute of Medicine reviewed several studies and found no links between SIDS and any of the childhood vaccines. Therefore, parents and doctors can be confident vaccinations will not lead to SIDS.

What factors can be linked to SIDS? A baby's sleep position is the most important factor found so far. After the American Academy of Pediatrics recommended that babies be put to sleep on their backs in 1992, the rate of SIDS dropped 40%. Studies have also linked SIDS to a baby's exposure to cigarette smoke.

Parents and caregivers can put this research into action. Vaccines prevent serious childhood diseases and do not cause SIDS.

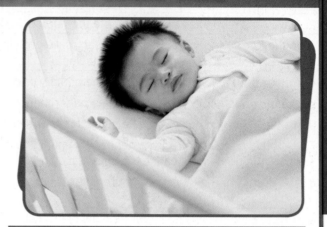

Thinking Critically

1. Do the benefits of vaccines outweigh the risks? Explain your answer.
2. How can parents and caregivers reduce a baby's exposure to cigarette smoke?
3. Two events that occur about the same time are said to be *correlated*. But this does not mean that one event causes the other event. Which correlated events caused some people to believe that vaccines cause SIDS?

Sometimes, diapers irritate a baby's skin, causing *diaper rash*. Diaper rash can be prevented by changing diapers soon after they become soiled, giving babies warm baths, and applying diaper ointment. A severe rash that lasts more than three days may need a doctor's attention.

Bathing the Newborn

Babies should be bathed regularly and gently because their skin is vulnerable to infections, but sensitive to chemicals and soaps. Until the umbilical cord falls off and the naval (belly button) heals, babies should receive sponge baths. A baby can be given a sponge bath while lying on a towel in a warm room or on a changing table.

Once the naval heals, a tub bath can be given using no more than three inches of warm water. A bathtub, sink, or baby bath tub can be used. First wash the baby's eyes with a soft washcloth dipped in clean, warm water. Wipe each eye from the inner to outer corner with a clean area of the washcloth. After rinsing the cloth, wash the baby's ears and nose. Baby shampoo or baby soap should be added to the water. Gently wash the baby's face and head, followed by all of the skin, and ending with the baby's genitals and bottom. Gently pat the skin dry.

Circumcision and Umbilical Cord Care

The circumcision wound and umbilical cord require cleaning and care. Some redness around the wound is normal as it heals. If redness increases and the wound produces pus, it may be infected and need a doctor's attention.

The umbilical cord area should not be immersed in water until the cord falls off and the naval area heals. In the meantime, the naval area can be cleaned with a cotton ball dipped in rubbing alcohol. However, some doctors recommend not disturbing the area until it heals completely. The cord usually falls off by three weeks and the area heals in four weeks, after which tub baths can begin.

Medical Care

Parents often choose a *pediatrician*, a doctor who specializes in babies and children, to care for their baby. Depending on the newborn's health, the pediatrician may want to see the baby at one to two weeks of age. During these visits, the doctor can answer parents' questions and monitor the baby's growth and development. The doctor may give the baby vaccines or follow up on test results.

Immunizations

Babies need *immunizations* (vaccinations) to protect them from common, contagious, and dangerous infections. If babies are breast-fed, they acquire temporary resistance to some infections through their mothers' breast milk. However, this resistance does not last long and does not protect them from many serious infections. Immunizations cause babies to develop their own longer-lasting protection from infections.

Immunizations also protect people in the community and children in schools from infectious disease. When a large fraction of a population is immunized, the infectious disease cannot easily infect people. For example, measles and whooping cough are both serious respiratory infections that can be prevented with immunization. In communities with good immunization programs, measles and whooping cough do not occur.

Some vaccinations are given in a single inoculation, while others require additional doses called *boosters*. The booster shots increase the body's immune response and improve protection against infections. For example, the hepatitis B vaccine is given in three doses. Some doctors give the baby a first dose of hepatitis B vaccine shortly after birth; other doctors do this vaccination along with other immunizations at two months of age. So, many babies begin hepatitis B immunization at around two months, receive a booster or second dose at four months, and a third dose at six months.

Before beginning school, children should also be immunized against chicken pox, measles, mumps, and rubella (Figure 21.10). These highly contagious diseases are transmitted in respiratory droplets. Chicken pox, measles, and mumps can cause severe

pediatrician
a medical professional who specializes in treating infants and children

Figure 21.10

The girl pictured here has rubella, or *German measles*, a disease characterized by rashes, mild respiratory distress, and a low fever. *How do you think a parent can best protect his or her child from this disease?*

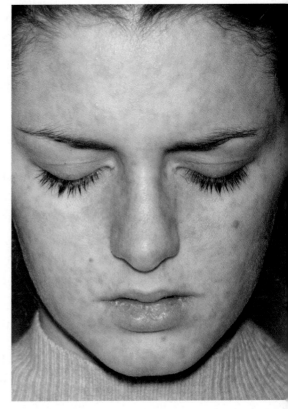

problems, even brain damage, in some children. Rubella normally causes mild illness, but can cause birth defects in the developing fetus of a pregnant woman.

Vaccinations can cause mild side effects such as fever, irritability, or soreness at the injection site. These temporary side effects usually subside within a few days. A doctor should be called if the side effects persist or become severe.

Parents and caregivers should be on alert for other medical issues commonly affecting newborns and infants. Certain signs and symptoms, or anything out of the ordinary, could signal minor medical problems or more serious diseases.

Signs of Illness

Fever is a common indicator of disease. A doctor should be called if a baby has a temperature above 100.4°F. Touching a baby's skin or using an oral thermometer is not an accurate way to measure his or her temperature. A baby's temperature should be read using a digital thermometer designed to be inserted in the outer ear canal or in the rectum. In babies three months and older, temperature can be measured using an infrared thermometer that scans the side of the forehead.

Doctors should also be contacted whenever skin rashes, red eyes, and white or yellow discharges from the eyes or nose occur. Call the emergency number if an infant or child is showing any of following signs of a possible medical emergency:

- difficulty breathing
- uncontrolled vomiting or diarrhea
- low levels of urine production
- unconsciousness

If a baby loses muscle tone, has difficulty sucking, or becomes twitchy or floppy, the baby should be taken to the doctor or emergency room immediately.

Lesson 21.2 Review

Know and Understand Assess

1. What is a *fontanel*?

2. List four ways to help prevent sudden infant death syndrome.

3. Discuss the advantages and disadvantages of disposable and cloth diapers.

4. List three ways to prevent diaper rash.

5. List three signs of a possible medical emergency in a baby.

Analyze and Apply

6. Compare and contrast the right and wrong ways to place a newborn's car seat in a vehicle.

7. Explain the procedure for giving a baby a tub bath.

8. Develop a presentation on the necessity of immunization for parents who are skeptical.

Real World Health

List all of the responsibilities involved in caring for a newborn, including those outlined in this lesson and additional tasks you know about. Next to each responsibility, write whether it is the job of the mother, the father, or both. After completing your list, pair up with a classmate of the opposite gender and share lists. Are your lists similar or different? Discuss why you assigned each responsibility as you did. If the two of you were caring for a newborn, how would you communicate about and compromise on any differences? Write a summary of your conclusions.

Newborn Nutrition, Growth, and Development

Lesson Objectives

After studying this lesson, you will be able to

- describe advantages and disadvantages of breast-feeding;
- summarize advantages and disadvantages of formula-feeding; and
- discuss newborns' rate of growth.

Warm-Up Activity

Breast-Feed or Formula-Feed?

Pediatricians recommend that infants be breast-fed for the first six months of life. Some women, however, decide to formula-feed their babies with infant formula. What factors influence this decision for a mother? Who can help her with this decision? How much does infant care depend on the individual needs of the baby and family? Write a short reflection responding to these questions.

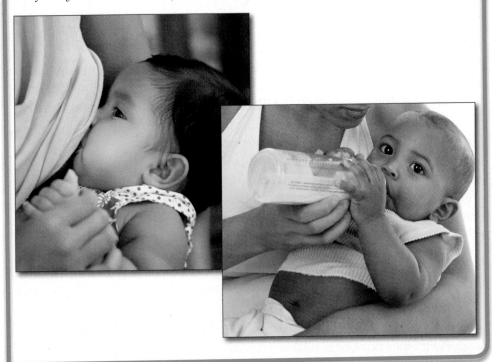

Key Terms E-Flash Cards

In this lesson, you will learn the meanings of the following key terms.

colostrum

lactation consultant

rooting reflex

Before You Read

Reading with Images

Before reading, look at the figures in this lesson. Based on what you see, write predictions about what will be discussed in the lesson. Include examples of one or more figures for each prediction. After reading the lesson, go back to your predictions. Were you correct or incorrect? If you were incorrect, write what you learned.

colostrum

a protein- and antibody-rich substance secreted in a mother's breasts for a few days after she gives birth

lactation consultant

a healthcare professional who counsels and assists new mothers as they breast-feed their babies

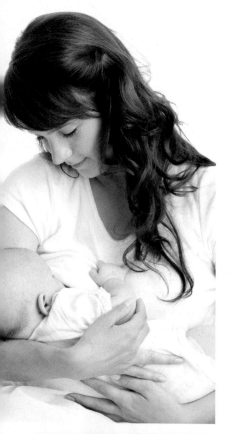

Figure 21.11

Because of the nutritious value of breast milk, pediatricians urge women to breast-feed their babies for the first six months of life.

Infants need proper nutrition and enough calories to sustain rapid growth and development. Both breast-feeding and bottle-feeding with infant formula will meet an infant's needs. Each has advantages and drawbacks. If desired, these methods can be used together. How do mothers decide which is best for their baby?

Breast-Feeding

At birth, a mother's breasts make **colostrum**, a nutritious, healthy liquid that is different from regular breast milk. It contains more protein and much less fat than regular breast milk. Colostrum also contains many antibodies that help the infant fight infections.

After birth, the dramatic change in the mother's hormones prompts milk production. Breast milk contains sugar, fat, protein, vitamins, minerals, and water in the right proportions for babies. Like colostrum, the milk contains antibodies. If possible, pediatricians recommend that breast-feeding be the only source of nutrition for infants during the first six months of life (Figure 21.11).

Advantages of Breast-Feeding

Breast-feeding has many advantages. Breast milk is the natural form of nutrition for babies and contains everything a baby needs to thrive. Later in life, breast-fed babies have lower risk for developing diabetes, asthma, allergies, and obesity. A nursing mother also benefits because breast-feeding helps her lose weight, causes her uterus to return to normal, and may reduce her risk for breast or ovarian cancer.

During the first six months, breast-fed babies do not need to drink juice or water, or eat any other foods. Pediatricians do recommend that babies receive a vitamin D supplement until they begin consuming vitamin-D-fortified cereals or milk after six months.

Breast-Feeding Issues

For various reasons, breast-feeding is not an option for all women. For example, mothers should not breast-feed if they are taking medications for cancer or if they have HIV/AIDS. Others may have a hard time breast-feeding because they work outside of the home. Some mothers have difficulty or are uncomfortable breast-feeding their babies.

If work schedules make breast-feeding difficult, mothers can express milk using a breast pump and refrigerate or freeze it for later feedings. A **lactation consultant** can assist mothers who are having trouble breast-feeding. If a mother cannot breast-feed, she should take comfort knowing that all of her baby's nutritional needs will be met with formula.

Although breast-feeding costs very little compared with formula feeding, it places many demands on the mother. For example, infants who are fed easily digested breast milk require feeding every two hours, around the clock. This can be exhausting for the mother during those first weeks until the baby grows larger, feeds more at each meal, and eats less frequently. To keep the milk flowing, the mother must be available to breast-feed or she must pump her milk.

Making milk requires calories, so nursing mothers need to eat more to make enough milk. Another obvious drawback to breast-feeding is that the father and other caregivers cannot feed the baby. This can be overcome if the mother pumps her milk and stores it in bottles so others can also feed the baby (Figure 21.12).

Formula-Feeding

Infant formula closely replicates the nutrients and caloric content of breast milk. While not identical to breast milk, formula provides complete infant nutrition.

Advantages of Formula-Feeding

Formula-feeding offers some advantages over breast-feeding. When formula-feeding, the mother can share feeding responsibilities with the father, family members, and other caretakers. These mothers do not have to pump milk when away from their babies.

Since babies digest formula more slowly than breast milk, they will feed less frequently, which allows caretakers more rest. Formula-feeding also allows mothers to monitor how much their babies are eating, which is difficult to determine when breast-feeding. Formula-fed babies should eat about two to three ounces at each feeding, and they will probably feed every two to four hours.

Infant Formula Issues

In addition to being more expensive than breast-feeding, formula feeding requires more planning. The baby's caretakers must always have formula on hand at home or when they are out. Formula requires prior preparation, refrigeration, and a steady supply of clean bottles. Refrigerated formula can be slightly warmed by running the bottle under warm water to make it more appealing to the baby.

Whether breast-feeding or formula-feeding, the mother and caretakers should feed the baby when the baby is hungry and stop when the baby is satisfied. Hungry babies often exhibit a ***rooting reflex***. They move their heads from side to side when something touches their faces, make sucking sounds, suck on their hands, and stick out their tongues. When babies become full, they turn their heads away from the bottle or nipple or suck weakly. Well-fed babies will regularly wet their diapers, have frequent bowel movements, and steadily gain weight.

It is normal for babies to spit up some food after eating, but they should not vomit after feeding. Most babies also swallow air when feeding, causing them to burp. Caregivers can encourage the passing of stomach gas by holding the baby upright and gently patting the baby's back. Babies should be burped once or twice during each feeding.

Newborn Growth

In the few days after birth, newborns lose up to 10 percent of their body weight, most of it fluids retained from birth. They regain the lost weight by

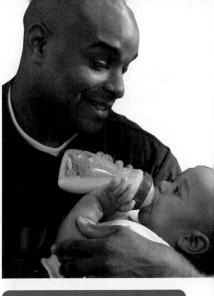

Figure 21.12

A mother may choose to express milk using a breast pump, allowing fathers and other caregivers to help feed the baby.

rooting reflex
an automatic muscle movement in which an infant turns his or her head and tries to suck when hungry

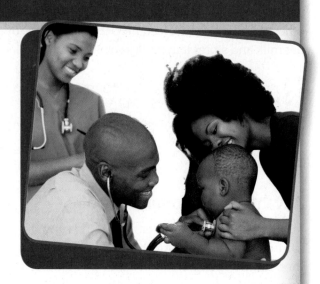

Suppose you are a pediatrician. A mother comes into your office with her baby. She recently gave birth to the baby boy and is breast-feeding him. She is concerned because the baby lost some weight after a few days at home, but slowly regained it. Now the baby breast-feeds frequently, about every hour. This has continued for nearly three weeks.

Thinking Critically

1. How would you explain the baby's early weight loss to the mother?
2. The mother wants to know if the baby is eating too little or too much. How can you learn the answer to this question?
3. What signs would you look for that would indicate that something is wrong with the baby?

two weeks, and then keep growing. The rate of growth is amazing. During their first 30 days, infants can gain an ounce each day. During the next two to three months, babies continue to grow at about the same rate, increasing in height as well—about one inch each month.

Most full-term newborns triple their birth weight in one year. Doctors track a baby's growth because it reflects a baby's general health. Slow growth could be a sign of underlying diseases or disorders. However, birth size and growth rates vary considerably.

Many factors influence a baby's birth weight and growth, but the most significant factor is the infant's nutrition. If an infant's intake of nutrients and calories are adequate and yet the baby still has growth problems, a disease or disorder is probably the cause.

Lesson 21.3 Review

Know and Understand

1. How does breast-feeding babies benefit them later in life?
2. List two reasons a woman may choose not to breast-feed.
3. What is the *rooting reflex*?
4. What is the major factor that influences an infant's growth after birth?

Analyze and Apply

5. How does colostrum differ from breast milk? How are they similar?
6. Why do newborns lose up to 10 percent of their body weight within the first few days after birth?

7. Compare and contrast breast-feeding and formula-feeding.

Real World   Health

Good nutrition and caloric intake are important to sustaining a newborn's rapid growth and development. Compare and contrast the nutritional values of breast-feeding and formula-feeding. Also, referencing the Warm-Up Activity for this lesson, consider which social, emotional, or practical factors might influence the effectiveness of these methods. Write and design a one-page flyer that lists the advantages and disadvantages of breast-feeding and formula-feeding.

Bonding, Communication, and Parenting Issues

Lesson Objectives

After studying this lesson, you will be able to

- explain how babies and parents bond;
- describe how babies communicate; and
- discuss the effects of shaken baby syndrome.

Key Terms E-Flash Cards

In this lesson, you will learn the meanings of the following key terms.

bond

sensory input

shaken baby syndrome

Warm-Up Activity

Bonding Activities

Based on what you've seen in your own life and in the media, what are four ways a parent or caregiver can bond with a new baby? Draw or find a picture of each bonding activity you've identified. In a chart like the one below, add pictures of the four bonding activities and answer the following question: How does this activity forge a connection between caregiver and child? When you are done, find a partner and share ideas. Then, pick your two favorite bonding activities and share them with the class.

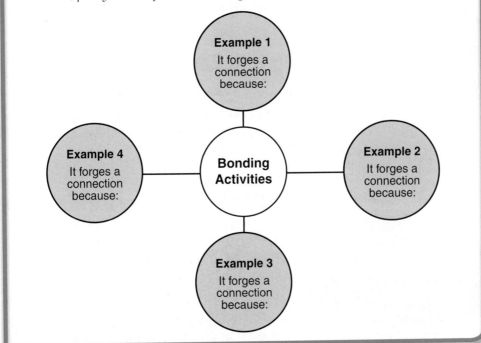

Before You Read

What You Know

Before reading, consider the title of this lesson. Brainstorm everything you know about bonding, communication, and parenting issues. Organize your thoughts in a chart like the one shown below. For each thought, identify whether it is the result of previous learning or personal experience. After reading the lesson, go back and write what you learned in the third column.

What I learned before	My own experience	This lesson

Newborn babies are born prepared to communicate and bond with adults. They are quite alert and quickly make a connection between their parents' faces and voices. These reactions are a newborn's first attempts at communication and bonding. Positive adult responses to these attempts will encourage communication and reinforce bonding.

Bonding with Babies

bond
to form an intimate, emotional attachment

Soon after birth, babies and their parents or caregivers **bond**—they form a close, intimate attachment. Communication and bonding promote closeness and affection, and encourage a sense of safety in babies. Recognition and response to the baby's needs help foster a baby's healthy social development.

How Parents and Babies Bond

Parents and caregivers can bond with babies by regularly holding them close, making eye contact, talking, and singing. Caregivers can take advantage of many other opportunities to bond. These include feeding, bathing, dressing, and playing with the baby (Figure 21.13).

Bonding with Adopted Children

Bonding requires trust between parent and child. Adoptive parents can encourage bonding by making their child feel safe and comfortable at their new home. Adoptive parents and child need time alone to have opportunities for trust to be tested and develop. Babies bond when their hunger and distress are met with parental attention and kindness. It may take more time for older children to bond, but in most cases, adoptive parents form loving, supportive attachment with their children.

Communicating with Babies

Babies first communicate primarily by crying. A baby's cry expresses hunger, stress, discomfort, or sleepiness (Figure 21.14). Over time, alert parents notice that babies develop different cries for different reasons.

Why Babies Cry

If a crying baby is not hungry and has a clean diaper, the parent or caregiver should carefully check for other possible problems. For example, babies easily overheat or become cold because they cannot effectively regulate their body temperature. Clothes or diapers can become tight or pinch, causing discomfort.

Figure 21.13

Caregivers can bond with their children through daily routines such as feeding, bathing, dressing, playing, or diapering. *What other ways could a caregiver bond with his or her child?*

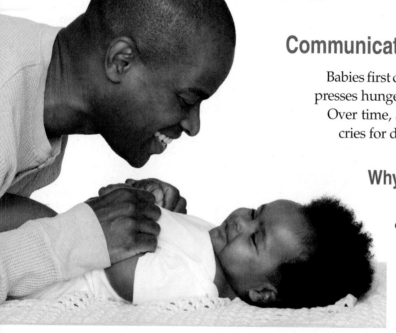

Babies also become overloaded with *sensory input*. Their new and stimulating world causes babies to tire easily, and so they may cry when sleepy. Babies also cry when they have gas or upset stomachs. It helps to burp the baby until this discomfort eases. Of course, a sick baby cries, too. Parents and caregivers should contact a doctor if their baby vomits, has diarrhea, or has a fever over 100.4°F.

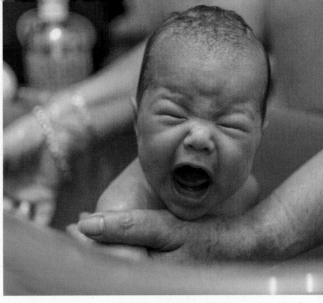

Responding to Crying

Parents and caregivers can respond to a crying baby with a soothing voice. Babies may respond by vocalizing, becoming quiet, moving their arms and legs in time with the voice, or turning their heads to find the parent or caregiver.

A baby's ability to communicate develops quickly to include vocalizing with gurgles, babbling, and giggles. Parents and caregivers should recognize and respond to these attempts at communication because it fosters the baby's healthy socialization and development.

These first conversations do not have to be complicated. Parents and caregivers can simply echo the baby's sounds and speak using adult sounds and words. During baths, feedings, and dressing the baby, parents can talk about what they are doing, what they see, and how they feel.

Figure 21.14

Babies cry for a number of different reasons, including hunger, stress, tiredness, or discomfort. In many cases, crying signals and communicates a baby's needs.

sensory input
the information that the brain receives related to sight, hearing, touch, and smell

Parenting Issues

Parenting is an enormous and stressful responsibility. It can be easier and more rewarding when shared with another loving adult. The important role of the mother in raising children is recognized, but sometimes the father's parental role and responsibilities are overlooked. Most fathers want to be involved in nurturing and caring for their children. Bonding between the infant and the father may develop more slowly than it does with the mother, especially if the baby is breast-feeding. Given time and regular interaction, however, fathers can and do form intimate bonds with their children.

Parents usually feel some degree of stress about pregnancy, parenthood, and its associated responsibilities. A father and mother need to openly discuss their concerns so they can focus on creating a nurturing, healthy environment for their child. Any friction or problems in their relationship should be addressed.

The Parents' Relationship

A baby demands much time and emotional energy from parents. As a result, the parents' relationship can suffer (Figure 21.15 on the next page). Intimacy may become difficult to achieve for parents who are tired, stressed, and moody. With time, open communication, and perhaps counseling, parents can maintain and restore intimacy as they adjust to parenthood.

Figure 21.15

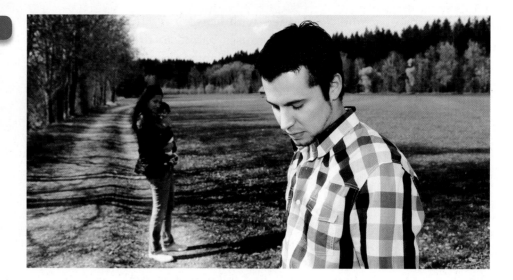

The physical and emotional demands of caring for a baby can sometimes take a toll on the parents' relationship. It is important that parents make time for intimacy and express their feelings in positive ways.

Anger

It is not unusual for parents to feel overwhelmed with responsibility, anxious about money, and frustrated about the relationship with their partner. It is important for parents to recognize these feelings, talk about them, and deal with them constructively. Uncontrolled anger creates an environment of chronic stress and anxiety for the baby.

shaken baby syndrome
trauma and brain damage caused by an infant being jostled or handled roughly

At worst, parents' anger can lead to physical abuse such as shaking or hitting, which can be deadly for a baby. **Shaken baby syndrome** is injury caused by shaking an infant in anger or frustration. Because babies have weak neck muscles and their skulls aren't fully formed, shaking a baby can cause brain trauma. The trauma may include spinal cord damage or bleeding in the brain or eyes. This can result in seizures, respiratory distress, permanent brain damage such as cognitive disabilities, and physical disabilities including blindness. Sometimes the consequences are fatal.

Shaking a baby is a form of child abuse. It is *never* appropriate to shake a baby under any circumstances. Parenting classes can help new parents learn ways to cope with the demands of parenting.

Lesson 21.4 Review

Know and Understand Assess

1. What are the effects of bonding and communication on caregivers and infants?
2. List four possible results of shaking a baby.

Analyze and Apply

3. Develop and evaluate a list of activities fathers could use to bond with their infants.
4. What sorts of first conversations can parents and caregivers use to help communicate with their infants?

Real World Health

Compared with the attention given to the mother's parental role, the father's parental role and responsibilities are often overlooked. Interview a father about his role in raising his child or children. How did he bond with his child or children? How involved is he in their lives? Using the information you gather from your interview, design a Father's Day card describing how that father bonded with and has parented his child or children.

Teen Parents

Lesson Objectives

After studying this lesson, you will be able to

- list challenges of teen parenting;
- describe responsibilities of teen fathers; and
- discuss reasons teen parents may choose to place their child for adoption.

Key Terms E-Flash Cards

In this lesson, you will learn the meanings of the following key terms.

child support
noncustodial parent
safe haven laws

Warm-Up Activity

Your Goals and Dreams

Imagine yourself in 10 years. Consider your goals and dreams for the future. Do you see yourself working in a particular field? Do you want to graduate from college? If you want to live in your own home, describe it. What kind of car will you drive? Do you want to travel and see the world? Are there any other interests you plan to pursue that will cost money? Do you want to be married? How much income will you need? Now, consider the responsibilities, time, and costs involved in caring for a baby. How would having a baby in the next few years affect your ability to pursue your goals and dreams? What would change in your life? Write a letter to yourself describing how teen pregnancy could affect the plans you have for your present and future.

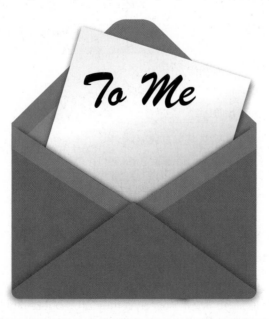

Before You Read

Reading with Objectives

Before reading this lesson, skim the lesson objectives. In a chart such as the one below, list the main topics you anticipate learning in the lesson. Beside each topic, write what you already know. Then, find a partner and share your knowledge. Write anything your partner teaches you in the third column of your chart.

Main topics	What I already know	What my partner knows

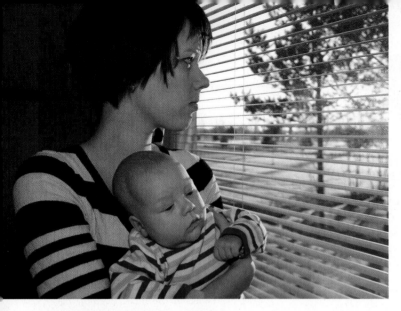

Teen parents often don't have access to the social and emotional support they need as they adjust to parenting. As a result, teen parents often feel isolated or excluded by their peers. *Why might teen parents not receive the emotional and social support they need?*

R aising a child can be a rewarding experience, but teen parents and their children face many challenges. Raising a child requires time, energy, and financial resources. It takes priority over school, career, and other personal goals.

Challenges of Becoming a Teen Parent

If pregnant teens decide to parent their child, they must prepare and learn everything they can about parenthood. Teen parents often cannot count on financial or emotional support of friends and family members (Figure 21.16).

Teens may find that some people withdraw and distance themselves when they learn about the pregnancy. Other people rally around and support the young parents. Some family members react in unexpected ways, perhaps because they are embarrassed or confused. Friends may drift away, leaving a teen parent feeling isolated and rejected. A tough time like this requires a teen to reach out to loving family members, good friends, and other trusted adults.

Parenting classes designed for teen parents teach the basics of infant care, feeding, sleeping, diapering, bathing, and child safety. Both the mother and father should attend these so they can each be prepared to share in childcare. Learning these basics is the first step in providing a positive future for the child. In general, the children of teenage parents face more challenges throughout life than children of adult parents (Figure 21.17).

Figure 21.17 Risks for Children of Teen Parents

Compared with children born to adult parents, the children of teen parents are

- less likely to have a father at home;
- less likely to graduate from high school;
- less likely to attend college;
- less likely to be employed after high school;
- more likely to become teen parents;
- less likely to receive attention for their medical needs;
- more likely to be abused, abandoned, or neglected;
- more likely to be placed in foster care;
- more likely to be convicted of a crime and sentenced to jail;
- two to three times more likely to run away from home; and
- ten times more likely to live in poverty if they drop out of high school.

Financial Challenges

Teen parents need to consider and plan for many issues that will arise as they begin parenting. Some high schools and community organizations offer child care or other assistance for teen mothers. Even with these resources, continuing high school is very difficult. Some teen parents work extra jobs or drop out of school to earn enough money to care for their baby.

Financial challenges of parenthood are substantial for teen parents in high school without significant earnings. The biggest expenses related to raising a child are child care, healthcare, and education. The parents need to decide who will care for the baby during and after school. The baby's grandparents might be available to help. Housing expenses may be small if the teens live with their parents. However, other expenses remain an enormous burden (Figure 21.18). This is why many teen parents must decide whether to stay in school or to drop out and begin working full time.

Most teen fathers would like to be involved with their child, but they also face financial and educational burdens. Even if the teen father does not marry the mother and is not involved with childrearing, most states require him to pay the mother *child support*. Unfortunately, many teen fathers are too poor to support themselves and pay child support.

Financial burdens are the main reason that teen parents should finish high school. Teen parents who graduate high school will have more opportunities for employment and better paying jobs than those who do not. This will allow them to better care for themselves and their baby.

Some high schools or community organizations offer services to help teen parents complete high school. These services include on-site child care in schools, babysitting after school, parenting classes, personal and family counseling, and career counseling.

child support
the financial contribution legally required of the noncustodial parent

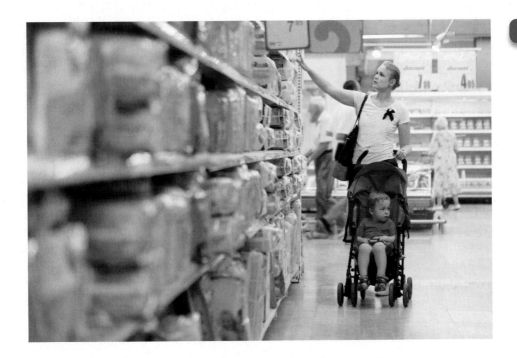

Figure 21.18

The many items needed to care for a baby can exert an enormous financial burden on all parents, and especially on teen parents.

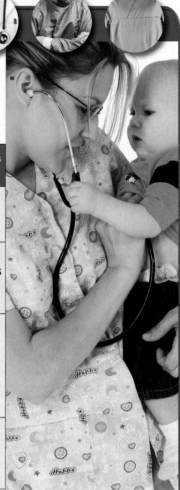

Careers Providing Care for Infants

You may want to explore the careers described below related to childbirth and the care of infants.

Career	Typical Education and Training	Typical Job Duties and Demands	Career Resources
Pediatric nurse	associate's degree or bachelor's degree	Delivers healthcare for newborns, infants, and children.	American Nurses Association
Certified Nurse-Midwife	college degree, graduate training, and certification	Provides prenatal care, assistance with pregnancy and delivery, and postnatal care.	American College of Nurse-Midwives
Obstetrician	bachelor's degree followed by a medical degree (M.D. or O.D.)	Provides pre- and postnatal care; deliver babies; diagnose and treat conditions related to pregnancy and childbirth.	American Medical Association, American Congress of Obstetricians and Gynecologists
Licensed Practical Nurse (LPN)	high school plus LPN certification/ license	Administers basic nursing care under direction of a registered nurse or physician.	National Federation of Licensed Practical Nurses

Exploring Careers

1. Think about your interests, strengths, and weaknesses. Which career described above appeals most to you? Which career does not interest you?

2. Do you know anyone who works in one of these careers? If so, ask this person why he or she chose this career and what he or she likes most and least about the work.

Responsibilities of Teen Fathers

Even though many teen parents will not marry, the mother and father must discuss how he will be involved. Too commonly, teen fathers do not take their parenting responsibility seriously, leaving child care and the associated costs to the mother and her family. In some cases, the teen mother's parents may be angry with the father. They may exclude him even when he wants to be involved with his child.

The teen father can help in many ways, beginning with prenatal care. He can attend prenatal and parenting classes with the mother and later support her by sharing child care duties. The father might not be able to contribute much financially, but his help with child care is important for both the child and the mother. His help can increase the chances of the mother completing high school.

If the parents are not married, the baby usually lives with his or her mother. When this is the case, the teen father is called the **noncustodial parent**. In some cases the baby lives with the father, and the mother is considered the noncustodial parent. The noncustodial parent has legal rights and a legal obligation to contribute financially to the care of the baby. The amount of child support varies and depends on the earnings of the noncustodial parent and his or her family.

noncustodial parent
a parent who does not provide primary care for a child, but has legal rights and responsibilities regarding a child

Placing a Child for Adoption

The decision about whether or not to raise a child should be made carefully by pregnant teens. Some girls feel that they will be unable to raise a child and decide to place their child for adoption.

Parents who choose this route may feel some grief and loss following adoption, but it may be best for their babies' future. By placing their babies for adoption, they may also be able to help couples have families that they could not otherwise have.

If someone is considering placing a child for adoption, he or she should learn what the adoption laws are in his or her state. In some states, the mother must obtain the consent of a birth father before an adoption can go forward.

When a pregnancy is unexpected, teens as well as adults can become desperate, depressed, and confused. In their confusion, some of them may consider abandoning their baby after the baby is born. Abandoned infants, however, are in great danger. Without regular feedings and a warm place to stay, the helpless babies can quickly become sick or die.

safe haven laws
laws that allow parents to leave their infant at designated locations if they wish to give up their child for adoption; age restrictions for the child vary by state; safe surrender laws

Every state has **safe haven laws** (also called *safe surrender laws*) that permit people to leave their babies at certain facilities with no questions asked. These laws protect innocent and vulnerable babies from the dangers of abandonment. Each state has age restrictions for a baby who is left at a safe haven. Safe havens include fire stations, police stations, and hospitals. The babies will be well cared for until they can be adopted.

Lesson 21.5 Review

Know and Understand

1. Why might a doctor recommend parenting classes designed for expectant girls and teen fathers?
2. What are the three biggest expenses related to raising a child?
3. What legal responsibility does the noncustodial parent have?
4. List three examples of safe havens for babies.

Analyze and Apply

5. Compare and contrast the financial challenges pregnant teens might face as compared to adults who are pregnant.

Real World Health

When teenage parents do not marry, a baby typically lives with the mother. The father is usually considered a noncustodial parent and spends less time with the baby. He does, however, still have legal rights and responsibilities regarding the baby. Using this textbook and outside sources, list the rights and responsibilities of a noncustodial father, according to the laws in your state. Finally, design an educational brochure outlining these rights and responsibilities. Also include websites and resources a noncustodial parent can view for additional information.

Childbirth and the First Days

Key Terms

adoption	dilation
Apgar test	epidural anethesia
birth plan	labor
birthing center	nurse-midwife
birthing room	oxytocin
cesarean section	reflex
(C-section)	vernix

Key Points

- Before delivery, parents-to-be must make decisions such as where to deliver and who will deliver the baby.
- The laboring process includes three main stages.
- A newborn's health is determined immediately after birth.
- Newborns share certain characteristics.
- Adoptive parents must also prepare for the arrival of their new child.

Check Your Understanding

1. A(n) _____ addresses the mother's preferences about the birth process, such as the location where she will give birth.

2. *True or false?* Epidural anesthesia can be administered immediately before the birth of a child.

3. The placenta is delivered in the _____ stage of labor.
   A. first
   B. second
   C. third
   D. fourth

4. In _____ adoptions, adopted children can have contact with their biological parents.

5. Infants who are born at _____ weeks of pregnancy or earlier are considered premature.

6. **Critical Thinking.** Explain what it means if a baby has an Apgar score of 9 when tested five minutes after birth.

Newborn Care

Key Terms

fontanel	sudden infant death
pediatrician	syndrome (SIDS)

Key Points

- Parents must learn the appropriate ways to handle their newborns.
- Newborn care includes learning about sleeping habits, bathing, and diapering.
- Immunizations will help prevent illness in infants.
- Parents and caregivers should be alert to signs of illness in infants.

Check Your Understanding

7. *True or false?* A newborn has relatively weak neck and shoulder muscles.

8. By around _____ months of age, babies begin sleeping through the night.

9. Which of the following actions will reduce the risk of SIDS?
   A. putting babies to sleep on their stomachs
   B. prohibiting smoking near babies
   C. using fluffy crib padding
   D. placing extra pillows in the crib

10. _____ cause babies to develop their own longer-lasting protection from infections.

11. **Critical Thinking.** Why should a child's car seat never be placed in the front seat of a vehicle?

Newborn Nutrition, Growth, and Development

Key Terms

colostrum	rooting reflex
lactation consultant	

Key Points

- Breast milk is a natural form of nutrition for babies.

- Parents may chose to formula-feed their babies for various reasons.
- Both breast-feeding and formula-feeding have their advantages and disadvantages.
- Infants grow quickly in the first year of life.

Check Your Understanding

12. At birth, a mother's breasts make a nutritious, healthy liquid called _____.

13. *True or false?* Pediatricians recommend that breast-feeding be the only source of nutrition for infants during the first six months of life, if possible.

14. *True or false?* Formula is identical to breast milk.

15. Hungry babies often exhibit a(n) _____ by moving their heads from side to side when something touches their faces, making sucking sounds, sucking on their hands, and sticking out their tongues.

16. Which of the following is *not* normal behavior for newborns?
    A. spitting up after eating
    B. vomiting after eating
    C. swallowing air when feeding
    D. burping during feeding

17. **Critical Thinking.** Summarize a baby's growth during the first year of life.

Lesson 21.4 — Assess

Bonding, Communication, and Parenting Issues

Key Terms

bond
sensory input

shaken baby syndrome

Key Points

- Newborns communicate and bond with their parents.
- Babies communicate by crying.
- Shaking a baby in anger and frustration can physically harm the baby and may even result in death.

Check Your Understanding

18. Babies _____ with parents when they form a close, intimate attachment.

19. *True or false?* Shaking a baby in frustration is a form of child abuse.

20. _____ overload may cause the baby to become overstimulated, tire easily, and cry.

21. **Critical Thinking.** Explain why babies cry.

Lesson 21.5 — Assess

Teen Parents

Key Terms

child support
noncustodial parent

safe haven laws

Key Points

- Teen parents face many challenges.
- Teen fathers have legal rights and responsibilities.
- Teens should be aware of state laws when considering placing their child for adoption.

Check Your Understanding

22. *True or false?* For teen parents, raising the child must be a priority over school, career, and other personal goals.

23. Children of teen parents are _____.
    A. more likely to graduate from high school
    B. less likely to attend college
    C. less likely to become teen parents
    D. more likely to be employed after high school

24. If the parents are not married and the baby lives with the mother, the father is called the _____.

25. *True or false?* Safe haven laws permit people to leave their babies at certain facilities after filling out government forms.

26. **Critical Thinking.** From a financial point of view, why do many teen parents drop out of high school?

Health and Wellness Skills

27. **Access Information.** Research safe haven laws for babies, why these laws exist, and how these laws are defined in your state. Draw a poster illustrating what places an unwanted baby can be left, if there are any age restrictions for the baby, and any other valuable information.

28. **Advocate for Health.** With a partner or in a small group, research resources for parents in your community or state, and find out what information and support they offer. Design a presentation covering this information and share it with your class.

29. **Comprehend Concepts.** In a small group, list 10 benefits of being a teenager. These should be benefits that disappear once someone is no longer a teenager. In a second column, list how these benefits would change if a teenager becomes a parent. Write a script for a television drama about a teenager who becomes a parent and experiences the loss of four of the items on your list.

30. **Make Decisions.** Based on what you've learned make a chart outlining the decisions that prospective parents must make about birthing plans. In addition, list people and groups that can serve as resources for prospective parents. Consider talking with your mother, or other close family member, about your own birth and early days. Once you've made your chart, outline your own personal birthing plan, whether for you or for your future partner.

Hands-On Activity
Flour-Sack Baby

Being a parent involves new responsibilities. For this activity, you will create and care for a flour-sack baby and document your days as a parent.

Materials Needed

- 5 lb. sack of flour (or sugar)
- markers to decorate the baby
- baby clothes (optional)
- materials to create a carrier for the baby
- camera
- scrapbooking supplies or slideshow/video technology

Steps for this Activity

1. Decorate your sack of flour, which is now considered your baby, and give your baby a name. Using cardboard or another sturdy material, create a carrier for your baby.

2. For one week, you are responsible for the care of your baby:

   - Your baby must stay with you at all times, unless you have made arrangements with another responsible caregiver. The baby should always be kept in its appropriate carrier or held.

   - Your baby is fragile and can make quite a mess if damaged. Report any abuse or injury to your teacher immediately.

   - Your baby will need to be fed and have its diaper changed. Every three hours, set aside 5–20 minutes to simulate these tasks. Create a log of the time you set aside.

   - During one night of caring for your baby, set an alarm to wake up around 2 a.m. for a "night-feeding." E-mail your teacher that you are feeding your baby.

3. Take pictures of your baby and how you have cared for it. At the end of the week, create a slideshow, photo album, or scrapbook, and write a page that describes your experience as a parent. Present your baby book to the class.

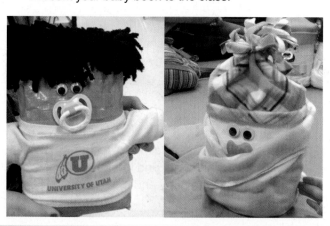

Core Skills

Math Practice

The following graphs show breastfeeding by birth year across a decade. Study the graph and then answer the questions.

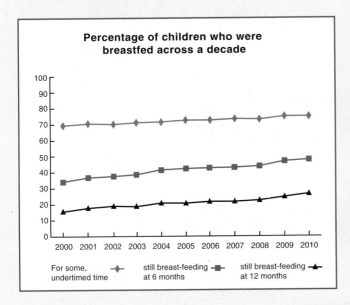

Percentage of children who were breastfed across a decade

Legend: For some, undertimed time ◆ still breast-feeding at 6 months ■ still breast-feeding at 12 months ▲

31. In 2000, what percentage of children had been breast-fed at some point?
    A. 70
    B. 40
    C. 30
    D. 10

32. In 2007, about how many more children had been breast-fed through six months of age than had been breast-fed through twelve months of age?
    A. 20 percent more
    B. 25 percent more
    C. 40 percent more
    D. 65 percent more

33. In 2010, how many more children had been breast-fed at all than were breast-fed at 12 months of age?
    A. 20 percent more
    B. 30 percent more
    C. 40 percent more
    D. 50 percent more

Reading and Writing Practice

Read the passage below and then answer the questions.

By law, infants must travel in a car seat every time they ride in a vehicle. Car seats reduce the chances for serious injury and death among children. A newborn should be placed in a rear-facing car seat in the back seat of the vehicle. Children seated in the front seat can be killed or severely injured if an air bag deploys. Parents should always check with their state's laws and guidelines regarding car seats. Parents can visit local fire or police stations with questions—many of them perform car seat inspections to ensure correct installation.

34. What is the author's main idea in this passage?
    A. Children riding in the front seat can be easily injured.
    B. State laws guide car seat regulations.
    C. Air bags can harm children.
    D. Car seats reduce the chance for serious injury among children.

35. Where should newborns be placed in cars?
    A. in a rear-facing car seat in the front seat
    B. in a rear-facing car seat in the back seat
    C. in a front-facing car seat in the back seat
    D. another passenger should hold the newborn

36. Write a paragraph about how you would install a car seat for an infant. Share your paragraphs in class.

37. Why can children sitting in the front seat be more seriously injured in an accident?
    A. Accidents usually cause more front-end damage.
    B. Car seats don't fit correctly in front seats.
    C. Air bags can deploy and cause injury or death.
    D. Engine fires are closer to the front seat.

38. Where can parents have their car seat installations inspected?
    A. police stations
    B. news stations
    C. hospitals
    D. libraries

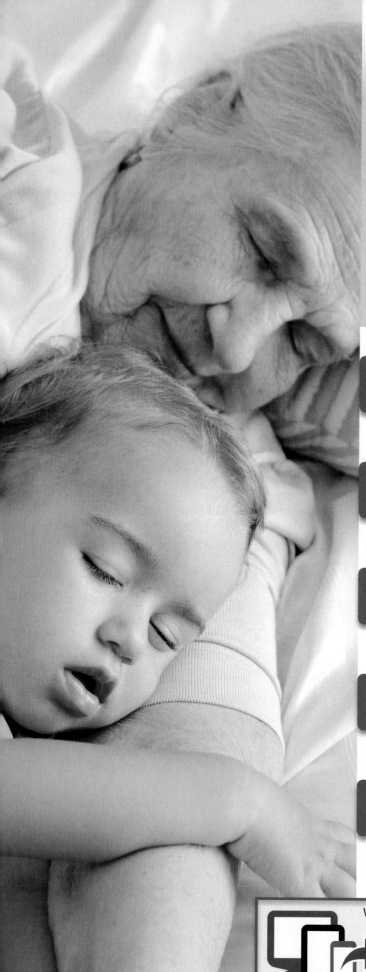

Chapter 22

Human Development across the Life Span

Lesson 22.1

Human Development: The Unfolding Self

Lesson 22.2

Infancy through the Preschool Years

Lesson 22.3

The School-Age and Adolescent Years

Lesson 22.4

Adulthood and the Nature of Aging

Lesson 22.5

The End of Life

While studying this chapter, look for the activity icon to:

- **review** vocabulary with e-flash cards and games;
- **assess** learning with quizzes and online exercises;
- **expand** knowledge with animations and activities; and
- **listen** to pronunciation of key terms in the audio glossary.

G-WLEARNING.com

www.g-wlearning.com/health/

What's Your Health and Wellness IQ?

Take this quiz to see what you do *and* do not *know about human development. If you cannot answer a question, pay extra attention to that topic as you study this chapter.*

1. *Identify each statement as* True, False, *or* It Depends. *Choose* It Depends *if a statement is true in some cases, but false in others.*
2. *Revise each* False *statement to make it true.*
3. *Explain the circumstances in which each* It Depends *statement is true and when it is false.*

Health and Wellness IQ Assess

1. Human development and human growth are the same process.	True	False	It Depends
2. Only genes control human life span.	True	False	It Depends
3. Children learn to walk before their first birthday.	True	False	It Depends
4. Toddlers do not easily share toys.	True	False	It Depends
5. School-age children think more abstractly than concretely.	True	False	It Depends
6. During puberty, most children grow to their adult height.	True	False	It Depends
7. Vision and hearing do not decline with age.	True	False	It Depends
8. There is no "typical" young adult in the United States.	True	False	It Depends
9. Adults can maintain a healthy, active life by adapting to changes caused by aging.	True	False	It Depends
10. Grief and loss are generally more common in older adulthood than in other stages of life.	True	False	It Depends

Setting the Scene

A human life is made up of stages like a book is made up of chapters. The opening chapter of a book sets the stage for the following chapters. The story of a life unfolds in the same way that chapters build on each other, and each new chapter brings new elements to the plot. From infancy through childhood, adolescence, and adulthood, people continue to develop and change in characteristic, fairly predictable ways.

In this chapter, you will learn about the stages of human life. You will also learn about grieving and coping with loss, especially at the end of a life. Although people of all ages experience the deaths of family members, friends, and even beloved pets, this type of loss occurs with growing frequency as people grow older and experience more stages of life.

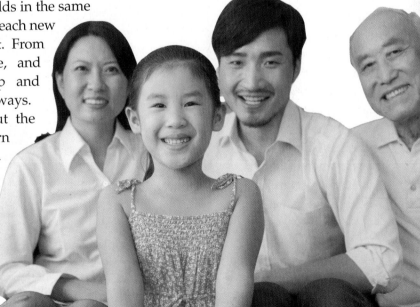

Human Development: The Unfolding Self

Key Terms E-Flash Cards

In this lesson, you will learn the meanings of the following key terms.

human life cycle
Individualized
    Education Plan (IEP)
Individualized Family
    Service Plan (IFSP)
interdependent
milestones

Before You Read

Mindmap
Create a visual chart to connect the information in this lesson with your prior knowledge about human development. In the center of your chart, write Human Development across the Life Span. *In surrounding circles, write the four sub-topics—* Human Life Cycle, Facets of Human Development, Developmental Delays, *and* Life Expectancy versus Life Span. *List as much information as you know about each sub-topic. After you read the lesson, go back and update your chart with the knowledge you have gained.*

Lesson Objectives

After studying this lesson, you will be able to

- summarize how growth and development are related but distinct processes;
- list the six developmental stages in the human life cycle;
- explain how physical, emotional, intellectual, and social development are related and interdependent;
- describe how genes and the environment interact to direct and influence human development; and
- recognize lifestyle choices that can reduce a person's life span.

Warm-Up Activity

The Stages of Life
Trace or draw the illustrations shown here and label each picture according to the stage of life it represents—infancy, toddlerhood, preschool, school-age, adolescence, or adulthood. Under each picture, list two to three qualities that you think are typical of that stage of life. After reading this lesson, revisit each stage and consider whether you would make any changes based on what you've learned.

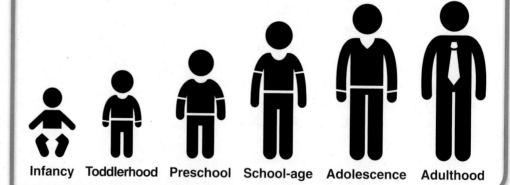

Infancy **Toddlerhood** **Preschool** **School-age** **Adolescence** **Adulthood**

L ooking at your baby pictures and school photos together would capture how dramatically you have changed since the day you were born. Thanks to continual growth and development, you hardly seem to be the same person. Growth and development are related, but distinct processes. *Growth* refers to increases in the size of the body and its parts. Increases in height and weight are examples of growth.

Human development includes many other critical changes in the body. Development produces new body structures and functions. This means that, in addition to growing physically, a person also acquires intellectual, emotional, and social abilities over time.

The Human Life Cycle

The *human life cycle* consists of a sequence of developmental stages. Each developmental stage is characterized by well-known, important events called **milestones**. Some people reach developmental milestones earlier or later than their peers. For example, a major developmental milestone is learning how to walk. The precise age at which a child reaches this milestone differs from one person to the next.

Overall, people pass through these life stages gradually. The most rapid, dramatic changes occur early in life, from infancy through adolescence. In this textbook, developmental stages will be defined by age because many people reach developmental milestones at about the same age. Remember that the boundaries between stages are not well-defined because people develop at different rates.

Developmental stages in the human life cycle include

- *infancy*—birth to one year of age;
- *toddlerhood*—one to three years of age;
- *preschool*—three to five years of age;
- *school-age*—five to 12 years of age;
- *adolescence*—12 to 19 years of age; and
- *adulthood*—20 years of age and older.

Types of Human Development

As you study human development, you will discover that people develop physically, intellectually, emotionally, and socially (Figure 22.1). These types of development are related and **interdependent**, meaning that they rely on each other.

- *Physical development*—includes growth of the body and body parts. The other aspects of human development build on the foundation of physical development. As the brain develops and grows more sophisticated in structure, a child is better able to process information, learn, and think in more sophisticated ways.

human life cycle
the sequence of developmental stages in a person's life span

milestones
significant events that mark each stage of human development

interdependent
the quality of one person or piece of information being reliant on another

Figure 22.1

Throughout their life spans, humans develop in a number of different ways—physically, emotionally, socially, and intellectually. *What are some examples of each type of development? How are these types of development measured?*

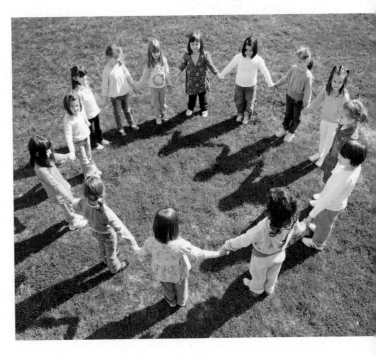

- *Intellectual development*—describes the maturation of an individual's thinking, information processing, and responsiveness to the world. This also includes the development of mature speech and language.
- *Emotional development*—refers to the achievement of individual identity, personality, independence, self-esteem, and other aspects of mental and emotional health. These aspects of emotional development normally arise in a healthy and safe environment as the brain matures.
- *Social development*—refers to the ability to interact with people in socially acceptable ways. Social and interpersonal skills develop throughout a person's life. Much of the foundation for these skills is laid, however, from infancy through childhood. While genes give people the capacity to develop these skills, family environment and education strongly influence their development.

Developmental Delays

Caregivers and pediatricians closely observe children's behavior, watching for changes that indicate healthy growth and development. Delays in development can represent an underlying problem that requires treatment.

A child with a developmental delay often needs help in school to be successful. Government-funded programs can provide this help. *Early intervention programs* provide special services for children from birth to three years of age who have developmental delays. These programs are run by teachers and staff with special training to teach children with developmental delays. These specialists can determine a child's needs and design daily activities to help him or her catch up developmentally.

For example, a child with speech and language delays will meet with a speech and language therapist during the day. Together they do activities and play games designed to encourage the development of language skills. These interventions are described in an ***Individualized Family Service Plan (IFSP)***. An IFSP is a formal document that outlines the special services needed to assist young children with developmental delays. If children still require special services after they reach three years of age, they are referred to resources at the local public school they will attend.

The public school staff works with parents to write an ***Individualized Education Plan (IEP)***. Some of the services provided in the early intervention program are continued. In addition, the IEP describes services the child needs in the classroom to be successful academically and socially. The IEP is revised as a child's needs change and may be discontinued if the child no longer needs assistance. If eligible for assistance, a child may receive the services of an IEP from 3 years of age to 21 years of age.

Life Expectancy versus Life Span

Life expectancy is the scientific estimate of the maximum length of life for people in a population. In the United States, the average life expectancy is 78 years of age. In contrast, *life span* refers to the number of years a specific individual actually lives.

Individualized Family Service Plan (IFSP)
an intervention program that outlines the special services a young child with a developmental delay will need

Individualized Education Plan (IEP)
a program that outlines the additional services a child with a developmental delay may require in a classroom setting

A person's life span can be less than or more than the life expectancy for the population of people born in the same year. An individual's life span and how the person ages depend on his or her genes, environment, and lifestyle. People age at different rates, which can affect their life spans. This is because aging carries with it risks for disease and disability that can shorten a life span. Certain changes that accompany aging are expected and occur in all people.

Genes and the Environment

Genes and the environment interact to direct and influence human development. Genes determine people's traits, such as eye color or skin color. Genes also instruct the body's cells to divide and reproduce. This cell division and reproduction causes the body's organs to grow and acquire new form and function over time. Genes that direct changes in the muscles and nerve cells of the body help people acquire muscle coordination and strength.

Genes, however, do not act alone. Genes are influenced by the environment of the developing body. Environmental toxins that enter the body affect genes and development. This is illustrated by how cigarette, alcohol, and drug use interfere with normal growth and development.

Lifestyle Choices

As you age, your body will show normal signs of wear and tear. Your knees may become sore from spending years playing sports or climbing up and down stairs. Making unhealthy lifestyle choices in the following areas will also leave their marks on your body and may take years off your life span.

- *Smoking.* Avoiding smoking can decrease a person's risk for diseases such as cancer, heart disease, stroke, chronic bronchitis, and emphysema. Deciding not to smoke can be one of the most important choices a person makes to prolong his or her life and health. Quitting smoking at any age immediately improves a person's health, and will significantly improve the quality of a person's life.

- *Nutrition.* Following a healthy diet throughout childhood and adolescence promotes a healthy adulthood. Good nutrition supports an active life and prevents weight gain. A healthy diet also reduces the risk for heart disease and hypertension, and helps the body maintain a strong immune system to fight infections. Healthy eating habits become especially important in older adulthood when people are more susceptible to the effects of a poor diet (Figure 22.2).

- *Physical activity.* Getting plenty of physical activity helps people maintain their strength and endurance, and improve their flexibility and balance.

Figure 22.2

Good nutrition promotes health for your present and future selves. Your eating habits now will impact your health as an adult. *What eating habits do you have now? Will these habits have a positive or a negative effect on your future health?*

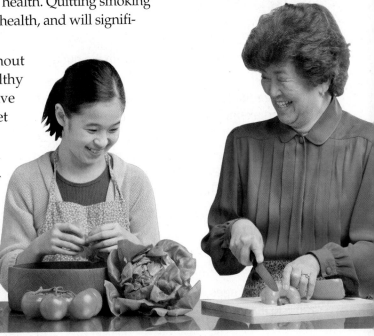

Being physically active can also help reduce depression and reduce the risk for a number of diseases, such as heart disease, diabetes, and osteoporosis. People who are not used to strenuous physical activity should consult a doctor before beginning a fitness program.

- *Sleep.* Lack of sleep causes people to have problems staying alert and active, and can also lead to memory problems and depression. Getting enough sleep each night is necessary to keep the body functioning at its best. Difficulties with sleeping may result from taking medications, drinking alcohol, smoking, or from anxiety and depression. A doctor should be consulted to help determine if a sleep problem is due to a disease.

Diseases and Disorders

When you are young, your body bounces back and heals after most illnesses and injuries. When you become an older adult, however, your body will be less able to repair itself. As a result, you will be more susceptible to diseases and disorders. These may include heart disease, stroke, cancer, respiratory disease, arthritis, osteoporosis, and infectious diseases.

The good news is that many of these diseases and disorders are preventable and can be avoided by living a healthy lifestyle. Begin those healthy habits now and you can reduce your chances of developing many of these age-related diseases.

People often keep many of the habits they develop in their youth. Therefore, your lifestyle choices today will influence your physical and mental fitness in the future as well as right now. Of course, you can always improve your habits and lifestyle during adulthood, and many adults do.

Lesson 22.1 Review

Know and Understand

1. List the six developmental stages in the human life cycle.

2. What are the four types of human development? Give an example of how these are related and interdependent.

3. What is the difference between an Individualized Family Service Plan (IFSP) and an Individualized Education Plan (IEP)?

4. Explain how genes direct and influence human development.

5. List four lifestyle choices that could affect a person's life span.

6. As a person ages, does he become more or less able to fight off and recover from diseases?

Analyze and Apply

7. Compare growth and development.

8. Explain the difference between life expectancy and life span.

Real World Health

The average life expectancy in the United States is 78 years of age. Search the Internet for two or three life expectancy calculators. Use these calculation tools to determine your projected life expectancy based on your genetics, lifestyle, and environment. Are you satisfied with the life expectancy you were given? Write a description of what you can do throughout your life, especially now, to extend your life expectancy. Share your thoughts with a partner.

Infancy through the Preschool Years

Lesson Objectives

After studying this lesson, you will be able to

- describe the physical development that occurs during early childhood;
- explain the development of gross- and fine-motor skills during early childhood;
- analyze children's intellectual development during early childhood; and
- describe emotional and social growth and development during early childhood.

Warm-Up Activity

Growing Like a Weed

When friends or relatives haven't seen an infant or preschooler for a long time, they are often amazed by the child's physical development and may say that he or she is "growing like a weed." Based on what you already know about early child development, what physical changes do you think infants and preschoolers undergo? Working with a partner, brainstorm a list of changes, then compare your list with your classmates' lists.

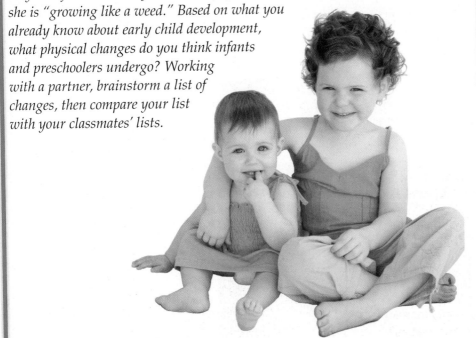

Key Terms E-Flash Cards

In this lesson, you will learn the meanings of the following key terms.

attachment
autonomy
fine-motor skills
gross-motor skills
motor development
object permanence
receptive language
separation anxiety
stranger anxiety
temper tantrum

Before You Read

Give One, Get One

Create a chart like the one shown here. In the "Give One" column, list what you already know about the topics discussed in this lesson. Then, as you read the lesson, list any new information you learn in the "Get One" column.

Give One (information you already know)	Get One (new information)

The first months of a person's life are characterized by dramatic adaptations to life outside the mother's body. Infants learn many new skills as they grow to become toddlers who are always on the move. Toddlers make great developmental strides as they grow into engaging and curious preschoolers. During the preschool years, children immerse themselves in life, soaking up everything they encounter, learning and growing faster than ever before.

In this lesson you will learn about the physical, intellectual, emotional, and social growth and development that occurs during these magical years of early childhood.

Physical Development

Physical changes seem to dominate the first months of infancy. During the first year of life, many babies triple their weight and grow about 12 inches in length. After babies reach their first birthday, their growth continues, but at a slower rate (Figure 22.3A).

Toddlers begin to leave their baby shapes and body proportions behind after reaching two years of age. They continue to lose baby fat and, as a result, their round faces and chubby legs. By the time children reach the preschool years, their bodies appear leaner, stronger, and taller.

Motor development refers to increased coordination and strength of muscles. Throughout early childhood, children grow increasingly strong and coordinated, relying less on reflex and more on purposeful, directed movements. Gross- and fine-motor skills develop quickly. **Gross-motor skills** involve

motor development
the increase in a person's coordination and strength of muscles

gross-motor skills
movements that use large muscles

Figure 22.3

From lying on their stomachs (A) to crawling (B) and walking (C), the first eighteen months of a baby's life are characterized by rapid physical development. *Why do you think babies develop so rapidly? Is there any other period in a person's life that is marked by this much change?*

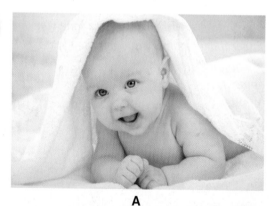
A

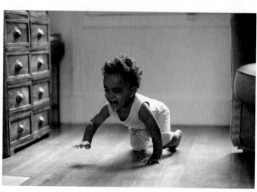
B

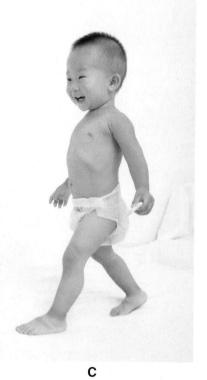
C

movements that use the large muscles of the body. *Fine-motor skills* involve movements that use the body's small muscles.

fine-motor skills
movements that use small muscles

Gross-Motor Skills

Children achieve many developmental milestones as their gross-motor skills improve. By their first birthday, most babies are able to roll over, sit up, crawl, and even grasp furniture or other objects to pull themselves up to a standing position (Figure 22.3B). As children enter the toddler years, they achieve a major developmental milestone, which involves taking their first steps and walking (Figure 22.3C).

Toddlers progress rapidly from walking to fairly complex movements. Motor milestones during the toddler years include the ability to run, kick and direct a ball, walk up and down steps alone while holding a railing or wall, sit in a chair, and stand on one leg.

By the time children enter the preschool years, their upper body and arm strength and greater coordination allow movements to become more refined and efficient. Improved strength and coordination also leads to the development of new skills. Preschoolers can run well, hop, and stand on one foot for a short time. They easily get around the house with no help, even up and down stairs. They can use their large muscles to throw, kick, and catch a ball. Physical coordination improves so much during this time that children can accurately imitate many adult movements by the end of the preschool years.

Fine-Motor Skills

Infants spend a lot of time playing with their hands to learn how they work and to develop dexterity and strength. As the months progress, hand coordination increases dramatically. By 12 months of age, children can grasp small objects with their index finger and thumb. This development of the *pincer grasp* is a sign that children are developing precise, refined muscle movements and coordination.

As small muscles continue to develop, eye-hand coordination improves (Figure 22.4). Toddlers become better at feeding themselves as they learn to hold cups and spoons. Toddlers also learn to string large beads, turn pages of books, and hold a crayon. Children may show a preference for their right or left hand as they become involved in more activities.

Fine-motor skills continue to improve during early childhood, which enables preschool children to do many activities that toddlers cannot. Preschoolers can use the small muscles of their hands to copy simple figures, draw some letters, and use child-size scissors. Preschool children are better able to dress and feed themselves than toddlers, although they may need occasional help from their caregivers.

Intellectual Development

During infancy, children rely heavily on touch, sight, sounds, and even taste to learn about the world.

Figure 22.4

As their smaller muscles grow and develop, toddlers practice and improve their fine-motor skills and coordination. These skills allow them to grasp objects and feed themselves. *What are some examples of fine-motor skills you use every day?*

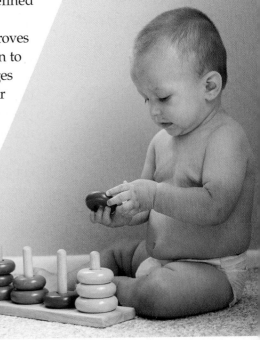

Infants show signs that they understand and think about what is happening around them. This is partly the result of a greater attention span and memory developing.

Toddlers and preschoolers build on these skills and learn many more important concepts as they grow. Language development also improves significantly during early childhood.

Concepts Learned

Infants enjoy shaking rattles, pushing toy cars, or repeatedly dropping stuffed animals out of their cribs. Through these actions, infants are learning the very important concept of *cause and effect*. Children are realizing that their actions result in reactions and changes in their environment.

As children approach the toddler years, their ability to sustain attention improves. Infants often play with a toy for only a couple of minutes, but toddlers can focus their attention on an interesting toy for a much longer period of time. Another milestone that occurs during the toddler years is development of the idea of **object permanence**. This is achieved when children understand that their world, and the objects and people in it, continues to exist even when they do not see it.

object permanence
the idea that objects and people are present even when they cannot be seen

By the preschool years, children develop keen *classification* skills, which enable them to sort toys and other objects by size, shape, and color. Preschoolers develop an understanding of time after experience with daily and weekly routines. By five years of age, many children can count and recognize differences in amounts and sizes. They can also recognize and assemble patterns using numbers, shapes, colors, and letters.

Language Development

receptive language
term for the understanding and processing of speech

Understanding and processing speech is called **receptive language**. During early childhood, language evolves from crying and cooing, to babbling and imitating sounds and words, to putting together simple sentences. Children begin speaking at various ages. Some children will say their first recognizable words by the end of infancy, while others may not speak until they are toddlers. Even though children may not be speaking, they often know the names of many objects and people and can understand many phrases. When children do say their first words, they have reached a major developmental milestone.

Throughout the toddler years, children's verbal communication skills expand as they add new vocabulary and more expressiveness. Toddlers often imitate the words and speech patterns of their caregivers and older children in their family. Simply by listening and talking to others, toddlers absorb many rules of grammar before entering preschool.

Preschoolers make considerable progress with their grammar, vocabulary, and pronunciation. Preschoolers can use language to describe objects as being the same or different. They can also tell stories and recall the main parts of stories they have heard or read with their caregivers. Other language milestones reflect cognitive milestones that continue to occur.

Emotional and Social Development

During infancy, children rely on their parents, caregivers, and other family members to meet their needs. As children grow and develop, they become more independent and learn more about themselves and others. Children require positive interactions with their caregivers and others to achieve healthy emotional and social development.

Interactions with Caregivers

Infants quickly become familiar with the comforting sights, sounds, and smells of their parents and caregivers. As caregivers respond promptly to an infant's smiling, crying, or other attempts to communicate, they reassure the baby that he or she is safe and loved. As a result, infants form a strong *attachment*, or emotional connection to their caregivers (Figure 22.5).

Around one year of age, children may become upset, shy, or afraid around unfamiliar people and in new situations. This is a normal developmental milestone called *stranger anxiety*. Caregivers can help children with stranger anxiety by gradually and patiently introducing them to new people and places.

Young children may also develop *separation anxiety*, meaning they become upset when they are away from their caregivers. Without a good understanding of time, children do not know how long these important people will be gone. Separation anxiety is normal and usually stops when a child is between two and three years of age.

The phrase *terrible twos* is often used to describe toddlers' behavior between two and three years of age. This age is characterized by the toddler alternating between displays of *autonomy* (self-directing freedom) and independence, and clinging, dependent behavior. Toddlers often react with frustration and anger—including yelling, crying, hitting, biting, or kicking—when they are prevented from doing what they want. This is called a *temper tantrum* (Figure 22.6). These reactions are normal and are simply the way toddlers test limits. Caregivers need to define limits and teach toddlers which behaviors (hitting, for example) are unacceptable. Toddlers will eventually learn these limits.

During the preschool years, children are more engaged with adults and seek to please others, especially parents, caregivers, family members, familiar adults, and friends. Preschoolers also begin to develop empathy. *Empathy* is a sense of how another person may be feeling. This is an emotional milestone because it prepares children to form healthy, close relationships, which are a cornerstone of social interaction.

attachment
an emotional connection, especially between a baby and his or her caregiver

stranger anxiety
fear of unfamiliar people or situations

separation anxiety
fear of being away from caregivers

autonomy
the freedom to direct one's self, independent of other influences

temper tantrum
a frustrated or angry reaction that includes crying, yelling, or mild physical violence

Figure 22.5

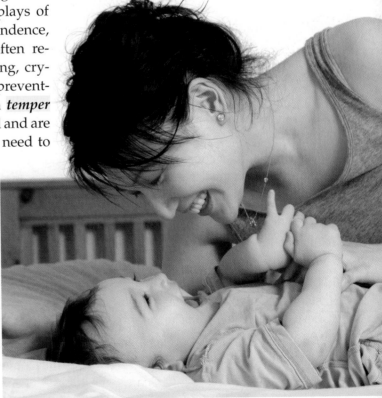

Babies develop an attachment to their caregivers when their caregivers respond promptly and positively to their needs. *Why is it important for babies and caregivers to form an emotional connection?*

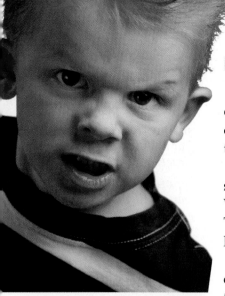

When toddlers throw temper tantrums, they often test their caregivers' patience. *What are some healthy ways a caregiver can deal with a toddler's temper tantrum?*

Interactions with Others

Toddlers enjoy watching other children play and like playing near other children. This type of play is called *parallel play* because it is neither cooperative nor interactive. Toddlers do not easily share toys, especially their favorite ones.

Because toddlers cannot understand empathy yet, they do not understand that they can hurt another child's feelings when fighting over toys. While this behavior may seem selfish, it is perfectly normal and common. Toddlers need guidance and occasional intervention from caregivers to learn how to handle friction and conflict with others.

When playing with other children, preschoolers move beyond the self-centered behavior of the toddler stage and engage in *cooperative play* rather than parallel play. Because preschoolers realize that others have feelings, they learn to cooperate, communicate, trade, and share when playing. Conflicts with other children occur less frequently. Children this age are forming their first friendships.

Preschool children have an active imagination with which they create imaginary, fantasy worlds. In this way, they play roles, express emotions, and try ideas to see how they work.

Many children create imaginary friends at this age. This type of play should be encouraged because it stimulates preschoolers' emotional growth and development. It is also normal for preschoolers to occasionally confuse their imaginary and real worlds. They can be confused and frightened by scary stories and movies. By the end of the preschool years, however, children are better able to tell the difference between fantasy from reality.

Lesson 22.2 Review

Know and Understand Assess

1. Explain the difference between gross- and fine-motor skills.

2. List two important concepts children learn during infancy and the toddler years.

3. Explain the importance of receptive language.

4. When do children typically experience stranger anxiety?

5. What does the term *autonomy* mean?

6. Do children develop empathy at the toddler stage or the preschooler stage? Why is the development of empathy important?

7. What is the difference between parallel play and cooperative play?

Analyze and Apply

8. Compare stranger anxiety and separation anxiety.

9. Explain how toddlers begin to display their autonomy and independence.

Real World Health

Most children love to have stories read to them. Reading to children teaches them about language and prepares them to read on their own. Choose a children's book and write a few paragraphs explaining why you chose that book, what age group the book is appropriate for, and why the book would fit that age group. Read the book to a small group of classmates and ask them to explain what age group the book is for and why. Take notes and add their comments to your written description.

Lesson 22.3

The School-Age and Adolescent Years

Lesson Objectives

After studying this lesson, you will be able to

- summarize the physical, intellectual, emotional, and social growth and development that occurs during the school-age years;

- compare the physical changes that occur in males and females during puberty;

- describe the intellectual, emotional, and social growth and development that occurs during adolescence; and

- identify common adolescent health and wellness issues.

Warm-Up Activity

Adolescent Changes

On a separate sheet of paper, create two columns and label them Male Changes *and* Female Changes. *Under each heading, brainstorm and list all of the physical, emotional, intellectual, and social changes associated with becoming an adolescent for that gender. Write a few paragraphs to compare and contrast the items on the two lists.*

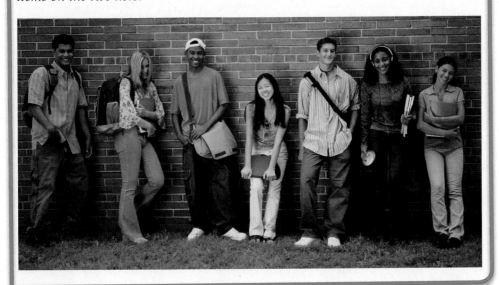

Key Terms E-Flash Cards

In this lesson, you will learn the meanings of the following key terms.

nocturnal emissions
primary sexual characteristics
puberty
secondary sexual characteristics

Before You Read

Linking Ideas
Your teacher will write the main headings in this lesson on chalkboards or dry-erase boards around the room. You will be asked to visit each board and briefly write what you know, or think you know, about each lesson heading without talking to your fellow classmates. You may comment on or add to other students' ideas and draw a line between your comment and theirs. After reading the lesson, go back around the room and add any new information you have learned under each lesson heading. Again, you may comment on or add to other students' ideas.

The school-age years are marked by gradual physical growth and maturation. Much intellectual, emotional, and social development also take place when children are between 5 and 12 years of age. Each year marks a single small step toward adolescence, which then brings the swift, dramatic changes that prepare children for adulthood.

In this lesson you will learn about the many ways in which children grow and develop as they progress toward becoming adults.

The School-Age Years

Most communities require children to begin school at a certain time, usually when children are five or six years of age. At this time, differences in children's development often become much clearer. Rates of development continue to vary throughout the school-age years and into adolescence. During these years, important physical, intellectual, emotional, and social growth and development take place.

Physical Development

"Slow and steady" describes children's growth during the school-age years. By the end of the school-age years, growth may alternate between periods of quick development and slow change. This is why the height and weight of children who are the same age can be very different, which is normal and expected (Figure 22.7).

Too many calories and not enough physical activity, however, can cause school-age children to become overweight or obese at an early age. Children who become overweight or obese often have a difficult time losing weight as they mature. Establishing healthful eating and physical

Figure 22.7

During the school-age years, children undergo periods of rapid development and periods of gradual change. Children in this age range vary dramatically in height and weight, though girls are usually taller than boys.

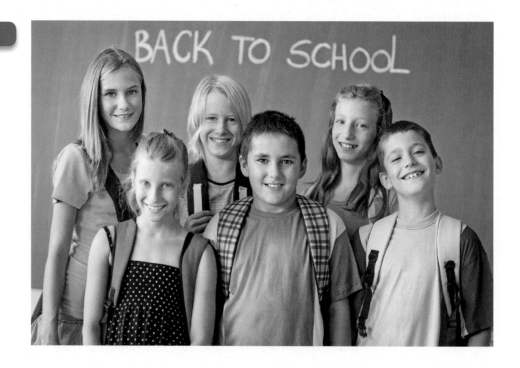

activity habits can help children maintain a healthy weight as they continue to grow and develop.

Being physically active also helps children improve their motor skills and increase flexibility and coordination. Children develop newfound interests as they engage in more physical activities. Many school-age children enjoy playing organized sports, such as baseball or soccer. Children who are active develop muscle strength and coordination faster than children who are less active.

Intellectual Development

Children encounter many new learning opportunities when they begin going to school. A greater emphasis on schoolwork and homework assignments increases language and problem-solving skills. School-age children become logical thinkers based on their previous experiences. They apply knowledge they have gained in the past to solve current problems.

During the school-age years, children think about their world in a concrete way. This means they think about the present and generally do not think about the future. School-age children cannot link today's actions to future effects. They have not yet developed the skill of planning ahead beyond the day because they are unable to think abstractly.

Most children do not view the world abstractly until the later years of adolescence. In addition, children generally think about issues as black or white, right or wrong, and good or bad. School-age children seek answers that are simple and straightforward, and do not see the complexity of problems very easily.

Emotional and Social Development

School-age children discover an expanding social network and begin learning about friendship. These years are characterized by the development of friendships and other relationships outside the family. Children make friends and learn how to be a good friend. During these years, children spend more time with others after school, on weekends, and during school vacations.

During the school-age years, children also develop their *self-esteem*, which is a sense of worth, purpose, security, and confidence. Healthy self-esteem develops with supportive family and friends, and with accomplishment and experience. Children can build their self-esteem as they successfully deal with mistakes, accomplish tough assignments at school, handle arguments with friends, and adapt to changes at home.

The Adolescent Years

A child's body and mind transform during the adolescent years. No longer children, but not yet adults, adolescents undergo changes that prepare their minds and bodies for adulthood. On their way to adulthood, adolescents experience many physical, intellectual, emotional, and social

primary sexual characteristics
physical features directly involved in sexual reproduction

secondary sexual characteristics
physical features that correspond with sexual development but are not directly involved in reproduction

puberty
the period during which levels of sex hormones increase and primary and secondary sexual characteristics develop

nocturnal emissions
ejaculations of semen while sleeping

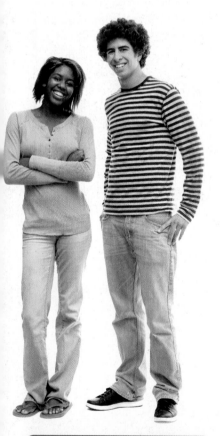

During adolescence, teenagers develop primary and secondary sex characteristics.

changes. These changes begin with puberty, when the reproductive system starts to mature.

Physical Development and Puberty

Physical changes are the trademark of adolescence. People complete most of their physical growth during adolescence, achieving their adult height and weight. The primary and secondary sexual characteristics also mature at this age (Figure 22.8). ***Primary sexual characteristics*** are the sex organs. In males, the primary sexual characteristics are the penis and testes. The female's primary sexual characteristics are the ovaries and vagina. ***Secondary sexual characteristics*** are other features that appear during puberty, such as body hair, a deep voice, or breast development.

Sex hormones drive the physical and emotional changes of **puberty**. Before puberty occurs, sex hormones are present at lower levels. Puberty is triggered when brain hormones affect the testes in males and the ovaries in females.

In males, testosterone triggers growth and development of the testes, penis, and other sexual characteristics. The testes respond by increasing the secretion of testosterone. In females, estrogen triggers growth and development of the ovaries, breasts, and other sexual characteristics. The ovaries respond by producing higher amounts of estrogen.

Puberty in Males. Puberty begins in males around 10 to 16 years of age with enlargement of the *testes*, the organs that produce sperm and testosterone. During puberty, males grow taller and gain weight quickly. Their growth rate may even double and males can grow 4 inches in one year. By the time puberty ends, a male may have grown 14 inches and gained 40 pounds. The male's secondary sexual characteristics that appear during puberty include pubic, facial, and body hair; deep voice; broad shoulders; and muscle mass.

During puberty, males also experience other changes, such as increased oil production on the skin and scalp. This extra oil can lead to acne on the face, shoulders, and chest. Sometimes males experience swelling in their breasts, a development that is normal and usually subsides as adolescence continues. Males experience erections and sexual excitement during puberty. They might also have ***nocturnal emissions***, which are the ejaculation of semen during the night while sleeping. Along with these physical changes, males become curious about sex and they may feel sexually attracted to another person.

Puberty in Females. Females begin puberty earlier than males. The first sign of puberty in females is breast development, which occurs around 8 to 14 years of age. During puberty, a female's body grows quickly, up to 3 inches per year. By the end of puberty, a female may have grown 10 inches and gained 25 pounds. In females, the secondary sexual characteristics include breast development, pubic and underarm hair, wide hips, and fat at the hips and buttocks.

During puberty, females also begin menstruating. The *menarche*, or first menstrual period, may be upsetting to a young female. Parents or a doctor can help the female understand what menstruation means and how to pre-pare for this monthly cycle. Like males, females experience increased oil secretion on the skin and scalp, so they may also develop acne. With these physical changes, females also grow curious about sex and may experience sexual attraction.

Intellectual Development

During adolescence, the brain is still developing and many changes in intellectual development occur. Young adolescents still think in con-crete terms, as they did in childhood. They often view the world in simple terms—black and white, with few shades of gray. They may fail to see the complexity of many situations and are unable to imagine future conse-quences that could arise from their actions. As a result, younger adoles-cents may act without thinking and take risks.

Research in Action

The Adolescent Brain

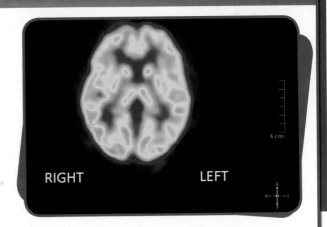

RIGHT   LEFT

Teenagers are known to be impulsive and emotional, and these traits are linked to risky behavior that can range from reckless driving to illegal drug use, or even sexual activity. Neuroscientists who study how the brain works have found that the adolescent brain is different from the adult brain. These differences may explain why many adolescents take the risks they do.

Brain activity can be studied using scans called *MRIs* and *PET*. These scans reveal the structure of the brain and pinpoint which areas are active and which are inactive under different conditions. For example, these scans can show which part of the brain is working while a person reads, listens to music, or speaks.

Scans of adolescent brains reveal that their brains are still immature and are not fully developed. On closer examination, scientists note that two specific parts of the brain develop at different rates. One part is the *amygdala*, a small structure deep in the brain that is responsible for emotions, aggressive behavior, and instinctual, emotional reflexes. The amygdala matures fairly early and is well-developed in adolescents.

The second part of interest is the *prefrontal cortex*, a region near the forehead. This area of the brain regulates attention, impulses, and abstract thinking. The prefrontal cortex allows for planning and for predicting consequences. The prefrontal

cortex, which also regulates the amygdala, has not yet developed in the adolescent brain.

Because the amygdala matures earlier than the prefrontal cortex, the adolescent brain is strongly influenced by emotion and impulsiveness without any regulation. This explains the risk-taking, impulsive behavior observed in adolescents.

Thinking Critically

1. What are some examples of adolescent behavior that is risky and impulsive?

2. Since the adolescent brain is not fully developed, does this mean that teenagers are not responsible for their impulsive behavior? Why or why not?

3. What role do a teenager's friends play in his or her risky behavior?

As adolescents mature, however, they develop the ability to think more abstractly and see the complexity of issues. This permits them to handle more challenging situations. Even older adolescents, however, may occasionally fail to predict the consequences of their actions and still take risks.

Intellectual development can be a stimulating part of adolescent life. The ability to comprehend concepts and ideas develops during adolescence. This means that adolescents develop the ability to think about abstract concepts apart from the concrete, real matters of daily life.

Emotional and Social Development

Adolescents feel the need to establish their independence, to be on their own, and to rely on their own judgment. School activities, friends, and work offer plenty of opportunities for adolescents to gain independence. This independent time for making decisions and exploring life is important for adolescents' emotional growth.

Some adolescents emphasize their independence by distancing themselves from their parents. Adolescents might not be as affectionate as they were in childhood, which can be upsetting to parents. They might talk less about their day at school to maintain privacy and to remind their parents of their independence.

The social world of the adolescent expands beyond family and close friends and becomes increasingly important to them. Adolescents' relationships will include new friends, friends of the opposite sex, boyfriends or girlfriends, teachers, and coaches. As their social life grows, adolescents get a taste of what adult life is like (Figure 22.9).

Adolescents are typically concerned about being accepted by their peers. They may seek their peers' approval and try to fit into a peer group. Peers can be a source of support and fun. Unfortunately, adolescents can also be negatively influenced by peers, which may cause them to engage in behaviors they might not otherwise choose.

Figure 22.9

Because of their expanding social worlds, teenagers experience both the benefits and challenges of relationships. Learning to manage their social worlds helps prepare teenagers for their adult lives. *What challenges and benefits have you experienced as your social world expands?*

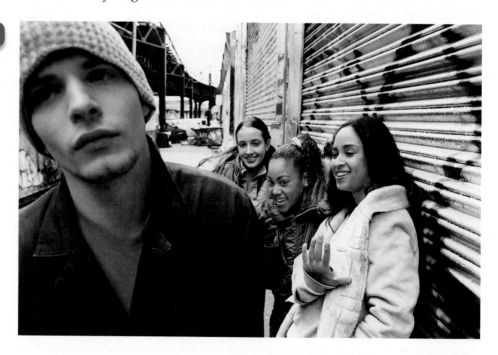

Healthy Adolescence

Strategies that can help you understand healthy adolescent development include the following:

- Learn where to find reliable information about adolescence.

- Understand the physical changes that occur during puberty.

- Understand the intellectual, emotional, and social changes that occur during adolescence.

- Develop methods for handling peer pressure regarding smoking, drinking, drugs, and sex.

- Learn about the harmful effects of tobacco, alcohol, and drugs on the body.

- Practice good communication skills with parents and other trusted adults.

- Learn how to manage your time so that you can balance school, work, athletics, and recreation.

- Develop and maintain healthy friendships and relationships with family.

- Learn about sexuality and human reproduction so you can remain healthy and avoid pregnancy.

Health and Wellness Issues

Adolescents face health and wellness issues that are not common in childhood and are not usually associated with adulthood. Some of these issues arise because of newly acquired independence, such as the ability to drive. Other health and wellness issues come with new pressures from peers to engage in risky behaviors. Their developing brain also makes adolescents vulnerable to risk-taking behavior, which can cause health and wellness issues.

Important health and wellness concerns that may affect adolescents include injuries, overweight and obesity, substance abuse, reproductive health, mental illness and suicide, and homicide, all of which you have studied throughout this text.

Lesson 22.3 Review

Know and Understand Assess

1. Why is it important for children to establish healthful eating and physical activity habits during the school-age years?

2. Do school-age children think in abstract or concrete terms? Explain your answer.

3. What are the primary sexual characteristics of males and females?

4. Explain the difference between primary and secondary sexual characteristics.

5. List three health and wellness concerns that may affect adolescents.

Analyze and Apply

6. Explain how children can develop healthy self-esteem during the school-age years.

7. Explain how personal relationships with friends and family might change during adolescence.

Real World (Health

Some cultures and religious groups celebrate a young person's entrance into adulthood with a ceremony or ritual. Use the Internet to research coming-of-age ceremonies and rituals and choose one that interests you. Write about your chosen tradition and answer the following questions: At what age do young people come of age in this tradition? What occurs during the ritual or ceremony you have chosen? How do aspects of the ritual or ceremony symbolize the transition from childhood to adulthood? After coming of age, what new rights and responsibilities do the young people have? Develop a presentation that summarizes your findings and present it to the class.

Adulthood and the Nature of Aging

Key Terms 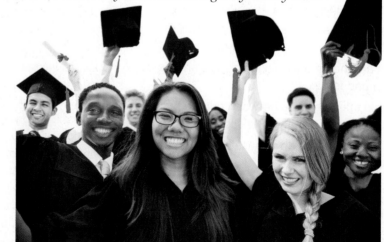 E-Flash Cards

In this lesson, you will learn the meanings of the following key terms.

dementia

incontinence

middle adulthood

older adulthood

sandwich generation

young adulthood

Before You Read

3, 2, 1

As you read this lesson, take notes about facts you discover, concepts you find interesting, and information you still question. After you have finished reading, fill in a chart like the one shown here with three of the facts you discovered, two of the concepts you found interesting, and one piece of information you still question.

3 facts I discovered	1. 2. 3.
2 concepts I find interesting	1. 2.
1 piece of information I still question	1.

Lesson Objectives

After studying this lesson, you will be able to

- assess various definitions of adulthood;
- identify and describe the stages of adulthood;
- summarize health changes that occur in the sensory organs and body systems during adulthood; and
- describe how people can adapt to the changes that occur during aging.

Warm-Up Activity

When Does Adulthood Begin?

In the United States today, the transition from childhood to adulthood is not clearly defined. How do you define adulthood and know when you've reached it? Are there events and milestones, such as high school graduation, that mark a person's passage into adulthood? When does a person become an adult according to the government and the legal system? What rights and responsibilities are given to people once they become adults? What does your family expect from you once you reach adulthood? Do all people reach adulthood at the same age? Write a paragraph that answers these questions. Once you have read this lesson, revisit your answers and add any additional thoughts you may have.

How do you know when you have become an adult? Do you become an adult when you reach a certain age—18 or 21, for example? Does a particular event such as getting a driver's license, graduating from high school or college, or getting married make you an adult? Do you become an adult when your body is fully developed and capable of reproduction?

In this lesson you will learn about adulthood and what to expect as you grow older. Some health changes that occur in adulthood are inevitable, but others can be avoided by making healthful choices today and throughout life.

The Mature Adult

Adulthood is defined in various ways. In the United States, state and federal governments recognize that most people experience the milestones of adulthood when they reach 18 years of age (Figure 22.10). Therefore, in most states, people are able to vote, purchase tobacco products, and marry without their parents' permission once they reach 18 years of age. When a person turns 18, he or she can also be treated as an adult in a court of law. People are unable to purchase alcohol until they reach 21 years of age.

Another definition of adulthood is based on the physical maturity of the body. The young adult's brain and body have reached physical maturity and peak function. Young adults have achieved their mature height and weight, possess their greatest physical strength and endurance, and enjoy their sharpest cognitive ability.

Many teenagers have developed mature reproductive systems and are physically able to create and have children. Adolescents must mature in many other ways, however, to be considered adults. Perhaps most importantly, adolescents must still achieve emotional and cognitive maturity. What are the indicators of maturity? People who are emotionally and cognitively mature possess the skills they need to

- plan ahead;
- make good, informed decisions regarding their own welfare;
- consider the impact of decisions on other people and events;
- communicate their feelings; and
- maintain healthy friendships and relationships.

Stages of Adulthood

Adults continue to change and develop through various stages of adulthood. *Young adulthood* occurs from 20 to 40 years of age, *middle adulthood* (*middle age*) occurs from 40 to

young adulthood
a stage of adulthood that occurs from 20 to 40 years of age

middle adulthood
a stage of adulthood that occurs from 40 to 65 years of age

Figure 22.10

Although teenagers can get their driver's license when they are 16, the age of adulthood is 18. At 18 years of age, teenagers can vote, be treated as adults in court, and make independent decisions regarding marriage and money.

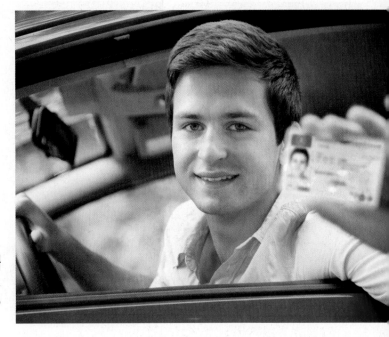

65 years of age, and **older adulthood** is considered 65 years of age and older. Adults in each stage share many experiences, rewards, and challenges.

Young Adulthood

People achieve full physical maturity during young adulthood. Adults who are 20 to 40 years of age possess their greatest strength, endurance, and cognitive abilities. Their sensory organs and reflexes have reached peak performance. As a group, young adults are healthy and active.

In the United States, young adults are expected to be fully responsible for their lives, which means having a job and living independently. There is no "typical" young adult in the United States. Young adults may be single, married, or divorced, and not all young adults have children. Some live alone or with their parents, and some live with other young adults.

Marriage and divorce are major life-changing events for young adults. In the United States, the age of marriage has risen steadily. Today, many adults are not married, and those adults who do marry wait until they are older and more mature. Statistics show that many men typically wait to marry until they are at least 29 years of age, while many women wait until they are 27 years of age.

Divorce can occur during any stage of adulthood. About one-half of marriages end in divorce. A divorce alters many aspects of a person's life, including income, living arrangements, and home ownership. Divorce also causes relationships with children, extended family members, and friends to change. Unmarried young adults in long-term relationships may experience break-ups that can be as difficult as a divorce.

Middle Adulthood

In the United States, adults who are 40 to 65 years of age tend to be fairly healthy (Figure 22.11). As a group, middle-aged adults remain active,

Figure 22.11

During middle adulthood, people remain fairly healthy but begin to experience declines in coordination, vision, and hearing. *Think of the people you know who are between 40 and 65 years of age. What challenges do they face?*

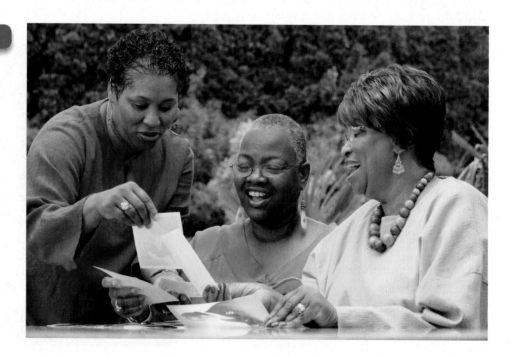

but their physical strength, coordination, and endurance gradually decline over time. Their reflexes slow, but their thinking skills and memory remain intact. Some loss of hearing and vision occurs during middle adulthood.

Middle-aged adults may have adolescent or adult children. This may cause financial and emotional stress. Middle-aged adults often have increased work responsibilities at about the same time that they have increased family demands.

One such family demand may involve caring for aging parents who need medical and financial help. This is a difficult burden for adults, especially those who also have children. Adults who care for their parents as well as their own children are called the *sandwich generation*. In recent years, the population of older adults has increased and more middle-aged adults—and some younger adults—are finding themselves caring for aging parents. Balancing personal and professional responsibilities can be a source of stress for middle-aged adults.

Older Adulthood

Advancing age brings joy and new life, as well as loss and grief. When older adults retire from work, they find time to start new jobs, pursue hobbies and interests, and make new friends. Older adults may enjoy the company of grandchildren and begin new relationships with their own adult children. However, older adults also experience declining health and independence, reduced income, and loss of friends and family.

After retirement, older adults need to maintain a social life, feel productive, and remain active, especially if they have lost their spouse and live alone. Retired adults can fulfill these needs by working part-time jobs; volunteering at schools, hospitals, or museums; or taking courses at local community colleges.

Health Changes during Adulthood

What can you expect to experience as your body ages? Obvious signs of aging include wrinkled skin, slower movement, and vision and hearing loss. A number of changes are expected during aging, but these changes are not necessarily diseases or disorders. It is normal for many body functions to decline as the body grows older (Figure 22.12).

Sensory Organ Changes

Skin is the largest sensory organ in the body, and it shows the first outward, obvious signs of aging. The development of wrinkles, age spots, and skin tags is a good example of this. Age spots are flat, brown spots on areas

sandwich generation
term that describes adults who care for their parents as well as their children

As adults age, they may experience wrinkled skin, slower movements, and other physical setbacks. They may rely more on help from people younger than them. *What physical changes have you seen older adults experience?*

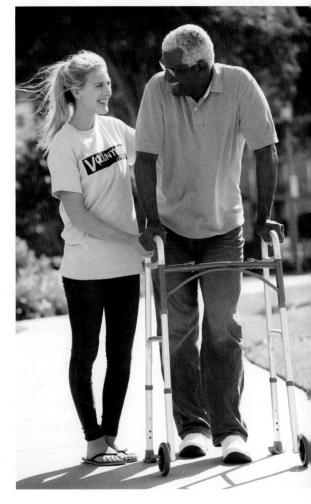

of exposed skin. Skin tags are small, raised growths of skin on the face, eyelids, neck, and elsewhere.

Other changes in the sensory organs occur so gradually that many people do not notice them until several years have passed. In middle age, vision-related changes often make it more difficult for people to focus on close objects or read small print. Hearing loss is also a common health problem as adults get older. Older adults may have difficulty hearing the TV or radio, and they may not hear the phone ring.

Certain medications can alter a person's ability to taste and smell food. Loss of these senses causes some people to lose their appetite, which can cause weight loss and malnutrition. Others may develop a preference for unhealthy foods that are high in salt or fat. People can handle this problem by adding pepper, seasoning, spices, or herbs to food to improve flavor without adding calories from salt and fat.

Body System Changes

Changes in the sensory organs and skin are easy to notice. Aging also affects other organs and areas of the body in ways that cannot easily be seen. These changes typically occur within the body systems.

The Digestive System. Aging affects all parts of the digestive system, from the mouth to the large intestine. Less saliva is produced as people age, which causes dry mouth. This means that bacteria do not get washed from the mouth. As a result, older adults are at risk for developing cavities and inflammation of the gums, known as *gingivitis*.

The lining of the intestines thins as people grow older, which slows digestion and absorption. The muscles in the intestinal walls act more slowly, causing waste, known as *feces*, to remain in the intestine longer. This dries the feces and makes it difficult to pass waste, a problem called *constipation*.

Liver function also declines with age. Because medications and toxins are normally made inactive by the liver, older adults with declining livers are more sensitive to a dose of medication. Older adults are also more likely to experience side effects of certain medications (Figure 22.13). The liver makes clotting factors that stimulate blood clotting to control blood loss. Since those clotting factors may not be as abundant, older adults can lose a lot of blood from minor injuries.

The Urinary System. With age, the kidneys become less efficient filters and excrete too much water from the body. Loss of extra water puts older adults at risk for dehydration. The muscles controlling urination also weaken with age. This causes **incontinence,** or the inability to prevent urination when urine accumulates in the bladder.

In addition, the muscle of the urinary bladder weakens, so the bladder does not completely empty anymore. Urine does not thoroughly wash bacteria from the bladder and urethra, which can lead to urinary tract infections. Older adults should drink plenty of fluids to stay hydrated (Figure 22.14).

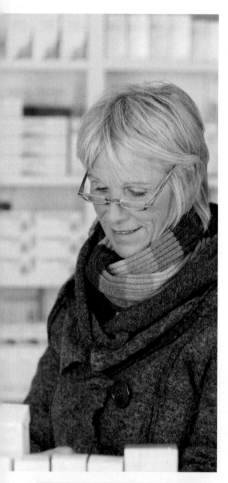

Figure 22.13

As people age, they are more likely to need various medications. Unfortunately, this increased need coincides with their body's declining ability to metabolize medicines.

incontinence
the inability to prevent urination when urine accumulates in the bladder

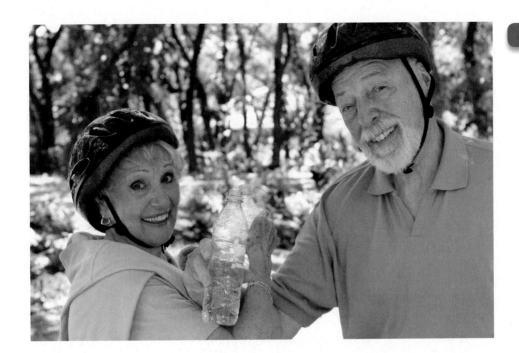

Figure 22.14

Older adults should make sure to drink plenty of fluids to prevent dehydration and urinary problems. *How might staying well-hydrated prevent urinary problems?*

The Cardiovascular System. Blood vessels stiffen and narrow with age, causing high blood pressure, or *hypertension*. Smoking, high-fat diets, and inactive lifestyles speed up the hardening and narrowing of blood vessels, which puts pressure on the heart muscle. This means older hearts are weaker than younger hearts and circulate blood less efficiently. Cardiovascular aging means older adults are at an increased risk for heart disease.

The Respiratory System. The respiratory system works with the cardiovascular system to obtain oxygen and deliver it to the blood. The ability to do so decreases with age as the chest and rib muscles become less flexible and the lungs become less elastic. Therefore, older adults get tired more easily and run out of breath sooner than younger adults.

The membrane that lines the respiratory system also thins with age. The respiratory membrane produces less mucus and does not protect from bacteria as well as before. That is why older adults have an increased risk for lung infections, such as influenza and pneumonia.

The Reproductive System. Women typically begin menopause in their late 40s to middle 50s. During menopause, egg production and menstruation stop because estrogen levels drop. Men's hormones decline too, but not as rapidly as estrogen does in women.

The *prostate* is a walnut-sized organ that surrounds the urethra below the urinary bladder. Sometimes the prostate begins enlarging in middle age. This enlargement is common and usually is not due to prostate cancer. An enlarged prostate blocks urine flow, making it difficult to urinate. This causes men to have a greater chance of developing urinary infections.

Muscles and Bones. Muscles lose mass and strength with age, especially when they are not regularly exercised. These changes cause older adults to become tired more quickly than younger people. Additionally, bones lose strength, mass, and density with age. As bones become more fragile, older adults become susceptible to fractures.

The skeleton consists of bones that are held together at joints. Some joints, such as the shoulder, elbow, and knee, are held together by strong bands of tissue called *ligaments*. *Cartilage* is a spongy pad that covers the surfaces of bones that meet at many joints. Both ligaments and cartilage wear with age, making joints stiff and sometimes painful. *Arthritis*, or inflammation of the joints, is a common condition among older adults.

The Nervous System. The most noticeable nervous system changes occur in the brain and spinal cord. Memory may slip up more often with age, but it usually remains intact unless a person develops **dementia,** which is a condition of mental deterioration. Reflex and reaction time slow as people get older, reflecting an aging spinal cord and nerves. Major changes in personality or language are signs of a nervous system disorder, including dementia.

dementia
a condition of mental deterioration

Adaptations to Aging

By adapting to the changes caused by aging, adults can maintain an active, healthy life. Adaptations include technologies that compensate for reduced abilities. Hearing aids and telephone amplification devices assist older adults with impaired hearing. Eyeglasses with extra lenses, called *bifocals*, improve reading. Large print books and larger fonts on computer monitors make reading easier for older adults.

Older adults can also adapt to reduced mobility, strength, and balance. Canes, wheelchairs, and other assistive devices enable adults to remain mobile. At home, ramps can replace steps, which may be difficult to climb. Physically disabled adults can share car rides with friends and family or use public transportation. The home can be modified to minimize falls.

Adults can continue to be physically active by adapting as they age. Instead of running, older adults can walk, bike, or swim to reduce impact on joints and bones. If endurance becomes a problem, older adults can be active more frequently, but for shorter periods of time.

Lesson 22.4 Review

Know and Understand

1. What are the three stages of adulthood? Include each stage's age range in your answer.
2. List two major life-changing events that may occur during young adulthood.
3. Define the term *sandwich generation*.
4. List two technologies that adults can use to adapt to reduced hearing and vision abilities.

Analyze and Apply

5. Explain how overall health commonly changes from young adulthood through older adulthood.

Real World Health

People who make up a generation typically share certain characteristics because of their similar experiences based on what is happening in the world as they are growing up. Research the different generational names and characteristics beginning in the early 1900s through present day. What influence did families, media, cultural traditions, and economic factors have on each generation's human development? Write a report about your findings. In small groups, compare what you learned with other students' findings.

The End of Life

Lesson Objectives

After studying this lesson, you will be able to

- summarize types of care people may need as they approach the end of life;

- identify transportation and housing options for older adults;

- describe financial and medical issues people may face at the end of life; and

- explain the stages of grief and how people can cope with grief and loss.

Key Terms E-Flash Cards

In this lesson, you will learn the meanings of the following key terms.

beneficiaries
hospice care
last will and testament
living will
palliative care

Warm-Up Activity

With Sympathy

When someone is grieving, words cannot stop the pain. However, words may bring comfort during a time of need. Pretend that someone you know has lost a loved one. Write a sympathy letter to this person, reflecting your sadness for his or her loss. As you write your letter, think about what words or thoughts might help you feel better in a time of grief or sadness.

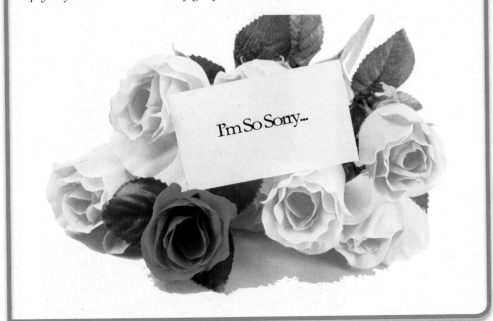

I'm So Sorry...

Before You Read

KWL Chart: End of Life

Create a chart like the one shown here to map what you know, what you want to know, and what you have learned about the end of life. In the first column, list facts you already know about death and dying. In the second column, list what you want to know. After reading the lesson, use the third column to outline what you learned.

K What you **Know**	W What you **Want to** know	L What you have **Learned**

A t your age, death feels distant and unfamiliar. It is a reality for the very old and sick, but not for you. Older adults once felt that way, too. As people age, life's end grows closer and the inevitability of death becomes more real. What do people face near life's end?

Caring for Older Adults

Many older adults can live independently as long as they remain healthy. Some older adults need minimal assistance, such as a ride to the doctor's office. Adults with serious health issues, however, require a great deal of medical and emotional care. This can include help with dressing, eating, hygiene, and using the bathroom, as well as specialized medical treatment and physical therapy. Older adults who require a great deal of care often cannot live alone and families might not have the expertise and time to care for them. Luckily, there are healthcare options to help take care of these older adults.

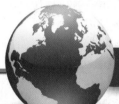

Local and Global Health
Worldviews on Older Adult Care

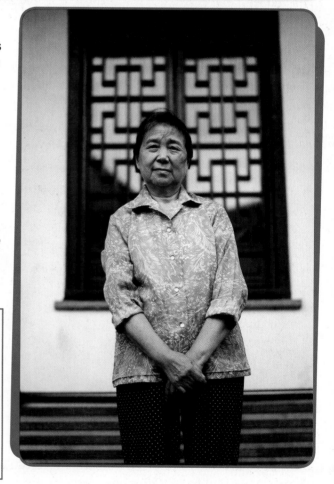

The type of care provided for older adults differs from country to country. In Asia, the family assumes most of this responsibility. In the United States, older adults are expected to plan and financially prepare for their own care. No US laws or cultural conventions require the family to contribute to older adult care. In contrast, Chinese cultural attitudes about the aging population emphasize respect for parents and ancestors in many family matters.

Even so, increased global travel and business have been drawing more Chinese young people away from their homes and their older relatives. In response, the Chinese government enacted an elder care law in 2013 that requires people to provide care for and to regularly visit with their older relatives.

Thinking Critically

1. How are the older adults cared for in your family? How does this reflect the ways in which your family views aging and older adulthood?

2. Should the US government enact a law to enforce the care of older adults, as China did?

3. Who will care for you in your old age? What role do you hope your family will play in your care?

Transportation Options

Someone who wants to work and live independently usually requires transportation. Many communities lack well-developed public transportation systems, and most adult drivers wish to continue driving as they age. More aging drivers are on the roads today than ever before and many are capable, safe drivers.

If driving seems unsafe, however, older adults have several alternatives. If buses, trains, subways, and other forms of public transportation are available, they often provide reduced rates for older adults. Community centers, religious organizations, city governments, and senior citizen organizations often provide free or affordable buses for older adults. Family members, friends, and neighbors may also be able to provide transportation.

Housing Options

Many forms of housing are available for older adults. These housing and assistance options include the following:

- *Family home.* Older adults may have a family member move in with them or they may move in with their family. This option works well if the family has enough time, space, and skills to care for the older adult.
- *Foster care.* In some communities, families provide foster care for older adults who have no family or friends and need help with some activities. This arrangement works well if the older adult can help with some of the foster family's expenses.
- *Retirement community.* Older adults who are healthy, independent, and have enough financial resources may choose to live in a retirement community. These communities consist of apartments or homes that might have common dining areas and housekeeping services. Retirement communities that provide independence along with a variety of forms of healthcare and end-of-life care are the fastest-growing housing options for older adults.
- *Assisted living facility.* Assisted living is available for older adults who need assistance with daily activities, but do not need regular skilled nursing care (Figure 22.15). The residents of assisted living facilities get help with food preparation, self-care skills, housekeeping, and laundry. Social activities may be offered.
- *Nursing home.* A nursing home is for older adults who have serious medical problems and require regular, skilled nursing care and assistance with daily living activities. When adults recover from their medical problems, they can move back to their own home, to their family's home, or into an assisted living facility.

Hospice and Palliative Care

The goal of ***palliative care*** is to bring comfort and pain relief to patients who are being treated for diseases or disorders. Palliative care is given in addition to treatment and is aimed at reducing symptoms such as pain, discomfort, depression, or anxiety. Palliative care can be given at home, in an assisted living facility, in a nursing home, or in the hospital.

palliative care
healthcare designed to bring comfort and relief to those being treated for diseases or disorders

Figure 22.15

Older adults who are relatively healthy but who require help with daily tasks such as bathing, dressing, or cleaning may reside in assisted living facilities. In these facilities, nurses and other workers attend to the needs of the residents and monitor progressing health issues.

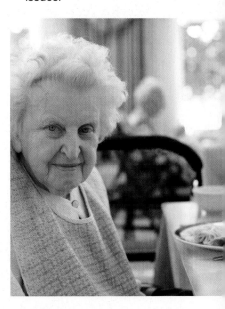

When Samantha's grandfather died after a long illness, her 74-year-old grandmother was shocked and took the loss pretty hard. She cried for days, did not eat very much, would not see anyone, and could not sleep. Now, six months later, Samantha's grandmother does not want Samantha to visit. When Samantha drops in to see her, she looks like she has not slept for days, her house is a mess, and her refrigerator is empty. Samantha is worried. She has never seen her grandmother in this condition.

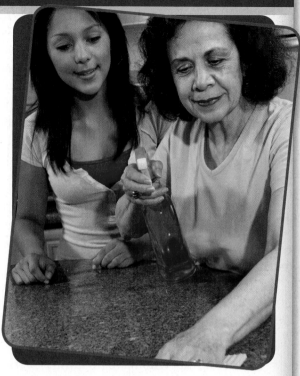

Thinking Critically

1. Grief after the death of a loved one is normal. Why would an older adult, such as Samantha's grandmother, have such a hard time after the death of her spouse?

2. In what ways is Samantha's grandmother putting her health at risk?

3. What can Samantha and her family do to help her grandmother cope with her grief?

hospice care
healthcare designed to provide comfort for terminally ill patients and their families

The goal of **hospice care** is to provide comfort for terminally ill people and their families. During hospice care, a dying person does not receive specific treatment for their disease. For example, cancer patients would enter hospice care when their cancer is untreatable. In hospice, patients receive pain relief, emotional support and comfort, care for their basic needs, and the opportunity to visit with family and friends. Hospice care can be given at home, in a nursing home, in a special hospice facility, or in the hospital.

Financial and Medical Issues at the End of Life

Medical care is expensive for adults with disabilities or adults near life's end. Adults who are 65 years of age and older may use *Medicare* insurance for some of these costs. Adults with disabilities who are unable to work can use disability insurance, which covers the loss of pay caused by their inability to work. Without this financial assistance, the adult children of older adults might pay for these costs, or the adults who are disabled may have to pay for the costs themselves.

At the end of life, a dying or terminally ill person may be unable to make financial and medical decisions. Under these circumstances, it is helpful for a designated person to have legal power to make healthcare decisions for the individual. This is called a *durable power of attorney for healthcare*. It is also helpful for another person to have *durable power of attorney for finances*. Adults can consult an attorney about how to arrange these legal powers ahead of time so that they are ready if something happens. Adults may also consider writing a *living will*, which directs a person's healthcare when the person becomes too sick to do so themselves. People write a *last will and testament* to determine how their money and property will be divided among beneficiaries. *Beneficiaries* are people or organizations that receive a person's money and property after that person's death.

Grief and Loss

Try to place yourself in the shoes of many older adults. Their own parents are gone, their brothers and sisters are aging and may have died, and some of their friends may also have died. As difficult as these losses are, the loss of a spouse or life partner can be the most painful. Older adults may experience more loss and grief than younger adults, but grief affects people of all ages.

Grief is a complex emotional experience that includes a profound sense of loss and sadness. A grieving person experiences many kinds of feelings following the death of a family member, spouse, or friend. People who are grieving need love and support from their family and friends. Some people may also need professional help to cope with their loss. When people do not get the help they need, they are at risk for developing major depression, which is a serious condition.

Stages of Grief

Every person experiences grief, loss, death of a loved one, and eventually their own death. These emotional experiences are personal and unique. Even so, people generally pass through certain stages when they are grieving (Figure 22.16).

- *Denial*—It is normal for some people to deny sad news. People may ignore the facts and try to carry on as though nothing has changed. Not all people experience denial, but those who do are protecting themselves from emotional pain. Most people move past denial at some point.

living will
an advanced directive that outlines what healthcare a person desires, to be used in the case that he or she is too sick to communicate his or her desires

last will and testament
an arrangement outlining how possessions, land, and property are to be divided upon a person's death

beneficiaries
people or organizations that will receive a person's property and money upon that person's death

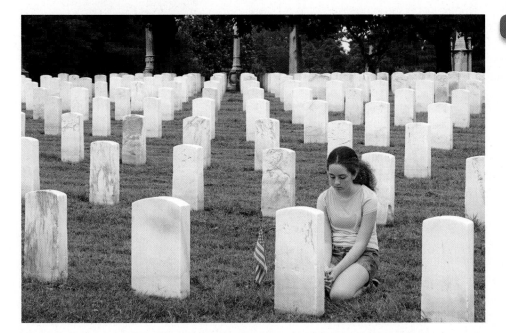

Figure 22.16

The last stage of grief is acceptance, during which a person moves on from the loss and emerges from depression. *Why do you think some people fail to experience this stage? How could a person get help in reaching this stage?*

- *Anger*—Some people become angry at the person who died. When facing a terminal illness, a person might become angry at doctors, family members, or friends. Most people understand that no one is at fault in these situations, and so they feel guilty about their anger. Although this stage is also temporary, it may last a long time, and a person's anger may push family and friends away.
- *Bargaining*—People feel out of control and helpless in the face of loss, terminal illness, and death. It is not unusual to react to these situations by trying to make deals and bargains as a way to regain control. A dying person might make promises in exchange for a chance to regain health or postpone death.
- *Depression*—Deep sadness comes with the reality of the loss. This depression is normal and can last several months.
- *Acceptance*—Not all people experience this stage. When they do, they accept the loss as real and begin to move on.

Spotlight on Health and Wellness Careers

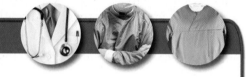

Older Adult Care

You may want to explore these rewarding careers related to the care of older adults.

Career	Typical Education and Training	Typical Job Duties and Demands	Career Resources
recreational therapist	bachelor's degree and certification	plans, directs, and coordinates recreational activities for older adults; should be organized, patient, and a good communicator	American Therapeutic Recreation Association
nursing assistant or orderly	state-approved education program and competency exam, on-the-job training	provides basic care and assistance for activities of daily living, such as bathing, dressing, and preparing meals for people in hospitals or in nursing homes; should have good physical stamina and be able to stand for most of the day	National Association of Health Care Assistants
geriatric social worker	master's degree	helps older adults solve problems of daily living and obtain medical, psychological, and financial assistance; should have good listening and communicating skills	National Association of Social Workers
rehabilitation counselor	master's degree and state license	assists older adults with the physical and emotional problems associated with recovery from disabilities and diseases	American Rehabilitation Counseling Association

Exploring Career

1. Think about your interests, strengths, and weaknesses. With these in mind, which career described above appeals most to you? Which career does not interest you?

2. Do you know someone who works in one of these careers? If so, ask this person why he or she chose this career and what he or she likes most and least about the work.

Counselors and health professionals recognize that these stages may not occur in order, and people may not experience all of the stages. Understanding these stages, however, can help people cope with grief.

Coping with Grief and Loss

How can people cope with loss and move on with their lives? How can you help others who are grieving? Grieving is a normal and healthy process. People should be allowed to grieve through whatever means they feel is right. They might need to feel very sad and cry for a long time. They might need to mark the loss with a ritual. Some rituals are private ceremonies held in the family home or in the community. Some people commemorate a death with a religious ceremony, such as a funeral. Friends, family, and coworkers often attend the funeral to support the surviving family members. Other people mark a death with a nonreligious memorial service, where family and friends share their grief and loss.

While grieving people might like some time alone, too much isolation is unhealthy. People who are grieving often find that sharing their feelings with someone—family, friends, a religious advisor, or a professional counselor—can help them heal.

People who are grieving should be discouraged from making difficult decisions. They should avoid life changes that bring additional stress, such as moving, changing jobs, or making large purchases. If necessary, such decisions should be made after consulting close family members who can help the person think through the decision carefully. Grief causes great physical and emotional stress. A grieving person may need help taking care of himself or herself during this difficult time. Good nutrition, physical activity, and adequate sleep help the body and mind face the challenges of grieving.

Lesson 22.5 Review

Know and Understand Assess

1. List two transportation options for older adults who are unable to drive.
2. List three housing options that are available for older adults.
3. What does it mean when a person has durable power of attorney for healthcare?
4. What is a living will?
5. Describe the stages of grief people may experience.

Analyze and Apply

6. Compare palliative care and hospice care.
7. Choose two online or print articles about coping with grief and the loss of a loved one to share with the class. As a class, analyze the articles and identify effective ways of coping with grief.

Real World Health

Older adults need to be prepared in case they become seriously ill. Talk with your parents or guardians, and with your grandparents, if possible, to find out what types of medical insurance they have in case they become ill or injured. Do they have extra insurance coverage such as life, disability, or long-term care insurance? Also find out if they have last will and testaments or living wills, including durable powers of attorney for healthcare and finances.

Write a paragraph or two about what you have discovered. What arrangements were most important to the people you interviewed? At what age did they make these arrangements? What were their reasons for making the arrangements they did?

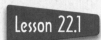
Human Development: The Unfolding Self

Key Terms

human life cycle
Individualized Education
  Plan (IEP)
Individualized Family
  Service Plan (IFSP)

interdependent
milestones

Key Points

- People pass through several developmental stages in the human life cycle, but the starting point and duration of each stage differs from person to person.
- Physical, intellectual, emotional, and social development are related and interdependent.
- Children with developmental delays often need help in school to be successful.
- Genes and the environment interact to direct and influence human development.
- Unhealthy lifestyle choices, such as smoking, poor nutrition, lack of physical activity, and lack of sleep, can take years off a person's life span.

Check Your Understanding

1. Each developmental stage is characterized by well-known, important events called _____.
2. The achievement of individual identity is a part of _____ development.
   A. social
   B. emotional
   C. physical
   D. intellectual
3. *True or false?* Delays in development can represent an underlying problem that requires treatment.
4. **Critical Thinking.** Think about the current life expectancy in the United States. What risk factors might contribute to decreasing life expectancy for people in a population?

Infancy through the Preschool Years

Key Terms

attachment
autonomy

fine-motor skills
gross-motor skills

motor development
object permanence
receptive language

separation anxiety
stranger anxiety
temper tantrum

Key Points

- Throughout early childhood, children grow increasingly strong and coordinated, relying less on reflex and more on purposeful, directed movements.
- Children learn many important concepts and progress significantly in language development from infancy through the preschool years.
- Children need to have positive interactions with their caregivers and others for healthy emotional and social development.

Check Your Understanding

5. _____ development refers to the increased coordination and strength of muscles.
6. Children understand the important concept of _____ when they realize that their world and the people in it continue to exist even when they do not see them.
   A. attachment
   B. cause and effect
   C. classification
   D. object permanence
7. *True or false?* Children who become upset, shy, or afraid around unfamiliar people and in new situations are experiencing separation anxiety.
8. **Critical Thinking.** As a caregiver, how would you respond to a toddler's temper tantrum?

The School-Age and Adolescent Years

Key Terms

nocturnal emissions
primary sexual
  characteristics

puberty
secondary sexual
  characteristics

Key Points

- Rates of development continue to vary throughout the school-age years and into adolescence.
- Physical changes during adolescence begin with puberty, when the reproductive system starts to mature.

- Adolescents refine the ability to think about abstract concepts apart from the concrete matters of daily life.
- Establishing independence and making decisions is important for adolescent emotional growth.

Check Your Understanding

9. *True or false?* Children who are less active develop muscle strength and coordination faster than children who are more active.

10. In males, the first sign of puberty is _____.
    A. hair growth on the face and under the arms
    B. pubic hair growth around the genitals
    C. nocturnal emissions
    D. enlargement of the testes

11. In females, the first sign of puberty is _____.
    A. menarche
    B. breast development
    C. hair growth under the arms
    D. pubic hair growth around the genitals

12. **Critical Thinking.** Explain changes in intellectual development that occur during the adolescent years.

Lesson 22.4   Assess

Adulthood and the Nature of Aging

Key Terms

dementia   older adulthood
incontinence   sandwich generation
middle adulthood   young adulthood

Key Points

- The stages of adulthood are young adulthood middle adulthood, and older adulthood.
- Changes in the sensory organs and body systems occur naturally as people age and more health problems arise as a result.
- By adapting to the changes involved with aging, adults can maintain an active, healthy life.

Check Your Understanding

13. In the United States, state and federal governments recognize that most people experience the milestones of adulthood after _____ years of age. (See top of next column.)

A. 16
B. 18
C. 21
D. 25

14. Flat, brown spots on areas of exposed skin are called _____.

15. The _____ is a walnut-sized organ that surrounds the urethra below the urinary bladder in men.

16. **Critical Thinking.** As you learned in this chapter, adulthood is defined in various ways. How would you define adulthood? Explain your answer.

Lesson 22.5   Assess

The End of Life

Key Terms

beneficiaries   living will
hospice care   palliative care
last will and testament

Key Points

- Some older adults need minimal assistance, while other older adults require a great deal of care.
- At the end of life, a dying or terminally ill person may need to appoint someone to help make important medical and financial decisions.
- Grief is a complex emotional experience that includes a profound sense of loss and sadness.

Check Your Understanding

17. A(n) _____ is a housing option for older adults who need regular, skilled medical care and assistance with daily living activities.

18. *True or false?* The goal of hospice care is to bring comfort and pain relief to patients who are being treated for diseases or disorders.

19. *True or false?* People who are grieving should be discouraged from making difficult decisions, such as changing jobs.

20. **Critical Thinking.** Compare a living will and a last will and testament.

Health and Wellness Skills

21. **Comprehend Concepts.** Use information from this chapter and your prior knowledge and experiences to create a timeline or infographic that charts the milestones reached during each stage of life. For each milestone, include a picture and a short description, including what it is and why it is important.

22. **Communicate with Others.** Many older adults enjoy visits from and conversations with younger people. In small groups, find a senior center or assisted living facility in your community that would welcome visitors. Plan some activities for your visit, such as talking to seniors, serving a meal, singing holiday carols, or leading a game. Set up a time at the facility and then visit. Afterward, share your experience with the rest of the class.

23. **Make Decisions.** Many American adults are part of the *sandwich generation*, meaning that they must care for their aging parent(s) as well as their own children. Find and interview someone who is part of this generation. How has this person's life changed since he or she took on these two responsibilities? What kinds of decisions does this person make for those under his or her care? How do the two caretaking roles differ? After interviewing the person and recording your information, film a short documentary reporting what you found.

24. **Practice Healthy Behaviors.** Chances are that you have experienced the grieving process, either firsthand or through someone you know. Think of a time you experienced loss or witnessed a friend or family member go through the stages of grief. Write a poem, letter, reflection, or song about the experience. Include how the loss felt, how grief was processed, and how the experience changed you or the other person.

Hands-On Activity
Birthday Party

In this activity, your class will be divided into small groups. Each group will plan a birthday party for someone in a particular age group. When the planning is finished, each group will host a Party Day during class to present their ideas and explain why these ideas are age-appropriate.

Materials Needed
- craft supplies to make invitations
- supplies for party activities
- party food

Steps for This Activity

1. Decide whose birthday you will be celebrating. If possible, choose a person—real or fictional—who does not belong to your age group. Choose a party theme that is age-appropriate for the guest of honor and which follows school rules.

2. Design a paper or electronic invitation to the party. Consider what is appropriate for the birthday guest when choosing the date, time, and location of the party.

3. Plan two to three age-appropriate activities or games for the party. Be prepared to have someone in your group play or lead each of these activities on Party Day.

4. Plan a party menu consisting of two to three party foods, such as a birthday cake or popcorn. Use your knowledge of what is healthy or age-appropriate for your birthday guest. Be prepared to serve a sample of one of these foods on Party Day.

5. When your group's Party Day arrives, present a description of your guest of honor, a sample invitation, the activities, the menu, and a sample party food to the class. Also explain why your group chose these items for your birthday guest. What makes your choices age-appropriate?

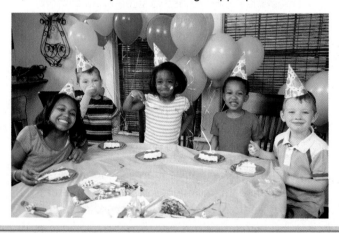

Core Skills

Math Practice

The following graph shows the occurrence of obesity among children and adolescents between 2 and 19 years of age and in three sub-groups of that age range. The statistics are organized by sex and age groups. Study the graph and then answer the questions.

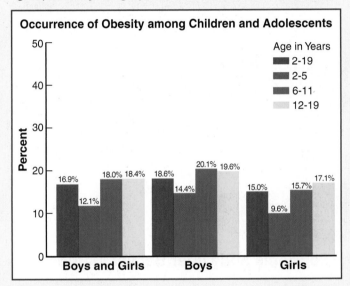

Occurrence of Obesity among Children and Adolescents

25. If there are 12,750 boys and girls between 6 and 11 years of age in the sample, how many are obese?
   A. 2,810
   B. 2,260
   C. 2,295
   D. 2,422

26. If there are 3,500 girls between 2 and 5 years of age in the sample, how many are obese?
   A. 325
   B. 336
   C. 342
   D. 350

27. What is the approximate percentage difference of 2–19 year-old girls who are obese as compared to boys in the same age group who are obese?
   A. 6.5%
   B. 3.6%
   C. 2.0%
   D. Insufficient information is provided to answer this question.

Reading and Writing Practice

Read the passage below and then answer the questions.

Toddlers enjoy watching other children play and like playing near other children. This type of play is called parallel play *because it is neither cooperative nor interactive. Toddlers do not easily share toys, especially their favorite ones.*

Because toddlers cannot understand empathy yet, they do not understand that they can hurt another child's feelings when fighting over toys, causing friction. While this behavior may seem selfish, it is perfectly normal and common. Toddlers need guidance and occasional intervention from caregivers to learn how to handle conflict with others.

28. What is the author's main idea in this passage?
   A. Toddlers do not like to share toys.
   B. Toddlers do not yet understand how to interact appropriately with other children and need guidance from caregivers.
   C. Caregivers need to make a list of inappropriate behaviors to share with toddlers.
   D. Toddlers are selfish.

29. In this passage, the term *friction* means _____.
   A. the act of rubbing items together
   B. a force that causes a moving object to slow when it touches another object
   C. disagreement between people
   D. the ability to understand what another person is feeling

30. From context, the word *empathy* in this passage means _____.
   A. selfish behavior
   B. being sensitive to others
   C. bullying
   D. fear of failure

31. Write a brief story for toddlers to explain that they can hurt other children's feelings by not sharing. Share your stories in class.

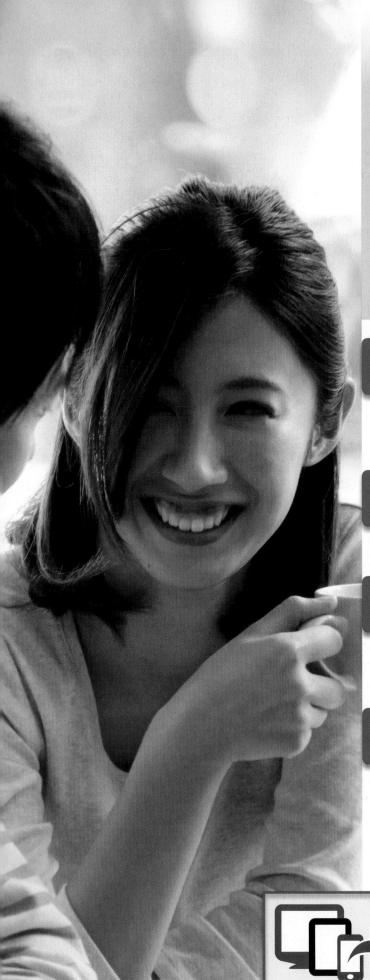

Chapter 23

Pregnancy Prevention

Lesson 23.1

Family Planning and the Role of Abstinence

Lesson 23.2

Condoms and Other Barrier Methods

Lesson 23.3

Hormonal Methods, IUDs, and Emergency Contraception

Lesson 23.4

Natural Methods and Sterilization

While studying this chapter, look for the activity icon to:
- **review** vocabulary with e-flash cards and games;
- **assess** learning with quizzes and online exercises;
- **expand** knowledge with animations and activities; and
- **listen** to pronunciation of key terms in the audio glossary.

G-WLEARNING.com

www.g-wlearning.com/health/

Take this quiz to see what you do *and* do not know about planning and preventing pregnancy. If you cannot answer a question, pay extra attention to that topic as you study this chapter.

1. Identify each statement as True, False, *or* It Depends. *Choose* It Depends *if a statement is true in some cases, but false in others.*

2. Revise each False *statement to make it true.*

3. Explain the circumstances in which each It Depends *statement is true and when it is false.*

Health and Wellness IQ Assess

1. A woman can't get pregnant the first time she has sex.	True	False	It Depends
2. No contraceptive method is 100% effective.	True	False	It Depends
3. A man must take male hormones after getting a vasectomy.	True	False	It Depends
4. A woman cannot become pregnant if she has sex during her menstrual period.	True	False	It Depends
5. When a woman is sterilized, a doctor removes her ovaries.	True	False	It Depends
6. The birth control pill works by stopping ovulation.	True	False	It Depends
7. If a man is allergic to latex, he cannot use a condom.	True	False	It Depends
8. You need a doctor's prescription to buy a condom at the drugstore.	True	False	It Depends
9. The birth control pill reduces the risk of both pregnancy and STIs.	True	False	It Depends
10. A woman can't get pregnant if a man withdraws his penis before he ejaculates.	True	False	It Depends

Setting the Scene

About 80% of teenage pregnancies are unplanned. In spite of the decades-long decline in teen pregnancy rates in the United States, the US teen birthrate is still among the highest in the industrialized world. The US teen birthrate is double what it is in Canada and France, three times higher than in Germany, and five times higher than in Japan.

Pregnancy and parenting at a young age take an enormous toll on the parents, their children, their extended families, and society. One of the most important steps you can take to achieve your life goals and reach your full potential is to avoid an unplanned pregnancy. The only 100% effective way to do this, and to avoid contracting an STI, is to abstain from sexual activity.

In this chapter, you will read about various contraceptive methods that temporarily block ovulation or fertilization. Surgical sterilization, the only permanent contraceptive method for adults, will be described. This chapter also explains how these methods work, their effectiveness, side effects, costs, and other advantages and disadvantages.

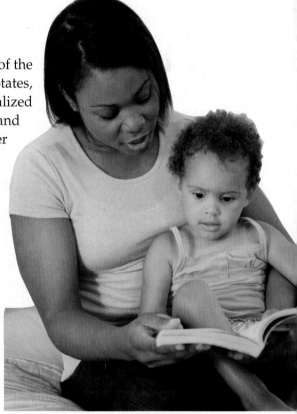

Family Planning and the Role of Abstinence

Key Terms
E-Flash Cards

In this lesson, you will learn the meanings of the following key terms.

contraception

family planning

Before You Read

KWL Chart: Pregnancy Prevention

Create a KWL chart like the one shown here to map what you know, what you want to know, and what you have learned about family planning, teen pregnancy, and abstinence.

K What you **K**now	W What you **W**ant to know	L What you have **L**earned

Lesson Objectives

After studying this lesson, you will be able to

- discuss family planning;
- explain the challenges of teen parenthood;
- identify the benefits of continuous abstinence;
- recognize pregnancy prevention facts and myths; and
- identify factors to consider when choosing a birth control method.

Warm-Up Activity

Family Planning

You may have heard the term family planning *in the media or in your own family. What does the term mean to you? What specifically comes to mind when you hear the term* family planning*? What does* abstinence *mean? What are some possible benefits of remaining abstinent? Write a paragraph containing your answers to these questions.*

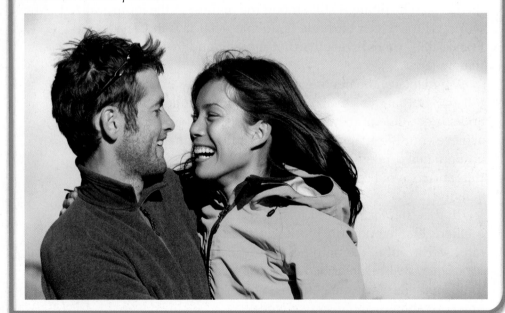

P regnancy, raising children, and family life can be among the most rewarding and meaningful experiences in a person's life. Many young people dream of someday having their own families. Experienced parents know, however, that pregnancy and family life demand attention, finances, time, and emotional maturity. Many couples plan their first pregnancy at a time when they are mature and best prepared to raise children.

Family Planning

A growing number of married couples choose to remain childless. Some of these couples worry that they will be unable to care for children for emotional, financial, or health reasons. A few are concerned about passing along a hereditary disease to their biological offspring. Some people may feel that having children is not necessary to lead a fulfilling life. In these situations, people want to know how to prevent pregnancy.

Other people want to raise children, but wish to postpone parenthood. They may want to have fewer children than their parents had, or wish to wait until they are financially self-sufficient and independent to have children. For these people, having the means to prevent pregnancy is vitally important.

Some people think family planning is the same as pregnancy prevention, but family planning is more than birth control. *Family planning* includes choosing when to have children, the number of children, the spacing of children, or whether or not to have children. Planning a family allows people to gather financial resources so they can provide their future children with adequate housing, food, healthcare, childcare, and education. By planning pregnancies, people can space their children so they are a certain number of years apart in age, if they feel it is important to do so. Family planning requires that a person thoroughly understands how pregnancy occurs and how pregnancy can be prevented.

Teen Parenthood: A Difficult Road

As you read in earlier chapters, sexual activity, pregnancy, and childbirth pose serious health risks to teenagers and their children. For the following reasons, teenagers should reduce their risk of pregnancy:

- **Physical Health Risks for the Mother.** Teenage mothers, as compared to adult mothers, are at higher risk for physical health problems caused by pregnancy and childbirth (see pages 614–615). Early sexual activity by teenagers also increases their risk of contracting STIs. An adolescent girl's immature cervix is more susceptible to chlamydia infection than an adult woman's cervix.

- **Physical Health Risks for the Child.** Teenage mothers are more likely than adult mothers to give birth to infants with a low birth weight. This is a concern because babies with a low birth weight

family planning
the process of making choices about having children, including number of children and spacing between them

Personal Profile

Is Someone You Know at Risk for Pregnancy?

The questions below can help people assess whether they are at risk for pregnancy. If you know someone who may be at risk for pregnancy, suggest that he or she answer the following questions.

I practice sexual abstinence.
yes no

We use a condom each time we have sex. **yes no**

My partner or I use birth control pills. **yes no**

I avoid alcohol and drugs.
yes no

I understand how pregnancy occurs. **yes no**

I know how to get birth control and information about birth control. **yes no**

I understand how to use birth control correctly. **yes no**

I understand how birth control methods work. **yes no**

Add the number of yes answers to assess risk for pregnancy. Even one no answer means a higher risk than if all answers were yes. The more no answers, the higher the risk for pregnancy.

are more likely to become ill or die than babies with a normal birth weight. As a whole, the children of teenage mothers tend to have more health problems and a lower overall quality of life than the children of adult mothers. These children are also more likely to become teen parents themselves.

- **Financial Burden.** Children require food, clothing, housing, childcare, and education. Estimates show that raising a child costs between $10,000 and $15,000 per year, or more, depending on the area in which the family lives. These are expenses that few teenagers can afford. To provide for their children's needs, teenage parents often become financially dependent on relatives and government agencies. Money that most teenagers spend on new clothes and going out with friends must be spent on diapers, baby food, and other needs of the child.

- **Disrupted Education.** The pressure to earn money and care for a child makes it difficult for teenage parents to complete high school (Figure 23.1). Only one out of three teenage mothers completes high school. Only 1.5% of teenage mothers complete college by age 30. To provide for their children, teenage fathers must sometimes drop out of school and work full time, making it extremely difficult for them to continue their education.

- **Economic Consequences.** Without a high school diploma or a certificate or degree from a college or technical school, teenage parents have limited job opportunities. The jobs they qualify for are time consuming, have difficult hours—including weekends and holidays—and often pay minimum wage. When they have jobs, they are usually low-wage jobs. Teen mothers and their children are more likely to live in poverty than adult parents and their children. In addition, evidence shows that children raised in such conditions are more likely than other children to continue this pattern of having children at an early age and, therefore, living in poverty.

- **Social and Emotional Health Risks.** Raising a child is often stressful and can take a toll on the emotional and social health of a teen parent. The responsibilities of parenthood leave little time and money for "hanging out" with friends or dating.

Abstinence

Only continuous abstinence works 100% of the time to prevent pregnancy. Even more important, continuous abstinence is also 100% effective at preventing the transmission of sexually transmitted infections (STIs). A person who was once sexually active may choose to stop having sex and become abstinent. Reasons why teenagers would choose to be abstinent include the following:

- *Abstinence prevents pregnancy.* They do not want to carry a child or become a parent.

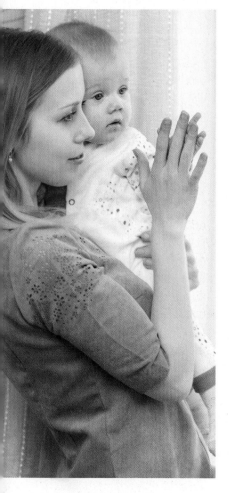

Figure 23.1

Teen parents face many challenges, including keeping up with schoolwork and struggling to pay for their baby's needs. *What are some physical risks that this young girl and her baby might face?*

Figure 23.2: Teens and Risky Sexual Behavior

41% of teens have had sexual intercourse at least once.
6% of teens had sexual intercourse for the first time before 13 years of age.
12% of teens have had sexual intercourse with four or more persons.
43% of teens did not use a condom the last time they had sexual intercourse.
70% of teens did not use birth control pills, or a related hormonal birth control method, before they last had sexual intercourse.
21% of teens drank alcohol or used drugs before they last had sexual intercourse.

- *Abstinence prevents STIs and HIV/AIDS.* They understand that sexual activity puts them at risk for STIs and HIV/AIDS.

- *Abstinence increases enjoyment of non-sexual activities.* They want to enjoy a romantic relationship, which can become complicated by sexual activity.

- *Abstinence allows time for other parts of life.* They are committed to important goals like education, career, and other personal interests.

- *Abstinence is a key component of their value system.* Abstinence supports their values or religious beliefs. A number of religions teach that couples should practice abstinence before marriage.

- *Abstinence allows for emotional growth and maturity.* Sexual relationships require emotional maturity, intimacy, closeness, and trust. Many teenagers feel they are not emotionally capable of handling a sexual relationship or the possibility of becoming a parent (Figure 23.2).

Birth Control Methods

A method for preventing pregnancy is called **contraception**, or *birth control*. Many birth control methods exist, and each couple must choose the method that works best for them.

contraception
a method or substance that helps to prevent pregnancy; also known as birth control

SKILLS FOR HEALTH AND WELLNESS

Practicing Abstinence

The strategies listed below can help you practice abstinence.

- Remember the reasons you decided to be abstinent. Teens choose abstinence for various reasons. Their religion may teach abstinence, or they may not feel emotionally ready for sex. Others want to avoid pregnancy and STIs.

- Remember the consequences of having sex. Pregnancy and complications from STIs, such as infertility, will have serious, long-lasting effects on your health and well-being.

- Decide to be abstinent now, when you are not in a sexual situation, and when you are emotionally calm. It is more likely that you will stick with your decision if you do so before putting yourself in a sexual situation.

- Avoid situations that can affect your decision to be abstinent. Do not use alcohol or drugs and do not attend parties where they are used. Do not attend unsupervised parties. Do not go anywhere alone with someone you do not know well.

- Discuss your decision with your boyfriend or girlfriend and explain why it is important to you to remain abstinent.

- Remind yourself of the benefits of abstinence.

People can consult a healthcare professional if they have questions about selecting a birth control method. A healthcare professional, and the manufacturer's instructions accompanying the product or device, provide information about how contraceptives should be used.

Some people in committed relationships choose not to use birth control because their religion's teachings oppose contraception. Other people think birth control is too expensive, inconvenient, or unreliable. Many contraceptive methods do not protect people from STIs and HIV/AIDS. Instead of birth control, some of these people choose abstinence, the only contraceptive method that is 100% effective in preventing pregnancy and STI transmission.

Myths and Facts about Pregnancy Prevention

Many myths exist about how pregnancy occurs. The best way to guard against falling for myths is to learn the facts about reproduction and pregnancy (Figure 23.3). The following are some myths and facts about pregnancy.

Myth #1: If a woman urinates after having sex, she won't get pregnant.

Fact: Urinating after sex does *not* prevent pregnancy.

Myth #2: If a woman douches, or cleans the inside of her vagina, after having sex, she won't get pregnant.

Fact: Douching after sex does *not* prevent pregnancy. In fact, douching can actually increase the likelihood of pregnancy by pushing semen deeper into the vagina. In addition, douching does *not* prevent the transmission of STIs and HIV/AIDS (Figure 23.4).

Figure 23.3

People often think they are being helpful and giving good advice when they are actually spreading myths. If you are unsure, talk to a doctor or other reproductive health expert to get accurate information about birth control.

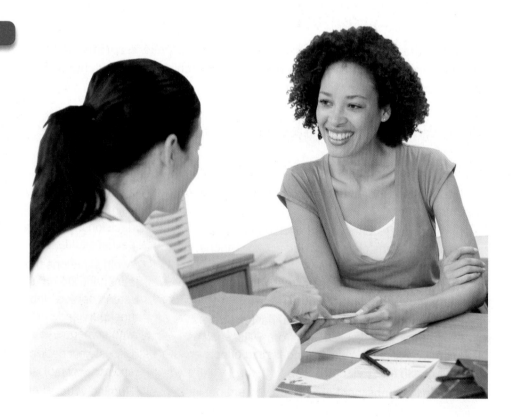

Myth #3: A woman cannot become pregnant the first time she has sex.

Fact: A woman *can* become pregnant the first time she has sex. If she has unprotected sex, or uses a form of birth control that is not 100% effective, she can become pregnant and acquire an STI or HIV/AIDS any time she has sex, including the first time.

Myth #4: A woman cannot become pregnant during her period.

Fact: A woman *can* become pregnant during her period. It is unlikely but possible. Women with regular cycles of 28 to 32 days will typically not become pregnant during their period. Many women, however, have irregular periods. Some women have shorter cycles (24 days, for example) and some ovulate earlier than the usual 14th day. These women can become pregnant during their period.

Myth #5: A woman cannot become pregnant if her partner withdraws or "pulls out" before he ejaculates.

Fact: A woman *can* become pregnant even if a man withdraws before ejaculation. Oftentimes, sperm is released from the penis before ejaculation. *Withdrawal*, which is covered later in this chapter, is the least effective method of birth control.

Myth #6: A woman cannot become pregnant if she stands up during or after sexual intercourse.

Fact: A woman *can* become pregnant no matter what position she is in during and after sexual intercourse. Standing up during sex will not prevent pregnancy.

Myth #7: Girls younger than 18 years of age cannot become pregnant.

Fact: Girls younger than 18 years of age *can* and *do* become pregnant. After a girl has begun menstruating, she can become pregnant no matter how old she is.

Myth #8: It is impossible for people to contract an STI or HIV/AIDS if they use a condom.

Fact: If used properly and consistently, latex and polyurethane condoms can reduce—but not eliminate—a person's risk of contracting an STI or HIV/AIDS.

Myth #9: A woman cannot become pregnant if she or her partner uses birth control.

Fact: Using a birth control method reduces, but does not completely eliminate, the risk of pregnancy. A woman's chances of becoming pregnant depend on the birth control method used—some methods have a greater percentage of effectiveness than others. The risk of pregnancy also depends on whether or not the birth control method is used consistently and correctly. Abstinence is the only way to avoid pregnancy completely.

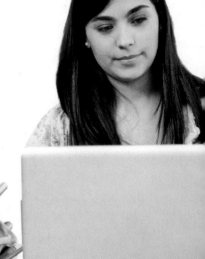

Figure 23.4

Your future is too important to risk on questionable advice or information—especially when accurate, reliable information is just a few mouse clicks away. *Can you name two or three reliable websites for information about reproduction and pregnancy?*

Factors to Consider When Selecting a Birth Control Method

Each birth control method has its advantages and disadvantages. A person should consider his or her goals when selecting a method. Is the goal to prevent pregnancy and have protection from STIs and HIV/AIDS? Certain methods, such as the latex male condom, can reduce the risk of pregnancy, STIs, and HIV/AIDS. Other methods, such as hormonal birth control, reduce the risk of pregnancy but do not protect from STIs and HIV/AIDS.

Cost and availability should also be considered. Some methods, such as the female condom or contraceptive sponge, are inexpensive and can be obtained without a doctor's prescription. Other methods, such as the IUD (intrauterine device), require a doctor's visit. If a woman is using the birth control shot, she must visit her doctor regularly.

Some people want to use a reversible method of birth control so that they can choose to have children in the future. Others, however, would prefer a method that is permanent. Surgical sterilization is permanent and practically irreversible. You will learn more about surgical methods of birth control later in the chapter.

The ease of use for each birth control method should also be considered. Each method is effective only when used correctly every time, which may not always be convenient or possible. Some people cannot use certain types of birth control, such as the hormonal methods, because of medical conditions. In the next three lessons, you will learn about the effectiveness, correct use, and pros and cons of several types of birth control.

Lesson 23.1 Review

Know and Understand Assess

1. What is the annual, estimated cost of raising a child?
2. Explain the economic consequences of teenage parenthood.
3. Which form of contraception is 100% effective for preventing pregnancy, STIs, and HIV/AIDS?
4. What are three factors to consider when choosing a birth control method?
5. Is sterilization reversible or permanent?

Analyze and Apply

6. How does family planning relate to pregnancy prevention?
7. Why do teenage parents have trouble completing high school?

Real World Health

Maria has just found out that she is pregnant. While this is great news, she has also just lost her job and no longer has health insurance. Use the Internet to research the different items that are needed for the first year of a baby's life. List the items and their costs on a piece of paper or in a spreadsheet. Add up the cost of all the items you listed. Remember that there are also medical costs involved in having a baby. Since Maria has recently lost her job and does not have health insurance, research and include healthcare costs that she might have and add those to your total. What is the final cost of having a baby and caring for it during the first year of life? Write a one-page paper describing what you have learned from this activity.

Condoms and Other Barrier Methods

Lesson Objectives

After studying this lesson, you will be able to

- explain how barrier methods are used to prevent pregnancy;
- understand how to use male and female condoms; and
- describe various methods of contraception.

Warm-Up Activity

Barrier Methods

Create an acrostic poem for the term barrier methods *using a template like the one shown here. For each letter, list a type of barrier method, advantage or disadvantage of using barrier methods, or something that you associate with barrier methods. After you and your classmates have created your poems, hang them up around the classroom. Discuss similarities and differences you see between your poem and your classmates' poems.*

B_____   M_____

A_____   E_____

R_____   T_____

R_____   H_____

I_____   O_____

E_____   D_____

R_____   S_____

Key Terms   E-Flash Cards

In this lesson, you will learn the meanings of the following key terms.

barrier methods

cervical cap

condoms

contraceptive sponge

diaphragm

spermicide

Before You Read

Male and Female Condoms

Create a Venn diagram comparing and contrasting the male condom and the female condom. What do they have in common? How are they different?

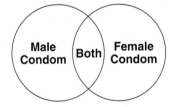

condom

a contraceptive product that fits over an erect penis or inside a woman's vagina, where it catches sperm and prevents them from reaching the ovum

barrier methods

contraceptive methods that physically block fertilization by preventing sperm from reaching the ovum

T he rate of teen births in the United States has been declining. Surveys show, however, that risky sexual behaviors remained about the same during that time period as they had previously—except for one behavior. During that time, condom use increased among sexually active teens. This data shows that using contraception can reduce teen pregnancy. Evidence suggests, however, that teens can still improve their knowledge and use of contraception, which would further reduce the number of unplanned teen pregnancies.

Condoms are one of several barrier methods of birth control. *Barrier methods* physically block fertilization by preventing sperm from reaching the ovum. Each barrier method has its advantages and disadvantages. For example, some methods protect users from contracting STIs and HIV/AIDS, while other methods do not.

It is important to keep in mind, however, that no barrier method is 100% effective in preventing STI transmission. For example, a person with the herpes virus or the human papillomavirus (HPV) may not have visible sores on the skin. The virus may be present on the skin not covered by a condom, however, and can be transmitted to a partner.

Men and women say that some barrier methods work well for them, but find others to be less "user friendly." Barrier methods of birth control include male condoms, female condoms, the diaphragm, the cervical cap, and the contraceptive sponge.

The Male Condom

Male condoms are worn on the penis during sexual intercourse. There are several types of male condoms:

- latex condoms—made from a form of natural rubber derived from the sap of rubber trees
- polyurethane condoms—made from various forms of plastic
- sheepskin, or lambskin condoms—made from the walls of sheep intestines. These condoms are sometimes called *natural*. The use of these condoms is *not* recommended because they contain small pores through which disease-causing organisms can pass into the vagina. Although these condoms reduce the risk of pregnancy, they do *not* prevent STIs and HIV/AIDS.

How it Works

The male condom is designed to fit over the erect penis (Figure 23.5). Condoms must be applied before the penis touches the sexual partner's genitals. This is important because fluids containing sperm, and possibly microorganisms that cause STIs, can be released from the penis prior to ejaculation.

spermicide

a substance that inactivates sperm; often applied to condoms and other contraceptive products

Condoms prevent pregnancy by catching the semen released during ejaculation and preventing sperm from reaching the ovum. In addition, some condoms are coated with *spermicide*, a substance that inactivates the sperm. Condoms cannot be reused; a new condom must be used each time intercourse occurs.

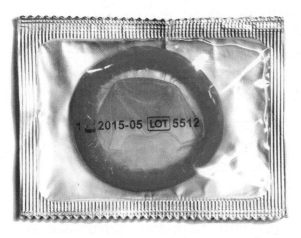

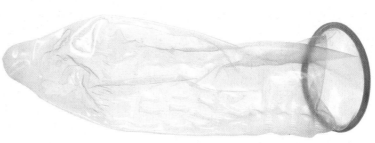

Condom use has no health-related side effects unless one partner has a latex allergy, which can trigger an allergic reaction if latex condoms are used. People who have a latex allergy should use a different type of condom, or a different method of birth control.

Condoms become dry, brittle, and ineffective over time. The expiration date on condoms should always be checked, and expired condoms should be discarded. Condoms should not be stored in hot or cold places (like cars) or in wallets, where they can be damaged or punctured.

How to Use a Male Condom

Using a male condom is easy, but care should be taken to open, apply, and remove the condom properly to prevent spilling semen in the vagina. It's a good idea to practice applying and removing a condom before having sex. People can practice applying a condom by applying a condom over an object shaped like a penis.

Applying a Male Condom

- Gently tear open the condom package at its edge. Teeth or scissors should never be used to do this. If the package is wet or sticky, it may have opened and the condom should be discarded. Each condom is rolled into a ring within its package.

- Determine which way the condom unrolls.

- Pinch the condom tip to remove air. This prevents breakage when the condom fills with semen. Leave a small amount of space at the tip of the condom to collect semen.

- Place the condom at the tip of the erect penis.

- The condom won't roll if it's placed incorrectly on the penis. Once the condom is positioned correctly, roll it to the base of the penis.

- Apply some water-based lubricant if the condom is not lubricated. *Always use water-based lubricants or lotions.* The label on a bottle of lotion should state whether it is safe to use with latex condoms. Never use petroleum-based lotions or lubricants such as Vaseline with a latex condom. These substances will break down the latex barrier.

Figure 23.5

The male condom is designed to fit over an erect penis. Condoms are effective at preventing pregnancy if used properly (see figure on pages 716 and 717). Condoms can also prevent the transmission of STIs. *What are the different types of male condoms?*

Removing a Male Condom

- Remove the penis from the partner's genitals before it softens. Otherwise, the condom can fall off and spill semen.
- Hold the base of the condom at its ring while withdrawing to keep the condom from coming off the penis.
- Pull off the condom and dispose of it in the trash. Wash your hands.
- Never reuse a condom. Always use a new condom for each erection.

The Female Condom

A female condom is a device similar to a pouch, which the woman inserts into her vagina (Figure 23.6). Female condoms are made of plastic so they do not cause allergic reactions in people allergic to latex. Each end of the female condom has a flexible ring to help the woman insert it into her vagina, and to hold it in place while the penis is inserted in the vagina. The effectiveness of female condoms can be improved by adding spermicide to the inside or by withdrawing the penis before ejaculation.

How It Works

The female condom must be inserted before the penis touches the woman's genitals. The female condom prevents pregnancy by catching semen and preventing sperm from entering the vagina. The female condom also forms a barrier to STIs.

How to Use a Female Condom

Care should be taken to insert a female condom and remove it properly to prevent semen from spilling in the vagina.

Inserting a Female Condom

- Apply spermicide to the end of the condom that will face the cervix.
- Squeeze the inner ring at the closed end of the condom and push it into the vagina as deep as it will go. The outer ring should rest about one inch outside the vagina.
- The woman or her partner can hold the outer ring against the woman's vaginal opening, while the penis is inserted. The penis should not slide outside of the female condom.

Removing a Female Condom

- Hold the outer ring and twist the end of the condom to trap semen inside and prevent spillage.
- Pull the condom out of the vagina and discard it in the trash. A female condom can only be used once. A new condom must be used each time a person has sexual intercourse.

Figure 23.6

Female condoms are inserted into a woman's vagina. The effectiveness of these condoms can be increased by adding spermicide cream or jelly. *How do female condoms prevent pregnancy?*

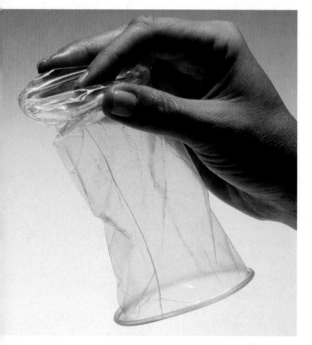

Contraceptive Sponge

The ***contraceptive sponge*** is a barrier birth control method that blocks sperm from entering the uterus. The sponge also contains spermicide, which stops sperm from swimming.

The contraceptive sponge is made of plastic foam and is about two inches in diameter (Figure 23.7). The sponge is inserted into a woman's vagina and is positioned to cover her cervix. A sponge can be inserted several hours before sexual intercourse occurs and it can be left in place for 30 hours.

Unlike the condom, the sponge does not have to be replaced each time a couple has intercourse. The same sponge can be used more than once during a 30-hour period. The sponge has a small loop that enables a woman to pull it out with her finger.

The contraceptive sponge does not protect women from contracting STIs and HIV/AIDS, so the woman's partner should always wear a condom. Sponges are less effective in preventing pregnancy than male and female condoms. The contraceptive sponge is more effective in preventing pregnancy for women who have never given birth, as compared to women who have given birth.

Diaphragm

The ***diaphragm*** is a flexible, cup-shaped disk that covers the cervix and blocks sperm from entering the uterus (Figure 23.8). Unlike condoms and sponges, a diaphragm requires a doctor's exam and prescription. During the exam, the doctor checks the health of the cervix and uterus and prescribes the correctly sized diaphragm. Diaphragms can be purchased with a prescription at drugstores. Diaphragms are made of silicone, a material that usually does not cause discomfort.

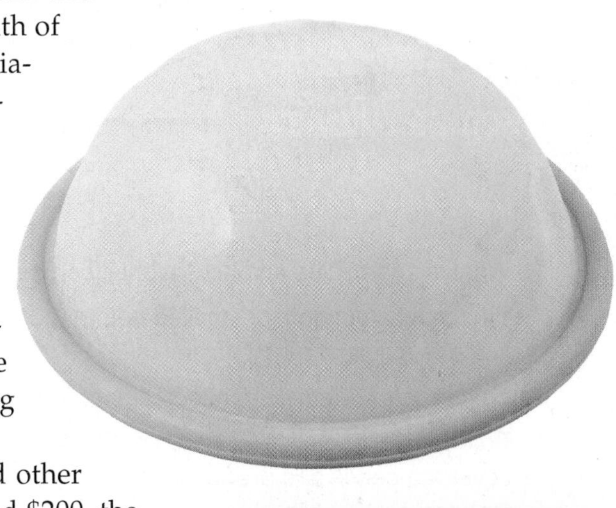

A woman must read and follow the package's directions for the correct insertion, removal, and care of the diaphragm. It must be inserted several hours before intercourse and must be used each time a woman has intercourse. A diaphragm is usually covered with spermicide before it is inserted. This causes the sperm to stop moving and prevents them from entering the uterus.

A diaphragm costs more than a condom, sponge, and other barrier methods. The doctor's exam costs between $50 and $200, the diaphragm costs from between $15 and $75, and the spermicide cream costs between $8 and $17 per tube. The diaphragm can, however, be used multiple times and for much longer than other barrier methods. Therefore, while initial costs are relatively high, the diaphragm is inexpensive for long-term contraception.

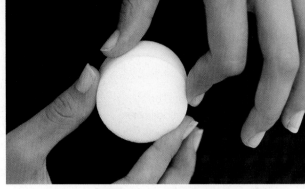

Figure 23.7

The contraceptive sponge blocks sperm from entering the uterus and contains spermicide to inactivate sperm. *Can the contraceptive sponge be used more than once?*

contraceptive sponge
a birth control method that blocks sperm from entering the uterus

diaphragm
a flexible, cup-shaped contraceptive product that covers the cervix and blocks sperm from entering the uterus

Figure 23.8

The diaphragm—a flexible, cup-shaped disk—covers the cervix and blocks sperm from entering the uterus. *What are some major differences between diaphrams and condoms?*

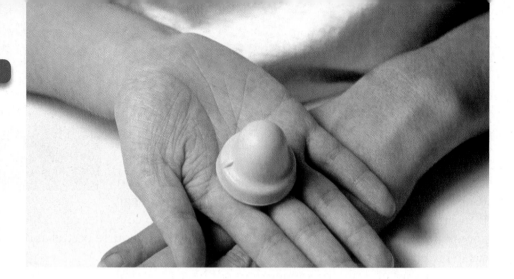

cervical cap
a flexible, silicone contraceptive product that covers the cervix and prevents sperm from entering the uterus

Cervical Cap

The *cervical cap* is a flexible cup that covers the woman's cervix (Figure 23.9). Like the diaphragm, the cervical cap is made of silicone and works by blocking sperm from entering the uterus. The cervical cap is smaller than a diaphragm and may be more difficult for a woman to position correctly. Because childbirth changes the size of a woman's cervix, women who have given birth will need to see a doctor to be fitted for a new cervical cap. The cap works best for women who have never given birth.

A woman must read and follow the package's directions for the correct insertion, removal, and care of the cervical cap. The cap must be covered with spermicide and inserted six hours before intercourse.

As with a diaphragm, women must see a doctor and obtain a prescription for a cervical cap. The doctor checks the health of the cervix and uterus and prescribes the correct size. The doctor's exam typically costs between $50 and $200, the cervical cap costs between $60 and $75, and the spermicide cream costs between $8 and $17 per tube.

Lesson 23.2 Review

Know and Understand

1. What is spermicide and how might it be used?

2. Why must a condom be applied before the penis touches a sexual partner's genitals?

3. *True or false?* Female condoms are reusable.

4. Both the _____ and _____ are flexible cups that cover the cervix and prevent sperm from entering the uterus.

5. Why are sheepskin or lambskin condoms unable to prevent STI transmission?

Analyze and Apply

6. What are some advantages and disadvantages of using barrier methods to prevent pregnancy?

7. Why is it important to practice properly applying and removing a condom before having sex?

Real World (Health

People's attitudes about teen sexual activity are often influenced by their cultures or religions. Consider what beliefs and cultures have shaped your attitude toward teen sexual activity. To do this, research the different cultures, religions, and ethnicities that make up who you are. Then, identify the corresponding beliefs about teen sexual activity for each of these groups. On a separate piece of paper, describe what you find and reflect on how these attitudes have influenced your personal opinions on teen sexual activity.

Hormonal Methods, IUDs, and Emergency Contraception

Lesson Objectives

After studying this lesson, you will be able to

- identify hormonal birth control methods;
- explain the use of oral contraceptives;
- describe two types of intrauterine devices (IUDs); and
- evaluate the use of emergency contraception.

Key Terms E-Flash Cards

In this lesson, you will learn the meanings of the following key terms.

emergency contraception
intrauterine device (IUD)
oral contraceptive

Warm-Up Activity

The Impact of Hormones
In a chart like the one shown here, identify the different ways that hormones affect our body functions. For example, the hormone prolactin stimulates breast milk production in new mothers.

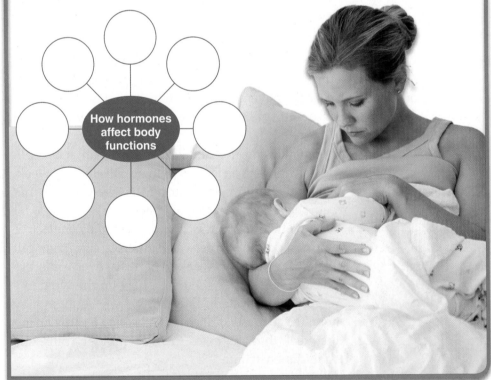

How hormones affect body functions

Before You Read

Important Terms
Scan this lesson and list any terms you can't define on a separate sheet of paper. Then, create a table like the one shown here. List the unfamiliar terms in the first column of your chart. In the second column, describe what you think the terms mean. As you read the chapter and learn what a term actually means, write its definition in the third column.

Term	What I Think It Means	What It Really Means

Hormones control many body functions, including reproduction. When used medically, as prescribed by a doctor, the female hormones estrogen and progesterone can stop ovulation, which is the release of an ovum. In this way, a doctor can help a woman control her reproductive cycle when she has severe menstrual pain, endometriosis, or another reproductive disorder. Because they block ovulation, these hormones can also prevent pregnancy.

Oral Contraceptives: The Birth Control Pill

oral contraceptive
a contraceptive substance that contains hormones that thicken cervical mucus and prevent ovulation; also known as the birth control pill *or the* pill

Oral contraceptives are usually referred to as the *birth control pill*—or just *the pill* (Figure 23.10). Birth control pills contain hormones that reduce the likelihood of pregnancy. The pill is taken by mouth, or *orally*, and should be taken at about the same time every day. Oral contraceptives do not prevent STIs, HPV, or cervical cancer.

Birth control pills prevent ovulation, which means that there is no ovum for sperm to fertilize. The pill also thickens cervical mucus, which slows down sperm's movement into the uterus.

Doctors need to examine all women using hormone-based birth control methods because women with certain medical conditions should not take the pill. The pill is effective at preventing pregnancy if taken *exactly as prescribed by the doctor*. Skipping even one pill increases the chance of becoming pregnant. Some research suggests that women who use birth control pills have an increased risk of contracting STIs.

The pill comes in two basic forms—the combination pill and the progesterone-only pill. Research is ongoing to identify options for male oral contraceptives.

Figure 23.10

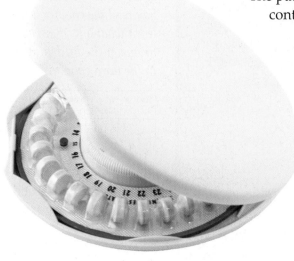

Birth control pills reduce the likelihood of pregnancy. These pills may contain a combination of estrogen and progesterone, or progesterone alone.

Combination Pill

Most women take the combination pill, which contains the hormones estrogen and progesterone. The combination pill comes in a pack of 21, 28, or 91 pills. All packs have *active pills*, which contain hormones. The packs of 28 and 91 pills also have *inactive pills*, which do not contain hormones.

A woman using the 21-pill pack takes an active pill every day for three weeks and then no pills for one week. Her period should begin during that week. After that week, she starts a new 21-pill pack.

A woman using the 28-pill pack takes one active pill each day for three weeks, then one inactive pill every day for one week. The last seven pills are placebo pills—they have no effect on the woman's reproductive system. She takes them because they help her keep the daily habit of taking a pill. During the week that she takes these "reminder" pills, she should menstruate.

A woman using the 91-pill pack only menstruates once every three months. She takes active pills for 12 weeks and then takes inactive pills for one week.

Progesterone-Only Pill

Some women take a form of the pill that contains only progesterone—no estrogen is included. The progesterone-only pill comes in a 28-pill pack; all the pills contain active hormones. This pill should be taken around the same time every day so it is not forgotten.

Birth Control Patch

The birth control patch (often called the *patch*) is a thin, 2- to 3-inch, plastic patch applied to the skin like a bandage (Figure 23.11). The patch contains the hormones estrogen and progesterone.

The patch works like the birth control pill, except the hormones are absorbed from the patch across the skin and into the blood. Like the pill, the birth control patch prevents ovulation and thickens cervical mucus, slowing down sperm's movement into the uterus.

One patch is applied to the skin for one week and then removed. It is replaced with a new patch for the second week. After removing the second patch, a third patch is worn for the third week and then discarded. No patch is worn during the fourth week (during menstruation).

Women should follow the package's directions for applying and removing patches. The directions should also state what women should do if a patch falls off, or if they forget to replace one.

Vaginal Ring

The vaginal ring is a small, flexible ring containing estrogen and progesterone (Figure 23.12). The ring works by releasing hormones that inhibit ovulation and thicken cervical mucus.

The ring is inserted in the vagina and used for three consecutive weeks. Exactly three weeks after insertion, the ring should be removed, ideally at the same time as it was inserted. The ring is then discarded, and no ring is used during the fourth week (during menstruation). Women should follow the package's directions about proper storage, insertion, and removal of the ring.

Birth Control Shot

A woman who receives the birth control shot, such as *Depo-Provera*, gets an injection of the hormone progesterone. The progesterone in the shot inhibits ovulation and thickens cervical mucus. She must see her doctor for a shot every three months. Depending on the type of shot, it can be given in the arm, the buttocks, or under the skin.

The birth control shot is highly effective in preventing pregnancy if injections are received according to schedule.

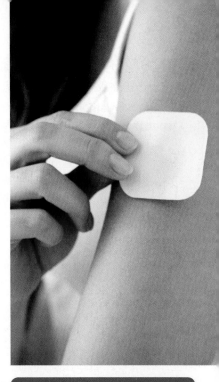

Figure 23.11

The birth control patch contains estrogen and progesterone, which are absorbed across the skin and into the blood. *For how long is the birth control patch worn?*

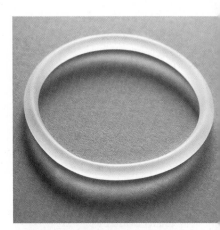

Figure 23.12

The vaginal ring releases low doses of estrogen and progesterone over the course of three weeks.

Figure 23.13 Birth Control Methods

When no method is used, 85 out of 100 women will become pregnant within one year.

Methods	Number of women (per 100) experiencing unintended pregnancies within first year of use		Factors to Consider
	Typical use	Perfect use	
Abstinence (continuous)	none	none	• 100% effective in preventing pregnancy • 100% effective in preventing STIs and HIV/AIDS • no medical side effects • free • no prescription needed
Male and female sterilization	fewer than 1	fewer than 1	• lasts a lifetime; rarely reversed • must undergo surgery • expensive • must use condom to protect from STIs and HIV/AIDS
Birth control implant (*Implanon*)	fewer than 1	fewer than 1	• does not have to be replaced for three years • must use with condom to protect from STIs and HIV/AIDS • must be inserted and removed by doctor; can be expensive • can cause scarring of tissue around implant site
Intrauterine device (IUD) (*Paraguard* and *Mirena*)	fewer than 1	fewer than 1	• lasts 5 to 12 years; the copper IUD (*Paraguard*) lasts longer • requires almost no care • must use with condom to protect from STIs and HIV/AIDS • must be inserted and removed by a doctor • initial cost from $500 to $1000, but long-term cost is low • abnormal bleeding and cramping can occur
Birth control shot (*Depo-Provera*)	3	fewer than 1	• easy to use • no need to remember to take a pill • must use with condom to protect from STIs and HIV/AIDS • frequent doctor visits for injections • use for two or more years causes reduced bone density
Vaginal ring (*NuvaRing*)	8	fewer than 1	• easy to use • must use with condom to protect from STIs and HIV/AIDS • requires doctor's visit and prescription • costs about $15 to $80 per month • increases risk for blood clots
Birth control patch (*Evra* patch)	8	fewer than 1	• safe for most women • easy to use • must be used with condom for STIs/HIV/AIDS protection • requires doctor's visit and prescription • costs about $15 to $80 for a one-month supply • increases risk for blood clots
Birth control pill	8	fewer than 1	• easy to use/ must remember to take it exactly as prescribed • few side effects for most women • must be used with condom for STI and HIV/AIDS protection • cannot be used by women with certain medical conditions • requires doctor's exam and prescription • combination pills raise the risk of forming blood clots • progesterone-only pills increase risk for gestational diabetes

Figure 23.13 Birth Control Methods *(Continued)*

Method			Details
Male condom (latex and plastic)	15	2	• provides protection from STIs and HIV/AIDS • inexpensive or free • easy to use; no prescription needed • can be used with other birth control methods • latex condom can cause allergic reaction in some people • can break or slip off during sexual intercourse • can expire, dry out, tear • must be removed immediately after ejaculation • can only be used once • more effective if used with spermicide
Female condom	21	5	• provides protection from STIs and HIV/AIDS • relatively inexpensive • easy to use; no prescription needed • can be used with oil-based or water-based lubricating lotions • can break or slip out of place during intercourse • must be removed immediately after ejaculation • can expire • can only be used once • more effective if used with spermicide
Diaphragm (with spermicide)	16	6	• can be used multiple times • initially costs more than other barrier methods • inexpensive for long-term use • must use condom for STIs and HIV/AIDS protection • must be used with spermicide • requires doctor's exam and prescription
Sponge Used by women who have given birth Used by women who have never given birth	 32 16	 20 9	• easy to use; no prescription needed • relatively inexpensive • need not be replaced each time a couple has intercourse • can be used again during a 30-hour period • must be used with condom for STI and HIV/AIDS protection • can cause infections and toxic shock syndrome if left in vagina too long
Fertility awareness methods ("rhythm methods")	25	5	• require detailed knowledge of the menstrual cycle • require record-keeping and daily attention • effectiveness depends on consistent and correct use
Withdrawal "Pull out"	27	4	• not recommended for birth control • often not used correctly • no protection from STIs and HIV/AIDS
Cervical Cap Used by women who have given birth vaginally Used by women who have never given birth	 32 16	 26 9	• not effective protection against STIs and HIV/AIDS • must be used with a condom • requires a doctor's exam and prescription
Spermicides	29	18	• not very effective when used alone • best used with a barrier method • available over-the-counter

This form of birth control costs about \$35 to \$75 per injection, and each doctor's visit will cost between \$20 and \$40, or more depending on a person's health insurance. Research about male contraceptive shots, including one recent study, is ongoing.

Birth Control Implant

The birth control implant is a flexible, toothpick-sized rod containing progesterone. The implant is inserted by a doctor under the skin of the upper arm, where it releases progesterone. The progesterone inhibits ovulation and thickens cervical mucus. The implant can be left in place for three or four years, during which time it gradually releases its dose of progesterone.

Intrauterine Device (IUD)

intrauterine device (IUD)
a T-shaped contraceptive product that is inserted into the uterus, where it helps prevent pregnancy

An **intrauterine device (IUD)** is a small, T-shaped device that is inserted into the uterus by a doctor (Figure 23.14). Two types of IUDs exist—copper IUDs (*ParaGard*) and hormonal IUDs (*Mirena, Liletta, Skyla, Kyleena*).

IUDs work in different ways to prevent pregnancy. The copper *ParaGard* IUD is thought to interfere with sperm movement, fertilization, and implantation. Hormonal IUDs inhibit ovulation and cause mucus in the woman's cervix to thicken, making it difficult for sperm to reach the uterus.

Hormonal IUDs last for years and can reduce menstrual cramps and significantly lighten or even stop a woman's period. Both copper and hormonal IUDs can be removed if a woman wants to become pregnant and can be used during breast-feeding. The advantage of the *ParaGard* IUD is that it can be left in place for 12 years and it does not affect a woman's hormone levels. The *ParaGard* IUD can also be used as a form of emergency contraception.

Emergency Contraception

Even when partners agree to use birth control and try to use it correctly, mistakes can happen. For example, a male condom can break, leak, or slip off. A female condom might leak or slip out of position. A woman might forget to insert a diaphragm or take the pill.

An IUD is a safe and effective way to prevent pregnancy, but it does not protect against STIs. *What is the difference between an IUD and a birth control implant?*

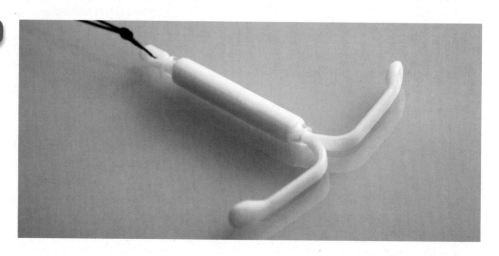

In these cases, *emergency contraception* can be used to prevent pregnancy. One type of emergency contraception is the *ParaGard* copper IUD. If inserted within five days of unprotected sex, it is the most effective method of emergency contraception. Several types of emergency contraceptive pills are also available, including *ella* and *Plan B*. These pills contain female hormones, which prevent ovulation and thicken cervical mucus. Emergency contraception is similar to other hormone-based birth control methods, but it contains a greater amount of the same hormones. Emergency contraception prevents fertilization; it does not stop or interrupt a pregnancy that has already occurred.

Most emergency contraceptive pills are available at drugstores without a prescription, and anyone can buy them, regardless of age. *ella* requires a doctor's prescription and is the most effective emergency contraceptive pill.

Emergency contraceptive pills can reduce the chance of pregnancy by up to 89% when used within five days of a woman having unprotected sex. The earlier it is taken, the more effective a pill will be. While effective as a back-up method, the 89% effectiveness rate of emergency contraception makes it less effective than the standard birth control pills and several other methods described in this chapter. Emergency contraception does not reduce the risk of the transmission of STIs and HIV/AIDS.

Emergency pills are not intended for regular use, and should not be used as regular birth control for several reasons. Long-term use can cause irregular and unpredictable periods. In addition, other forms of contraception are much less expensive and much more effective than the emergency pills.

Emergency contraceptive pills cost between $25 and $75. The cost of a doctor's visit, if needed, can be more expensive.

emergency contraception
contraceptive method that can be used to prevent pregnancy if other birth control fails or has been used incorrectly

Lesson 23.3 Review

Know and Understand

1. When used medically, which two hormones can stop ovulation?
2. What are the two forms of oral contraceptives?
3. In terms of location, how are birth control implants and IUDs different?
4. Describe the proper use of a vaginal ring for birth control.
5. Which hormone is contained in the birth control shot?
6. *True or false?* Emergency contraception protects against STI infection.

Analyze and Apply

7. Why might birth control pills be a poor option for someone who is forgetful?
8. Compare and contrast the two types of birth control pills.

Real World Health

Identify a person in your community who is an expert on birth control methods. This person could be a gynecologist or a therapist or counselor who specializes in reproductive health. Schedule an interview with this person and during your interview, ask about the hormonal birth control options that are available. For each type of birth control, ask the following questions:
- What are the short-term side effects?
- What are the long-term side effects?
- Are teenagers more likely to suffer from these side effects than people in their 20s, 30s, and 40s?
- How much does it cost?
- What are the advantages and disadvantages of using this contraceptive?
- How old do you have to be to purchase this contraceptive?

Natural Methods and Sterilization

Key Terms 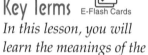 E-Flash Cards

In this lesson, you will learn the meanings of the following key terms.

abortion

fertility awareness method (FAM)

sterilization

tubal ligation

vasectomy

withdrawal

Before You Read

Understanding Topics

Scan the main headings in this lesson and create a chart like the one shown here. List the main headings in the first column and write what you think each heading describes in the second column. As you read the lesson, list what each section heading really describes in the third column.

Heading	What I Think It Describes	What It Really Describes

Lesson Objectives

After studying this lesson, you will be able to

- describe the fertility awareness method (FAM);
- identify natural methods for tracking an ovulation cycle;
- explain why the withdrawal method is ineffective;
- summarize reasons for choosing or avoiding sterilization; and
- determine what options are available when contraception fails.

Warm-Up Activity

Natural Methods

What are some natural methods for preventing pregnancy? Why do you think these methods are described as natural? Why might a couple decide to use natural methods? Why might they not *decide to use natural methods? Write a paragraph that includes your responses to these questions.*

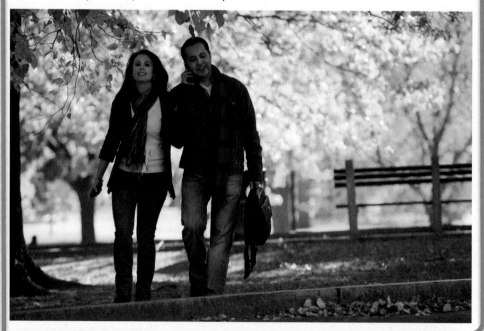

N atural methods of birth control do not use hormones, medicines, or barriers. Instead, they use techniques such as the fertility awareness method (FAM) and withdrawal.

In this lesson, you will read about various natural methods of birth control and about the only permanent method—sterilization.

Natural Methods

Some people prefer natural methods of contraception. This preference might be a result of religion prohibiting the use of contraceptive barriers, medicines, or hormones. Other people cannot use contraceptives for medical reasons. Additionally, the cost of contraceptive devices or medicines may mean some people cannot afford these methods. In each of these cases, people may choose to use natural birth control methods.

Fertility Awareness Method (FAM)

The *fertility awareness method (FAM)* is considered a natural birth control method because it takes advantage of the natural rhythm of a woman's fertility. Couples using FAM learn when the woman ovulates and which days the ovum is capable of being fertilized. FAM is extremely useful for planning a pregnancy, but it is only somewhat helpful for preventing pregnancy. There are several types of FAM and they all rely on monitoring a woman's cycle of fertility (Figure 23.15 on the next page).

You learned about the male and female reproductive systems in Chapter 20, *Reproduction and Pregnancy*. Reviewing that chapter, especially the section on *Ovulation and Menstruation* on pages 600–601 will help you understand how FAM works.

The Cycle of Fertility. As you read earlier in this textbook, a sperm must meet an ovum in the fallopian tube for fertilization to occur. This is possible during certain days of the menstrual cycle and impossible on other days.

The menstrual cycle ranges from 21 to 40 days, with the average span being about 28 days. In general, sexual intercourse on just 7 of those 28 days can result in an ovum being fertilized. This is because an ovum lives for about one day, while sperm can live for three to five days. This means it is possible for a woman to become pregnant if she has intercourse three to five days before ovulation, on the day of ovulation, and on the first—and possibly second—day after ovulation. If a woman wishes to become pregnant, she should have sexual intercourse on those days. If she wishes to avoid pregnancy, she should *not* have sexual intercourse on those days.

The best way to find out which days a woman can become pregnant is to determine which day she ovulates. Once she knows the day of ovulation, she will know the approximately seven days that she is capable of becoming pregnant. A woman can use several methods to determine when she is ovulating.

fertility awareness method (FAM)
a natural birth control method in which couples plan sexual intercourse for times when a woman is least fertile and avoid sexual intercourse during times of high fertility

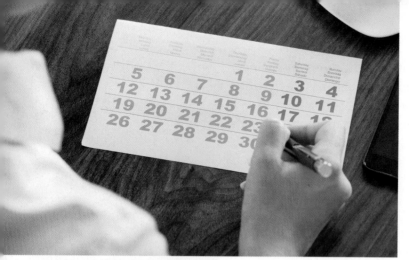

Figure 23.15

All of the different types of FAM involve keeping track of the woman's menstrual cycle each month. To do this effectively she needs to be detail-oriented, precise, consistent, and careful. Some women can do this more effectively than others.

Temperature Method. A woman can determine when she ovulates by measuring her body temperature. Her body temperature rises slightly after ovulation and stays higher than normal for most of the remainder of that menstrual cycle. Her temperature drops back to normal near the end of her cycle, when her period begins.

If she wants to prevent pregnancy, a woman should not have sex until three days after her body temperature rises (remember—the ovum lives for about one day, so wait three days to be safe). She can have sex from this point until her temperature declines, which is about the time she begins her next period and menstrual flow.

To avoid pregnancy, a woman must make sure no sperm are in her body in the days leading up to ovulation. A woman's temperature can tell her when an ovulation has just happened, but it cannot predict when the next ovulation will occur. To reduce her chances of becoming pregnant, a woman should have sex only in the interval described above: from three days after her temperature rises until the day her temperature declines.

The practice described above will reduce a woman's risk of pregnancy only if the woman correctly and precisely measures her body temperature. Women using FAM need to measure their *basal body temperature* (resting temperature) every morning when they wake up. During ovulation, a woman's temperature rises only by small amounts, just tenths of a degree. Because the change is so small, women should use a special basal temperature thermometer, which can be purchased at a drugstore for about $10. She should record her daily temperatures on a chart to track the changes and the pattern.

Women should record several months of temperature readings so that they can recognize their natural variations, and understand how different factors might affect their basal temperature (Figure 23.16). For example, one woman might notice that stress affects her body temperature. Another might discover that lack of sleep or alcohol consumption affects her body temperature. Because of these sorts of variations and uncertainties, most women combine the temperature method with another FAM, such as the cervical mucus method described below.

Cervical Mucus Method. Mucus is a thick, watery secretion that is present in many parts of the body, including the throat, intestines, stomach, lungs, and the vagina and cervix. The consistency of cervical mucus changes during the menstrual cycle. These changes include the following:

- *during period (menstrual flow)*: mucus cannot be observed because of the blood flow

- *a few days after flow*: there is little or no mucus ("dry" days)

- *as follicle and ovum ripen*: the amount of mucus increases and appears at the opening of the vagina; mucus is yellow or cloudy, and sticky

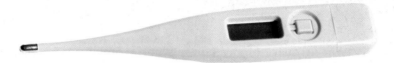

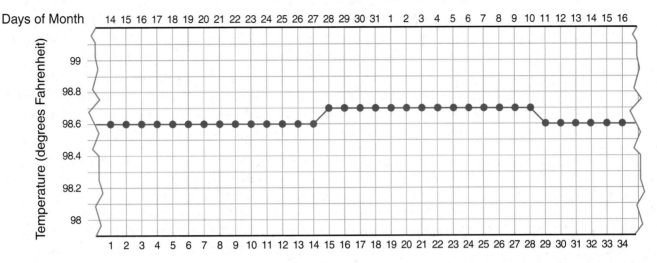

Days of Month 14 15 16 17 18 19 20 21 22 23 24 25 26 27 28 29 30 31 1 2 3 4 5 6 7 8 9 10 11 12 13 14 15 16

Days of Menstrual Cycle (the first day of menstruation is day 1; ovulation begins on day 14)

- *just before ovulation*: the most mucus is produced; mucus is clear and slippery ("slippery" days); may last four days; sexual intercourse during these days is most likely to result in a pregnancy
- *after four slippery days*: mucus reduces and becomes cloudy, and then turns dry again

According to the cervical mucus method, a woman can become pregnant two or three days before slippery mucus begins, for about three days after slippery mucus reaches its greatest amount, and possibly, but not likely, on a day at the end of her period. Using this method, a woman *cannot* become pregnant when the slippery mucus begins to decline, when it becomes sticky or cloudy, and during the dry days that follow this decline.

Women can examine their cervical mucus by placing their fingers inside their vagina or by examining mucus discharged on their underwear. Women should see their doctors for advice on how to assess their mucus.

Once a woman is confident that she knows her cycle and her cervical mucus, she can combine this information with her basal temperature to plan for or prevent pregnancy. Generally, if her cycle is regular and she can reliably identify her mucus, a woman can have sex during the "dry days" and avoid becoming pregnant.

The cervical mucus prevention method requires practice and some advice from a doctor. If used regularly and correctly, only about 3 out of 100 women will become pregnant.

Calendar-Based Methods. Several different calendar-based methods are used to reduce the risk of pregnancy. In general, a woman marks the day she begins her period and then marks the days on the calendar that she may and may not become pregnant. If her cycle is regular, and occurs every 26 to 33 days, she can use this method to predict when she is most likely to become pregnant.

Figure 23.16

Using a basal temperature thermometer and a chart like this one, a woman can record changes in her body temperature. Doing this regularly and precisely over a period of time can help her determine (but not guarantee) when she is ovulating. *Why would a woman want to know when she is ovulating?*

In place of a calendar, some women use beads on a string, called *cycle beads*, to keep track of these days. Generally, women cannot become pregnant during the six days that follow the beginning of their period, and during days 19–32 after their period begins (Figure 23.17). However, a woman's cycle can change at any time due to illness or stress.

Of the women with regular cycles who use this method regularly and correctly, about 5 out of 100 will become pregnant. The calendar method is not precise; it only predicts days that are likely or unlikely for pregnancy. It is especially unreliable for women with irregular periods.

Disadvantages of FAM. The FAM has several drawbacks and is not appropriate for everyone. FAM requires attention and record keeping and is subject to many mistakes. It requires cooperation with a woman's sexual partner. Many couples who use FAM do not use the methods regularly and correctly. As a result, about 25 out of 100 couples become pregnant, which is a very high rate of pregnancy compared with the other birth control methods discussed in this chapter.

Furthermore, FAM does not prevent STIs. FAM is best for couples who are married or in a committed, monogamous relationship. For these reasons, FAM is not recommended for teens.

Withdrawal

withdrawal
an unreliable birth control method in which a man pulls his penis out of a woman's vagina before he ejaculates; also known as pulling out

Withdrawal, or *pulling out*, is the most commonly used birth control method. A man using withdrawal pulls his penis out of the woman's vagina before he ejaculates. This may keep sperm out of the vagina and reduce the risk of pregnancy.

Withdrawal is *not* an effective method of birth control for several reasons. Withdrawal is difficult to time correctly and requires self-control. It is not easy for the man to withdraw during intense sexual excitement. In addition, before ejaculation, it is common for fluid containing sperm to leak from the penis. This pre-ejaculate fluid is known to cause pregnancy. Withdrawal results in many pregnancies and does not protect people from STIs.

Research shows that when withdrawal is used correctly every time, about 6% of women become pregnant. If not always performed correctly almost 30% of women become pregnant. This is a very high rate of pregnancy compared to the other birth control methods mentioned in this chapter.

Figure 23.17

Women using the *cycle beads* method described above use a chart like this one to keep track of the days that they can and cannot have sexual intercourse. The days shaded in blue are considered "safe." Sexual intercourse on the days shaded in yellow can result in pregnancy.

Period Begins

0	1	2	3	4	5	6
7	8	9	10	11	12	13
14	15	16	17	18	19	20
21	22	23	24	25	26	27
28	29	30	31	0	1	2

Period Begins

Sterilization

sterilization
a surgical contraceptive method in which a person is rendered permanently unable to conceive children

Sterilization is the only permanent birth control method. Sterilization procedures performed by a medical doctor prevent the sperm and ova from uniting to form a fertilized egg. Sterilization may be the best choice for adults who know they do not want children or any more children. However, sterilization is not appropriate for everyone. Reversing surgical sterilization is difficult and often unsuccessful. Therefore, people considering surgical sterilization must be sure they do not ever want children.

Couples choose sterilization because other contraceptive methods are, for various reasons, not acceptable. For example, hormonal birth control methods can be medically risky for women who have certain health conditions.

Some couples find that other birth control methods do not do enough to reduce the risk of pregnancy. For some women, pregnancy is simply too dangerous for health reasons, and they do not want to accept any risk of becoming pregnant.

Couples for Whom Sterilization Could Be the Best Choice

Sterilization could be the best choice for the following groups of people:

- *Adults who know they do not want to have children.* Adults who have had children may not want more. Other adults do not want to have children at all. Some adults would rather adopt children who need families.

- *Adults who find other birth control methods unacceptable for various reasons.* Hormonal methods may be risky or have too many side effects for some women. The risk of becoming pregnant using barrier methods may be too high for some people.

- *Adults who have a hereditary illness.* An adult who knows he or she has inherited a disease or disorder may not want to risk passing along this illness to children.

- *Adults who feel they are emotionally or financially unable to raise a family.* Not everyone has the stability necessary for raising a child. Some people may never feel "ready" for children.

Couples for Whom Sterilization Is Not a Good Choice

Sterilization is considered permanent, although people may attempt to undo the procedure and reestablish their fertility. This involves complicated, expensive surgery that is often unsuccessful, and sometimes impossible. Couples should choose sterilization for good reasons. Sterilization is *not* a good choice for some adults, including the following groups:

- *Adults who might want children.* If there is any chance people might someday want children, they should select a birth control method other than sterilization.

- *Adults who are being pressured.* Adults should not choose sterilization because of pressure from family or friends. Adults who are considering sterilization should make their own decisions since they are the ones who will live with the consequences of the decision.

- *Adults reacting to other personal problems.* Adults experiencing financial or personal stress might choose sterilization. They may not want to have children, who could compound their stress. Financial and personal stresses may be short-term, however. In these cases, non-permanent types of birth control should probably be used.

Vasectomy: Male Sterilization

vasectomy

a sterilization surgery in which a man's vas deferens is cut, preventing sperm from leaving the testes

Men can be sterilized through a procedure called *vasectomy*, a surgery performed by a doctor. During a vasectomy, two tubes called the *vas deferens* are closed, preventing sperm from leaving the testes. A vasectomy is usually done in the hospital and most men who have the surgery return home the same day.

The surgery involves a small incision or puncture in each side of the scrotum, through which the vas deferens is clipped, tied, or blocked (Figure 23.18). Vasectomy is nearly 100% effective, making it the most effective and permanent method of birth control for men.

Most men recover quickly with no side effects. Some men experience bruising, swelling, and discomfort after the procedure. After a vasectomy, the prostate and seminal vesicles continue to function. Men can ejaculate normally and continue to produce semen. The testes continue to make testosterone and men can have an erection and have sex, as they did prior to the operation. Couples should know that vasectomies are far less expensive than female sterilization.

Tubal Ligation: Female Sterilization

tubal ligation

a sterilization surgery in which a woman's fallopian tubes are cut, making it impossible for sperm to reach the ova

Women can be sterilized by cutting the fallopian tubes and sealing them with surgical thread, a surgery called *tubal ligation*. The tubes can also be closed with clamps, clips, or rings (Figure 23.19 on the next page). A section of each tube can also be removed. Each of these procedures makes it impossible for sperm to reach the ova, which means that tubal ligation is nearly 100% effective in preventing pregnancy.

Figure 23.18

In a vasectomy, the vas deferens are cut and sealed to stop the release of sperm. *Does a vasectomy affect a man's ability to have sex?*

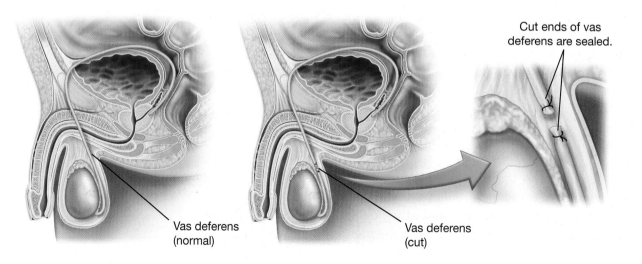

Cut ends of vas deferens are sealed.

Vas deferens (normal)

Vas deferens (cut)

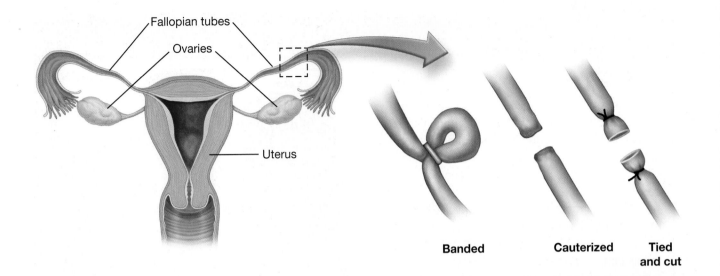

Banded   **Cauterized**   **Tied and cut**

Figure 23.19

In a tubal ligation procedure, the fallopian tubes are cut and sealed to stop sperm from reaching an ovum. *Which sterilization procedure is more expensive—a vasectomy or a tubal ligation?*

Some types of sterilization are done by a doctor in a hospital, while others are done in an outpatient surgery clinic. Depending on the type of surgery, some women return home the same day, while others recover in the hospital.

Three months after surgery, doctors must view an X-ray to confirm that the tubes were successfully blocked. During those first three months, a woman must use an alternative form of birth control.

Sterilization does not affect the function of the ovaries. A woman continues to make female hormones and ovulate after this procedure. Sterilization does not affect a woman's sexual characteristics, sexual arousal, or her ability to have sex. The procedure cannot cause menopause. If financial costs are a concern, couples might decide for the man to get the less expensive vasectomy.

Remember that sterilization prevents pregnancy by preventing sperm from reaching the ovum. People who have been sterilized must still use a condom to reduce the risk of STI transmission.

When Contraception Fails

As you know from reading this chapter, only one method of contraception is 100% effective—abstinence. That means that if couples use other contraceptive methods, and use them correctly, some women may still become pregnant. Unplanned pregnancies can also occur because couples fail to use any contraceptives or have medical complications, and in situations involving sexual abuse. When faced with an unplanned pregnancy, what options does a woman have?

Of course, the woman can decide to give birth and raise the child. As you read in chapter 21, some women decide to give birth, but then give the child up for adoption for emotional, medical, or financial reasons. Other women decide to end the pregnancy with a surgical procedure called **abortion**.

It is important to realize that abortion is not a type of birth control. Birth control methods—the methods you have read about in this chapter—are

abortion
a surgical procedure that ends a pregnancy

Long-Term, Reversible Contraceptives for Men

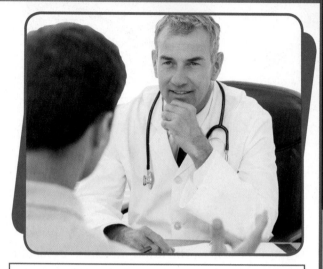

Women have had access to long-term and reversible birth control methods for many years. These methods include birth control pills, shots, patches, rings, and the diaphragm. Each method reduces the risk of pregnancy and each one is easily reversed.

No such methods have been available for men, until now. A procedure first used in India should be available in the United States in 2018. In this simple procedure, a doctor injects a substance called *Vasalgel* through the scrotum, into each vas deferens. Vasalgel works by breaking apart sperm cells.

The use of Vasalgel has several advantages over a vasectomy. The procedure takes only fifteen minutes, and men recover from the procedure quickly. Studies in India found it to be 100% effective. Perhaps the biggest advantage is that the procedure can be easily reversed. An injection in the vas deferens that inactivates the Vasalgel can restore sperm production in a few weeks.

Thinking Critically

1. Why is it important to have long-term birth control methods available to men as well as women?
2. Do you think this procedure will be more affordable than a vasectomy? Explain your answer.
3. Would you recommend this procedure for monogamous couples? Explain your answer.

designed to prevent a pregnancy from happening. Abortion is a procedure used to end a pregnancy that has already begun.

A woman who decides to have an abortion should do so at the earliest possible date. The further she is into the pregnancy, the more risk to her health should she decide to have an abortion. In general, abortions performed in the first three months are of minimal risk.

You are probably aware that abortion is a controversial topic. Many people are strongly opposed to abortion. Others believe it is a personal choice. For mature adults, deciding whether or not to have an abortion can be difficult. This decision will likely involve a person's religious beliefs, values, and strong emotions.

For teens, an unplanned pregnancy presents an especially difficult situation, as discussed in chapter 21. If considering abortion, these teens can benefit from a strong family support system. Counseling from doctors and spiritual advisors can also be helpful.

Helpful Resources

Having read this chapter, you should know more about different types of birth control, how they work, and their advantages and disadvantages. However, you may have more questions about birth control. Where will you turn for reliable information? How will you decide which sources to use and which information is correct?

You can ask these questions to determine the credibility of a source's information:

- *Does the source have medical expertise?* Birth control is based on human anatomy and physiology. A person or organization must have medical and scientific expertise to describe birth control. For example, a reliable source might be a medical organization, such as the Mayo Clinic, a hospital and research facility. A source like the Mayo Clinic employs doctors with MD degrees and expert researchers with PhD or MS degrees.

- *What is the mission or objective of the source?* The organization's mission should be easily found on its website. The mission describes the organization's purpose and goals. Your source must be dedicated to promoting the physical and mental health of teens. Their employees should have medical and scientific expertise.

- *Does the source describe alternatives?* Birth control is complicated. Many methods are available, and some may not be right for certain couples. Therefore, a source should offer information about several options, and their advantages and disadvantages. This allows couples to make a good decision about which birth control method is best for them.

- *Is the source a profit-making organization?* Some organizations are businesses with the goal of making money. The information these organizations present may be biased. For example, a company that makes a certain type of birth control may present incomplete or misleading information about abstinence or other birth control methods in an effort to make you choose their birth control option.

Lesson 23.4 Review

Know and Understand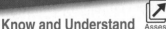

1. *True or false?* The FAM method is more effective for preventing a pregnancy than planning a pregnancy.

2. How long is the average menstrual cycle?

3. Explain the use of the temperature method.

4. _____ is the only permanent method of birth control.

5. What is a vasectomy?

Analyze and Apply

6. Why might natural methods be preferable to barrier methods, medicines, or hormonal methods?

7. Why are calendar-based birth control methods especially unreliable for women with irregular periods?

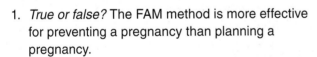

Use the Internet to research the sterilization options available for men and women. For each sterilization procedure, list what the procedure does, when and where the procedure is performed, how much the procedure costs, advantages and disadvantages of the procedure, and how effective it is. After gathering your information, create an informative pamphlet or brochure that details the sterilization methods you researched. Present your final product to the class.

Family Planning and the Role of Abstinence

Key Terms

contraception   family planning

Key Points

- Family planning allows couples to decide how many children they would like to have and when.
- Teen parenthood results in a variety of challenges including increased health risks, financial burdens, and disrupted education.
- Continuous abstinence is the only method of birth control and STI prevention that is 100% effective.
- Examining the pros and cons of different contraceptives can help a couple choose the method that works best for them.
- Understanding reproduction facts and myths will help guard against unplanned pregnancy.
- Cost, effectiveness, ease of use, and expense are some factors to consider when choosing a method of birth control.

Check Your Understanding

1. Identify five reasons to choose abstinence.
2. Which of the following is an effective method for preventing pregnancy?
   A. urinating after sex
   B. using the pull-out method
   C. standing up after sex
   D. None of the above
3. *True or false?* Girls younger than 18 years of age cannot become pregnant.
4. Which of the following is a consequence of teen parenthood?
   A. disrupted education
   B. physical health risks
   C. financial burden
   D. All of the above
5. What health risks are associated with teenage pregnancy and parenthood?
6. *True or false?* A woman cannot become pregnant during her menstrual cycle.
7. **Critical Thinking.** How might a couple benefit from family planning?

Condoms and Other Barrier Methods

Key Terms

barrier methods   contraceptive sponge
cervical cap   diaphragm
condoms   spermicide

Key Points

- Barrier methods physically prevent sperm from reaching the ovum.
- No barrier method is 100% effective in preventing STI transmission.
- Condoms can only be used once, must be stored appropriately, and disposed of once expired.
- Applying or removing a condom incorrectly may cause it to be less effective.
- Female condoms, contraceptive sponges, diaphragms, and cervical caps are forms of birth control inserted into the vagina prior to intercourse.

Check Your Understanding

8. How do barrier methods prevent pregnancy?
   A. by stopping ovulation
   B. by stopping sperm
   C. by stopping hormones
   D. by stopping menstruation
9. *True or false?* It is safe to store condoms in a car or wallet.
10. How should a male condom be removed?
11. Male condoms can be made of _____.
    A. polyurethane
    B. sheepskin
    C. latex
    D. All of the above
12. What is a cervical cap?
13. *True or false?* A contraceptive sponge will prevent STI transmission.
14. How do condoms prevent pregnancy?
15. Which barrier method can be used more than once over the course of a 30-hour period?
16. **Critical Thinking.** What are some strategies for increasing condom use among sexually active teenagers?

Hormonal Methods, IUDs, and Emergency Contraception

Key Terms

emergency contraception   oral contraceptive
intrauterine device (IUD)

Key Points

- Estrogen and progesterone are used in hormonal contraceptives to prevent ovulation.
- Oral contraceptives prevent ovulation and thicken cervical mucus, which slows down sperm.
- The birth control patch contains hormones that are absorbed through the skin and into the bloodstream.
- Progesterone injections given every three months are a highly effective form of birth control.
- Birth control implants and IUDs have high initial costs but last for several years.
- When taken within five days of unprotected sex, emergency contraception can prevent ovulation.

Check Your Understanding

17. How do birth control pills prevent pregnancy?

18. What is the difference between combination birth control pills and progesterone-only birth control pills?

19. *True or false?* The birth control patch should be worn continuously for four weeks, and then discarded.

20. How do hormones in the birth control patch enter a woman's body?

21. *True or false?* Oral contraceptives also prevent STI transmission.

22. How often must the birth control shot be administered to be effective?

23. Which two hormonal contraceptives must be inserted by a doctor?

24. *True or false?* Emergency contraception prevents ovulation and thickens cervical mucus.

25. **Critical Thinking.** Why should hormonal contraception be combined with a barrier method such as a condom?

Natural Methods and Sterilization

Key Terms

abortion
fertility awareness method (FAM)
sterilization

tubal ligation
vasectomy
withdrawal

Key Points

- Natural birth control methods do not use hormones, medications, or barriers.
- The fertility awareness method (FAM) uses the natural rhythm of a woman's fertility cycle to prevent pregnancy.
- Ovulation dates can be identified using the temperature method, cervical mucus method, or calendar-based method.
- Withdrawal, or *pulling out*, is not an effective method of birth control.
- Sterilization is the only permanent method of birth control.
- A vasectomy is the surgical procedure used to sterilize males; women are sterilized through tubal ligation.
- Abortion is a procedure used to end a pregnancy; it is not a method of birth control.

Check Your Understanding

26. Sexual intercourse on _____ days of a woman's 28-day cycle can result in fertilization.

27. *True or false?* A woman's body temperature drops slightly after ovulation.

28. According to the cervical mucus method, on which days can a woman become pregnant?

29. What are three disadvantages to using the FAM method?

30. *True or false?* Withdrawal is an effective method of birth control.

31. _____ is the only permanent method of birth control.

32. **Critical Thinking.** Why is the FAM method more appropriate for monogamous, adult couples than teens?

Health and Wellness Skills

33. **Communicate with Others.** Contact a person you know who had a baby early in his or her life, preferably before or during college. List several questions that you would like answered and then interview this person about his or her experience. After the interview, write an essay describing what you learned.

34. **Set Goals.** Create a timeline for your life. What are your goals for the next five years? the next ten years? Do you want children? Remember that to reach your goals, you also need to set restrictions. Identify what events or pressures might deter you from living the life you have planned, and describe how you might avoid these obstacles.

35. **Analyze Influences.** How do you think the media portrays teen pregnancy? Write a short paragraph in response to this question. Be sure to provide specific examples that support your beliefs.

36. **Advocate for Health.** The number of teen pregnancies in the United States has declined over the past two decades. However, the number of pregnant teenagers in the United States is still extremely high compared to other industrialized countries. Plan an event within your school or community that will outline the potential outcomes of sexual activity during the teenage years and explain why abstinence is a positive choice. In your event, also compare contraceptive options to avoid pregnancy.

Hands-On Activity
The Cost of Birth Control

Contraception can seem expensive to those who are buying it often or are considering buying it. The costs of purchasing contraception are minimal, however, in comparison to the costs of giving birth to and caring for a baby. In this activity, you will research online or visit local stores to compare the cost of purchasing contraception for one year versus the cost of having and caring for a baby for one year.

Materials Needed

pad of paper, calculator, camera, computer

Steps for this Activity

1. Choose two contraceptive products discussed in this chapter. The products you choose should be available at a store. Research or estimate how often a person might need to purchase these products if he or she were sexually active.

2. Develop a comprehensive list that includes all the products a person would need to purchase to care for a newborn baby. Include cribs, carriers, baby clothes, and repeat purchases such as diapers, wipes, and food. Also research and record the cost of giving birth to a baby at your local hospital. You may use the information you gathered in Lesson 1's Real World Health activity for this step.

3. Now, calculate the costs of the items on your list. Use your computer to do your price checking online, or go to local stores. If you do your research at a local store, take a camera. First, find the contraceptive products you chose and find their prices. Take screen shots or print pictures of the products if you are working online. Take pictures if you are in a store. Then, locate all of the items on your list and record their prices. Take pictures of all these items, or print screenshots from your computer.

4. Multiply the costs of the contraceptive products you chose by the number of times a person would purchase them in one year of being sexually active. Record this number on a piece of paper. Then, add up the prices of the items a person would need to care for a newborn baby for one year. Make sure to multiply the cost of repeat purchases such as diapers. Finally, add the cost of giving birth to a baby. Record your total.

5. Compare the two numbers you recorded. How big is the difference between the cost of using contraception for one year and the cost of birthing and caring for a baby? On a poster, write both numbers and attach pictures of all the items a person would purchase in each situation. Present your poster to the class.

Core Skills

Math Practice

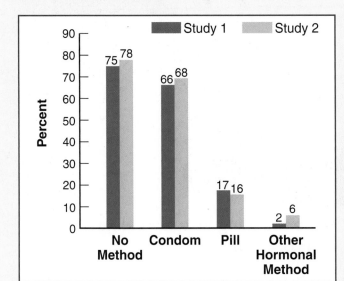

The graph above shows the use of birth control among females between 15 and 19 years of age the first time they had sex, as determined by two different studies. Study the graph and then answer the questions.

37. What percentage of teenage girls were not using any method of birth control in the first study?
    A. 22%
    B. 75%
    C. 25%
    D. 78%

38. Approximately what percentage of girls were using a hormonal method in the second study?
    A. 2%
    B. 20%
    C. 16%
    D. 6%

39. Assuming 100 girls responded to each survey, how many more girls were relying on condoms for contraception than the pill in the second study?
    A. 16
    B. 17
    C. 52
    D. 49

Reading and Writing Practice

Read the passage below and then answer the questions.

Oral contraceptives are usually referred to as the birth control pill—or just *the* pill. *Birth control pills contain hormones that reduce the likelihood of pregnancy. The pill is taken by mouth, or orally, and should be taken at about the same time every day. Oral contraceptives do not prevent STIs, HPV, or cervical cancer.*

Birth control pills prevent ovulation, which means that there is no ovum for sperm to fertilize. The pill also thickens cervical mucus, which slows down sperm's movement into the uterus.

Doctors need to examine all women using hormone-based birth control methods because women with certain medical conditions should not take the pill. The pill is effective at preventing pregnancy if taken exactly as prescribed by the doctor. Skipping even one pill increases the chance of becoming pregnant. Some research suggests that women who use birth control pills have an increased risk of contracting STIs.

The pill comes in two basic forms—the combination pill and the progesterone-only pill.

40. How do oral contraceptives prevent pregnancy?
    A. by speeding up ovulation
    B. by thinning the cervical mucus
    C. by preventing ovulation and thickening the cervical mucus
    D. by killing sperm in the uterus

41. Why is a medical exam required to obtain a prescription for oral contraception?
    A. to determine the length of the woman's cycle and how many pills she will need
    B. to prevent girls under 18 years of age from taking the pill
    C. because women with certain medical conditions should not take the pill
    D. None of the above.

42. Do oral contraceptives prevent STIs, HPV, or cervical cancer? Why or why not?

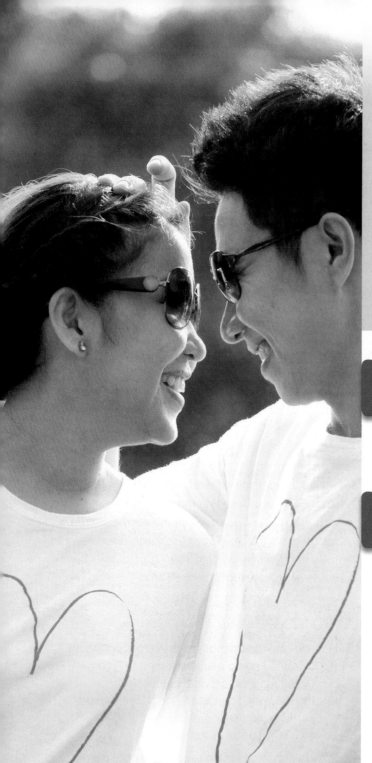

Chapter 24
Understanding Sexuality

Lesson 24.1

Understanding Sexual Feelings and Behavior

Lesson 24.2

What Is Sexuality?

While studying this chapter, look for the activity icon 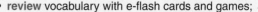 to:
- **review** vocabulary with e-flash cards and games;
- **assess** learning with quizzes and online exercises;
- **expand** knowledge with animations and activities; and
- **listen** to pronunciation of key terms in the audio glossary.

G-WLEARNING.com

www.g-wlearning.com/health/

Take this quiz to see what you do and do not know about sexuality. If you cannot answer a question, pay extra attention to that topic as you study this chapter.

1. *Identify each statement as* True, False, *or* It Depends. *Choose* It Depends *if a statement is true in some cases, but false in others.*
2. *Revise each* False *statement to make it true.*
3. *Explain the circumstances in which each* It Depends *statement is true and when it is false.*

Health and Wellness IQ Assess

1.	Sexual thoughts and feelings are normal during puberty.	True	False	It Depends
2.	Most teens are not sexually active.	True	False	It Depends
3.	A baby's biological sex is obvious at birth.	True	False	It Depends
4.	Gender identity is assigned at birth and never changes.	True	False	It Depends
5.	It is possible for a person to embody the extremes of femininity or masculinity.	True	False	It Depends
6.	Many teenagers who are homosexual are comfortable with their sexual orientation.	True	False	It Depends
7.	Sexual activity requires mutual consent.	True	False	It Depends
8.	Masculinity means that all men must possess aggression and strength.	True	False	It Depends
9.	Ejaculation occurs during orgasm.	True	False	It Depends
10.	Gender is determined by a person's genes.	True	False	It Depends

Setting the Scene

Sexuality is a natural and important part of human biology and behavior. During puberty, sexual development speeds up. As a result, adolescents experience physical changes and unfamiliar, intense drives and emotions. It is normal for adolescents to become curious about sex, sexual development, and romantic relationships at this point in their lives.

These new thoughts and emotions can be confusing. You probably have many questions, which is only natural. Your thoughts, questions, and emotions are the result of human biology unfolding during puberty.

For a happy and healthy transition to adulthood, you need to have reliable information and develop effective skills for dealing with sex, sexuality, and relationships. This chapter should answer some of your questions and help you develop the skills you need to address these important topics.

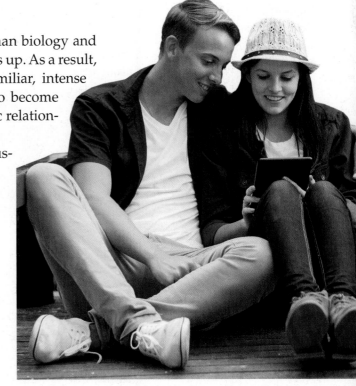

Understanding Sexual Feelings and Behavior

Key Terms
E-Flash Cards

In this lesson, you will learn the meanings of the following key terms.

estrogens

human sexual response cycle

masturbation

orgasm

Before You Read

Understanding the Lesson

Skim the headings and subheadings in this lesson and consider what questions you have about sexual feelings and behavior. List three to four of these questions, especially those that you expect will be answered in this lesson. After reading the lesson, revisit your questions and answer them, if possible. If they have not been answered, research answers to your questions or ask an adult in your life about them.

Lesson Objectives

After studying this lesson, you will be able to

- identify the physical and hormonal changes associated with puberty;
- list the phases of the human sexual response cycle;
- explain the impact of sexual relationships; and
- explore the benefits of abstinence and strategies for dealing with sexual pressure.

Warm-Up Activity

You Want To Talk About Sex?

Being curious about sex is a normal part of a teenager's development. Understanding good sexual health and practices is important, not only for your adolescent years, but also for your lifetime. Why is it important to talk about this subject? Why do you think some people have a hard time talking about sex? Who might you need to talk to about sex? If you have a hard time discussing this subject, what might make it easier? Think about answers to these questions and then share your thoughts with a classmate.

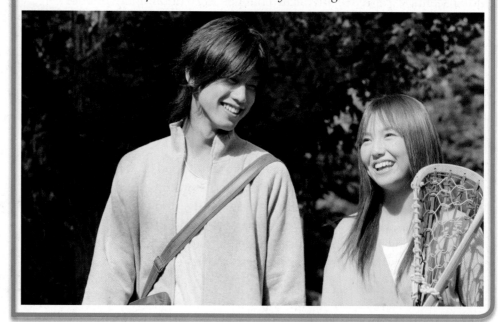

C an you remember when your peers—who once hung out in same-sex groups—begin to pair off into couples? Do you remember when you began having sexual feelings and thoughts?

In this lesson, you will learn about the sexual feelings that develop during adolescence and how the body responds to them. You'll also learn why entering sexual relationships in response to these feelings carries risks and responsibilities that teenagers can find difficult to handle.

Puberty

Puberty plays a major role in your sexual development. In chapter 22, you read about the physical changes that occur as children go through puberty and adolescence on their way to adulthood. You read briefly about the hormones that transform your body from that of a child into that of an adult. These hormones also trigger powerful sexual feelings and drive the physical and emotional changes of puberty. Because these changes are so important to your sexuality, this lesson will examine puberty more closely.

The Importance of Sex Hormones

Hormones are specialized chemical messengers produced by glands and released into the blood. Because hormones travel through blood, they can carry their messages to nearly every cell in the body. Each type of hormone affects the activity of only specific target tissue. For example, the hormone known as *growth hormone* affects only bone, muscle, and connective tissue. A hormone called *oxytocin* affects only the uterus and the mammary glands.

Before puberty, sex hormones are present in the body, but at low levels. Puberty is triggered when the brain releases *gonadotropin-releasing hormone*, which specifically affects the pituitary gland located in the brain. The pituitary gland controls many other glands in the body. The gonadotropin-releasing hormone signals the pituitary gland to begin producing *follicle-stimulating hormone* and *luteinizing hormone* (Figure 24.1).

These hormones affect the testes in boys and the ovaries in girls. The testes respond by increasing the secretion of testosterone, and the ovaries respond by producing higher amounts of hormones called *estrogens*. In boys, testosterone triggers growth and development of the testes, penis,

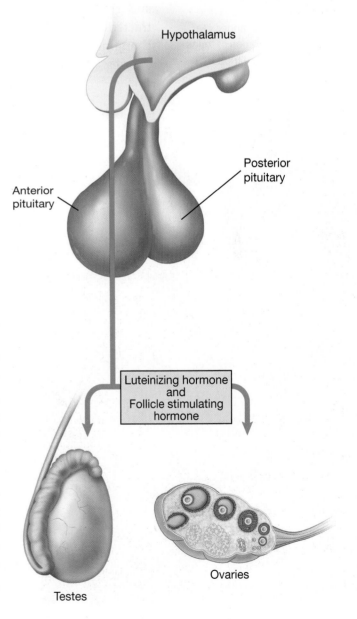

Figure 24.1

Luteinizing hormone and follicle-stimulating hormone are released by the pituitary gland and stimulate the testes and ovaries. *What hormones do the testes and ovaries release in response to this stimulation?*

Hypothalamus

Posterior pituitary

Anterior pituitary

Luteinizing hormone and Follicle stimulating hormone

Ovaries

Testes

estrogens
hormones that trigger the development of the ovaries, breasts, and other sexual characteristics in females

and other sexual characteristics. In girls, **estrogens** trigger growth and development of the ovaries, breasts, and other sexual characteristics.

What Changes Can You Expect?

As you know if you read chapter 22, both boys and girls should expect dramatic physical and emotional changes during puberty. Some changes occur abruptly, and others happen gradually. Some teens experience a growth spurt in which they quickly grow taller, repeatedly outgrowing their pants and shoes. The growth spurt is the most obvious external change that occurs during puberty, and it can be embarrassing for teens who grow faster or slower than most of their friends.

Other physical changes include some weight gain. In boys, this is due to muscle development. In girls, weight gain is due to the development of both body fat and muscle.

Elevated hormone levels also affect the brain and may cause both boys and girls to become sensitive, emotional, easily angered, and sexually attracted to others. It is also normal for boys and girls to worry about their changing bodies and feelings. Questions commonly fall into these categories: "Am I normal?" and "Should I feel this way?" Both the physical changes and emerging sexual feelings of puberty are expected and perfectly normal.

During puberty, boys and girls develop primary and secondary sexual characteristics. Primary sexual characteristics pertain to the sex organs. Secondary sexual characteristics pertain to other parts of the body and are signs that the body is maturing (Figure 24.2).

In boys, the testes and penis grow. Boys' shoulders broaden, muscles develop, their voices deepen, and they grow facial hair and more body hair, especially under the arms and around the genitals. Acne often develops on the face, shoulders, chest, and back. The sweat glands under the arms and around the genitals produce thicker, odorous sweat. Boys will also notice *erections*, the lengthening and hardening of the penis in response to sexual excitement or for no reason at all. Along with these physical changes, boys become curious about sex, and they may feel sexually attracted to another person.

In girls, the ovaries, vagina, and labia mature and grow. Girls' bodies change shape, hips widen, and body fat develops, especially at the hips and breasts. Breasts and nipples grow, sometimes becoming temporarily asymmetrical or sore. Menstruation begins about 2 years after the breasts develop. Vaginal secretions increase. Hair develops under the arms and around the genitals. With these physical changes, girls also grow curious about sex and may experience sexual attraction.

Figure 24.2

The development of secondary sexual characteristics changes the physical appearance of teens as they go through puberty.

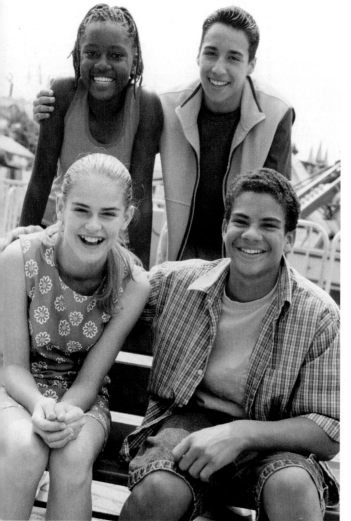

Early Sexual Feelings

If you're around children—even very young children—you may notice that they frequently touch their own genitals. From an early age, children are curious about their bodies and derive pleasure and comfort from touching themselves.

As you have just read, curiosity about sex is a sign of normal development during the teenage years. Sexual excitement, or *arousal*, is also normal, and can be caused by sexual thoughts, daydreams, or images that originate in the brain. Many teenagers find themselves thinking about sex often or having sexual dreams and fantasies about celebrities or people they know. Teenage boys may also experience erections and nocturnal emissions. A nocturnal emission, or *wet dream*, is ejaculation that occurs during sleep.

During adolescence, both boys and girls might begin masturbating in response to the sexual arousal caused by their dreams and fantasies. *Masturbation* is self-stimulation of the sex organs and is a common, normal response to sexual excitement. Masturbation is a sexual activity that allows people to safely release sexual tension. During adolescence, masturbation may culminate in orgasm, which you will read about later in this section.

Some teenagers feel embarrassed or guilty about masturbating because they've been led to believe that masturbation is wrong or shameful. They may have heard that masturbation can cause acne, blindness, or other problems. These beliefs are myths—masturbation does not cause these problems. Teens who are uncertain about how to respond to these impulses can talk about masturbation with a doctor, nurse, parent, or other trusted adult.

masturbation
self-stimulation of the sex organs in response to sexual excitement

Human Sexual Response Cycle

Feelings of sexual attraction accompany sexual development during puberty. The sex organs and brain produce hormones that influence sexual development and feelings. You may already be experiencing these feelings; if not, you probably will before too long. This combination of romantic and physical attraction is new, complicated, and intense, as well as a normal part of human biology.

Physical attraction often leads to sexual excitement. When a person becomes sexually aroused, physical changes occur in the body. The physical changes occur in four phases—excitement, plateau, orgasm, and resolution. Together, these phases are referred to as the *human sexual response cycle*.

human sexual response cycle
term for the four phases of physical changes that occur when a person is sexually aroused; includes the excitement phase, plateau phase, orgasmic phase, and resolution phase

Excitement Phase

The excitement phase begins with increased blood flow to the sensitive sex organs. In females, the clitoris responds by elongating and swelling. The labia swell, flush with color, and separate. In males, the penis responds by lengthening and hardening.

Sexual stimulation of the female causes increased vaginal secretions, which lubricate and prepare the vagina for sexual intercourse. Blood flow increases to the vagina, labia, and clitoris, causing a warm sensation. The breasts swell and become sensitive.

Sexual stimulation of the male causes blood to flow into the erectile tissue of the penis, and results in an erection. The erect penis becomes hard, elongated, and capable of being inserted into the vagina for sexual intercourse. The heart rate and blood pressure increase in both males and females.

Plateau Phase

During the plateau phase, heart rate and blood pressure continue to rise. In females, blood flow increases to the vaginal wall, the labia continue to swell and flush with color, and the clitoris withdraws under tissue called a *hood*. In males, the penis becomes fully erect and the testes swell.

orgasm
the climax of sexual excitement, characterized by pleasurable sensations in the genital area

Orgasmic Phase

Sexual excitement may increase and proceed to the orgasmic phase. *Orgasm* is the climax of sexual excitement, characterized by pleasurable sensations in the genital area. This phase is marked by rhythmic muscular contractions in the sex organs and throughout the body.

In males, orgasm usually accompanies ejaculation. Ejaculation occurs when muscular contractions forcefully eject semen out of the urethral opening of the penis. Orgasm in females occurs as rhythmic vaginal contractions. During orgasm, both males and females experience an intense sense of pleasure and release.

Resolution Phase

During the resolution phase, blood pressure lowers and heart rate slows down. Less blood flows to the sex organs. In females, the labia and clitoris reduce in size and return to their unexcited state. Males lose their erection and the testes return to their unexcited size and position.

Impacts of Sexual Relationships

For adults in committed relationships, sexual feelings lead to sexual activities that can facilitate physical and emotional intimacy. Sexual feelings solidify these relationships and bring people closer.

Sexual activity does not play the same role in relationships between teenagers. Sexual activity can bring intense emotion and stress to romantic teen relationships and can complicate lives in ways that teenagers are unprepared for (Figure 24.3). You may want to review Chapter 18, Lesson 3, *Healthy Dating Relationships*, which describes factors involved in both healthy and unhealthy relationships.

Figure 24.3

Sexual activity can complicate teenage relationships, creating intense emotion and even conflict.

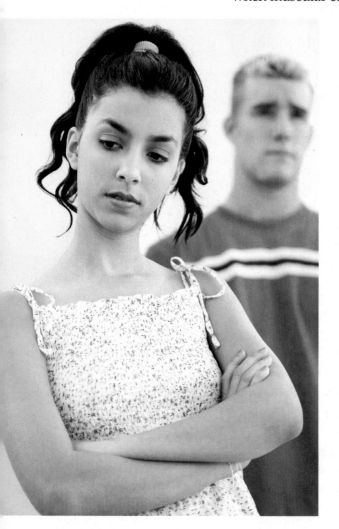

In addition to the risk of pregnancy and the risk of contracting sexually transmitted infections, sexually active teens face emotional and social challenges that can have unfortunate consequences. While teens are developing the desire and capability for having sex, experts agree that many teens are not emotionally mature enough to handle the consequences of sexual activity. The following scenarios illustrate just a few of the problems that can occur:

- *Trust*—After having sex with his girlfriend, Miles finds out that she told her friends. He feels betrayed that she shared something that he considered private with others. Miles' girlfriend doesn't seem to think this is a big deal. This type of breach in trust can end a relationship.

- *Individual Growth*—Matt and Jane have been dating for a while and decide to have sex. This decision makes their relationship more intense, and Matt and Jane soon find they are focusing only on their relationship to the exclusion of other relationships and their own personal growth. Their schoolwork begins to suffer, Matt even misses a few football practices, and Jane finds herself turning down invitations from her friends to hang out. Venturing into sexual activity for the first time can create an intensity in teen relationships that makes it difficult to focus on individual growth.

- *Jealousy*—After Robert began having sex with his girlfriend, he noticed a change in her. She is now possessive and jealous; she calls and texts him constantly. She gets upset if he talks to another girl or if he is out with friends. If Robert's girlfriend believes that sex should lead to marriage, and he does not, this may make her anxious. The more she pushes, the more he withdraws, and the more unstable the relationship becomes.

Health in the Media

Portrayal of Sex in the Media

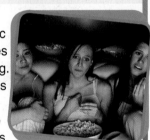

Sexual images are used in television programs, movies, music videos, and music to get audiences interested and keep them watching. The portrayal of sex in the media is often a fiction. In fact, the media often sends potentially destructive messages about sex to consumers. Some programs portray men or women as objects for sexual activity. Others associate sexual activity with aggressive behavior or violence. Research shows that, as media exposure increases, teens are more likely to accept sex role stereotypes as realistic.

For this activity, view a music video or popular television program that features young adults or teen performers. Evaluate the video (decide *yes* or *no*) according to each of the following statements about sex or sexual behavior. Then answer the questions that follow.

- People are often portrayed as sex objects.
- People often wear revealing clothes.
- Physical appearance of men or women seems more important than other personal qualities.
- Kissing and sexual activity are important parts of the story or plot.
- Most of the dialogue focuses on discussions about romantic and sexual relationships or sexual activity.
- Most scenes that portray romantic relationships show or imply sexual activity.
- Abstinence or birth control use is not shown, implied, or discussed.

Thinking Critically

1. How do these media images differ from your real-life experiences?
2. What is wrong with portraying men or women as sexual objects?
3. Do you think any of these images and messages influence teenagers' views on sex? Explain your answer.

Before a couple chooses to be sexually active or to enter a sexual relationship, they should do the following:

- *Discuss* their views on sex. This discussion should occur early in the relationship, before people become sexually involved or sexually aroused. People should be able to give their views openly and honestly, knowing that their partner will listen and understand. If a person is undecided about sex, he or she needs to make a decision before beginning a romantic relationship. It takes maturity to share, communicate honestly, and to trust.

- *Respect* the other person's decision about sex. Before having sex, each person must consent to sex. One person cannot make the decision for the other person or assume that the other person will go along.

- *Agree* on the methods that will be used for birth control and the prevention of STIs. If the decision is to engage in sexual activity, both people should agree on the method of protection they will use. These methods are summarized in chapter 23.

- *Share* their sexual histories. If either person is infected with an STI, the couple must discuss this and take steps to prevent transmission of the infection to the uninfected partner.

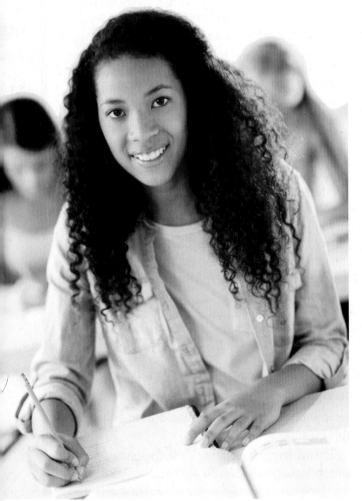

Choosing abstinence allows a teen to focus on personal growth. *What are some other benefits of choosing abstinence?*

Choosing Abstinence

Throughout this text, you have read that abstinence is recommended for teenagers for many reasons. Important reasons for choosing abstinence include avoiding pregnancy and avoiding the transmission of sexually transmitted infections. Because sexually active teens often focus on their relationships at the expense of their individual growth, abstinence can also be beneficial to a person's growth and self-esteem. Immature teens involved in sexual relationships can experience reduced intellectual, social, and emotional growth, while their peers who choose abstinence continue to mature and grow in all of these aspects of health and wellness (Figure 24.4).

Teenage romantic relationships can be fun and rewarding without sex. Knowing the reasons you want to abstain will help you stick to your decision. Be clear in your own mind about the reasons you will abstain from sex so that you can explain your decision to your boyfriend or girlfriend.

You should avoid situations that will make abstinence difficult. These situations could include alcohol or drug use and unsupervised parties.

If you feel confused about how to make a decision about a sexual relationship, talk to a trusted adult—a parent, adult sibling, doctor, or teacher (Figure 24.5).

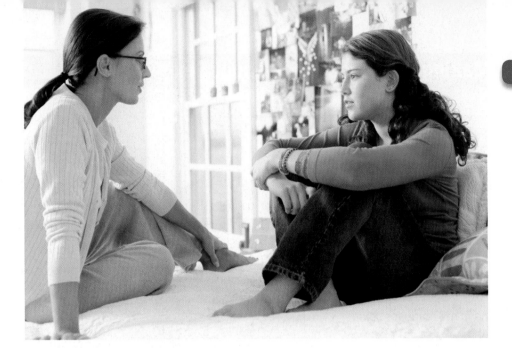

Figure 24.5

Sharing your concerns about sex with a parent or adult sibling can help you make an informed decision.

These people can help you understand your concerns so that you can make a well-reasoned decision. Your decision to abstain from sex is entirely your own, and is a sign that you are strong, in control of your body, and focused on your goals and the future.

Dealing with Sexual Pressure

Teenagers who choose abstinence may encounter many outside pressures and conflicting messages about sex. Boyfriends or girlfriends may pressure them to have sex. Their friends and peers may tell them "everyone is doing it." However, this is not true. In reality, most teenagers are not having sex.

Many of these conflicting messages come from the media. Advertisements, films, and other media often portray teenagers and young adults involved in sexual relationships. The implied message is that sex is a common part of teen relationships. In the media, sexual relationships seem casual, involving little or no responsibility, risk, or emotional fallout. While these scenes create interesting storylines, the messages they convey are not realistic.

SKILLS FOR HEALTH AND WELLNESS

Resisting Sexual Pressure

Certain situations can put you at risk for unwanted sexual activity. These may be situations that involve sexual pressure, so refusal skills are important. You have read about refusal skills on pages such as 385 and 386 in this textbook. Here are some strategies that will help you resist pressure to engage in sex and avoid unwanted sexual activity.

- Practice what you would say if pressured to engage in sexual activity.

- Surround yourself with like-minded people who will help you resist unhealthy peer pressure.

- Go out with a group instead of only the person you are interested in.

- Use your words to strongly refuse any sexual pressure—say "no" and mean "no" if that's how you feel.

- If you continue to be pressured after verbally refusing, leave the situation.

- Carry money for a cab, or call a parent, caregiver, or friend if you need to get away from someone.

- Remember why you want to remain abstinent. Reminding yourself of those reasons will help strengthen your ability to refuse pressure.

Marie and Craig have been dating for three months. After a concert, Craig asks Marie to hang out at his house. Craig's parents are not home, and after he and Marie begin kissing, he tells Marie that he wants to have sex. Craig and Marie have not been having sex, and they have not yet discussed sex. Marie does not want to have sex, and she is not sure what to do.

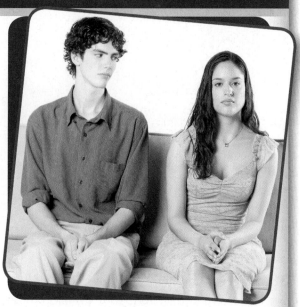

Thinking Critically

1. Marie is in an uncomfortable situation. What do you think she should say and do?

2. If Marie tells Craig she is not ready for sex, what should he say and do?

3. How could Marie and Craig have avoided placing themselves in this difficult situation?

If you find yourself in a situation that makes abstinence difficult, there are several things you can do to resist sexual pressure. Practice the words and actions you would use if faced with pressure to engage in sexual activity. Knowing what you would say and do will make dealing with sexual pressure easier. Remember that verbally refusing may not be enough; you may have to physically leave the situation or walk away from people who are pressuring you. It can also be helpful to find a group of supportive people—friends and trusted adults—who understand your decision to remain abstinent and can help you resist sexual pressure.

Lesson 24.1 Review

Know and Understand Assess

1. What are hormones?

2. Which hormone triggers the start of puberty?

3. List three changes boys experience during puberty and three changes girls experience.

4. _____ is self-stimulation of the sex organs.

5. What is the human sexual response cycle?

6. *True or false?* A couple should reveal their sexual histories before beginning a sexual relationship.

Analyze and Apply

7. Why might sexual activity create feelings of jealousy in a relationship?

8. Why should a couple discuss their views on sex before becoming sexually active?

Real World Health

When it comes to sex, people sometimes say that "everyone is doing it." The media may support this belief by portraying teens and young adults who are involved in casual sexual relationships with no responsibilities attached. Research the latest statistics on teenagers and sexual activity. How many teenagers are actually sexually active? Are these sexual relationships really casual, with no responsibilities attached? Record a short infomercial or PSA discussing the phrase "everyone is doing it."

What Is Sexuality?

Lesson Objectives

After studying this lesson, you will be able to

- recognize the different aspects of sexuality;
- explain the concept of biological sex;
- describe how gender is identified and expressed;
- summarize the differences between masculinity and femininity;
- identify various sexual orientations; and
- understand the challenges associated with homophobia.

Warm-Up Activity

Word Swap

List the terms masculine *and* feminine *on a separate sheet of paper, leaving space below each term. Write the first thing you think of when you hear each term. Then exchange papers with as many students as you can in the time given by your teacher. Write something new for each term on your classmates' papers; do not repeat any comments from previous students. When the time is up, get your own paper back and read what your classmates wrote. Share your notes with the class.*

Masculine	Feminine

Key Terms E-Flash Cards

In this lesson, you will learn the meanings of the following key terms.

biological sex

bisexual

heterosexual

homophobia

homosexual

intersex

sexual orientation

sexuality

transgender

Before You Read

Using the SQ3R Method
Use the **SQ3R** *method of comprehension to survey and then thoroughly read and understand this lesson. First,* **S**urvey *this lesson by glancing through it. Then, rewrite the headings and subheadings as* **Q**uestions *that might be answered within the text. Third,* **R**ead *the lesson to find answers to your questions.* **R**ecite *the information and write it in your own words. Finally,* **R**eview *to make sure you didn't miss anything.*

Survey
Questions
Read
Recite
Review

sexuality
the expression of a person's gender through behavior and mature anatomy and physiology

biological sex
a person's sex—male or female—as determined by chromosomes

intersex
a condition characterized by ambiguous biological sex at birth

Figure 24.6

A doctor can determine a baby's biological sex by analyzing an ultrasound image.

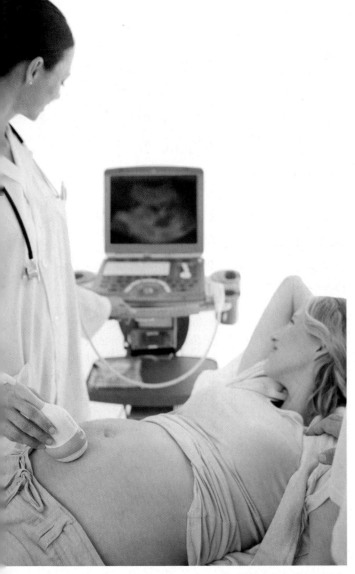

A person's **sexuality** has to do with anatomy, and with being male or female. As you'll learn in this chapter, however, a person's sexuality is about much more than his or her chromosomes and body parts, or whether the person is sexually active. Sexuality develops with maturation and is the expression of a person's gender through behavior and mature anatomy and physiology.

Your sexuality is an important part of your identity that includes how you look, feel, think, and behave. It affects how other people perceive and treat you, and the roles you play in your family and in society. Your sexuality includes

- your biological sex;
- your gender—how you experience and express emotions such as love and intimacy, your gender roles, and your gender identity (masculinity and femininity for example);
- your sexual orientation; and
- your sexual experiences and thoughts.

You'll read more about each of these aspects of sexuality in this lesson.

Biological Sex

As you learned in chapter 20, your **biological sex** is determined by your sex chromosomes. Boys inherit a Y chromosome from their fathers and an X chromosome from their mothers. Girls inherit an X chromosome from each parent. These chromosomes direct the development and growth of sex organs and other sexual characteristics. Much of this growth and development occurred before you were born.

At about the seventh week of embryonic development, a person's biological sex is determined. After the 18th week of development, the sex organs of a fetus can be seen using ultrasound (Figure 24.6). At birth, biological sex is usually obvious by observation of the external sex organs. According to this observation, the baby is either a boy or a girl.

Intersex

While most babies are easily identified as either boys or girls, some babies are born with an ambiguous biological sex. This condition is called *intersex*. Scientists recognize that some degree of intersex is relatively common, occurring in about 1 in 2,000 live births.

Intersex babies have external sex organs that are not obviously male or female. This doesn't mean that intersex babies possess both male and female organs. Instead, the organs have not developed fully and can't be identified. For example, male organs may appear smaller or resemble female organs. Due to this ambiguity, some babies cannot be assigned a sex at birth based on their anatomy alone.

Other Biological Differences

In other cases, the external sex organs do not match the baby's chromosomal sex. That is, some babies with XY chromosomes are born with female characteristics, and some babies with XX chromosomes develop male characteristics.

Other sex chromosome combinations cause ambiguous sexual development. For example, babies with *Turner Syndrome* have XO chromosomes, one X chromosome from one parent and no sex chromosome from the other parent. *Klinefelter Syndrome* describes the presence of two X chromosomes and one Y chromosome in boys.

Babies with Turner Syndrome or Klinefelter Syndrome do not show signs of ambiguity at birth. Instead, their sexually ambiguous traits appear during puberty. These observations indicate that being male or female is more complicated than possessing certain sexual anatomy or sex chromosomes.

Local and Global Health
The Evolving View of Gender

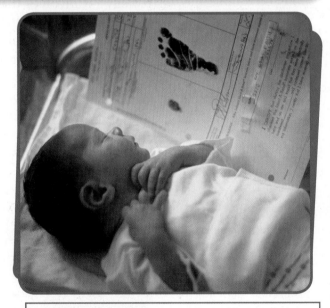

The United States officially recognizes two genders— male and female. Medical professionals have long known that a small percentage of children are born intersex. These children may face problems as they grow and mature if their assigned gender conflicts with their own gender identity.

Other countries have taken action to help protect the intersex minority. In 2013, Germany enacted a law that allows parents to avoid designating a gender to their baby on the birth certificate if the baby is born intersex. The parents can assign *male* or *female*, or they can select *neither*. Note that these babies are not assigned to a third gender. This system is intended to allow these children to select their gender, should they wish to, at a later date.

Germany joins Nepal and Sweden in recognizing non-traditional genders. In Sweden, parents may assign a third gender to their child. Boys are called *han*, girls are called *hon*, and an intersex child is called *hen*, a Swedish word recently coined for the third gender. Australia recently enacted a law that protects intersex people from discrimination. Australia is also considering taking further steps to recognize the intersex gender.

Thinking Critically

1. What is the advantage of allowing intersex individuals to select their gender when they grow up?

2. Do you think a person should be required to select a gender? Please explain your answer.

3. What kind of discrimination might an intersex person face?

Gender

You learned about gender and its relationship to mental health in chapter 15. As you know, *gender* refers to the characteristics a society associates with a particular biological sex. Sex is a legal status that is written on a birth certificate. *Male* and *female* are the sexes assigned to babies in the United States.

Within seconds, you usually know if a person is male or female. Think about how you know whether a person is a boy or a girl. You may rely on a person's physical traits, such as height and build, to determine gender. However, gender and being male or female encompass more than a person's anatomy.

Your perception of a person's gender is also influenced by behavior and other aspects of appearance, such as clothing and accessories. For example, what gender would you associate with someone dressed in pink and carrying a purse? How about someone wearing a baseball cap and a three-day beard? If you grew up in North America, you'd probably say the first person is female and the second a male.

Despite what most people think, masculinity and femininity are not defined by a person's sex chromosomes. Instead, they are defined by a person's gender expression, gender role, and gender identity.

Gender Identity and Expression

As you learned in chapter 15, gender identity has to do with more than biology—it involves the way people feel about and express their gender. Gender identity develops very early in life, with most three-year-olds easily identifying themselves as a boy or girl. A child's sense of his or her gender becomes well-established around five years of age.

Most boys will play with other boys, and girls will play with other girls. This may be a way for children to solidify and support their own sense of gender identity. It is normal, however, for some children to occasionally role-play as the opposite sex or to prefer playing with children of the opposite sex (Figure 24.7).

Figure 24.7

Although most children play with members of their same gender, it is normal for some to prefer playing with the opposite gender. *When you were a child, did you play with other children of your own gender or the opposite gender?*

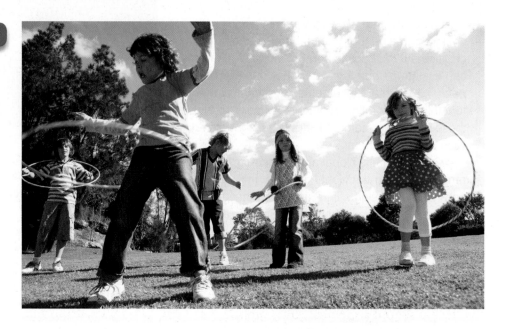

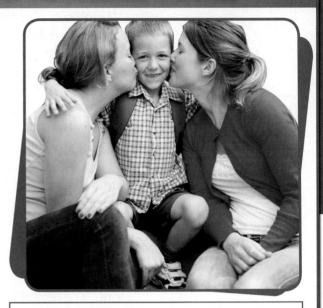

About 200,000 children are raised by gay and lesbian couples in the United States. Many of these couples are legally married.

Some people question whether a child should be raised by gay or lesbian couples. The American Academy of Pediatrics (AAP), which is the nation's leading organization engaged in the scientific study of healthcare for children, has studied this topic. The AAP reviewed more than 30 years of scientific research pertaining to the well-being of children in families with same-sex parents. The AAP concluded that the parents' sexual orientations had no effect on the emotional or physical health of their children.

In addition, the parents' genders were found to have no effect on the children's well-being. Children fare as well with two male parents as they do with two female parents. The AAP found no evidence that same-sex marriage causes harm to children. They suggest that the stability of family life, and not the gender of the parents, is the most important factor for children's welfare.

Thinking Critically

1. Why do you think some people question the welfare of children raised by homosexual parents?

2. In the United States, people once questioned the welfare of children raised by one parent. Single parents rarely face that stigma today. Why do you think the view of single parents has changed?

Gender identity is both assigned and chosen. That is, parents assign gender to a baby when the baby's biological sex is identified at birth. Parents raise the baby as a boy or a girl, and the child learns to identify himself or herself as a boy or girl.

During adolescence or adulthood, some people realize that they are not comfortable with the gender assigned to them. This happens for many reasons. For example, an intersex person with female external organs may be raised as a female, but later in life may feel she is a male, regardless of her anatomy or chromosomes. She may choose to identify herself as male and assume the role and behaviors associated with males. This person is considered to be *transgender*.

Transgender people identify with the gender opposite their biological, anatomical sex. A transgender female is born with male sexual anatomy, but identifies with the female gender. A transgender male is born with female sexual anatomy, but identifies with the male gender. Because of social and cultural gender expectations, some transgender people are confused about their gender identity for many years before they are able to understand themselves.

Transgender people cope differently, but most face discrimination, difficulties at school and work, and complicated social lives. Some choose to

transgender
term that describes a person who identifies with the gender opposite his or her biological sex

change their appearance, clothing, and name to match the gender they feel they really are. A few transgender people undergo expensive reconstructive surgery to match their organs with their gender.

If children are confused about their gender or convinced that they are the opposite gender, parents should be supportive and try to help them understand their feelings. Sexual identity is *inborn*, or present at birth; children cannot help their sense of sexual identity.

Masculinity and Femininity

A society expects certain traits and behaviors to be exhibited by males and females. Masculinity and femininity are not defined by a person's sex chromosomes, biological sex, or assigned gender. Masculinity and femininity are expectations defined by a society.

The definitions of masculinity and femininity vary among societies and cultures, and change over time. Characteristics commonly described as masculine or feminine are generally extreme opposites. For example, a trait commonly considered masculine is "strong"; its corresponding feminine trait is "weak." The feminine trait "graceful" has the masculine counterpart "clumsy." The masculine "aggressive" becomes the feminine "passive."

Naturally, it is impossible to be completely aggressive or completely passive. Most people's behavior lies somewhere in between these two extremes. In addition, no person possesses only masculine traits or only feminine traits. People exhibit both masculine and feminine traits, and their personalities contain aspects of both.

For these reasons, the expression of masculinity and femininity can be a source of insecurity for teens. Because they are still developing emotionally, physically, and socially, teens are often insecure about the way others perceive them. They think they are supposed to be "masculine" or "feminine," not realizing that these are just descriptions, or stereotypes, and not something that exists in real individuals (Figure 24.8).

Figure 24.8

Many boys feel they should exhibit masculine traits, while girls may feel pressured to be feminine. *Can you recall a time when you felt pressure to be more masculine or feminine?*

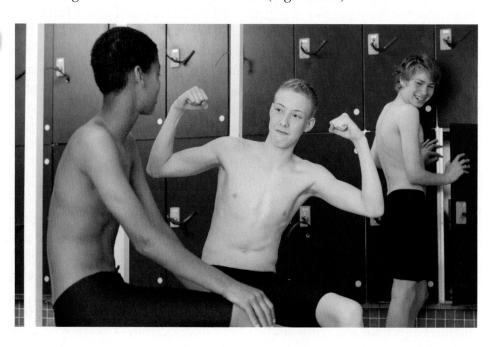

Movies, advertisements, and other media present unrealistic, exaggerated images of masculinity and femininity. In some cases, the media imply that extreme masculinity and femininity are normal and desirable. Realistically, however, no person exhibits these traits to the extreme, and no one can attain them to the degree portrayed by the media.

Sexual Orientation

Sexual orientation refers to the gender to which a person is romantically and physically attracted. The different types of sexual orientation include heterosexual, homosexual, and bisexual.

- **Heterosexual.** People who are *heterosexual* are romantically and physically attracted to people of the opposite gender. Heterosexuals are sometimes called *straight*.

- **Homosexual.** People who are *homosexual* are romantically and physically attracted to people of their own gender (Figure 24.9). The term *gay*, can refer to both homosexual men and women. Gay women also refer to themselves as *lesbian*. Results of the CDC's National Health Interview Survey found that about 1.6% of US adults identify themselves as gay or lesbian.

- **Bisexual.** People who are *bisexual* are romantically and physically attracted to people of both genders. About 0.7% of US adults say they are bisexual according to the CDC report.

People of all three sexual orientations can be found in all races, ethnicities, cultures, countries, and social and economic backgrounds. Many factors, some unknown, influence the development of a person's sexual orientation. Known factors include a person's genes, environment, and experiences. Early in puberty, some teenagers have already developed an awareness that they are homosexual or bisexual. Some may have known since childhood.

LGBT, which stands for *lesbian*, *gay*, *bisexual*, and *transgender*, is a common abbreviation used to identify people of these sexual orientations or gender identity. LGBT is sometimes expanded to include *Q, I,* and *A* (Q for those who are questioning their sexuality, I for intersex, and A for allies of the gay community). Some people argue that, despite efforts to make this abbreviation more inclusive, it still does not represent every sexual orientation or gender identity. Some people also argue that they do not want to be defined by an abbreviation. As the LGBT community continues to evolve, so will the terminology used to describe it.

sexual orientation
term that describes which gender a person is attracted to

heterosexual
the quality of being romantically and physically attracted to members of the opposite gender

homosexual
the quality of being romantically and physically attracted to members of the same gender

bisexual
the quality of being romantically and physically attracted to members of both genders

Figure 24.9

Some homosexuals develop an awareness of their sexual orientation during adolescence.

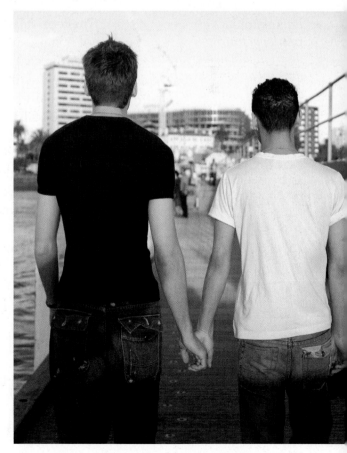

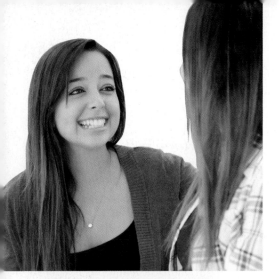

Figure 24.10

Developing a "crush" on a member of the same sex is fairly common among adolescents and is not necessarily an expression of homosexuality.

homophobia
irrational fear, discrimination, and anger directed at homosexuality and LGBT individuals

Questions about Sexual Orientation

Whether straight, gay, or bisexual, teenagers often have questions about their emerging sexuality. It is not unusual for some teenagers to be unsure of or confused about their sexual orientation.

At times during adolescence, some heterosexual boys and girls develop romantic or physical attraction to people of the same gender. This does not necessarily mean, however, that they are homosexual or bisexual. For example, a girl might develop a "crush" on another girl in her school or on a female celebrity (Figure 24.10). This type of generalized sexuality and sexual curiosity is fairly common while adolescents are maturing, due in large part to increased hormone levels that occur during puberty. In time, most teenagers sort out their feelings as they discover and understand their sexual orientation.

While heterosexual teens are exploring their sexuality and sexual orientation, LGBT teens are doing the same. LGBT teens think about and want to discuss their romantic feelings, dating experiences, and sexuality, just as heterosexual teens do. LGBT teens often feel, however, that they must hide this part of themselves from others.

From a young age, LGBT teens notice that most people are straight, or heterosexual, and that straight sexual behavior is considered the norm. In much of society, LGBT teens are expected to be straight, and their sexual identity is expected to match their biological sex.

Coping with Homophobia

The term *homophobia* was first used in 1969 to describe an irrational fear of homosexuality. Today, homophobia describes discrimination, anger, and fear directed at homosexuality and LGBT individuals. LGBT teens may have to deal with other people's negative attitudes and actions, in some cases on a daily basis. Some of the people exhibiting this negative behavior may be the LGBT teen's own family members.

LGBT individuals are accepted more widely today than in the past. However, LGBT individuals still experience varying degrees of prejudice, rejection, bullying, sexual harassment, and violence. Compared with heterosexual teenagers, LGBT teens are at a greater risk for developing depression and anxiety, and for dropping out of school and running away from home. To avoid harassment, many LGBT people hide their sexual orientation or transgender identity, although it can be difficult and painful to deny this basic part of who they are.

Despite the discrimination that is still present, many LGBT teens, especially those who have good support systems, do feel comfortable with themselves. Many "come out" and tell trusted family members and friends about their sexual orientation or transgender identity.

Support for LGBT Youth

It is important for LGBT teens to have a supportive and accepting group of people around them (Figure 24.11). To create such a group, many schools have created student organizations for LGBT students and the students who support them. Governments have also passed laws to protect LGBT individuals from discrimination and persecution. Federal laws, including the Civil Service Reform Act of 1978 and the Civil Rights Act of 1991, prohibit workplace discrimination against employees because of their sexual orientation.

You read briefly about hate crimes in chapter 19. Hate crimes are criminal acts motivated by the offender's bias against the victim's actual or perceived race, religion, disability, ethnicity, or sexual orientation. Many hate crimes are committed by teenagers. LGBT teenagers and adults are frequent victims of these crimes.

The Matthew Shepard and James Byrd, Jr. Hate Crimes Prevention Act protects people from crimes that target people because of their sexual orientation and race. Matthew Shepard was a young man who was murdered because he was gay. James Byrd was killed by a white supremacist because he was African-American.

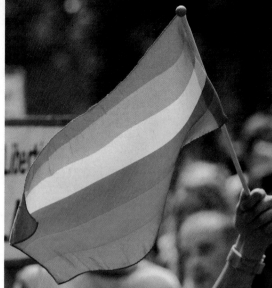

Same-Sex Marriage

Same-sex marriage is the legal marriage between two people of the same sex. On June 26, 2015, the United States Supreme Court decided that same-sex couples have the right to marry. Therefore, all states must issue marriage licenses to same-sex couples, and states must recognize same-sex marriages legally performed in other states. The Court's decision was based on the Fourteenth Amendment of the United States Constitution, which guarantees all people have the rights given to all other US citizens.

Lesson 24.2 Review

Know and Understand

1. What are four aspects that define a person's sexuality?
2. Which chromosome combination results in a male biological sex? Which results in a female biological sex?
3. What does it mean to be born intersex?
4. _____ people feel strongly that their gender is the opposite of their biological, anatomical gender.
5. What does the acronym *LGBT* stand for?
6. What is homophobia?

Analyze and Apply

7. Does gender determine a person's masculinity or femininity? Explain your answer.
8. How do prejudice and discrimination based on gender nonconformity affect the LGBT community?

Real World Health

People come in all varieties, with all different types of characteristics. Spend some quality time observing and watching different types of people. This people-watching activity can be done at school, at the mall, or in any area where many people are coming and going. What qualities do you immediately notice about the people you see? How do your observations vary based on the person's gender? What do you notice about yourself and your attitude toward certain types of people? What stereotypes might be influencing how you see people? Write a reflection about the qualities, behaviors, and attitudes you observed. What do these observations tell you about gender, sexuality, and cultural attitudes toward these concepts? What do they tell you about yourself?

Understanding Sexual Feelings and Behavior

Key Terms

estrogens
human sexual response
  cycle

masturbation
orgasm

Key Points

- Puberty plays a major role in sexual development.
- Hormones released during puberty affect physical and emotional development.
- Curiosity about sex and feelings of arousal are part of development during adolescence.
- Masturbation is a common response to sexual excitement and a safe way to release sexual tension.
- The human sexual response cycle includes four stages—excitement, plateau, orgasmic, and resolution.
- Sexual activity can complicate teenage relationships and create intense emotion and stress.
- Before engaging in sexual activity, a couple should have an honest conversation about sex.
- Choosing abstinence allows teenagers to focus on individual growth, self-esteem, and the future.

Check Your Understanding

1. What are estrogens?

2. How do hormones travel through the body?

3. *True or false?* Hormones affect only a specific target tissue.

4. Puberty is triggered when the brain releases _____ hormone.
   A. follicle-stimulating
   B. oxytocin
   C. gonadotropin-releasing
   D. luteinizing

5. During puberty, girls and boys develop _____ and _____ sexual characteristics.

6. A(n) _____, or *wet dream*, is ejaculation that occurs during sleep.

7. _____ is a normal response to sexual excitement.

8. What are the four stages of the human sexual response cycle?

9. During the _____ phase, heart rate and blood pressure continue to rise.
   A. orgasm
   B. excitement
   C. resolution
   D. plateau

10. List the physical changes that males and females experience during the excitement phase.

11. _____ is the climax of sexual excitement.
   A. Orgasm
   B. Masturbation
   C. Arousal
   D. Plateau

12. List three potential problems that might occur as a result of sexual activity in teen relationships.

13. *True or false?* Couples should not discuss their views on sex.

14. Another term for sexual excitement is _____.
   A. wet dream
   B. masturbation
   C. arousal
   D. nocturnal emission

15. *True or false?* Teen romantic relationships can be fun and rewarding without sex.

16. Provide two examples of situations that might make abstinence difficult.

17. *True or false?* The media often presents accurate portrayals of teenage sexual relationships.

18. **Critical Thinking.** Why might choosing abstinence improve individual growth?

What Is Sexuality?

Key Terms

biological sex
bisexual
heterosexual
homophobia
homosexual

intersex
sexual orientation
sexuality
transgender

Key Points

- Sexuality is defined by sexual orientation and experiences, as well as biological sex and gender.
- Biological sex is determined by your sex chromosomes.
- Some children are born intersex, meaning their biological sex is ambiguous.
- Transgender people feel as though their actual gender is the opposite of their anatomical gender.
- Masculinity and femininity are expectations defined by society.
- Heterosexuality, homosexuality, and bisexuality are three types of sexual orientation.
- Homophobia describes the discrimination, anger, and fear directed at LGBT individuals.

Check Your Understanding

19. *True or false?* Sexuality is defined only by gender.
20. Which of the following is not an aspect of sexuality?
    A. sexual orientation
    B. hormonal balance
    C. biological sex
    D. sexual experiences
21. What is gender?
22. Which biological sex is indicated by a chromosome pair of *XY*?
    A. male
    B. intersex
    C. female
    D. Turner syndrome
23. When do the sexually ambiguous traits begin to appear in children with Turner Syndrome or Klinefelter Syndrome?
24. *True or false?* Intersex individuals are born with an ambiguous biological sex.
25. Which of the following terms describes people who strongly feel their gender is the opposite of their biological, anatomical gender?
    A. intersex
    B. bisexual
    C. heterosexual
    D. transgender

26. *True or false?* While heterosexual teens are exploring their sexuality, LGBT teens are doing the same.
27. In which year was the term *homophobia* first used?
    A. 2010
    B. 1969
    C. 2000
    D. 1943
28. Identify three types of sexual orientation.
29. *True or false?* People of all three sexual orientations can be found in all races, ethnicities, and cultures.
30. People who are _____ are attracted to people of their own gender.
    A. bisexual
    B. heterosexual
    C. intersex
    D. homosexual
31. *True or false?* Your gender determines your masculinity or femininity.
32. A child's sense of gender becomes well-established around _____ years of age.
    A. two
    B. ten
    C. five
    D. three
33. *True or false?* It is not possible to embody extreme masculinity or femininity.
34. Masculinity and femininity are expectations defined by _____.
    A. society
    B. nature
    C. birth
    D. biological sex
35. *True or false?* People do not know their sexual orientation until they reach adulthood.
36. What is homophobia?
37. *True or false?* The LGBT acronym represents every sexual orientation and gender identity.
38. When was same-sex marriage legalized in the United States?
39. **Critical Thinking.** Is gender identity chosen or assigned? Explain your answer.

Health and Wellness Skills

40. **Access Information.** Learning about sex from unreliable sources can lead to teenagers believing myths and misconceptions about sex. Research places you could go to get *credible* information on topics related to sex. These places may be online or in your community. Create an infographic or one-page handout listing the resources you found and describing what makes them credible.

41. **Advocate for Health.** Research and define the term *homophobia*. In what year did the term originate? What views does homophobia include? Do these views exist in your community? in your school? In small groups, list some examples of homophobia, including physical, mental, emotional, sexual, and verbal abuse, or cyberbullying. Next, discuss actions you could take to help someone experiencing these types of bullying. As a group, come up with a positive message that could take the place of the homophobic message a bully might communicate. Share your work with the class.

42. **Make Decisions.** In this chapter, there is a Case Study about Marie and Craig. After a concert, they go to Craig's house, and Craig tells Marie he wants to have sex. Marie doesn't want to have sex, and she isn't sure what to say. The Case Study ends with the reader uncertain about whether Marie and Craig have sex, but it is clear that Marie and Craig have put themselves in a risky situation. Rewrite this story, using all of the knowledge and skills you have learned so far regarding healthy relationships for teens, and add a definite ending in which Marie and Craig make a healthy decision about whether to have sex or remain abstinent.

43. **Practice Healthy Behaviors and Reduce Health Risks.** Abstinence is the only guaranteed way to prevent pregnancy and avoid sexually transmitted infections. If you are unsure about your decision to remain abstinent, whom can you talk to in your personal support network? Choose one of these people and write a role-play scenario illustrating how you might approach him or her and start a conversation.

Hands-On Activity
Personal Action Plan

In this chapter, and in other chapters, you have learned about healthy teen relationships, the risks of having sex as a teenager, and the benefits of remaining abstinent. In this activity, you will formulate a *Personal Action Plan* that you can use when faced with challenges to your own sexual values and decisions.

Steps for this Activity

1. On a separate sheet of paper or on your computer, create a chart as described in the following steps.

2. Consider your current goals and dreams. In a box labeled *Now*, list your short-term goals. Where do you hope to be in one year? What are your current dreams and hobbies? What do you enjoy about your life? In a box labeled *Later*, list your long-term goals and dreams. Where do you hope to be in 10 years? What do you want your life to look like? What do you want to achieve?

3. Explore your own personal values. What beliefs are important to you and why? Could you defend these values and beliefs, if challenged? How do these values and beliefs fit into your present and future goals and dreams? How do your values and beliefs affect your sexual behavior and your reaction to challenges of a sexual nature? At the bottom of your chart, list your most important values and beliefs and how they relate to challenges of a sexual nature.

4. In boxes between *Now* and *Later*, formulate pledges or promises to yourself that will help you reach your *Later* goals. These pledges are personal oaths or statements you can use when faced with sexual challenges. The pledges could range from not drinking alcohol, to only kissing, to communicating your limits and wishes to your partner. As you formulate these pledges, think about the different challenging situations you might face. How far would you be willing to go sexually if someone asked you? How might alcohol or being in a bedroom affect your decisions?

5. When complete, keep your *Personal Action Plan* in a place where you can reference it or change it, if needed.

Core Skills

Math Practice

The pie chart shown below breaks down the 6,216 single-bias hate crimes reported by the FBI in one year by types of groups targeted. Study the pie chart and then answer the questions. Round decimals to the nearest whole number.

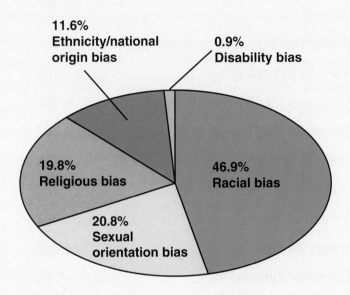

11.6%
Ethnicity/national origin bias

0.9%
Disability bias

19.8%
Religious bias

46.9%
Racial bias

20.8%
Sexual orientation bias

44. How many sexual orientation bias hate crimes were reported?
  A. 1,293
  B. 56
  C. 1,200
  D. 846

45. How many racial bias hate crimes were reported?
  A. 721
  B. 3,108
  C. 2,003
  D. 2,915

46. How many more sexual orientation bias crimes were reported than religious bias crimes?
  A. 60
  B. 62
  C. 1
  D. 51

Reading and Writing Practice

Read the passage below and then answer the questions.

While heterosexual teens are exploring their sexuality and sexual orientation, teens who are lesbian, gay, bisexual, or transgender (often abbreviated as LGBT) are doing the same. LGBT teens think about and want to discuss their romantic feelings, dating experiences, and sexuality, just as heterosexual teens do. LGBT teens often feel, however, that they must hide this part of themselves from others.

From a young age, LGBT teens notice that most people are straight, or heterosexual, and that straight sexual behavior is considered the norm. In much of society, LGBT teens are expected to be straight, and their sexual identity is expected to match their biological sex.

The term homophobia was first used in 1969 to describe an irrational fear of homosexuality. Today homophobia describes discrimination, anger, and fear directed at homosexuality and LGBT individuals. LGBT teens may have to deal with other people's negative attitudes and actions, in some cases on a daily basis. Some of the people exhibiting this negative behavior may be the LGBT teen's own family members.

47. People who are "straight" are also known as
  _____.
  A. bisexuals
  B. homosexuals
  C. heterosexuals
  D. transgender

48. What does the abbreviation *LGBT* stand for?

49. The term homophobia _____.
  A. describes the discrimination, anger, and fear directed at LGBT individuals
  B. was introduced in 1969
  C. was first used to describe an irrational fear of homosexuality
  D. All of the above.

Background Lessons

On the next several pages you will find information and activities on key health and wellness topics. The material is presented concisely so that you can quickly access the information you need. For many of these topics you will be refreshing your memory from lessons you have studied in other courses.

These lessons are divided into two main parts, which are listed below with their individual lessons.

Body Systems

Safety and First Aid

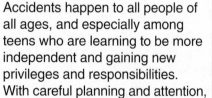

Background Lessons Video

Safety and First Aid Videos

Accidents happen to all people of all ages, and especially among teens who are learning to be more independent and gaining new privileges and responsibilities. With careful planning and attention, however, many accidents can be avoided, and even in those that can't, teens can learn to manage the situation and help those at risk.

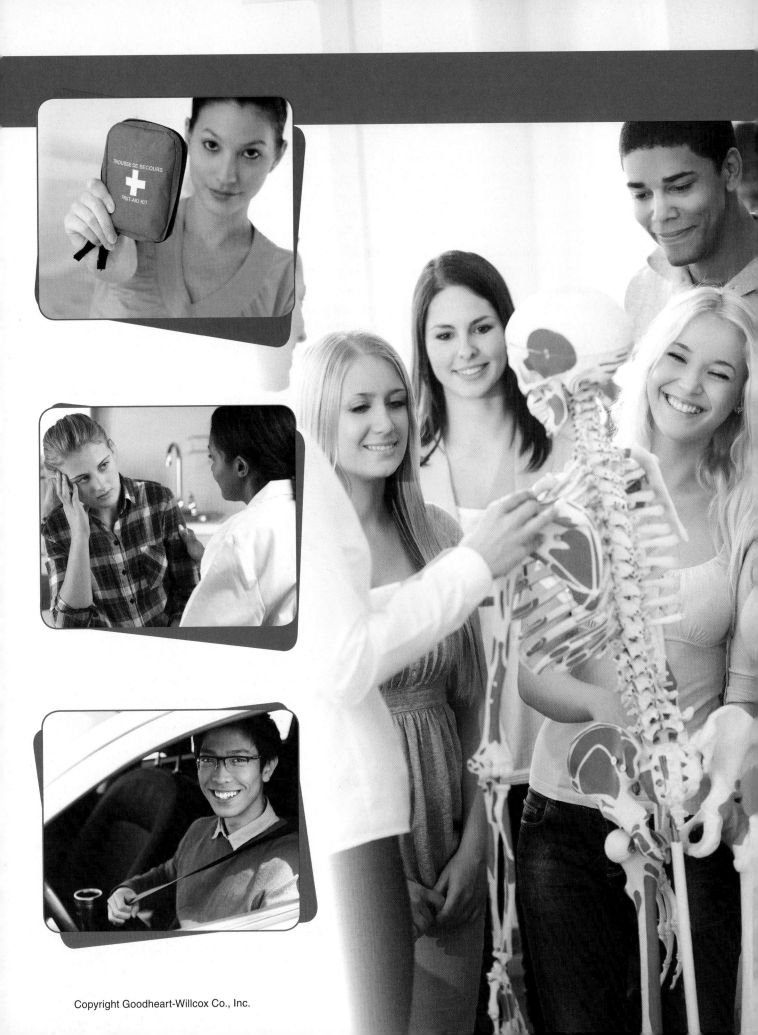

The Human Body and Its Systems

How does your body temperature stay constant at about 98.6°F, even on hot and cold days? How does willing your body to do something—walk across a room or jump for a fly ball, for example—cause it to happen? How does your hand know to pull back from a hot stove? How is a slice of pizza or an apple broken down into the energy your body needs to function?

These are just a few of many tasks your body accomplishes every day that enable you to function and stay alive. Each task requires the monitoring, coordination, and cooperation of multiple cells, tissues, and systems throughout your body.

Cells are the microscopic building blocks that make up your body. Your body consists of trillions of cells—red and white blood cells, brain cells, liver cells, skin cells, and so forth. Cells come together to form tissues. The cells in a particular type of tissue have a similar structure and function. Examples of the many types of tissues in the body include bone tissue, muscle tissue, nerve tissue, and connective tissue.

After cells and tissues, the next level in the organization of the body is the organ level. An organ is a body part that performs a particular function. The heart, lungs, liver, brain, and kidneys are a few of the organs in your body. Each organ consists of several types of tissues (Figure BL1.1).

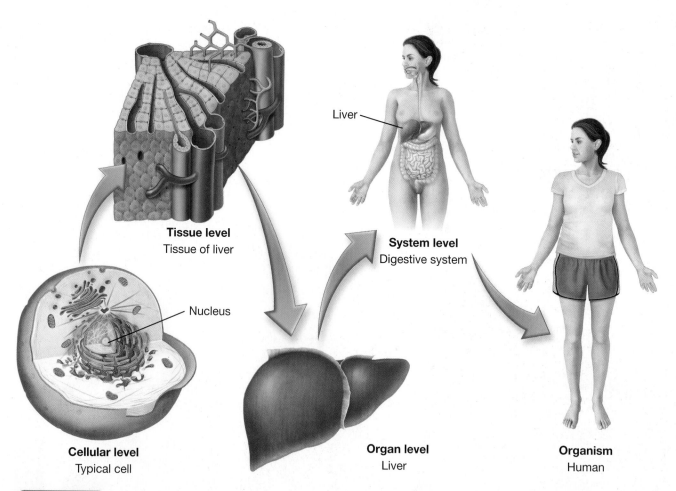

Tissue level
Tissue of liver

Nucleus

Cellular level
Typical cell

System level
Digestive system

Organ level
Liver

Organism
Human

Liver

Figure BL1.1 Your body consists of trillions of cells, which are organized into complex tissues. Similar tissues go together to form organs, and related organs combine to make up body systems. These body systems perform specific functions, but work together to create a special type of organism, a human being.

To better understand how the body works, scientists have found it helpful to divide the body up into various organ systems, also called *body systems*. Each body system includes two or more organs that work together. Examples of body systems include the nervous system, the respiratory system, and the cardiovascular (*circulatory*) system.

Although these systems, for the most part, are presented as separate entities, they are highly integrated. They work together in complex and ingenious ways to maintain homeostasis. Homeostasis is the process of maintaining an internal state of physiological balance. A small adjustment or imbalance in one system often has a ripple effect through other systems and the body as a whole. Through homeostasis, the body seeks to rebalance itself.

Why doesn't your body temperature shoot up to 100°F on a hot day, or drop below 98.6°F on a cold day? The hypothalamus in the brain is the body's thermostat. It works like a thermostat in a home. If you set the thermostat at a particular temperature—perhaps 68°F—when the temperature drops, the heating system will automatically turn on to warm the home. When the temperature exceeds the set point of 68°F, the heating system automatically turns off.

Like the thermostat, the hypothalamus monitors body temperature (Figure BL1.2). When body temperature drops below the hypothalamic set

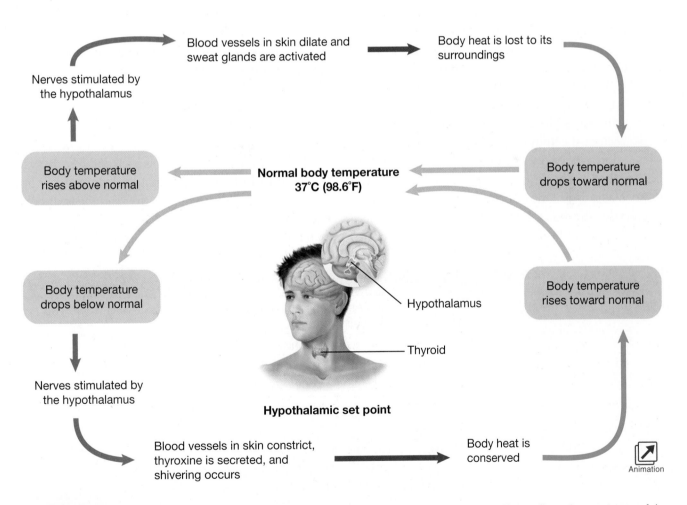

Figure BL1.2 For you to stay alive and healthy, all the parts of your body—from the smallest cells to the most powerful muscles—work together to maintain homeostasis. The regulation of body temperature is just one example of how the body accomplishes homeostasis.

point of 98.6°F, the hypothalamus responds in several ways that raise body temperature. The hypothalamus

- releases hormones that act on the thyroid gland, which in turn releases a hormone that raises the body's metabolic rate, producing heat;
- commands the nervous system to send signals to the body to initiate shivering, which raises body temperature; and
- decreases blood flow to the skin, conserving body heat.

When the hypothalamic set point is reestablished, the hypothalamus signals the thyroid gland to stop releasing the hormone that raises the metabolic rate. The hypothalamus also signals the body to stop shivering and restore blood flow to the skin.

On the other hand, when the body temperature rises above the hypothalamic set point of 98.6°F—when you are hot—the hypothalamus works to lower it. In order to cool the body, the hypothalamus

- stimulates the sweat glands to increase the production of sweat;
- increases blood flow to the skin; and
- causes the thyroid gland to decrease the secretion of hormones that raise body temperature.

Another example of how the body maintains homeostasis is in the monitoring and regulation of glucose, the body's fuel source. The pancreas, which is part of both the digestive and endocrine systems, contains cells that secrete hormones. These hormones regulate the concentration of glucose in the blood. The hormone glucagon raises blood glucose levels, while the hormone insulin reduces blood glucose levels. The two hormones in the pancreas work together to keep the level of blood glucose constant—not too high and not too low.

However, if the pancreas stops secreting enough insulin, the cells of the body become starved because they cannot absorb needed glucose. This is what occurs in people who have the disease type 1 diabetes mellitus. This serious disease is a leading cause of kidney failure, limb amputation, and blindness. Diabetes is also a major cause of heart disease and stroke.

As you know from reading this textbook, diseases and disorders are associated with various risk factors. These risk factors may include those that are inherited, part of the environment, and factors resulting from peoples' behavior or lifestyle. The good news is that people can often influence what happens in their bodies. Eating a healthful diet, exercising regularly, and avoiding hazardous substances and activities (such as tobacco and alcohol use) can go a long way toward reducing the risks of many diseases and disorders.

The next ten lessons discuss each of the body systems and include detailed, anatomic drawings. You can refer to these drawings as you read the textbook. The following table indicates which chapters cover material associated with particular body systems.

Body System	Chapters
Nervous	Sleep, Alcohol, Medications and Drugs, Managing the Stress in Your Life, Mental Illnesses and Disorders
Cardiovascular	Physical Fitness, Noncommunicable Diseases
Respiratory	Physical Fitness, Tobacco
Skeletal	Nutrition, Body Weight and Composition, Physical Fitness
Muscular	Body Weight and Composition, Physical Fitness
Digestive	Nutrition
Urinary	Reproduction and Pregnancy
Endocrine	Managing the Stress in Your Life, Reproduction and Pregnancy, Noncommunicable Diseases
Lymphatic (Immune System)	Infectious Diseases
Reproductive	Sexually Transmitted Infections and HIV/AIDS, Reproduction and Pregnancy, Childbirth and Parenting Newborns

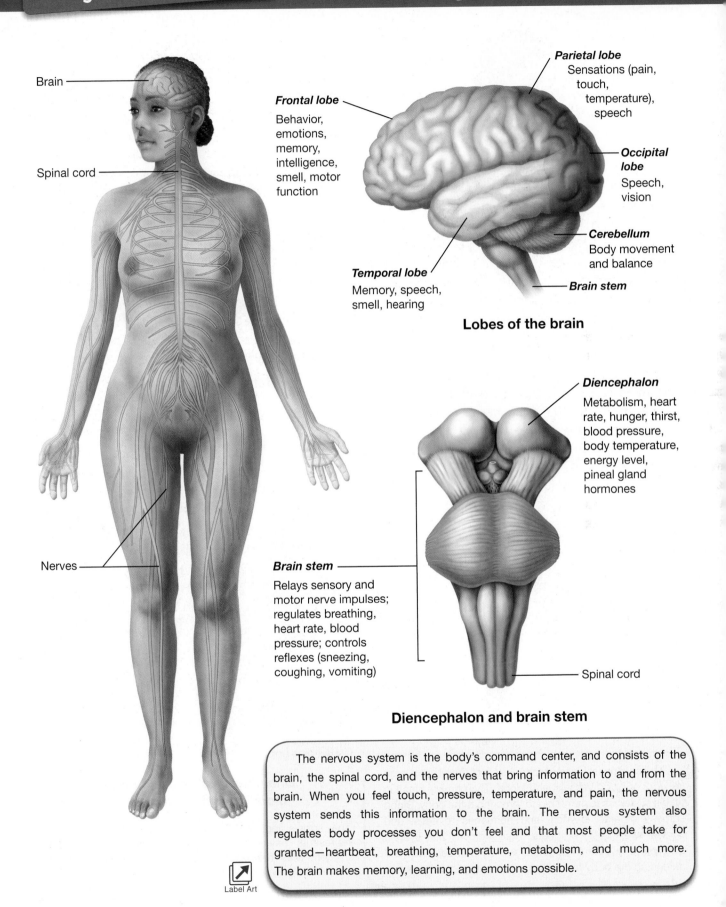

Brain

Spinal cord

Nerves

Frontal lobe
Behavior, emotions, memory, intelligence, smell, motor function

Parietal lobe
Sensations (pain, touch, temperature), speech

Occipital lobe
Speech, vision

Cerebellum
Body movement and balance

Brain stem

Temporal lobe
Memory, speech, smell, hearing

Lobes of the brain

Diencephalon
Metabolism, heart rate, hunger, thirst, blood pressure, body temperature, energy level, pineal gland hormones

Brain stem
Relays sensory and motor nerve impulses; regulates breathing, heart rate, blood pressure; controls reflexes (sneezing, coughing, vomiting)

Spinal cord

Diencephalon and brain stem

The nervous system is the body's command center, and consists of the brain, the spinal cord, and the nerves that bring information to and from the brain. When you feel touch, pressure, temperature, and pain, the nervous system sends this information to the brain. The nervous system also regulates body processes you don't feel and that most people take for granted—heartbeat, breathing, temperature, metabolism, and much more. The brain makes memory, learning, and emotions possible.

Label Art

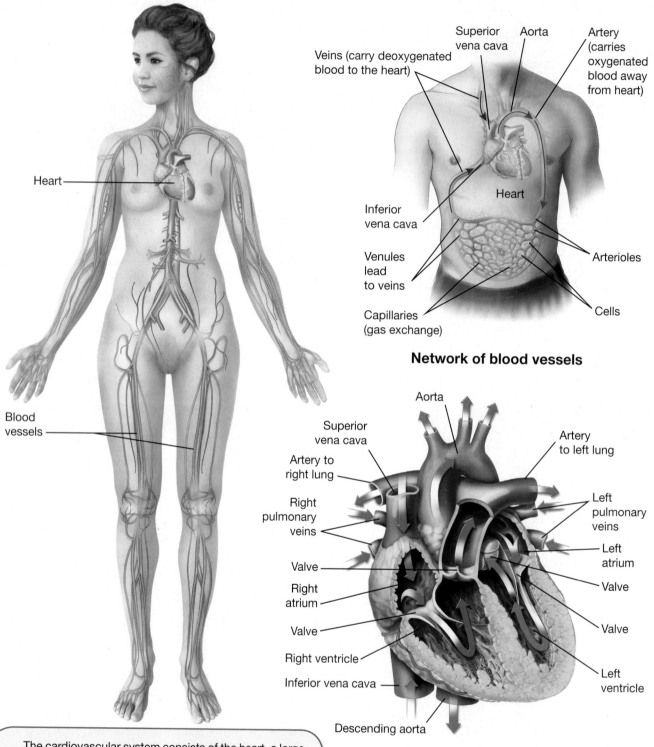

Network of blood vessels

Chambers, valves, and large blood vessels of the heart

The arrows indicate the direction of blood flow. Red represents oxygenated blood, or blood that contains oxygen. Blue represents deoxygenated blood, or blood depleted of oxygen.

The cardiovascular system consists of the heart, a large network of blood vessels, and blood. The primary function of this system is to pump blood throughout the body. Blood carries nutrients, oxygen, and hormones to cells, and carries away waste products. The cardiovascular system also plays a role in regulating body temperature and defending the body from disease-causing microorganisms.

Animation   Label Art

The respiratory and cardiovascular systems work together to deliver oxygen to cells and carry away carbon dioxide, a waste product. Lung tissue contains millions of alveoli clusters—each of which consists of many alveolar sacs. When you breathe, the alveolar sacs fill with air. The thin alveolar sac walls allow oxygen to pass, or diffuse, from the alveolar sacs to the red blood cells in the capillaries. Carbon dioxide diffuses in the opposite direction and is expelled through the lungs. This process is called gas exchange.

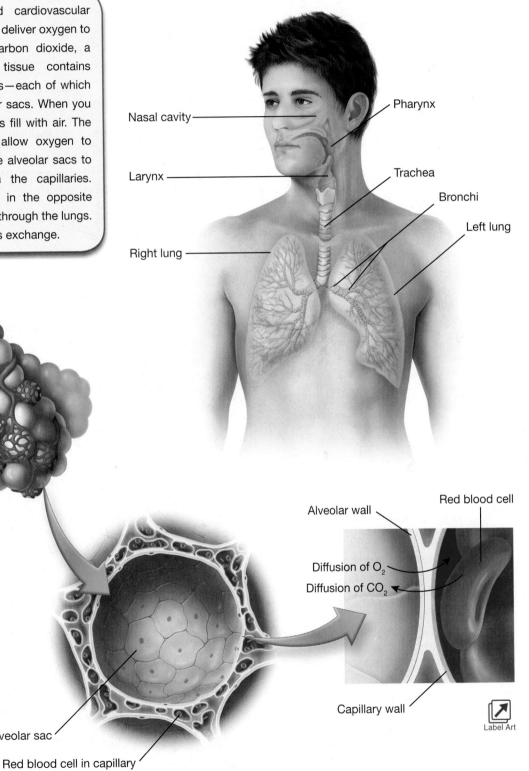

Nasal cavity

Pharynx

Larynx

Trachea

Bronchi

Left lung

Right lung

Cluster of alveoli

Red blood cell

Alveolar wall

Diffusion of O_2

Diffusion of CO_2

Capillary wall

Label Art

Alveolar sac

Red blood cell in capillary

Gas exchange

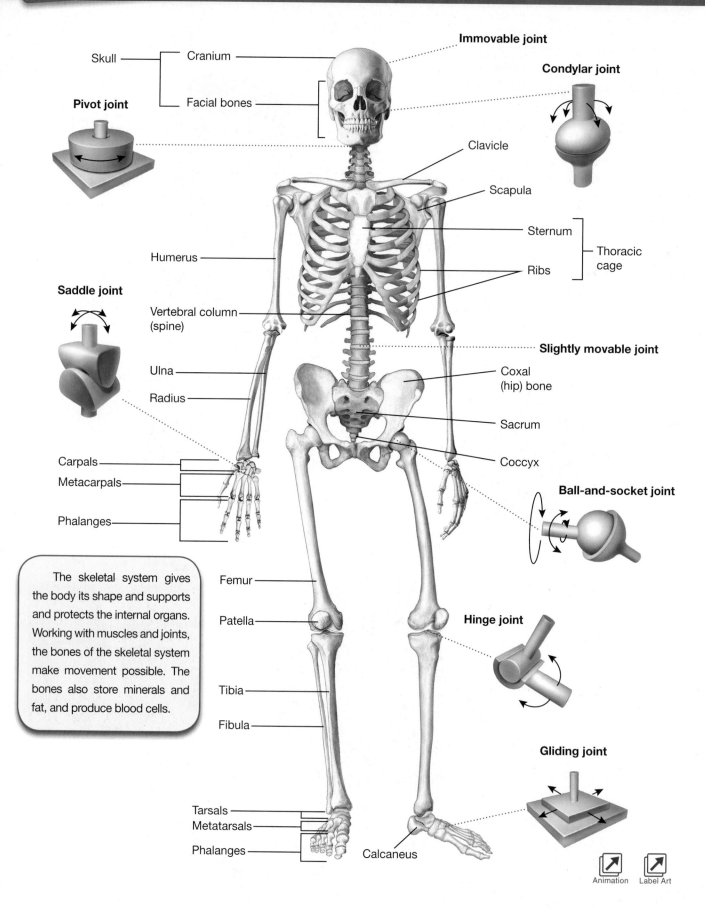

Immovable joint

Condylar joint

Skull — Cranium

Pivot joint

Facial bones

Clavicle

Scapula

Sternum

Humerus

Thoracic cage

Ribs

Saddle joint

Vertebral column (spine)

Slightly movable joint

Ulna

Coxal (hip) bone

Radius

Sacrum

Carpals

Coccyx

Metacarpals

Ball-and-socket joint

Phalanges

The skeletal system gives the body its shape and supports and protects the internal organs. Working with muscles and joints, the bones of the skeletal system make movement possible. The bones also store minerals and fat, and produce blood cells.

Femur

Patella

Hinge joint

Tibia

Fibula

Gliding joint

Tarsals

Metatarsals

Phalanges

Calcaneus

Animation   Label Art

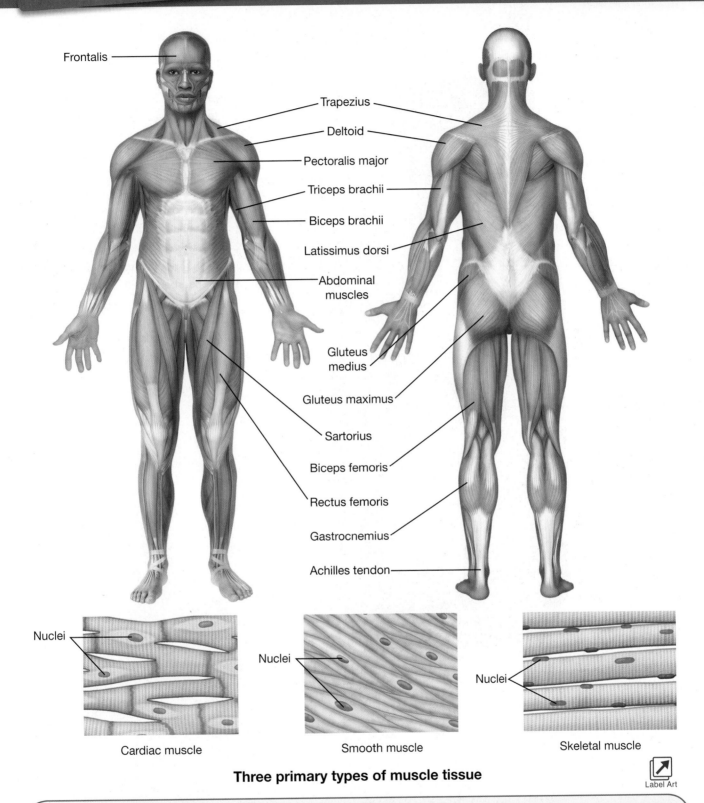

Frontalis

Trapezius

Deltoid

Pectoralis major

Triceps brachii

Biceps brachii

Latissimus dorsi

Abdominal muscles

Gluteus medius

Gluteus maximus

Sartorius

Biceps femoris

Rectus femoris

Gastrocnemius

Achilles tendon

Nuclei

Cardiac muscle

Nuclei

Smooth muscle

Nuclei

Skeletal muscle

Three primary types of muscle tissue

Label Art

The muscular system consists of three types of muscles: cardiac, smooth, and skeletal. Cardiac muscles pump blood through the heart and body. Smooth muscle is found in the walls of many internal organs. For example, smooth muscle moves food through the gastrointestinal tract. Skeletal muscles are attached to bones. When these muscles contract, or shorten, they pull on bones and make movement possible.

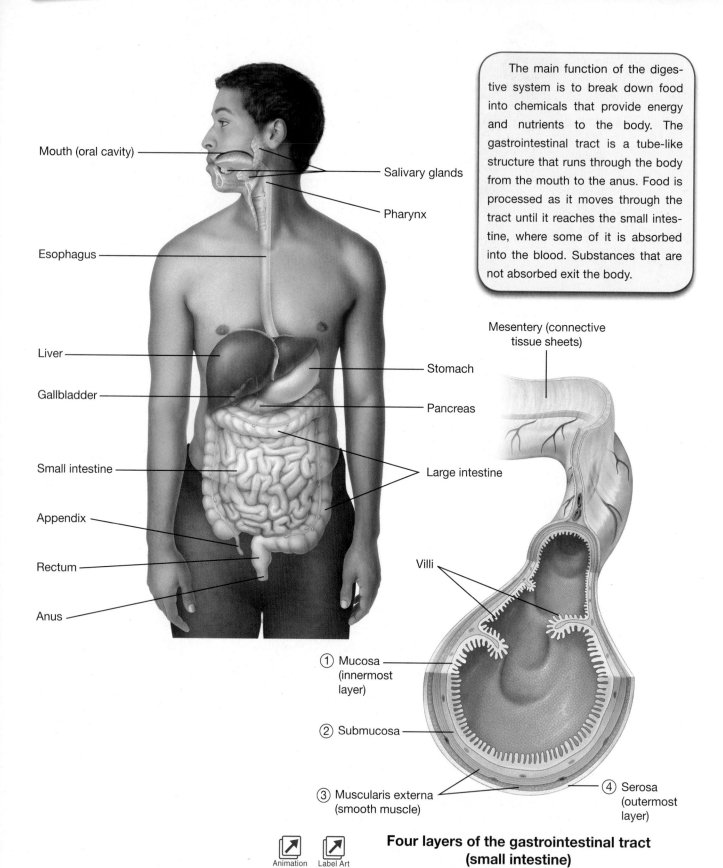

Mouth (oral cavity)

Salivary glands

Pharynx

Esophagus

The main function of the digestive system is to break down food into chemicals that provide energy and nutrients to the body. The gastrointestinal tract is a tube-like structure that runs through the body from the mouth to the anus. Food is processed as it moves through the tract until it reaches the small intestine, where some of it is absorbed into the blood. Substances that are not absorbed exit the body.

Liver

Gallbladder

Small intestine

Appendix

Rectum

Anus

Stomach

Pancreas

Large intestine

Mesentery (connective tissue sheets)

Villi

① Mucosa (innermost layer)

② Submucosa

③ Muscularis externa (smooth muscle)

④ Serosa (outermost layer)

Animation   Label Art

Four layers of the gastrointestinal tract (small intestine)

The urinary system includes two kidneys that filter waste from the blood. The liquid waste is held in the bladder and eventually eliminated as urine. This system also monitors and helps regulate the volume of water in the body and the concentrations of sodium, chloride, and other elements in the blood.

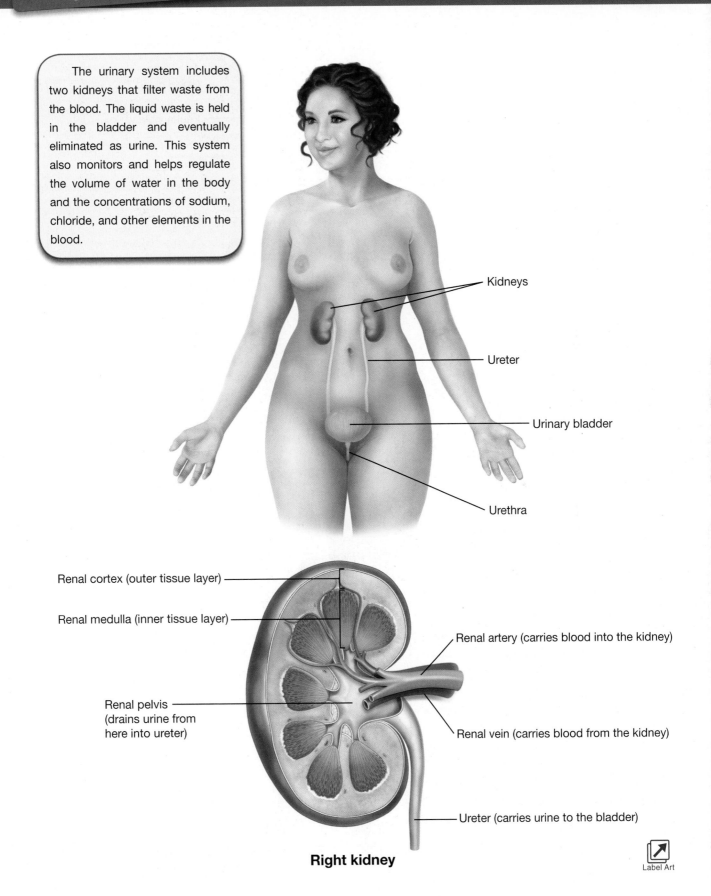

Kidneys

Ureter

Urinary bladder

Urethra

Renal cortex (outer tissue layer)

Renal medulla (inner tissue layer)

Renal pelvis
(drains urine from
here into ureter)

Renal artery (carries blood into the kidney)

Renal vein (carries blood from the kidney)

Ureter (carries urine to the bladder)

Right kidney

Label Art

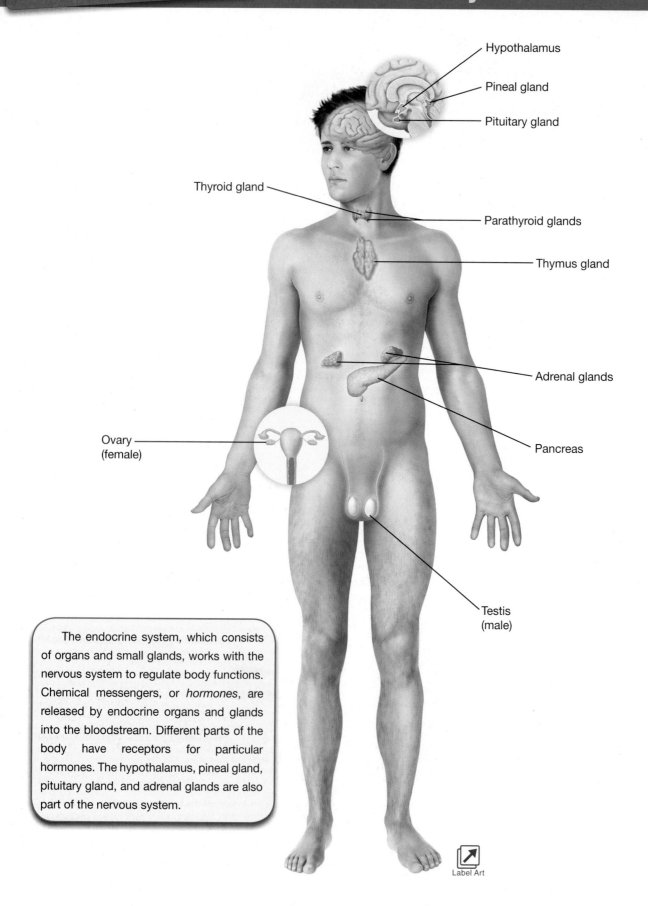

Hypothalamus

Pineal gland

Pituitary gland

Thyroid gland

Parathyroid glands

Thymus gland

Adrenal glands

Ovary
(female)

Pancreas

Testis
(male)

Label Art

The endocrine system, which consists of organs and small glands, works with the nervous system to regulate body functions. Chemical messengers, or *hormones*, are released by endocrine organs and glands into the bloodstream. Different parts of the body have receptors for particular hormones. The hypothalamus, pineal gland, pituitary gland, and adrenal glands are also part of the nervous system.

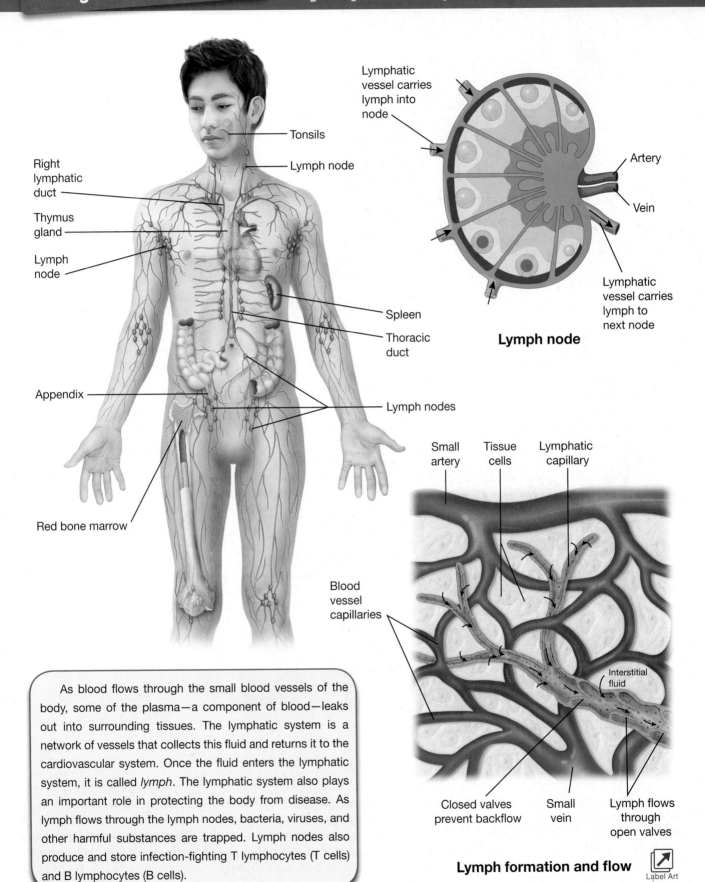

Tonsils

Lymph node

Right lymphatic duct

Thymus gland

Lymph node

Appendix

Red bone marrow

Spleen

Thoracic duct

Lymph nodes

Lymphatic vessel carries lymph into node

Artery

Vein

Lymphatic vessel carries lymph to next node

Lymph node

Small artery

Tissue cells

Lymphatic capillary

Blood vessel capillaries

Interstitial fluid

Closed valves prevent backflow

Small vein

Lymph flows through open valves

Lymph formation and flow

Label Art

As blood flows through the small blood vessels of the body, some of the plasma—a component of blood—leaks out into surrounding tissues. The lymphatic system is a network of vessels that collects this fluid and returns it to the cardiovascular system. Once the fluid enters the lymphatic system, it is called *lymph*. The lymphatic system also plays an important role in protecting the body from disease. As lymph flows through the lymph nodes, bacteria, viruses, and other harmful substances are trapped. Lymph nodes also produce and store infection-fighting T lymphocytes (T cells) and B lymphocytes (B cells).

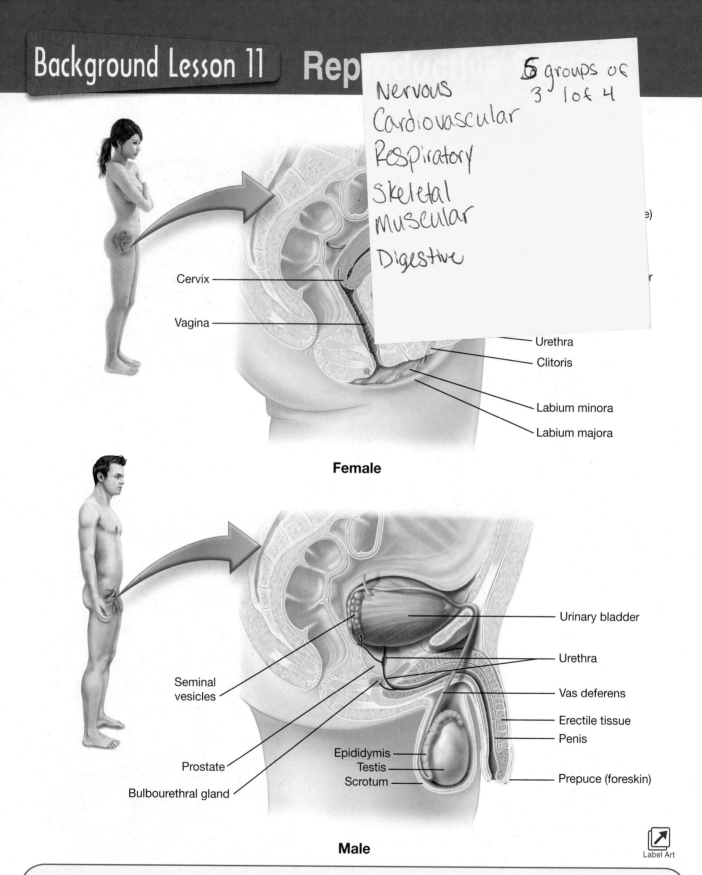

Handwritten note:

6 groups of
3   1 of 4

Nervous
Cardiovascular
Respiratory
Skeletal
Muscular
Digestive

Cervix

Vagina

Urethra

Clitoris

Labium minora

Labium majora

Female

Seminal
vesicles

Urinary bladder

Urethra

Vas deferens

Erectile tissue

Penis

Epididymis

Testis

Scrotum

Prepuce (foreskin)

Prostate

Bulbourethral gland

Male

Label Art

The reproductive system consists of a group of organs that work together to allow for the creation of new life. Unlike other body systems, the reproductive system is different in males and females. The male reproductive system creates sperm and the female reproductive system creates eggs. Fertilization occurs when sperm and egg unite. Other functions of the female reproductive system include nourishing the developing embryo and fetus, giving birth, and producing breast milk. Unlike other body systems, the reproductive system does not begin to function at birth, but at puberty.

Body Systems Review and Assessment

Know and Understand

1. _____ is the process of maintaining an internal state of physiological balance.

2. After cells and tissues, the next level of organization in the body is the _____ level.
   A. organ
   B. system
   C. human
   D. organism

3. The _____ system consists of the brain, spinal cord, and nerves.
   A. lymphatic
   B. endocrine
   C. cardiovascular
   D. nervous

4. List the four lobes of the brain.

5. *True or false?* The diencephalon is responsible for metabolism, heart rate, hunger, and thirst.

6. _____ carry oxygenated blood away from the heart.

7. _____ carry deoxygenated blood to the heart.

8. *True or false?* The cardiovascular system plays a role in regulating body temperature.

9. Which two body systems work together to deliver oxygen to cells and dispose of carbon dioxide?

10. Where does the process of gas exchange occur?

11. _____ is a waste product expelled through the lungs.
    A. Serosa
    B. Alveoli
    C. Oxygen
    D. Carbon dioxide

12. The _____ system gives the body its shape, protects internal organs, and makes movement possible.
    A. skeletal
    B. muscular
    C. endocrine
    D. digestive

13. The _____ is an example of a ball-and-socket joint.
    A. jaw
    B. metatarsal
    C. hip
    D. patella

14. *True or false?* Bones store minerals and fat and produce blood cells.

15. *True or false?* The thoracic cage is composed of the ribs and scapula.

16. The joints between vertebrae in the spine are called _____.
    A. freely movable joints
    B. slightly movable joints
    C. gliding joints
    D. hinge joints

17. Identify the three primary types of muscle tissue.

18. _____ muscle is found in the walls of many internal organs.

19. *True or false?* Smooth muscle makes movement possible.

20. _____ muscles pump blood through the heart and body.

21. What is the main function of the digestive system?

22. *True or false?* The mouth is also known as the *oral cavity*.

23. Which of the following correctly lists the four layers of the gastrointestinal tract, starting with the innermost layer?
    A. submucosa, mucosa, serosa, muscularis externa
    B. mucosa, submucosa, muscularis externa, serosa
    C. mucosa, serosa, muscularis externa, submucosa
    D. serosa, muscularis externa, submucosa, mucosa

24. The _____ is a tube-like structure that runs through the body from the mouth to the anus.
    A. esophagus
    B. mesentery
    C. small intestine
    D. gastrointestinal tract

25. Liquid waste is filtered from the blood and expelled from the body by the _____ system.
    A. cardiovascular
    B. urinary
    C. respiratory
    D. endocrine

26. *True or false?* The digestive system helps regulate the volume of water in the body.

27. *True or false?* The renal medulla is the outer tissue layer of the kidney.

28. The _____ carries urine from the kidney to the bladder.
    A. renal pelvis
    B. renal artery
    C. urethra
    D. ureter

29. Which body system consists of organs and small glands that regulate body functions?
    A. endocrine system
    B. nervous system
    C. immune system
    D. urinary system

30. *True or false?* The endocrine and nervous systems work together.

31. *True or false?* The pancreas is part of both the digestive and endocrine systems.

32. *True or false?* The ovaries and testes are part of the endocrine system.

33. Chemical messengers called _____ are released by the endocrine organs and glands to regulate body functions.

34. *True or false?* The lymphatic system is the *only* organ system that defends the body from disease-causing microorganisms.

35. Once fluid enters the lymphatic system, it is called _____.

36. Which body system includes a network of vessels that collects leaking plasma from tissues surrounding blood vessels
    A. endocrine system
    B. urinary system
    C. cardiovascular system
    D. lymphatic system

37. _____ produce and store infection-fighting T cells and B cells.
    A. Capillaries
    B. Lymph nodes
    C. Tonsils
    D. Lymphocytes

38. Which is the only body system that begins to function at puberty rather than birth?
    A. respiratory system
    B. lymphatic system
    C. reproductive system
    D. endocrine system

39. The epididymis and two testes are held in the _____.

40. _____ occurs when sperm and egg unite.

41. Which of the following are functions of the female reproductive system?
    A. creating eggs
    B. nourishing the embryo and fetus
    C. producing breast milk
    D. All of the above

Analyze and Apply

42. Identify two body systems that work together and explain how these systems are integrated.

43. What are possible consequences if the body fails to maintain homeostasis?

44. Do you think the process of gas exchange occurs rapidly or slowly? Explain your answer.

45. Explain the importance of the lymph nodes in fighting infection.

46. Compare and contrast the functions of the male and female reproductive systems.

Body Systems **Skill Development**

47. **Comprehend Concepts.** Do a sit-up, push-up, and then a squat. Using Lesson 6 as a reference, identify the muscles you used to complete each movement.

48. **Access Information.** Choose one of the body systems discussed in Lessons 3–11. Research three diseases and disorders associated with that system. Then, create a presentation identifying each disease or disorder, any risk factors, symptoms, and treatments. Share your findings with the class.

49. **Communicate with Others.** Research a career associated with each of the ten body systems discussed in these lessons. Create a digital presentation describing the educational requirements, salary, responsibilities, and job outlook for each career. Be sure to explain the connection between the body system and career. As you complete your research, you should also identify the career that appeals to you the most and explain why in your presentation. Share your presentation with the class, discussing the benefits and challenges of each position.

Motor vehicle crashes are the leading cause of death among adolescents, accounting for about 70% of the deaths associated with unintentional injuries. Many of these fatalities occur among pedestrians involved in the accidents.

Safety in Motor Vehicles

Immaturity and inexperience at the wheel contribute to the high prevalence of vehicle fatalities in teens. Most fatal car crashes involve driving at an unsafe speed or exceeding the legal speed limit. Poor driving habits, including cell phone use and texting while driving, are also to blame. Teen drivers are often distracted by their cell phones while they are in the car. Texting is especially dangerous because it distracts vision and thinking (Figure BL12.1).

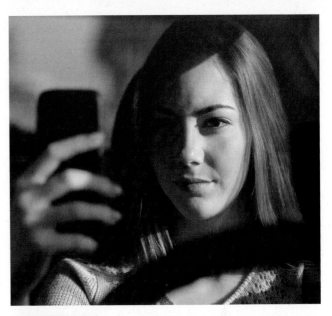

Figure BL12.1 Texting while driving is a dangerous behavior that diverts a driver's sight and attention from the road. Losing attention for even a few seconds can lead to a serious, possibly fatal, car crash. *What actions could you take to minimize your temptation to text and drive?*

Fast Fact

The National Highway Traffic Safety Administration reports that drivers take their eyes off the road for nearly 5 seconds during an average text. At 55 miles per hour, a car can travel the distance of about one football field in 5 seconds.

Safe Driving

As a responsible driver, you must take care to obey the rules and regulations of the road. These rules are in place to maintain a safe community, and it is your job as a driver to avoid accidents and drive responsibly. A more detailed discussion of these specific rules and regulations should be covered in your driver's education course.

Driving experience has been recognized as an important element in preventing vehicle crashes. As a result, many states have implemented Graduated Driver Licensing (GDL) for teen drivers. GDL gives younger drivers time to establish driving experience before they receive full licensing. A specific set of regulations apply to these young drivers as they complete their GDL.

After completing driver's education, the driver permit stage, and licensing, teen drivers should follow these policies:

- Do not use any illegal drugs. Do not drive while using prescription or over-the-counter drugs that can impair alertness, reflexes, or coordination.
- Do not use alcohol while driving and do not get into a car with a driver who has been using alcohol. You cannot legally operate a vehicle while under the influence of drugs and alcohol.
- Never use a cell phone while driving.
- Never text while driving.
- Do not drive with passengers under 18 years of age until the driver is 18 years of age.
- All passengers and the driver must wear seat belts at all times.
- Driving after 10:00 p.m. is not allowed during the first six months of licensing.

Passenger Safety

Taking responsibility for your safety means that you do not get into a car driven by someone who does not practice safe driving policies. Reckless, drowsy, and distracted drivers put the safety of their passengers at risk. Never get in the car with a driver who does not have a driver's license, carries more passengers than the law allows, or has been using drugs or alcohol.

Always get permission from your parents to ride in a car driven by another teenager. Let your parents know who is driving or if commuting plans change.

Pedestrian Safety

As a pedestrian, always look in every direction to locate drivers who may be nearby. You can improve your safety as a pedestrian by taking the following precautions:

- Always assume that drivers cannot see you. Never assume that drivers will stop or avoid you, even when you have the right-of-way.
- Walk where drivers would expect you to walk, which is on sidewalks if possible.
- Make eye contact with drivers at intersections to be sure you see each other.
- Obey traffic signals and use designated pedestrian crosswalks.
- If you must walk on a road, always walk as far to the side as possible, facing traffic.
- Avoid walking near traffic at night or when visibility is poor.
- If you must walk at night, wear bright clothing or carry a flashlight.

Cycling Safety

Cycling is good exercise and a fun, inexpensive form of transportation. Take basic precautions for a safe ride:

- Always wear a properly fitted helmet.
- Know and obey all traffic rules.
- Ride on the right side of the road and with traffic, never facing traffic.
- Ride with companions in a single file.
- Signal your turns at intersections so drivers can anticipate your movements. With your left arm, point left to indicate a left turn and bend your forearm up to indicate a right turn.
- Always stop at red lights.
- Wear bright clothing during the day and reflective clothing at night.
- If you must ride after dark, use front and rear lights.

Lesson Activities

1. Research your state's laws about phone use while driving. Is it legal in your state to talk on a handheld cell phone and drive at the same time? Is it legal to talk with a hands-free device while driving? Is it legal to text and drive? After completing your research, create a presentation for your peers that details what you found.

2. Choose one healthy behavior from each of the three areas covered in this lesson and demonstrate these behaviors in your life. Take a picture or have someone take a picture of you. Then, write a caption advocating for the healthy behavior you are practicing for each picture.

Over half of all injury-related deaths occur in the home. If you know the risks, hazards, and injuries that are possible in the home environment, you can take steps to make your home safer.

Preventing Poisoning

The chemicals in household products can be poisonous if used in the wrong way. Post the national toll-free number for the Poison Control Center (800-222-1222) in a prominent location in your home. This phone number can be used throughout the United States and Canada to reach a center at any time. Poison control centers are run by hospitals, government agencies, or other medical organizations. The centers will answer questions about all types of poisonings, give first aid directions, and contact emergency services for you.

Many products used in and around the home can be hazardous if used improperly. These products include

- cleaning agents such as bathroom, toilet, oven, and floor cleaners; bleach; and furniture polish;
- automotive chemicals, such as antifreeze, engine oil, gasoline, and windshield wiper fluid;
- personal items, such as cosmetics, hairspray, nail polish remover, rubbing alcohol, hydrogen peroxide, antibiotic ointment, and mouthwash; and
- garden, yard, and home items, such as paints, paint thinner, stains, and varnishes; plant fertilizer; insect repellent; pesticides and insecticides; weed killer; and lighter fluid.

To prevent someone in your home from becoming ill or injured by these products, always follow these guidelines:

- Read and follow label directions for safe use (Figure BL13.1). Note label precautions regarding the product's flammability or hazardous fumes.

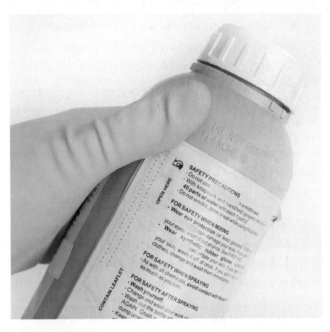

Figure BL13.1 Poisoning is often caused by the improper use of household chemicals. Before using any chemical substance in your house, you must read the label and safety instructions.

- Store all chemicals in their original containers and as described on the labels. Store hazardous chemicals away from food in a locked area that children and pets cannot access.
- Wear protective equipment required by the label (such as goggles, gloves, or mask).
- Read the label for first aid treatment of accidental skin exposure, eye exposure, or ingestion.
- Dispose of chemicals as described on the label.

Preventing Falls at Home

Most falls are preventable accidents. The following steps will help reduce the risk of falls in your home:

- Clear the floors and stairs of clutter.
- Keep electrical cords and telephone lines away from walkways.

- Cover slippery floors with nonslip rugs.
- Install handrails for stairs, in bathtubs, and near toilets for older adults.
- Ensure good lighting by replacing burned lightbulbs and using night-lights.
- Use step stools or ladders to reach high cabinets or shelves.
- Repair or replace worn carpet edges and seams.

Fast Fact

Unintentional falls lead to about 18,000 deaths each year in the United States.

Home Fire Prevention and Safety

You can help your family recognize and eliminate many hazards around your home to lower your chances of being injured in a fire.

Install Smoke Detectors

The installation and maintenance of smoke detectors can reduce your risk of injury and death from fire. The United States Fire Administration reports that having working smoke detectors more than doubles the chances of surviving a fire (Figure BL13.2). The following steps can ensure proper use of a smoke detector:

- Properly place detectors on every level of the home, including the attic and basement.
- Install a smoke detector outside all sleeping areas, in the kitchen, and near the furnace.
- Test your smoke detectors monthly.
- Replace smoke detector batteries at least once a year. A good time to do so is in October during Fire Prevention Week and before the heating season. If the smoke alarm chirps, promptly replace the battery.

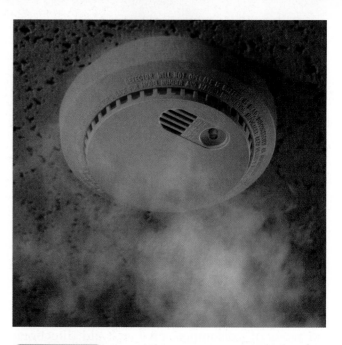

Figure BL13.2 Properly installed smoke detectors can decrease the risk of you and your family being harmed by fire. Smoke detectors should be maintained and tested monthly, to ensure consistent performance. *How often does your family test your smoke detectors?*

Prohibit Smoking Indoors

To greatly reduce the risk for fire, family members and guests should never smoke inside your home—especially in bed or on couches. Careless smoking is the leading cause of death from home fires. Fires can start if a smoker falls asleep with a lit cigarette, cigar, or pipe. If a family member smokes, quitting will reduce the risk of fire and bring many other health benefits.

Other Fire Prevention Steps

The following are other steps to take to prevent fires in the home:

- Never leave burning candles unattended.
- Keep flammable materials away from sources of heat and flames. These can be easily ignited by fire or a spark and burn rapidly. Store flammable paints, gasoline, and chemicals outside the home in a shed or garage.

- Use space heaters exactly as described by the manufacturer. They should turn off automatically if tipped over accidentally. Never use an extension cord with a space heater.

- Always clean grease buildup on stovetops, on burners, and in the oven.

- Clean the filter on clothes dryers after every use.

- If your home has a fireplace, dispose of coals and any fireplace waste in a nonflammable container. Chimneys should be cleaned and inspected regularly to remove flammable material that coats the inside of chimneys.

- Periodically check all electrical cords and discard worn electrical cords and wires. Never overload an electrical outlet with more plugs than it can receive. Unplug electrical appliances when they are not in use.

- Always turn off the power at the main supply before working on an electrical outlet or light fixture.

Devise a Fire Emergency Plan

An established emergency evacuation plan will help all family members get out of your home safely in case of a fire. Practice your plan once a year when you change the smoke detector batteries. Your plan should include several important precautions and procedures:

- Close bedroom doors when sleeping to keep out smoke and flames in the event of a fire.

- During a fire, feel doors with the back of your hand to determine if they are hot before opening. If the door is hot, escape through a window.

- Check that all bedrooms have a window that opens. Windows should be easy to unlock and open quickly.

- If you can, alert people in your home. Get out of the building and call 911 from a neighbor's home or cell phone.

- Crawl near the floor to escape dangerous smoke, toxic fumes, and heat.

- If your clothing catches fire, stop, drop, and roll to extinguish flames.

- Once outside, never go back into a burning building.

Everyone should know the location of fire extinguishers in the home. Fire extinguishers can control small fires and prevent them from causing damage or injury (Figure BL13.3 on the next page). A fire extinguisher should be available near the furnace, in the garage, and in the kitchen for grease and cooking fires. Everyone in the family who is old enough should learn how to use a fire extinguisher.

Chemical Hazards

Even a chemical that seems safe can become hazardous when the body is exposed to it in a particular way or in certain quantities. Some chemicals are skin, eye, and respiratory irritants that cause pain, inflammation, and allergic responses. Other chemicals cause breathing difficulty due to constricted airways. Chemicals known as *carcinogens* can cause cancer if they are handled improperly.

Aside from health problems, hazardous chemicals can also cause a situation to become unsafe. Flammable chemicals, for instance, will burn in the presence of sparks, flame, heat, friction, pressure, or other reactive chemicals. Other chemicals react with a violent release of energy in these conditions. Corrosive chemicals cause damage to other substances, including a person's skin. These chemicals pose a risk for serious injuries.

Radon

Radon is a colorless, tasteless, odorless, radioactive gas. It can seep from the ground and accumulate inside the basement and lower levels of homes, where it can cause damage before breaking down.

Figure BL13.3 Types of Fire Extinguishers

Fires	Type	Use	Operation
Class A Fires Ordinary Combustibles (Materials such as wood, paper, textiles.) *Requires... cooling-quenching* Old New	**Soda-acid** Bicarbonate of soda solution and sulfuric acid	Okay for use on **A** Not for use on **B C D**	Direct stream at base of flame.
	Pressurized Water Water under pressure	Okay for use on **A** Not for use on **B C D**	Direct stream at base of flame.
Class B Fires Flammable Liquids (Liquids such as grease, gasoline, oils, and paints.) *Requires...blanketing or smothering.* Old New	**Carbon Dioxide (CO_2)** Carbon dioxide (CO_2) gas under pressure	Okay for use on **B C** Not for use on **A D**	Direct discharge as close to fire as possible, first at edge of flames and gradually forward and upward.
Class C Fires Electrical Equipment (Motors, switches, etc.) *Requires... a nonconducting agent.* Old New	**Foam** Solution of aluminum sulfate and bicarbonate of soda	Okay for use on **A B** Not for use on **C D**	Direct stream into the burning material or liquid. Allow foam to fall lightly on fire.
Class D Fires Combustible Metals (Flammable metals such as magnesium and lithium.) *Requires...blanketing or smothering.* D	**Dry Chemical**	Multi-purpose type / Ordinary BC type Okay for: **A B C** / **B C** Not okay for: **D** / **A D**	Direct stream at base of flames. Use rapid left-to-right motion toward flames.
	Dry Chemical Granular type material	Okay for use on **D** Not for use on **A B C**	Smother flames by scooping granular material from bucket onto burning metal.

If inhaled, these radioactive particles can damage lung tissues. Homeowners should test for radon gas in their homes using inexpensive kits. Simple repairs will significantly reduce the amount of radon in your home. Have cracks sealed in basement floors and walls where radon enters your home. A qualified technician or plumber can install an exhaust system.

Fast Fact

Radon is formed from naturally occurring uranium that is found in small amounts throughout the earth's soil and rocks. As radon forms, it seeps to the surface and into the air.

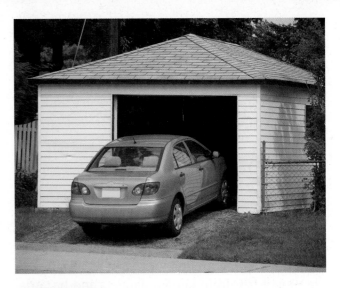

Figure BL13.4 Running a car or lawn mower in a closed garage can cause a buildup of carbon monoxide. To prevent carbon monoxide poisoning, run these machines outside.

Carbon Monoxide

Carbon monoxide is a toxic, odorless, invisible gas produced during combustion of gasoline, natural gas, oil, kerosene, charcoal, and other fuels. Carbon monoxide adheres to the hemoglobin in red blood cells, preventing the blood from transporting oxygen to the tissues. The result is potentially deadly carbon monoxide poisoning.

The signs and symptoms of carbon monoxide poisoning include extreme fatigue, sleepiness, nausea, confusion, dizziness, and headache. This condition can rapidly lead to coma and death. If carbon monoxide poisoning is suspected, leave the building immediately and go to an emergency room.

To prevent carbon monoxide poisoning, take the following steps:

- Install carbon monoxide detectors near furnaces, hot water heaters, and all sleeping areas.

- Never use barbecue grills indoors.

- Never use a gas stove or oven to heat the house.

- Never leave a vehicle's motor or a lawn mower running in a garage (Figure BL13.4).

- Use portable fuel-burning appliances such as space heaters and generators outside your home in well-ventilated areas.

Lesson Activities

1. When disposed of improperly, prescription drugs and medications can be harmful to the environment and present a danger. Research drug disposal programs in your area.

2. Create an illustration of a typical room at school or at home that contains 10–15 potentially hazardous objects or situations. Then, trade illustrations with a classmate to see if he or she can identify all the hazards and explain why they are hazardous.

3. Due to fire codes, buildings must meet standards that protect people and property from fire. Research past and present fire codes in your area. How do fire-code standards prevent and protect people from fires?

Having a job gives a teenager the chance to make new friends, gain independence, learn valuable skills and responsibilities, and earn money (Figure BL14.1). However, the workplace can also be a hazardous place if both employees and employers are not alert.

Workers' Rights

The US government has established laws that guarantee all workers certain rights pertaining to safety in the workplace. Employers are responsible for providing their employees with a working environment free from known dangers and hazards. The law that protects workers and gives them rights is called the *Occupational Safety and Health Act*, or OSH Act. This law is enforced by the Occupational Safety and Health Administration (OSHA), which is a specific branch of the Department of Labor.

The OSH Act includes several protections for workers:

- If known hazards are present in the workplace, employers must inform workers before they begin their work.

- Employers must train workers in the safe and correct execution of their duties.

- Employers must train workers to handle workplace emergencies and accidents.

- Employers must provide workers with equipment such as helmets, goggles, and earplugs if needed to work safely.

Workers have the right to refuse to do work that can cause them injury or illness. They cannot be fired or disciplined for reporting hazards and dangers in the workplace to their employers.

The government has established laws that require employers to provide medical care and certain benefits if an employee is injured at work. Under *workers' compensation*, an injured employee may receive pay, healthcare, or other benefits. In exchange for guaranteed benefits and some income, the injured employee is not permitted to take legal action against the employer.

In addition to these laws, teens should be aware of labor laws that specifically apply to teen workers. For example, certain types of jobs are too dangerous for teenagers. The law describes which jobs teens can and cannot do. These laws also describe permissible hours for teenage workers. Lastly, children under 14 years of age are only permitted to hold certain jobs, such as babysitting and delivering newspapers.

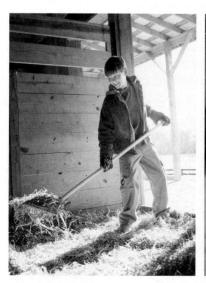 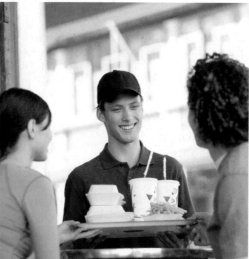 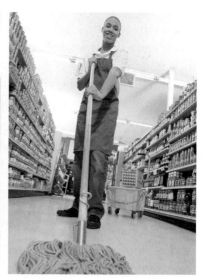

Figure BL14.1 Having a job provides teenagers with an opportunity to gain experience, earn money, and expand their social worlds.

Workers' Responsibilities

Workers should also take responsibility for their own safety on the job, as well as the safety of coworkers and customers. Workers are responsible for following the policies and procedures that are in place to protect their health and safety. They need to inquire about any hazards and dangers in the workplace. Workers must alert their supervisors to unsafe work practices or working conditions.

When training is provided, workers are responsible for learning and following safety procedures, and using any required safety equipment.

Ergonomics

Ergonomics is the study of how objects and environments should be designed and arranged so people can use them efficiently without endangering their health and safety (Figure BL14.2). These objects and environments include furniture, machines, and tools.

The goal of ergonomics is to create a safe, comfortable working environment.

Many kinds of work require repetitive, stressful movement that causes types of *repetitive strain injuries (RSIs)*. These injuries are due to repeated movement of muscles and joints, which can cause inflammation, pain, and disability. *Tendinitis*, inflammation of a tendon, is a type of repetitive strain injury. Another common injury is *carpal tunnel syndrome*, a painful swelling of a nerve in the wrist, which results from repeated motion of the wrist and fingers.

Lesson Activity

1. Draw two illustrations of a person sitting at a computer: one of the correct ergonomic position and one of an incorrect ergonomic position. Then, analyze your own habits while working at the computer. Which illustration more closely resembles your position?

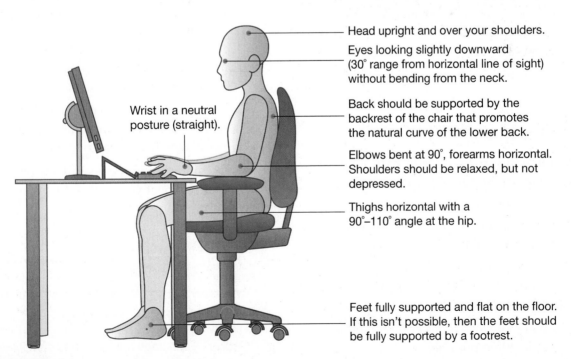

Wrist in a neutral posture (straight).

Head upright and over your shoulders.

Eyes looking slightly downward (30° range from horizontal line of sight) without bending from the neck.

Back should be supported by the backrest of the chair that promotes the natural curve of the lower back.

Elbows bent at 90°, forearms horizontal. Shoulders should be relaxed, but not depressed.

Thighs horizontal with a 90°–110° angle at the hip.

Feet fully supported and flat on the floor. If this isn't possible, then the feet should be fully supported by a footrest.

Figure BL14.2 Maintaining a good posture while working at a desk can help prevent health complications such as back pain, wrist pain, and eyestrain. *Assess your own work posture. What aspects of good posture do you already practice? What aspects can you improve?*

Personal Safety and Security

Whether you are on your own or with friends, you need to take steps to ensure your personal safety and security. This precaution applies even to the most familiar settings, such as school football games, field trips, dates, your own home, and around your neighborhood. Your attention to security is especially important when you are in unfamiliar areas or alone.

Staying Safe at School

School safety emerges from collaboration between school personnel, parents, and students. Students are expected to follow safety procedures and alert school staff to unsafe conditions and emergencies.

- Learn your school's rules regarding appropriate behavior and safety procedures. These rules will apply whenever you are on school property.

- Report problems you observe in and around your school as well as during extracurricular activities. If you are uncomfortable about what you see, tell a teacher, counselor, dean, or school security officer.

- Leave valuable items and jewelry at home.

Precautions in Public Places

The following steps can help reduce your risk of personal injury in public places:

- Tell your parents or guardian where you are going, how you will get there, and when you will be back.

- Take identification and only enough money for your needs. Carry a charged cell phone to call for a ride or help if you need it.

- Travel in well-lit areas and with other people when possible.

- If you are confronted by a thief who demands your valuables, hand them over without fighting.

Safety in Vehicles

If you have car trouble in an unfamiliar place or on the highway, stay in the car, lock the doors, and call 911 for assistance. Do not get out of the vehicle to meet people who stop to help you. Instead, roll the window down a bit and ask them to phone for assistance, or thank them and let them know you have already called for help. Do the same if you get into a minor accident in an unfamiliar place and you are not injured.

Precautions Online

Remember that there are risks to communicating online. You can protect your privacy and safety by following these online safety guidelines:

- Never give your personal information or the personal information of others to anyone without getting your parent's permission. Personal information such as your name, home address, school's name, or photographs can identify you and make it easy for someone you do not know to find you.

- Do not send anyone a photograph of yourself or anyone else in your family without permission from a parent or guardian.

- Do not agree to meet someone or ask them to meet you without your parents' permission.

Lesson Activity

1. Write an e-mail, text, or letter to a friend, giving him or her the information about personal safety and security that you learned in this lesson. Encourage your friend to practice these personal safety and security behaviors. How did your friend respond? How did it feel to be a peer educator?

Basic Emergency and First Aid Preparedness

You can prepare for different kinds of emergencies by assembling a first aid kit and emergency supplies. By learning and practicing first aid skills, you will be able to remain calm, think, and act rationally during the stress of an emergency.

A *medical emergency* is an urgent, life-threatening situation. Medical emergencies can involve health problems, such as a person having a heart attack. Medical emergencies also involve injuries, including severe bleeding, fractures, or burns. *First aid* is treatment given in the first moments of a medical emergency—usually before medical professionals arrive on the scene. First aid techniques can save lives and prevent emergencies and injuries from becoming worse during the wait for professional medical help.

First Aid Skills

Although there are many types of medical emergencies, the initial steps of first aid apply to most emergencies. If you encounter an emergency situation, first determine whether you can safely assist the victim (Figure BL16.1). You cannot help someone else if you are injured in the process. If you cannot physically get to the person because of his or her location or because of hazardous conditions, call 911 immediately. If you can safely help, then stay calm and perform these three key actions:

1. **Check the victim's condition.** Do a very quick assessment. If the victim exhibits one or more of the following conditions, he or she requires immediate first aid and medical care:
   - severe bleeding;
   - no breathing or difficulty breathing;
   - *shock*—a life-threatening condition in which the vital organs do not receive enough blood and oxygen; or
   - unconsciousness—the person passes out and cannot be awakened.

   Do not move the person unless you must leave a dangerous situation.

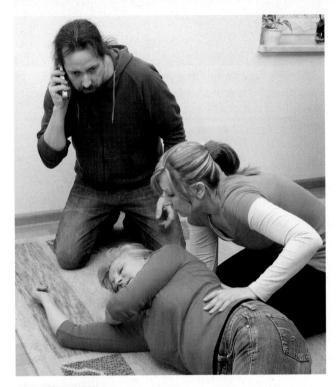

Figure BL16.1 If you witness a medical emergency, check the victim's condition and then call 911 immediately.

2. **Call 911.** As soon as you can, call 911 or your local emergency services, or tell a bystander to call while you administer first aid. The 911 dispatchers are trained to coach callers so the callers can give emergency first aid. Stay on the phone with the 911 dispatcher until emergency help arrives (Figure BL16.2). If you are at school, tell a teacher or coach about the emergency. They may be able to call 911 or help give first aid while you call 911.

3. **Give first aid.** If possible, obtain consent from the injured or ill person before you begin administering first aid. According to the law, you can administer first aid without consent under certain conditions:
   - The injured or ill person is unconscious or otherwise unable to give consent.
   - The person is a child whose parents are not present.

Figure BL16.2   Strategies for Communicating Effectively with Emergency Services

State your location and give the street address. If you do not know the address, ask a bystander to tell the 911 dispatcher while you begin first aid.

Tell the dispatcher why you called. Name the specific type of emergency.

Describe the victim's condition, age, and gender.

Give any other important information about the scene. For example, tell the dispatcher about downed power lines, poisons, or anything else that might help them understand the emergency.

If you have begun first aid, describe what you have already done.

Be prepared to listen to and follow the dispatcher's first aid directions.

Standard Precautions

Bloodborne pathogens such as HIV, hepatitis B, and hepatitis C can be transmitted in blood and body fluids contaminated with blood. You cannot know if the person you are helping is carrying these viruses. Therefore, when possible, take steps to protect yourself and handle each emergency as if infection is possible.

Standard precautions are infection control practices developed by the Centers for Disease Control and Prevention (CDC). Standard precautions apply when giving first aid to any person under any circumstances. Such practices include the following:

- Wear protective gloves when there is a risk of contact with blood or body fluids that may contain blood.

- If a respirator mouthpiece is available, use it when performing rescue breathing. Although rescue breaths may be given without a mouthpiece, it is better to take the precaution in case blood is present.

- Wash hands with soap and water after giving first aid.

First Aid Kit

A first aid kit should contain the supplies needed to treat most types of injuries and emergencies (Figures BL16.3 and BL16.4). You can put together your own kit or purchase a ready-made kit at most drugstores.

Your first aid materials should be enclosed in a clean, waterproof bag or box that is clearly labeled. The kit should be small enough to store in a car, a backpack, or a cabinet at home. The kit should be stored out of reach and out of sight of small children and away from family pets.

Figure BL16.3   First Aid Kit Essentials

- first aid manual
- phone numbers: Poison Control Center, family doctor, police, fire department

Supplies for treating wounds, such as

- gauze pads and assorted bandages to cover wounds;
- adhesive tape to fasten gauze and bandages;
- cotton balls and cotton swabs to apply antiseptics; and
- scissors to cut tape, gauze pads, or an injured person's clothing.

Supplies for preventing infections, such as

- antibiotic ointment for wounds and burns;
- antiseptic solution and antiseptic wipes;
- hand sanitizer to disinfect hands when handling wounds; and
- disposable latex or synthetic gloves to protect against bloodborne infections.

Supplies for treating various injuries, such as

- elastic wrap to treat sprains;
- instant cold packs to treat sprains, muscle strains, or bruises;
- tweezers to remove splinters or ticks; and
- sterile eyedrops or eyewash solution.

Over-the-counter medications, including

- pain relievers—ibuprofen or acetaminophen;
- hydrocortisone cream that reduces itching and swelling from poison ivy and other skin allergies; and
- antihistamines that reduce allergic response to ragweed, pollen, bee stings, and poison ivy.

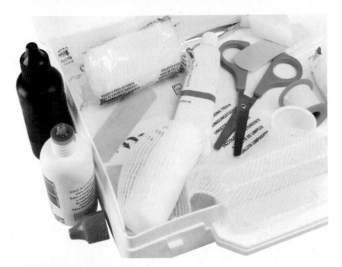

Figure BL16.4 A first aid kit should contain a manual, emergency phone numbers, supplies for treating wounds and infections, and a selection of over-the-counter medications. *List the items in the first aid kit above. Why do you think these items are included?*

Emergency Preparedness

With some simple preparation and the appropriate supplies, you can be ready to deal with emergencies at home or on the road. The types of emergencies you encounter will depend on where you live. Natural disasters and other emergencies could include

- weather-related emergencies (thunderstorm, flood, tornado, hurricane, or winter storm);
- power failure;
- landslide;
- fire or wildfire;
- earthquake; and
- terrorism.

Most emergency situations create common problems, such as exposure to the elements, loss of power, lack of sanitation, and contaminated water. Planning for these problems is part of emergency preparation. In emergencies, people also need to communicate and receive emergency information. Doing so improves your chances of staying safe during these dangerous situations.

Preparing Emergency Supplies

In addition to a first aid kit, a few other essentials will help you and your family stay safe during many kinds of emergencies (Figure BL16.5). Store these supplies in an easily accessible area of your home or car, and make sure everyone in your family knows where to find them. These supplies include

- a waterproof flashlight and extra batteries;
- candles and matches;
- blankets or sleeping bags for each person in your family;
- a waterproof tarp for shelter and to keep supplies dry;
- rope;
- a pocket knife or multitool;
- water/wind-resistant jackets and other warm clothing;
- nonperishable food;
- bottled water;
- water purification tablets or a portable water filter;
- a battery-powered or hand-crank radio;
- personal hygiene items such as toilet paper;
- a cell phone with chargers;
- extra cash; and
- a backpack to carry emergency items, first aid kit, and personal items.

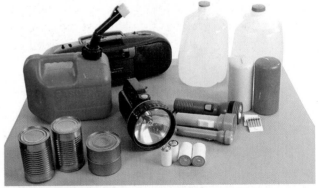

Figure BL16.5 Equally as important as a first aid kit is an emergency kit for situations such as hurricanes, tornadoes, or other disasters. These kits may contain flashlights, water, and canned foods.

Making an Emergency Plan

After assembling emergency supplies and a first aid kit, draw up a plan to follow during an emergency (Figure BL16.6). Different emergencies require different actions. Regardless of the type of emergency, an emergency plan should address the following issues:

- Where will you take shelter during this emergency? For example, go to a basement or a sturdy inner room such as a bathroom during a tornado. If you live in an area affected by hurricanes, know evacuation routes and shelters.

- How will you communicate with your family? Do you know how to reach a parent or guardian at work? Can you designate a contact person who lives outside of the area to relay information to all family members? How and where will you meet if you are separated?

- Who will you contact for emergency assistance, and how will you contact them? For example, know how to contact police, fire department, and paramedics in an emergency.

- What supplies and equipment will you need to get through the emergency? Where will the supplies be located? What do you need to do to make sure these supplies are available?

- How will you learn when the danger has passed?

Lesson Activities

1. Create a first aid kit for your home. Consider any special emergency supplies to include based on your locale. Do you live in an area prone to tornadoes or flooding? Make a list of each item you included in your kit.

2. Create an emergency plan for your family. As you draft your plan, consider the questions included in this lesson. Present your plan to the class.

3. Describe the difference between emergencies and nonemergencies. Give two examples of emergencies and two examples of nonemergencies.

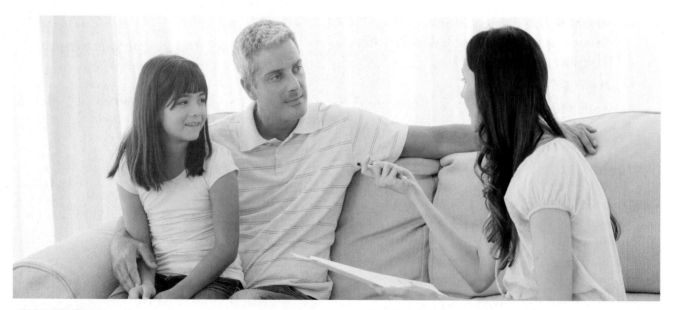

Figure BL16.6 Planning how to handle potential emergencies is a sure way of guarding against the chaos and panic that often accompanies emergency situations. *What plans does your family have in place for emergency situations?*

Medical emergencies in which a person's heart stops beating or the victim stops breathing are life-threatening. In these situations, first aid and medical care must begin as soon as possible to restore breathing and heartbeat. Quite a few medical conditions can cause breathing and heartbeat to stop.

Fast Fact

During a heart attack, the blood stops circulating, cutting off the brain's oxygen supply. Deprived of oxygen, the brain can survive for only about four minutes before irreversible damage occurs. The typical emergency crew response time from call to arrival is four to ten minutes. During the wait for medical help, quick action can save a life.

Cardiopulmonary Resuscitation (CPR)

The American Heart Association (AHA) and Red Cross recommend that Hands-Only™ cardiopulmonary resuscitation (CPR) be used to deliver blood circulation to a victim who suffered cardiac arrest (Figure BL17.1). To perform Hands-Only CPR

1. **call 911; and**
2. **do chest compressions.**

   - Position your hands over the center of the person's chest.
   - Push down hard at a rate of 100 times per minute.

Each time, the chest should be compressed at least two inches and then be allowed to rise completely before it is compressed again. Do this continuously without stopping, using your body weight to press straight down.

Don't slow down or stop compressions until emergency services arrives or an *automated external defibrillator (AED)* is available and ready for use (Figure BL17.2). This rescue device delivers a controlled, precise shock to the heart. An AED can restore the heart's electrical rhythm and heartbeat

Hands-Only CPR

1. Make sure the person is lying down.
2. Kneel next to the person's shoulder and neck. Place the heel of one hand on the center of the chest on the breastbone, between the nipples.
3. Place the heel of the other hand on top of the first hand, lacing your fingers together.
4. Keep your arms straight and position your shoulders directly over your hands.

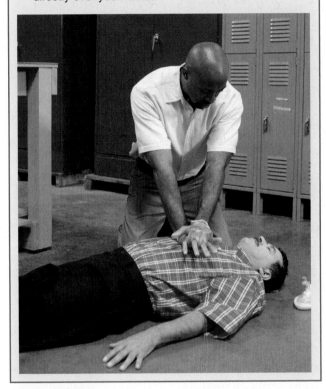

Figure BL17.1 Hands-Only CPR is performed to stimulate blood circulation in a victim who is experiencing cardiac arrest. By delivering chest compressions, someone practicing Hands-Only CPR can aid the victim's body in delivering oxygen to the body's organs.

in the event of a cardiac arrest. Hands-Only CPR and AEDs can be used even by people with little or no training.

Full CPR involves a combination of chest compressions *and* rescue breaths (called *mouth-to-mouth breathing*). Use this technique only if you are well trained in performing it. Training courses are available through the American Heart Association (AHA) and American Red Cross.

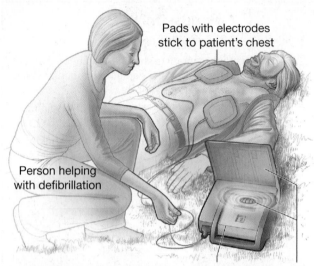

Pads with electrodes stick to patient's chest

Person helping with defibrillation

Automated external defibrillator (AED) (checks heart rhythm and can send electric shock to restore normal rhythm)

AED has written instructions and gives voice instructions

Figure BL17.2 AEDs deliver precise shocks to a victim's heart, in hopes of stimulating blood circulation. These machines contain written and auditory instructions, making them easy to use.

Shock

Shock is a life-threatening condition in which a person's body does not get enough blood and oxygen. If left untreated, shock can cause serious organ damage or death. Common signs and symptoms of shock include

- cold, clammy, pale, or gray skin;
- weak, rapid pulse;
- slow, shallow breathing or abnormally rapid breathing (hyperventilation);
- dilated (enlarged) pupils;
- weakness, confusion, agitation, or anxiety; or
- unconsciousness.

First aid for shock begins with calling 911 or the local emergency number. Have the person lie down with feet elevated about 12 inches higher than the head and heart. Doing this will move blood from the lower body toward the brain, heart, and organs of the trunk. This will also reduce stress on the heart.

Cover the person with a blanket and keep him or her warm. Do not give the person water or anything else to drink because this may cause choking or vomiting. Monitor breathing and pulse, and be prepared to begin CPR if needed (Figure BL17.3). Give first aid for any injuries or conditions that caused the shock. Do not move the person unless there is an immediate danger.

Choking

Choking is a medical emergency in which a foreign object blocks the airway. When people are choking, their oxygen supply is cut off.

Signs of Choking

Many people instinctively grab their throats with both hands when they are choking. Choking is marked by the inability to speak and breathe. A choking person

- cannot breathe normally;
- cannot talk or make noise;
- cannot cough or expel air forcefully;
- has blue skin, lips, and nails; and
- eventually becomes unconscious.

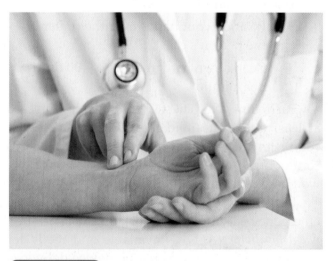

Figure BL17.3 While waiting for emergency medical professionals to arrive, monitor the pulse of the person experiencing shock.

"Five-and-Five" Method for Aiding Person Who Is Choking

1. Give five back blows.

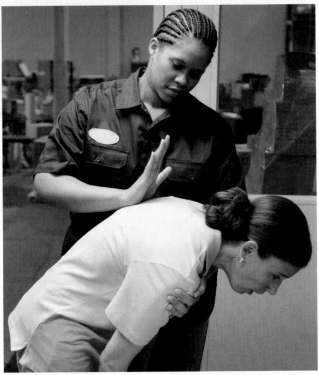

2. Give five abdominal thrusts.

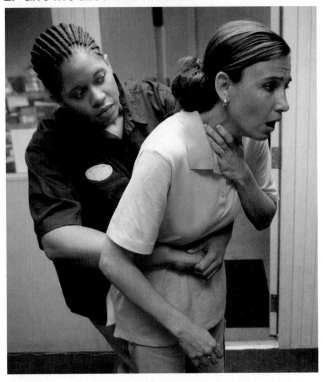

Figure BL17.4 The "five-and-five" method for helping a person who is choking includes delivering five back blows and then five abdominal thrusts.

General First Aid for Choking

The American Red Cross recommends the *"five-and-five" method* for aiding a person who is choking. This method involves the use of a series of back blows alternating with abdominal thrusts, which force air out of the choking person's lungs (Figure BL17.4). This should help push the stuck object out of the airway. Abdominal thrusts are also called the *Heimlich maneuver*. The following is the "five-and-five" method procedure:

1. Ask someone to call 911.
2. Perform five back blows. When you perform a back blow, hit the choking person's back between the shoulder blades using the heel of your hand.
3. Perform five abdominal thrusts:
   - Stand behind the person, wrap your arms around their waist, and clasp your hands together at the front.

- Bend the person forward slightly.
- Form a fist with one hand and press it against the abdomen. Hold your fist with your other hand.
- Push hard, in and up against the abdomen.

Make sure someone has called 911. Then continue with the "five-and-five" rescue method until the person is no longer choking or emergency services arrive. Be prepared to give CPR if necessary.

First Aid for Unconscious Choking Victims

If the choking person loses consciousness, check the mouth and throat for any foreign objects and sweep them out with your fingers. While doing this, be careful not to push anything further down the airway. Continue the "five-and-five" method and be prepared to perform CPR if needed.

Drowning

Water-related accidents are common. Most occur when children fall into a pool or are left alone in a bathtub. You can prevent accidents by learning and practicing water safety:

- Never leave children alone in or near water of any kind—including ponds, lakes, swimming pools, and beaches—even when lifeguards are on duty. A drowning can occur in minutes.
- Do not leave children alone in bathtubs.
- Empty standing water from tubs, pails, and other containers.

If you believe someone is drowning, call 911 or tell someone to call right away. The American Red Cross recommends that untrained rescuers avoid entering the water. Drowning people panic and will push you down. Instead, rescuers should reach for the drowning person or throw him or her a flotation device, life jacket, rope, or any object that will float (Figure BL17.5).

Once the person is out of the water, check his or her pulse and breathing as you do before giving CPR. If needed, give CPR. You must avoid moving drowning victims if their heads, necks, or backs are injured. Place rolled towels or cushions on either side of the head to keep it from moving.

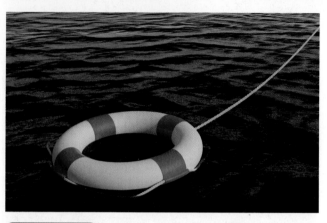

Figure BL17.5 Life preservers may be used to rescue a drowning person, particularly if the rescuer is untrained.

The signs and symptoms of electrical shock include numbness or a tingling sensation, muscle spasms, burns, unconsciousness, cardiac arrest, and respiratory failure. Take these first aid steps while waiting for emergency medical help to arrive:

- Call 911.
- Do not touch the person if they are in contact with electricity, such as a power line or wires.
- Turn off the electricity at the source if you can.
- If you must move a live electrical wire or appliance, push it away with a piece of wood, plastic, or cardboard. These substances do not conduct electricity.
- Check the person's pulse and breathing. Begin CPR if necessary.
- Treat the person for shock.

Fast Fact

About 3,600 people drown each year in the United States, with the highest death rate occurring among children under four years of age.

Electrical Shock

Electrical shock occurs when the body comes into contact with an electrical current. The shock could come from fallen power lines, a hazard that accompanies severe weather. People also get shocked when standing in flooded streets or basements. In these situations, the water conducts electricity to the body from electrical wires, outlets, or downed power lines.

Lesson Activity

1. Safety around water can reduce accidents. With a partner, list risks related to water and explain how to reduce these risks and resist pressure to engage in unsafe behaviors around water. Discuss safe alternatives to risky situations involving water and create a plan for ensuring water safety.
2. In small groups, research regulations about emergencies (for example, the Good Samaritan Law). Choose one law to study and report about it to the class.

Clotting factors in the blood stop bleeding caused by a minor injury and prevent major blood loss. Clotting factors are also triggered in the event of more severe wounds, but clots cannot easily seal injuries to large blood vessels. If a large artery is injured, a lot of blood may be lost before the blood's clotting response can effectively stop the bleeding. Immediate first aid for minor wounds can speed healing and prevent serious, sometimes life-threatening infections.

Severe Bleeding

The most important part of first aid for severe bleeding is the application of pressure to the wound. Other steps slow blood loss by careful positioning of the body and by reducing the victim's heart rate and blood pressure. Following are steps to take when providing first aid to someone experiencing severe bleeding:

1. Apply pressure to wound or squeeze arterial pressure points.
2. Position the wound higher than the heart.
3. Dress the wound.
4. Keep the victim calm.
5. Treat the victim for shock.

Major Cuts and Puncture Wounds

Although you can treat many minor wounds yourself, certain injuries must be treated by medical professionals. These injuries include

- deep or jagged cuts;
- deep puncture wounds;
- deep scrapes; and
- abrasions that cover a large area of skin.

A doctor needs to clean the wound in these cases because these injuries are prone to developing dangerous infections. People with these injuries may also need a vaccine to prevent *tetanus*, a serious bacterial infection associated with these types of wounds.

A deep cut will not close or heal well without stitches to hold together the wound's edges.

Deep cuts and puncture wounds may also contain debris that can cause a serious infection. The debris can be difficult to remove from the wound.

Puncture wounds—such as penetrating wounds from nails, thorns, or other sharp objects—usually bleed a small amount and appear to close up right away. The object that caused the puncture, however, can introduce bacteria deep into the tissues where it can become trapped and cause infections.

Until you get to a hospital, you can follow the following steps for first aid:

- Apply pressure to stop the bleeding.
- Cleanse the wound with clean water and remove any debris.
- Cover the wound.
- Tightly affix a bandage to hold the wound closed (Figure BL18.1).
- Elevate the wound.

Animal Bites

Being bitten by an animal, particularly a wild or unfamiliar animal, is cause for concern. Bite wounds that break or puncture the skin carry the

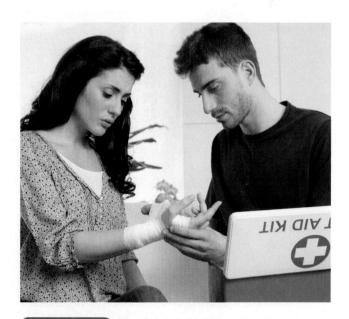

Figure BL18.1   Gently apply bandages to cuts and puncture wounds.

risk of infection. The most dangerous of these infections is the *rabies virus*, which infects the nerves, brain, and spinal cord. The disease is fatal if it is not treated immediately, before the virus reaches the brain and symptoms begin.

Animals that are infected with the rabies virus can spread the infection by biting humans and other animals. Always stay away from wild animals and avoid domestic animals when you do not know if they have been vaccinated for rabies (Figure BL18.2). Take care to avoid any animals that act aggressively, exhibit unusual behavior, or seem weak or sick.

All animal bites require a doctor's attention. Until you see the doctor, you can wash the wound with soap and water, cover it with a clean bandage, and elevate the affected area.

Minor Wounds and Bleeding

Most wounds result in some degree of bleeding. Although blood flow can flush foreign material and infectious agents from the wound, you must still control bleeding and protect the wound to allow it to heal and to prevent infection.

Before you touch the wound, wash your hands well with soap and water and dry them with a clean towel. Then take the following first aid steps:

1. Stop the bleeding. A minor wound should stop bleeding on its own, or you can apply gentle, direct pressure for up to 20 minutes. If necessary, elevate the area of the body that has been wounded.
2. Cleanse the wound by flushing the area with clean water. You can use soap to clean the skin around the wound, but not the wound itself because soap can cause irritation.
3. Apply an antibiotic cream or ointment (Figure BL18.3).
4. Cover the wound with clean adhesive bandages or gauze held in place by tape. Change the bandages daily.

Lesson Activity

1. Create a cartoon that illustrates how to treat minor wounds and bleeding. Draw a minimum of five panels in your cartoon.
2. Choose one injury you have experienced and describe it. Then trade descriptions with a partner and analyze how your partner's injury could have been prevented and how it was treated using first aid.

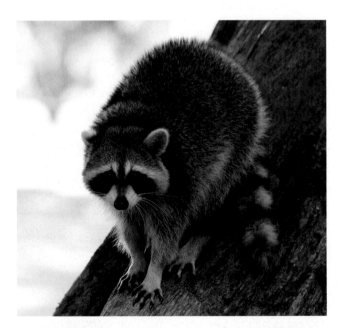

Figure BL18.2 Wild animals such as raccoons may be infected with the rabies virus.

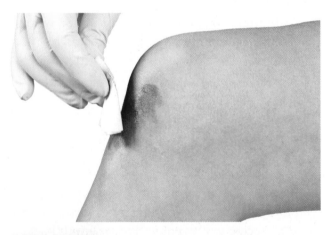

Figure BL18.3 Applying antibiotic cream or ointment helps prevent a wound from becoming infected. *Do you have antibiotic cream in your home? What are the active ingredients identified on the label?*

Burns, Poisons, and Insect Bites

Unfortunately, burns, accidental poisonings, and insect bites are extremely common among people of all ages. Learning how to treat these injuries is an important first aid measure.

Burns

Burns are common injuries that range from mild to life-threatening. A burn can be caused by exposure to any source of heat and energy including fire, burning or smoldering materials, steam, hot surfaces, or extremely hot gases and liquids. Burns can also be caused by other sources, including chemicals, electric current, and the sun.

All types of burns can seriously damage skin. Dangerous complications from burns include infection, shock, dehydration, pain, and immobility of the affected body part. First aid is essential for all burns. To give appropriate first aid, you need to identify the type of burn.

Fast Fact

According to the Centers for Disease Control and Prevention, 300 people under 20 years of age visit an emergency room each day for burn injuries.

Burn Classification

A burn is classified according to the level of damage caused. There are three levels of burn classifications—first degree, second degree, and third degree burns (Figure BL19.1).

First-degree burns are the least serious type of burn because only the outer layer of skin is damaged. Skin affected by a first-degree burn appears red and slightly swollen, and may be painful. First-degree burns include minor sunburns and burns caused by touching the skin to hot surfaces such as stoves, pots, and pans.

A second-degree burn affects the second layer of skin and is extremely painful. Skin damaged by a second-degree burn develops blisters (which are a source of infection), turns red, and swells. Burns affecting areas less than three inches in diameter are considered minor injuries. Second-degree burns affecting larger areas are considered medical emergencies and require emergency medical attention. Serious sunburns can become second-degree burns.

Third-degree burns are the most serious classification of burn, affecting all layers of skin, underlying tissue, muscle, fat, and even bone. A third-degree burn is considered a true medical emergency. Third-degree burns can lead to other serious medical problems including shock, infections, blood loss, dehydration, or unconsciousness.

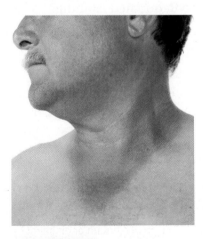 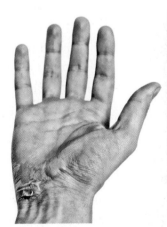 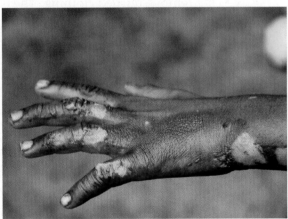

Figure BL19.1 First-degree burns, such as sunburns, affect only the outermost layer of skin (A). Second-degree burns are characterized by blisters and affect the first and second layers of skin (B). Third-degree burns affect all layers of skin and, in some cases, the underlying tissues (C).

First Aid for Minor Burns

The following steps should be used to treat first-degree burns and minor second-degree burns:

- Hold the burned skin under cool water for at least 10 minutes.

- Cover the burn with sterile gauze or bandage.

- Take a non-aspirin pain reliever, such as acetaminophen or ibuprofen.

First Aid for Serious Burns

Different steps need to be taken when treating more serious second-degree or third-degree burns:

- First, call 911 or a local emergency phone number.

- If the burn victim is unconscious, check for breathing and pulse and give CPR, if needed.

- Elevate the burned parts of the body above the level of the victim's heart, if possible.

- Cover the burned area loosely with moist, cool, sterile gauze; a bandage; or a clean cloth.

- Treat the burn victim for shock if necessary.

When treating major second-degree and third-degree burns, there are a few things you should *not* do:

- Do *not* remove burned clothing. The clothing may be adhered to burned tissue.

- Do *not* immerse these burns in cold water. This will cool the body and cause shock.

First Aid for Electrical Burns

When you find someone suffering from an electrical burn, call 911 immediately. Remember that first aid for an electrical burn begins with your own safety. You must first check for the source of the electrical current and carefully follow the steps discussed earlier to prevent yourself from receiving an electric shock. Check for breathing and pulse. The victim may need CPR or treatment for shock.

Poisoning

Poisoning is caused by exposure to or ingestion of a number of chemicals and fumes. These include household cleaning products, automotive chemicals, gasoline, and carbon monoxide.

If you suspect a person has been poisoned, call 911 or the Poison Control Center at 800-222-1222 to summon emergency help any time, day, and place in the United States. The kind of first aid to perform depends on the type of poisoning that has occurred.

If the person has swallowed something, take the following steps:

- Remove any substances left in the mouth.

- Read the label of the suspected container.

- Tell the Poison Control Center the name of the substance that you suspect was taken.

- Follow directions given by the Poison Control Center.

- If you cannot contact the Poison Control Center, follow any directions on the chemical container for the treatment of accidental poisoning.

- Check breathing and pulse, and give CPR if needed.

- Treat the victim for shock if necessary.

- Rinse spilled chemicals from skin and remove any contaminated clothing.

- Lay the person on his or her side with the head turned to the side to prevent choking on or inhalation of vomit.

- Do *not* induce vomiting without specific directions from the Poison Control Center.

Fast Fact

Hospital emergency rooms in the United States see more than 800,000 poisoning cases each year. Accidental poisoning kills around 37,000 people each year.

A. Poison Ivy Rash

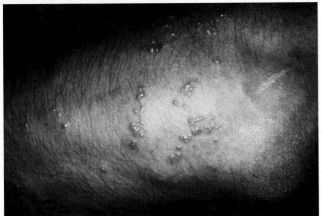

B. Poison Ivy

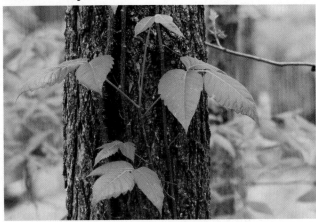

Figure BL19.2 — An itchy or painful rash can develop when skin comes in contact with poison ivy (A). Poison ivy can be found growing up from the ground or around trees (B).

Toxic Fumes

If carbon monoxide fumes or other toxic fumes are the suspected cause of poisoning, move the affected person from the building to an area with fresh air. Check the person's breathing and pulse, and give CPR if needed. Then treat the victim for shock if necessary.

Plant Toxins and Poison Ivy

A few plants produce *toxins*, or poisons that cause illness. If someone mistakenly eats berries or parts of an unknown plant, treat the situation as a possible poisoning. Contact the Poison Control Center, describe the plant, and follow the poison control center's directions.

Some plants produce poisons that affect any areas of the body that come into contact with the plants (Figure BL19.2). For example, poison ivy, poison sumac, and poison oak all cause watery, itchy blisters to develop where the plant touches skin. These plants grow in shady spots nearly everywhere in the United States. You may encouner these plants when hiking and camping, or even in parks and yards.

First aid for poison ivy exposure involves washing the affected area with soap and water, which serves to remove the plant's oils. Itching—a common symptom of poison ivy exposure—

can be treated with calamine lotion or hydrocortisone cream. Applying a cold cloth to the affected area can also reduce itching and pain. See a doctor at any sign of infection or anaphylaxis (allergic reaction).

Insect Bites

Common biting and stinging insects include bees, wasps, mosquitoes, and some types of ants. Mild reactions to insect bites include swelling or itching at the site of the bite. These reactions commonly follow mosquito bites and can be treated with cool cloths, calamine lotion, or over-the-counter hydrocortisone cream if the itching is severe.

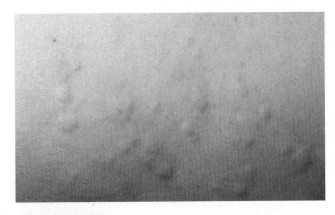

Figure BL19.3 — Some severe allergic reactions result in hives, a swollen rash that develops on the skin.

More severe reactions are typically associated with stings from bees, wasps, yellow jackets, and fire ants. The venom of these insects triggers pain, swelling, and redness. Some people also develop hives—a swollen, fluid-filled skin rash (Figure BL19.3 on the previous page). These stings can be treated with cold compresses or ice, pain reliever, elevation of the stung area, and rest. Use tweezers to remove any stingers stuck in the skin, wash the area, and apply hydrocortisone cream to relieve swelling and itching.

The most severe reactions need emergency care. A small number of people develop anaphylaxis. The signs and symptoms of anaphylaxis include

- nausea and vomiting;
- intestinal cramps and diarrhea;
- extensive swelling (baseball size or larger);
- hives;
- difficulty breathing;
- swelling of the throat, tongue, and lips;
- fainting;
- confusion; and
- rapid, shallow heartbeat.

First aid steps that should be taken if anaphylaxis occurs include the following:

- Call 911.
- Ask the person if they have medication such as the EpiPen® (Figure BL19.4).
- Give EpiPen® medicine as described by the package's directions.
- Loosen the person's clothing.
- Cover the person with a blanket and treat for shock.
- Lay the person on his or her side with the head turned to the side to prevent choking on or inhalation of vomit.
- Check breathing and pulse, and give CPR if needed.
- Do *not* give the person water or any other liquid.

Substances other than insect venom that may trigger anaphylaxis include peanuts, tree nuts

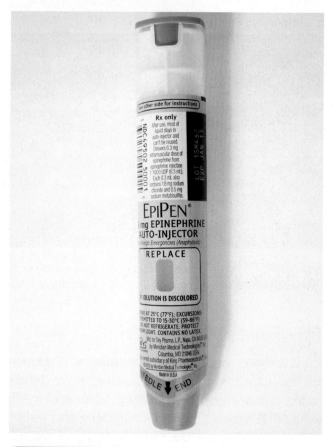

Figure BL19.4 Many people who know they have allergies carry an EpiPen®, an auto-injector containing medicine that will alleviate allergic symptoms. *Do you have any friends with severe allergies? If so, where do they keep their EpiPens®?*

such as cashews, fish, shrimp and other shellfish, cheese, and eggs.

Lesson Activities

1. With a partner, compose a short skit in which one character is burned and the other provides first aid for a minor or serious burn. Write the dialogue and actions for both characters. Be prepared to perform your skit for your classmates.

2. Research the toxic and poisonous plants found in your state. Do these plants grow year-round? Do they look different depending on the season? Create an informational pamphlet for visitors to your state detailing each plant and where it grows. Also include images for reference.

Movement places great stress on bones and joints, making them susceptible to injuries. Sports activities, falls, and motor vehicle accidents are common causes of fractures and related injuries.

Fractures

Fractures are broken bones. Any bone can break in a number of different ways (Figure BL20.1). In a compound fracture, broken bone protrudes from the body. All broken bones require medical attention. The goal of first aid for a fracture is to immobilize the fractured bone, keep the victim calm, and stop any bleeding that has occurred.

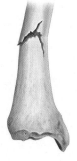

A. A *greenstick fracture* is incomplete. The break occurs on the convex surface of the bend in the bone.

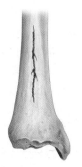

B. A *stress fracture* involves an incomplete break.

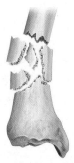

C. A *comminuted fracture* is complete and splinters the bone.

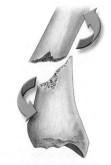

D. A *spiral fracture* is caused by twisting a bone excessively.

Figure BL20.1 Types of fractures include greenstick fractures (A), stress fractures (B), comminuted fractures (C), and spiral fractures (D).

First aid for a fracture involves the following steps:

- Call 911.
- Stop any bleeding with pressure and elevation.
- Immobilize the fracture with a splint, which can be made by gently tying a broken limb to a stiff board so the joint cannot move.
- Apply ice wrapped in a cloth to the fracture to control swelling.
- Administer a pain reliever.
- Treat the victim for shock.
- Do *not* move the victim.
- Do *not* realign a broken bone or push compound fractures back into place.

Dislocations

A *dislocation* is a condition in which bones move out of their normal position. Dislocations usually result from traumatic impact to the body, such as a fall or car crash. The severe pain and joint swelling require medical attention. Until a doctor is available, the dislocated joint and bones should be immobilized with a splint or an arm sling. Ice should be applied to the joints. If you experience a dislocation, never force the bones back into position yourself. This can seriously damage muscles, joints, and nerves.

Sprains

A sprain is an injury to tissues called *ligaments* that hold joints together. If a joint moves suddenly beyond its normal range of motion, the ligaments stretch and tear. The ankle, knee, and wrist are the most commonly sprained parts of the body.

Swelling and pain around the affected area are familiar signs of a sprain. First aid for a sprain follows the RICE treatment:

- **R**est the limb to allow recovery and healing.
- **I**ce the injury immediately for 10 minutes, and then four to eight times per day for two days to control swelling (Figure BL20.2).

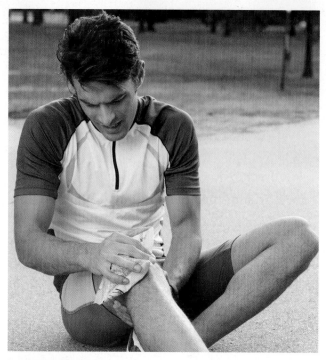

Figure BL20.2 Icing an injury helps reduce swelling and alleviate pain. *Why is it important to reduce the swelling that accompanies an injury?*

- **C**ompress the injury with an elastic bandage to immobilize it and reduce swelling.
- **E**levate the injury above the heart to control swelling.

To reduce pain and swelling, a person with a sprain should take acetaminophen or ibuprofen. You should see a doctor if the injury does not improve after two to three days, if swelling and pain worsen, or if the pain cannot be controlled with ice and medication.

Bruises

Bruises are caused by bleeding blood vessels within the skin. Bumps, blows, and falls commonly cause bruising. A bruise first appears as a purple color and later becomes green or yellow as the blood breaks down within the tissue. First aid treatment for a bruise includes applying ice or a cold cloth several times each day and resting the injured area.

Head Injuries

Consider every head injury to be a medical emergency for which you need to call 911. While waiting for medical help to arrive, give first aid for a head injury, including the following steps:

- Have the injured person remain lying down.
- Keep the injured person calm.
- Stop any bleeding.
- If the person is wearing a helmet, leave the helmet on.
- Check breathing and pulse, and begin CPR if necessary.
- Do *not* apply pressure to the skull if a fracture is suspected.
- Do *not* move the person at all— particularly the head or neck.

If the person is alert and responsive, have him or her rest quietly and remain still until emergency personnel arrive. The person could have sustained a concussion, which can be diagnosed and treated at the hospital.

Eye Injuries

Flushing with cool water is helpful for some minor eye injuries. One type of eye injury, a *corneal abrasion*, is a scratch on the outer covering of the eye. A corneal abrasion feels like sand in the eye and can be very painful. The best first aid treatment for an abrasion is to rinse the eye with cool water to wash out any foreign objects.

If a chemical is splashed in your eyes, it should be treated as an emergency. After calling 911 or telling someone to call, flush your eyes with clean water for 15 minutes while waiting for medical help.

Lesson Activity

1. Choose one of the injuries mentioned in this lesson. Create a poster or digital presentation outlining what to do and what not to do when providing first aid for this injury. Be prepared to share this information with your class.

Extreme weather conditions may cause safety and health emergencies requiring specific first aid.

Cold Weather Emergencies

Exposure to extreme cold causes two serious health issues that require immediate first aid and medical attention: frostbite and hypothermia.

Frostbite is a condition in which skin and underlying tissue freezes. Frostbite affects exposed skin and extremities, especially the nose, ears, fingers, and toes. If left untreated, frostbite can kill tissue and cause infection or loss of limbs. Signs of frostbite include

- white, gray, or yellow skin;
- cold and waxy skin;
- blistered, hardened skin; and
- numbness, burning, and itching.

The key to recovery is to warm the frostbitten areas gradually. Important first aid steps to take in case of frostbite include the following:

- Remove wet clothes.
- Immerse frostbitten hands or feet in warm (not hot) water.
- Cover ears, nose, or other cold areas with a warm blanket.
- Wrap in a warm blanket to preserve body heat and reduce stress.

Fast Fact

If the affected frostbitten area remains numb or painful after treatment, see a doctor immediately. There may be deep tissue damage or dead tissue.

Hypothermia is a medical emergency characterized by dangerously low body temperature. This condition occurs when the body is wet and exposed to cold or relatively cool air, even during summer (Figure BL21.1). Hypothermia can be fatal if untreated.

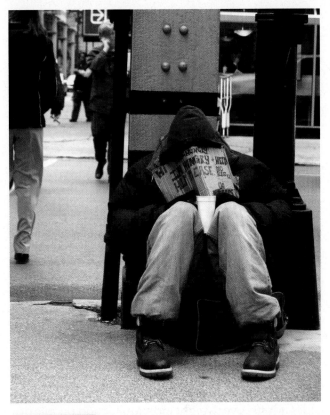

Figure BL21.1 Those who are homeless are often at risk for hypothermia, due to their frequent exposure to cool air and damp conditions.

Hypothermia can be recognized by these signs and symptoms:

- uncontrollable shivering
- slurred speech and loss of coordination
- abnormal, slow breathing
- extreme fatigue
- confusion or memory problems

If someone is showing signs of hypothermia, call 911 or the local emergency number and begin first aid immediately. Shock and cardiac arrest may occur. The following are important first aid procedures to remember:

- Move the person indoors. If you cannot get indoors right away, get into a car or move out of the wind. Use blankets, coats, or other padding to provide insulation from the cold ground.

- Remove the person's wet clothing and replace it with dry clothing or blankets. Cover the trunk of his or her body with as much warm clothing and blankets as possible.

- Give the individual warm drinks unless he or she is unconscious, too weak to swallow, or vomiting.

- Lie down with the person under a blanket to share body heat and warm him or her.

- Do *not* apply direct heat such as heating pads.

- Do *not* give the person alcoholic drinks.

- Do *not* massage or rub his or her skin.

Hot Weather Emergencies

Exposure to hot weather can tax the body's capacity to regulate its temperature. Heat and dehydration can cause *heat cramps*, or the more serious *heatstroke* and *heat exhaustion*. Infants, young children, older adults, overweight individuals, and people doing physical labor and or playing sports outdoors are susceptible to these heat-related illnesses.

Heat cramps are the mildest form of heat illness and typically affect muscles of the abdomen, arms, and legs. People can develop heat cramps during or after exercising or working outdoors in intense heat (Figures BL21.2 and BL21.3). This condition develops suddenly and is characterized by painful muscle cramps and spasms, especially in the legs. When experiencing heat cramps, it is important to rest, stay hydrated, and avoid strenuous activity for several hours. More serious conditions may develop if heat cramps are ignored.

Heat exhaustion, a more serious illness, is a sign that the body is having trouble handling extreme heat. It is important to treat heat exhaustion before it develops into a life-threatening condition called heatstroke. Heat exhaustion can be recognized by these signs and symptoms:

- cool and moist skin

- pale, gray, or flushed skin

- headache

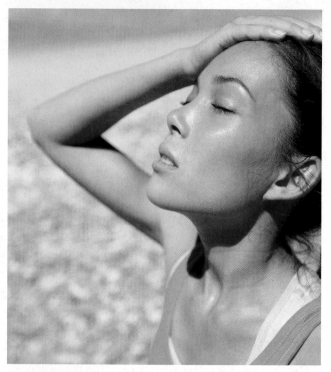

Figure BL21.2 Exercising in extreme heat can result in heat cramps, the mildest form of heat illness. *What should you do if you begin experiencing heat cramps?*

- nausea

- dizziness

- weakness and exhaustion

The first aid procedures for heat cramps and heat exhaustion are aimed at cooling and hydrating the person. If you encounter someone who appears to have heat cramps or heat exhaustion

- move the person to a shady, cooler environment, or indoors;

- remove as much of the person's clothing as you can;

- apply cold, wet towels to the skin on the trunk, back of the neck, and forehead;

- have the person sip cool drinks if he or she is conscious—do *not* give the person alcoholic or caffeinated beverages; and

- in the case of heat cramps, have the person gently stretch the cramping muscle.

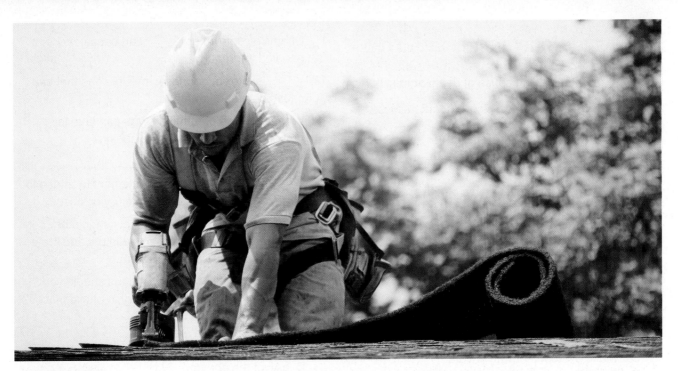

Figure BL21.3 Workers who spend time outdoors during periods of extreme heat are encouraged to wear light-colored clothing, take frequent breaks, and drink enough water so that they never become thirsty.

The person's condition should improve following these treatments. Call 911 if he or she does not recover, loses consciousness, or vomits. These symptoms mean the person might be developing heatstroke. Other signs of heatstroke include

- very high body temperature;
- red skin;
- altered consciousness or confusion;
- seizures; and
- rapid and weak pulse.

Fast Fact

Human body temperature varies throughout the day, but experts agree 98.6°F is the normal body temperature for healthy individuals. A body temperature of 104°F or higher is the main sign of heatstroke.

The key to surviving this dangerous condition is rapid cooling of the body. Take the following first aid steps for someone suffering from this condition:

- Call 911.
- Submerge the body in cold water up to the neck in a bathtub. Do not leave the person alone in the water.
- Have the person lie down with the feet elevated and soak him or her with a hose or shower.
- Cover the person's skin with towels soaked in ice-cold water or cover the victim with bags of ice.
- Monitor the person's body temperature and be prepared to give CPR or first aid for shock.

Lesson Activity

1. Risks due to extreme weather often accompany such activities as skiing or hiking on hot summer days. In small groups, discuss whether you think media portrayals of these activities are accurate and how these portrayals impact people's risk-taking behaviors. Write a short report detailing the risks involved in one extreme-weather activity.

Know and Understand

1. _____ are the leading cause of death among adolescents.
   A. Sports accidents
   B. Heart attacks
   C. Drug overdoses
   D. Motor vehicle accidents

2. *True or false?* Taking your eyes off the road for only five seconds is a safe driving practice.

3. Many states have implemented _____, allowing teen drivers to gain more experience before becoming fully licensed.

4. Which of the following is *not* a safe act for a pedestrian?
   A. When walking on a road, face traffic and walk as far to the side as possible.
   B. Make eye contact with drivers.
   C. Do not carry a flashlight when walking at night; this will distract drivers.
   D. Walk on the sidewalk whenever possible.

5. *True or false?* It is safest to ride your bike on the side of the road, facing traffic.

6. To signal a right-hand turn when riding your bicycle you should _____.
   A. Yell out, "turning right!"
   B. Stick your left arm out, bent up at the forearm.
   C. Stick your right arm out to the side.
   D. Point to the sky using your left arm.

7. *True or false?* When used improperly, cleaning products may be hazardous to your health.

8. If you have questions about a potentially poisonous substance, call the Poison Control Center at _____.

9. *True or false?* The installation and maintenance of smoke detectors can reduce your risk of injury or death from fire.

10. Which of the following is *not* a way to prevent fires in the home?
    A. Clean the filter on clothes dryers once a month.
    B. Always clean grease buildup off stovetops.
    C. Unplug electrical appliances when not in use.
    D. Never leave candles unattended.

11. Chemicals known as _____ can cause cancer if handled improperly.

12. _____ is a toxic, odorless, invisible gas that can cause coma and death.

13. What are three precautions you can take to prevent carbon monoxide poisoning?

14. What is the *OSH Act*?

15. *True or false?* Workers have the right to refuse to do work that can cause them injury or illness.

16. _____ is the study of how objects should be designed and arranged to avoid injury and create a safe, comfortable environment.

17. Which of the following precautions should you take to reduce your risk of injury in public places?
    A. Bring a charged cell phone.
    B. Travel in well-lit areas.
    C. Tell your parents where you are going.
    D. All of the above.

18. What are three precautions to always take when communicating online?

19. *True or false?* A 911 dispatcher will coach you through emergency first aid.

20. What are *standard precautions*?

21. What are the two steps involved in Hands-Only CPR?

22. The _____ involves a series of back blows and abdominal thrusts to aid a person who is choking.
    A. AED method
    B. Hands-Only CPR method
    C. "five-and-five" method
    D. Heimlich maneuver

23. *True or false?* When someone has a severe, bleeding wound, they may need to be treated for shock.

24. What is the difference between Hands-Only CPR and full CPR?

25. _____ is a serious bacterial infection associated with cuts and puncture wounds.

26. There are _____ levels of burn classification.
    A. two
    B. seven
    C. three
    D. four

27. How should poison ivy exposure be treated?

28. Signs of anaphylaxis include _____.
    A. swelling of the throat, tongue, and lips
    B. confusion
    C. hives
    D. All of the above.

29. *True or false?* Peanuts may cause anaphylaxis.

30. *True or false?* A greenstick fracture is a complete fracture.

31. What is the difference between a stress fracture and a comminuted fracture?

32. A(n) _____ is a condition in which bones move out of their normal position.

33. The RICE method can be used to treat _____.
    A. heatstroke
    B. fracture
    C. sprains
    D. infection

34. Signs of frostbite include _____.
    A. white, gray, or yellow skin
    B. numbness, burning, or itching
    C. cold and waxy skin
    D. All of the above.

35. _____ is a medical emergency characterized by dangerously low body temperature.

36. Heat cramps, heatstroke, and _____ are all types of hot weather emergencies.

37. *True or false?* The homeless are often at risk for hypothermia.

38. *True or false?* Covering a victim of heatstroke with bags of ice will help lower his or her body temperature.

Analyze and Apply

39. Do you think Graduated Driver Licensing (GDL) is a necessary policy for young drivers? Explain your answer.

40. Why is it important for a bicyclist to know and obey all traffic rules?

41. Why do labor laws restrict children and teenagers from holding particular jobs?

42. Sidney and her brother Jake are playing barefoot in their grandparents' backyard when Sidney steps on a rusty nail. The nail punctures her foot. What medical treatment should Sidney receive?

43. Think about the risks in your community, including risks related to technology, transportation, and high-risk behaviors. Make a list of five risks and describe how they affect safety. Then propose ways to protect yourself and others from these risks.

Safety and First Aid **Skill Development**

44. **Access Information.** Go through the closets, medicine cabinets, and cleaning cupboards in your home and make a list of any items that could be poisonous. You may need to read the item's label to determine if it might be hazardous. Post the list in a place where your entire family can see it. Were there any items on the list that surprised you?

45. **Communicate with Others.** Imagine you and a friend are involved in a situation that required emergency medical care. Perhaps your friend has choked on his or her lunch, or you have suffered a severe wound. Write and act out a short skit describing the scenario and the emergency medical care given.

46. **Practice Healthy Behaviors and Reduce Health Risks.** During a typical day, make a list of any unsafe behavior you see from drivers, bicyclists, and pedestrians. Are you guilty of committing any of these behaviors? In small groups, share your list and discuss alternative, safe behaviors.

47. **Demonstrate Skills.** Take a first aid or CPR certification class at your school or in your community. Using the mannequins provided in the class, role-play how to perform CPR, how to use an AED, and how to provide basic first aid. As you demonstrate these skills, have another student film you. Submit the film as well as a short essay reflecting on the experience to your instructor.

Body Mass Index for Boys

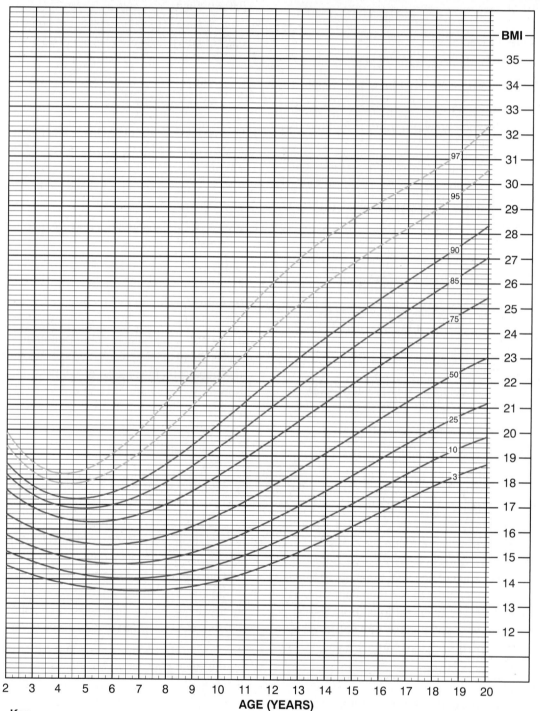

Weight Status Category	Percentile Range
Underweight	Less than the 5th percentile
Healthy weight	5th percentile to less than the 85th percentile
Overweight	85th to less than the 95th percentile
Obese	Equal to or greater than the 95th percentile

Key

SOURCE: Developed by the National Center for Health Statistics in collaboration with the National Center for Chronic Disease Prevention and Health Promotion

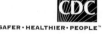

SAFER · HEALTHIER · PEOPLE™

Body Mass Index for Girls

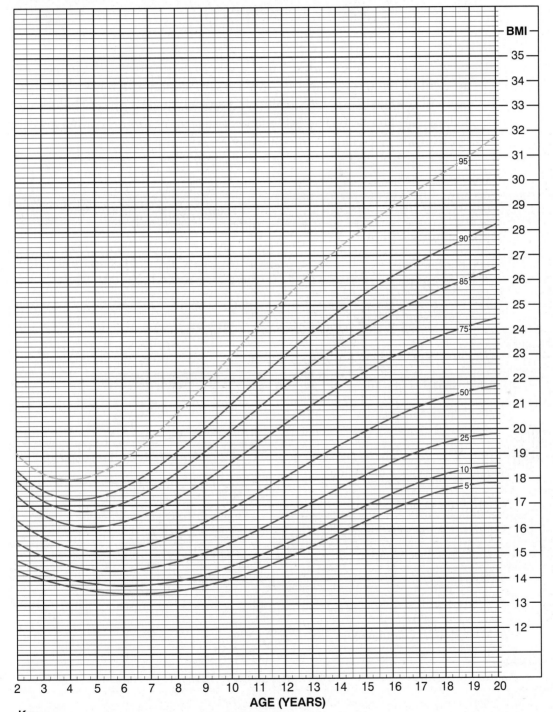

BMI

AGE (YEARS)

Key

Weight Status Category	Percentile Range
Underweight	Less than the 5th percentile
Healthy weight	5th percentile to less than the 85th percentile
Overweight	85th to less than the 95th percentile
Obese	Equal to or greater than the 95th percentile

SOURCE: Developed by the National Center for Health Statistics in collaboration with the National Center for Chronic Disease Prevention and Health Promotion

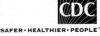

SAFER · HEALTHIER · PEOPLE™

Nutrient Content Claims

A claim on a food product that implies or directly states the level of a nutrient in the food—such as "low fat" or "contains 100 calories"— is a nutrient content claim. A Nutrition Facts panel must be present before such a claim can be made. The table shows several common claims and the appropriate criteria that must be met by a food product.

Nutrient Content Claims	
Claim	Definition (per serving)
Calorie free	Fewer than 5 calories
Low calorie	40 calories or fewer
Reduced or fewer calories	At least 25% fewer calories
Light or lite	One-third fewer calories or 50% less fat
Sugar free	Fewer than 0.5 grams sugars
Reduced sugar or less sugar	At least 25% less sugars
No added sugar	No sugars added during processing or packing, including ingredients that contain sugars, such as juice or dry fruit
Fat free	Fewer than 0.5 grams fat
Low fat	3 grams or fewer of fat
Reduced or less fat	At least 25% less fat
Saturated fat free	Fewer than 0.5 grams saturated fat and less than 0.5 grams *trans* fatty acids
Low saturated fat	1 gram or less and 15% less calories from saturated fat
Reduced/less saturated fat	At least 25% less saturated fat
Cholesterol free	Fewer than 2 milligrams cholesterol and 2 grams or fewer of saturated fat
Low cholesterol	20 milligrams or fewer cholesterol and 2 grams or fewer of saturated fat
Reduced or less cholesterol	At least 25% less cholesterol and 2 grams or fewer saturated fat

(Continued)

Nutrient Content Claims (Continued)	
Claim	**Definition (per serving)**
Sodium free	Fewer than 5 milligrams sodium
Very low sodium	35 milligrams or fewer sodium
Low sodium	140 milligrams or fewer sodium
Reduced or less sodium	At least 25% less sodium
Light in sodium	At least 50% less sodium

Health Claims

Health claims indicate a link between foods or nutrients and their ability to reduce the risk of contracting a disease or poor health condition. One such example is this: "Three grams of soluble fiber from oatmeal daily in a diet low in saturated fat and cholesterol may reduce the risk of heart disease. This cereal has 2 grams per serving." Health claims cannot state that a certain food or nutrient can prevent a disease.

A health claim can be used after approved by the FDA upon finding significant scientific agreement (SSA) to support it. The following table lists several common claims approved by the FDA and model statements that manufacturers can use on food labels.

Qualified Health Claims

Similar to health claims, qualified health claims also suggest a link between consuming certain foods or nutrients and reducing the risk of disease or poor health conditions. However, qualified health claims do not require the stronger support of the SSA.

Health Claims on Food Product Labels	
Approved Claim	**Model Claim Statement**
Calcium, vitamin D, and osteoporosis	Calcium and Osteoporosis: Adequate calcium throughout life, as part of a well-balanced diet, may reduce the risk of osteoporosis.
	Calcium, vitamin D, and osteoporosis: Adequate calcium and vitamin D, as part of a well-balanced diet, along with physical activity, may reduce the risk of osteoporosis.
Dietary fat and cancer	Development of cancer depends on many factors. A diet low in total fat may reduce the risk of some cancers.
Dietary saturated fat and cholesterol and coronary heart disease	While many factors affect heart disease, diets low in saturated fat and cholesterol may reduce the risk some types of cancer, a disease associated with many factors.

(Continued)

Approved Claim	Model Claim Statement
Fiber-containing grain products, fruits, and vegetables and cancer	Low-fat diets rich in fiber-containing grain products, fruits, and vegetables may reduce the risk of this disease.
Fruits, vegetables, and grain products that contain fiber, particularly soluble fiber, and risk of coronary heart disease	Diets low in saturated fat and cholesterol and rich in fruits, vegetables, and grain products that contain some types of dietary fiber, particularly soluble fiber, may reduce the risk of heart disease, a disease associated with many factors.
Sodium and hypertension (high blood pressure)	Diets low in sodium may reduce the risk of high blood pressure, a disease associated with many factors
Fruits and vegetables and cancer	Low-fat diets rich in fruits and vegetables (foods that are low in fat and may contain dietary fiber, vitamin A, or vitamin C) may reduce the risk of some types of cancer, a disease associated with many factors. Broccoli is high in vitamins A and C, and is a good source of dietary fiber.
Folate and neural tube birth defects	Healthful diets with adequate folate may reduce a woman's risk of having a child with a brain or spinal cord defect.
Dietary noncariogenic carbohydrate sweeteners and dental caries	Frequent between-meal consumption of foods high in sugars and starches promotes tooth decay. The sugar alcohols in [name of food] do not promote tooth decay.
Soluble fiber from certain foods and risk of coronary heart disease	Soluble fiber from foods such as [name of soluble fiber source and food product] as part of a diet low in saturated fat and cholesterol, may reduce the risk of heart disease. A serving of [name of food product] supplies _____ grams of the soluble fiber from [name of soluble fiber source] necessary per day to have this effect.
Soy protein and risk of coronary heart disease	(1) 25 grams of soy protein a day, as part of a diet low in saturated fat and cholesterol, may reduce the risk of heart disease. A serving of [name of food] supplies _____ grams of soy protein. (2) Diets low in saturated fat and cholesterol that include 25 grams of soy protein a day may reduce the risk of heart disease. One serving of [name of food] supplies _____ grams of soy protein.
Plant sterol/stanol esters and risk of coronary heart disease	(1) Foods containing at least 0.65 grams per reference amount of vegetable oil sterol esters, eaten twice a day with meals for a daily total intake of at least 1.3 grams, as part of a diet low in saturated fat and cholesterol, may reduce the risk of heart disease. A serving of [name of food] supplies _____ grams of vegetable oil sterol esters. (2) Diets low in saturated fat and cholesterol that include two servings of foods that provide a daily total of at least 3.4 grams of plant stanol esters in two meals may reduce the risk of heart disease. A serving of [name of food] supplies _____ grams of plant stanol esters.
Whole-grain foods and risk of heart disease and certain cancers	Diets rich in whole-grain foods and other plant foods and low in total fat, saturated fat, and cholesterol may reduce the risk of heart disease and some cancers.

(Continued)

Health Claims on Food Product Labels *(Continued)*

Approved Claim	Model Claim Statement
Whole grain foods with moderate fat content and risk of heart disease	Diets rich in whole grain foods and other plant foods and low in total fat, saturated fat, and cholesterol may help reduce the risk of heart disease.
Potassium and the risk of high blood pressure and stroke	Diets containing foods that are a good source of potassium and that are low in sodium may reduce the risk of high blood pressure and stroke.
Fluoridated water and reduced risk of dental caries	Drinking fluoridated water may reduce the risk of dental caries or tooth decay.
Saturated fat, cholesterol, and *trans* fat, and reduced risk of heart disease	Diets low in saturated fat and cholesterol, and as low as possible in *trans* fat, may reduce the risk of heart disease.
Substitution of saturated fat in the diet with unsaturated fatty acids and reduced risk of heart disease	Replacing saturated fat with similar amounts of unsaturated fats may reduce the risk of heart disease. To achieve this benefit, total daily calories should not increase.

One example of a qualified health claim is this approved statement for whole or chopped walnuts: "Supportive but not conclusive research shows that eating 1.5 ounces per day of walnuts, as part of a low saturated fat and low cholesterol diet and not resulting in increased caloric intake, may reduce the risk of coronary heart disease. See nutrition information for fat and calorie content."

Appendix D

Physical Activity Guidelines for Americans

Physical Activity Guidelines for Americans

Children and Adolescents (6–17 years)

- Should do 1 hour or more of physical activity every day.

- Most of the 1 hour or more of physical activity should be either moderate- or vigorous-intensity aerobic activity, and should include vigorous-intensity physical activity at least 3 days per week.

- Part of the daily physical activity should include muscle-strengthening activity on at least 3 days per week.

- Part of the daily physical activity should include bone-strengthening activity on at least 3 days per week.

Adults (18–64 years)

- Should do 2 hours and 30 minutes a week of moderate-intensity, or 1 hour and 15 minutes a week of vigorous-intensity aerobic physical activity, or an equivalent combination of moderate- and vigorous-intensity aerobic physical activity. Aerobic activity should be performed in episodes of at least 10 minutes, preferably spread throughout the week.

- Additional health benefits are provided by increasing to 5 hours a week of moderate-intensity aerobic physical activity, or 2 hours and 30 minutes a week of vigorous-intensity physical activity, or an equivalent combination of both.

- Should also do muscle-strengthening activities that involve all major muscle groups performed on 2 or more days per week.

Older Adults (65+ years)

- Older adults should follow the adult guidelines. If this is not possible due to limiting chronic conditions, older adults should be as physically active as their abilities allow. They should avoid inactivity.

- Older adults should do exercises that maintain or improve balance if they are at risk of falling.

Vitamin and Mineral Deficiency Disease

Vitamin and Mineral Deficiency Diseases

Vitamin	Deficiency Disease or Symptoms
A	Blindness (xerophthalmia), roughened skin, decreased resistance to infection
B_6 (Pyridoxine)	Microcytic hypochromic anemia, dermatitis, depression
B_{12} (Cyanocobalamin)	Anemia, tingling numbness, cognitive changes
C	Scurvy
D	Rickets (misshapen leg and breastbones), osteomalacia, osteoporosis
E	Premature hemolysis
K	Reduced bone density
Folate/Folic Acid/ Folacin	Inflammation of the tongue, digestive disorders, anemia (fatigue and weakness), increased risk of birth defects
Riboflavin	Shiny, inflamed tongue; painful, sore mouth; cracks in corner of mouth, lips; dermatitis
Thiamin	Beriberi (muscle weakness, loss of appetite, nerve degeneration)
Niacin	Pellegra (dementia, diarrhea, dermatitis)
Minerals	**Deficiency Disease or Symptoms**
Calcium	Osteoporosis
Magnesium	Weakness, heart irregularities, disorientation, seizures
Sodium	Cramps, nausea, vomiting
Potassium	Cramps, decreased appetite, heart malfunction, constipation, confusion
Iron	Anemia, fatigue, decreased appetite
Zinc	Delayed growth and sexual development (children); decreased appetite, resistance to infection, sense of smell and taste
Iodine	Goiter, impaired development of fetus
Selenium	Heart disease
Chromium	Impaired glucose metabolism

Photo Credits

Front Matter

Table of Contents Images   Plush Studios/Blend Images/Thinkstock.com, Yuganov Konstantin/Shutterstock.com, gbh007/iStock/Thinkstock.com, milias1987/Shutterstock.com, Alexander Raths/Shutterstock.com, takayuki/Shutterstock.com, Rido/Shutterstock.com, Dziurek/iStock/Thinkstock.com, luminaimages/Shutterstock.com

Unit 1 Opener   oliveromg/Shutterstock.com

Unit 1 Video Image   g-stockstudio/Shutterstock.com

Chapter 1

Figure 1.0   Maridav/iStock/Thinkstock.com; Ch 01 Setting Scene Image   Marijus Auruskevicius/iStock/Thinkstock.com; Lesson 1.1 Warm-Up Activity   YanLev/Shutterstock.com; Figure 1.1A   clsgraphics/iStock/Thinkstock.com; Figure 1.1B   sam74100/iStock/Thinkstock.com; Figure 1.1C   Stockbyte/Stockbyte/Thinkstock.com; Figure 1.1D   George Doyle/Stockbyte/Thinkstock.com; Figure 1.2   Denis Kuvaev/Shutterstock.com; Lesson 1.2 Warm-Up Activity   6493866629/Shutterstock.com; Figure 1.4   rbtl_00/Photodisc/Thinkstock.com; Figure 1.5   Plush Studios/Blend Images/Thinkstock.com; Ch 01 Case Study   Esperanza33/iStock/Thinkstock.com; Figure 1.8   Alexander Raths/iStock/Thinkstock.com; Lesson 1.3 Warm-Up Activity   michaeljung/Shutterstock.com; Figure 1.9   MANDY GODBEHEAR/Shutterstock.com; Lesson 1.4 Warm-Up Activity   emilie zhang/Shutterstock.com; Figure 1.10   Alexander Raths/iStock/Thinkstock.com; Figure 1.12   Pixland/Pixland/Thinkstock.com; Figure 1.13   BananaStock/BananaStock/Thinkstock.com; Figure 1.15   AlexRaths/iStock/Thinkstock.com

Chapter 2

Figure 2.0   Golden Pixels LLC/Shutterstock.com; Ch 02 Setting Scene Image   Jani Bryson/iStock/Thinkstock.com; Lesson 2.1 Warm-Up Activity   AJP/Shutterstock.com, Rohit Seth/Shutterstock.com, PT Images/Shutterstock.com; Figure 2.2   Alexander Raths/Shutterstock.com; Ch 02 Global Health   Ammit/iStock/Thinkstock.com; Figure 2.3   Jochen Schönfeld/iStock/Thinkstock.com; Figure 2.4   BananaStock/BananaStock/Thinkstock.com; Ch 02 Research in Action   Courtesy of the National Institute of General Medical Sciences; Figure 2.5A   Digital Vision/Digital Vision/Thinkstock.com; Figure 2.5B   Michael Blann/Digital Vision/Thinkstock.com; Figure 2.5C   Monkey Business Images/Monkey Business/Thinkstock.com; Lesson 2.2 Warm-Up Activity   Sean Locke Photography/Shutterstock.com; Figure 2.6   SurkovDimitri/iStock/Thinkstock.com; Figure 2.7   Jacek Chabraszewski/iStock/Thinkstock.com; Figure 2.8   XiXinXing/iStock/Thinkstock.com; Figure 2.9   Ingram Publishing/Thinkstock.com; Lesson 2.3 Warm-Up Activity   Lisa F. Young/Shutterstock.com; Figure 2.10   Todd Warnock/Photodisc/Thinkstock.com; Ch 02 Case Study   dotshock/Shutterstock.com; Figure 2.11   Iakov Filimonov/Shutterstock.com; Figure 2.12   moodboard/moodboard/Thinkstock.com; Lesson 2.4 Warm-Up Activity   Dudarev Mikhail/Shutterstock.com; Figure 2.13A   TimHesterPhotography/iStock/Thinkstock.com; Figure 2.13B   johnnorth/iStock/Thinkstock.com; Figure 2.13C   Anton Foltin/iStock/Thinkstock.com; Figure 2.14   gpointstudio/iStock/Thinkstock.com; Figure 2.15   Studio-Annika/iStock/Thinkstock.com; Hands-On Activity   bikeriderlondon/Shutterstock.com; Math Practice   Courtesy of Centers for Disease Control and Prevention, National Center for Health Statistics

Unit 2 Opener   Cathy Yeulet/Hemera/Thinkstock.com

Unit 2 Video Image   g-stockstudio/Shutterstock.com

Chapter 3

Figure 3.0   Monkey Business Images/Shutterstock.com; Ch 03 Setting Scene Image   Pekic/iStock/Thinkstock.com; Lesson 3.1 Warm-Up Activity   Sea Wave/Shutterstock.com, stockcreations/Shutterstock.com, Nattika/Shutterstock.com, CWA Studios/Shutterstock.com, KITSANANAN/Shutterstock.com, stockcreations/Shutterstock.com, Jacek Chabraszewski/Shutterstock.com, Diana Taliun/Shutterstock.com; Figure 3.1   MJTH/Shutterstock.com; Figure 3.2   ddsign_stock/iStock/Thinkstock.com; Figure 3.3   Jacek Chabraszewski/Shutterstock.com; Figure 3.4   aida ricciardiello caballero/iStock/Thinkstock.com; Figure 3.5   olvas/iStock/Thinkstock.com; Ch 03 Case Study   AntonioGuillem/iStock/Thinkstock.com; Figure 3.8   Christopher Futcher/Hemera/Thinkstock.com; Lesson 3.2 Warm-Up Activity   karelnoppe/Shutterstock.com; Figure 3.9A   pudi studio/Shutterstock.com; Figure 3.9B   ElenaGaak/Shutterstock.com; Figure 3.9C   Chiyacat/Shutterstock.com; Figure 3.9D   Elena Elisseeva/Shutterstock.com; Figure 3.9E   Goodheart-Willcox; Figure 3.9F   Stephen Mcsweeny/Shutterstock.com; Figure 3.9G   yelbuke/Shutterstock.com; Ch 03 Research in Action   Nuno Garuti/Hemera/Thinkstock.com; Figure 3.11A   Givaga/Shutterstock.com; Figure 3.11B   Carla Nichiata/Shutterstock.com; Figure 3.11C   zkruger/Shutterstock.com; Figure 3.13A   eurobanks/Shutterstock.com; Figure 3.13B   MSPhotographic/Shutterstock.com; Ch 03 Health in the Media   Irina Schmidt/Shutterstock.com; Lesson 3.3 Warm-Up Activity   Jean Valley/Shutterstock.com, Boarding1Now/iStock/Thinkstock.com; Figure 3.16   Courtesy of the FDA; Figure 3.17   Fuse/Thinkstock.com; Figure 3.19   Slawomir Fajer/iStock/Thinkstock.com; Figure 3.20   Purestock/Thinkstock.com; Figure 3.21A   gebai/iStock/Thinkstock.com; Figure 3.21B   Pakhnyushchyy/iStock/Thinkstock.com; Figure 3.21C   Igor Tarasyuk/iStock/Thinkstock.com; Figure 3.21D   Mark Tomline/iStock/Thinkstock.com; Figure 3.21E   illustrart/iStock/Thinkstock.com; Figure 3.21F   Petro Perutskyi/iStock/Thinkstock.com; Figure 3.21G   AlexRaths/iStock/Thinkstock.com; Figure 3.21H   cynoclub/iStock/Thinkstock.com; Hands-On Activity   Elena Itsenko/Shutterstock.com; Math Practice   Courtesy of the FDA

Chapter 4

Figure 4.0   Stock-Asso/Shutterstock.com; Ch 04 Setting Scene Image   Bine Å edivy/iStock/Thinkstock.com; Lesson 4.1 Warm-Up Activity   Paolo Bona/Shutterstock.com; Figure 4.1   Digital Vision/Photodisc/Thinkstock.com; Figure 4.2   airet/iStock/Thinkstock.com; Lesson 4.2 Warm-Up Activity   dionisvero/iStock/Thinkstock.com, yvdavyd/iStock/Thinkstock.com, LiuMeiLi/iStock/Thinkstock.com; Figure 4.3   Jason Stitt/Shutterstock.com; Figure 4.4   kzenon/iStock/Thinkstock.com; Ch 04 Research in Action   kzenon/iStock/Thinkstock.com; Figure 4.5   Layland Masuda/Shutterstock.com; Ch 04 Global Health   Adapted from the Centers for Disease Control and Prevention; Figure 4.6   Siri Stafford/Photodisc/Thinkstock.com; Lesson 4.3 Warm-Up Activity   DS011/iStock/Thinkstock.com, tarasov_vl/iStock/Thinkstock.com; Ch 04 Case Study   Monkey Business Images/Monkey Business/Thinkstock.com; Figure 4.7   bevangoldswain/iStock/Thinkstock.com; Figure 4.8   Yuganov Konstantin/Shutterstock.com; Figure 4.9   papa1266/Shutterstock.com; Figure 4.10   michaeljung/Shutterstock.com; Figure 4.11   Alliance/iStock/Thinkstock.com; Hands-On Activity   Image Point Fr/Shutterstock.com

Chapter 5

Figure 5.0   monkeybusinessimages/iStock/Thinkstock.com; Ch 05 Setting Scene Image   Galina Barskaya/Shutterstock.com; Lesson 5.1 Warm-Up Activity   InnervisionArt/Shutterstock.com; Lesson 5.1 Before You Read   wavebreakmedia/Shutterstock.com; Figure 5.1   wavebreakmedia/Shutterstock.com; Figure 5.2   Iv Mirin/Shutterstock.com; Ch 05 Research in Action   Jupiterimages/Stockbyte/Thinkstock.com; Figure 5.3   Ryan McVay/Photodisc/Thinkstock.com; Figure 5.4   Steve Pepple/iStock/Thinkstock.com; Ch 05 Global Health   Jose Gil/Shutterstock.com; Figure 5.5   Brian McEntire/iStock/Thinkstock.com; Lesson 5.2 Warm-Up Activity   Sarunyu_foto/Shutterstock.com; Figure 5.6   Viktor Neimanis/iStock/Thinkstock.com; Ch 05 Case Study   Elena Elisseeva/iStock/Thinkstock.com; Figure 5.7   Teguh Mujiono/Shutterstock.com; Figure 5.8   History of Medicine, The National Library of Medicine; Figure 5.9   Catherine Yeulet/iStock/Thinkstock.com; Figure 5.10   alexsokolov/iStock/Thinkstock.com; Figure 5.11   Lisa F. Young/iStock/Thinkstock.com; Ch 05 Health in the Media   Vladimir Gjorgiev/Shutterstock.com; Figure 5.12   AndreyKrav/iStock/Thinkstock.com; Hands-On Activity   sagir/Shutterstock.com

Unit 3 Opener   Gert Very/iStock/Thinkstock.com

Unit 3 Video Image   g-stockstudio/Shutterstock.com

Chapter 6

Figure 6.0   dotshock/Shutterstock.com; Ch 06 Setting Scene Image   Creatas Images/Creatas/Thinkstock.com; Lesson 6.1 Warm-Up Activity   Ermolaev Alexander/Shutterstock.com, JNP/Shutterstock.com; fotokostic/iStock/Thinkstock.com; Figure 6.1   Maria Teijeiro/Digital Vision/Thinkstock.com; Figure 6.2   Photodisc/Photodisc/Thinkstock.com; Ch 06 Research in Action   gbh007/iStock/Thinkstock.com; Figure 6.3   prudkov/Shutterstock.com; Figure 6.4   Jupiterimages/Creatas/Thinkstock.com; Ch 06 Health in the Media   Goodshoot RF/Goodshoot/Thinkstock.com; Figure 6.5   bikeriderlondon/Shutterstock.com; Figure 6.6   Goodluz/Shutterstock.com; Figure 6.7A   moodboard/moodboard/Thinkstock.com; Figure 6.7B   Ingram Publishing/Thinkstock.com; Figure 6.9   Monkey Business Images/Monkey Business/Thinkstock.com; Figure 6.10   Levente GyÅri/iStock/Thinkstock.com; Ch 06 Global Health   OlegD/Shutterstock.com; Figure 6.11   Gert Vrey/iStock/Thinkstock.com; Figure 6.12   Kzenon/Shutterstock.com; Figure 6.13   Maridav/iStock/Thinkstock.com; Figure 6.14   hanker81/iStock/Thinkstock.com; Ch 06 Case Study   Andersen Ross/Blend Images/Thinkstock.com; Figure 6.15A   Goodshoot/Goodshoot/Thinkstock.com; Figure 6.15B   Lilyana Vynogradova/Shutterstock.com; Figure 6.15C   Diego Barbieri/Shutterstock.com; Figure 6.16   Ingram Publishing/Thinkstock.com; Figure 6.18   Michael Blann/Photodisc/Thinkstock.com; Lesson 6.3 Warm-Up Activity   Fuse/Thinkstock.com; Lesson 6.3 Before You Read   Oleksiy Mark/Shutterstock.com; Figure 6.19   gbh007/iStock/Thinkstock.com; Figure 6.20   Nikolay Mamluke/iStock/Thinkstock.com; Figure 6.21   Action Sports Photography/Shutterstock.com; Figure 6.22   iofoto/Shutterstock.com; Figure 6.24   Peter Kim/Shutterstock.com; Hands-On Activity   CandyBox Images/Shutterstock.com

Chapter 7

Figure 7.0   Rommel Canlas/Shutterstock.com; Ch 07 Setting Scene Image   Myimagine/Shutterstock.com; Lesson 7.1 Warm-Up Activity   Vava Vladimir Jovanovic/Shutterstock.com; Figure 7.1   Fuse/Thinkstock.com; Figure 7.2   Blade_kostas/iStock/Thinkstock.com; Ch 07 Case Study   fotokostic/iStock/Thinkstock.com; Lesson 7.2 Warm-Up Activity   Monkey Business Images/Shutterstock.com; Figure 7.3A   oriontrail/Shutterstock.com; Figure 7.3B   Songchai W/Shutterstock.com; Figure 7.3C   TheYok/Shutterstock.com; Figure 7.3D   Wisut/Shutterstock.com; Figure 7.4   © Body Scientific International; Ch 07 Research in Action   AntonioGuillem/iStock/Thinkstock.com; Lesson 7.3 Warm-Up Activity   wavebreakmedia/Shutterstock.com; Figure 7.6   tab1962/iStock/Thinkstock.com; Ch 07 Global Health   Adrin Shamsudin/iStock/Thinkstock.com; Figure 7.7   Marcos Mesa Sam Wordley/Shutterstock.com; Figure 7.8   Fuse/Thinkstock.com; Figure 7.9   Amy Walters/iStock/Thinkstock.com; Lesson 7.4 Warm-Up Activity   Paul Matthew Photography/Shutterstock.com; Figure 7.10   Monkey Business Images/Monkey Business/Thinkstock.com; Figure 7.11   fatchoi/iStock/Thinkstock.com; Ch 07 Health in the Media   Thinkstock Images/Stockbyte/Thinkstock.com; Figure 7.12   gemphotography/iStock/Thinkstock.com; Hands-On Activity   Dudarev Mikhail/Shutterstock.com

Chapter 8

Figure 8.0   Digital Vision/Digital Vision/Thinkstock.com; Ch 08 Setting Scene Image   luanateutzi/iStock/Thinkstock.com; Lesson 8.1 Warm-Up Activity   Pixland/Pixland/Thinkstock.com; Figure 8.1   © Body Scientific International; Figure 8.2   roibu/iStock/Thinkstock.com; Lesson 8.2 Warm-Up Activity   karelnoppe/Shutterstock.com; Figure 8.3   © Body Scientific International; Figure 8.4   John Lund/Heather Hryciw/Blend Images/Thinkstock.com; Ch 08 Health in the Media   Accord/Shutterstock.com; Figure 8.5   Jason Stroja/iStock/Shutterstock.com; Figure 8.6   dmitryzubarev/iStock/Thinkstock.com; Lesson 8.3 Warm-Up Activity   zimmytws/Shutterstock.com; Figure 8.7   © Body Scientific International; Figure 8.8   © Body Scientific International; Ch 08 Case Study   Fuse/Thinkstock.com; Figure 8.9   bikeriderlondon/Shutterstock.com; Figure 8.10   © Body Scientific International; Figure 8.11   © Body Scientific International; Figure 8.12   © Body Scientific International; Ch 08 Research in Action   Sophie James/iStock/Thinkstock.com; Hands-On Activity   JJ Studio/Shutterstock.com

Unit 4 Opener   Comstock/Stockbyte/Thinkstock.com

Unit 4 Video Images   g-stockstudio/Shutterstock.com

Chapter 9

Figure 9.0   Dario Lo Presti/iStock/Thinkstock.com; Ch 09 Setting Scene Image   Lana K/Shutterstock.com; Lesson 9.1 Warm-Up Activity   David Koscheck/Shutterstock.com; Figure 9.1   rui vale sousa/Shutterstock.com; Figure 9.3   © Body Scientific International; Figure 9.4   Arthur Glauberman/Science Source; Figure 9.5   srdjan111/iStock/Thinkstock.com; Figure 9.6   Photo Works/Shutterstock.com; Figure 9.7   Elena Kouptsova-Vasic/Shutterstock.com; Ch 09 Case Study   Martin Allinger/Shutterstock.com; Figure 9.9   Martin Novak/iStock/Thinkstock.com; Lesson 9.3 Warm-Up Activity   Radu Razvan/Shutterstock.com, michaeljung/Shutterstock.com, Olena Zaskochenko/Shutterstock.com, My Good Images/Shutterstock.com; Figure 9.10   Courtesy of the Centers for Disease Control and Prevention; Figure 9.11A   jcjgphotography/Shutterstock.com; Figure 9.11B   bikeriderlondon/Shutterstock.com; Figure 9.12   Sergey Ash/Shutterstock.com; Ch 09 Global Health   VikramRaghuvanshi/iStock/Thinkstock.com; Figure 9.13   Lester Balajadia/Shutterstock.com; Figure 9.14   baur/Shutterstock.com; Ch 09 Research in Action   Courtesy of the Centers for Disease Control and Prevention; Figure 9.15   milias1987/Shutterstock.com; Hands-On Activity   vadimmmus/Shutterstock.com; Math Practice   Courtesy of the Centers for Disease Control and Prevention

Chapter 10

Figure 10.0   Brian McEntire/iStock/Thinkstock.com; Ch 10 Setting Scene Image   Roger Dale Pleis/Shutterstock.com; Lesson 10.1 Warm-Up Activity   Don Pablo/Shutterstock.com; Figure 10.1A   Neyro/Shutterstock.com; Figure 10.1B   VikaSuh/Shutterstock.com; Figure 10.1C   StudioSmart/Shutterstock.com; Figure 10.2   © Body Scientific International; Figure 10.3   Ridofranz/iStock/Thinkstock.com; Figure 10.4   East/Shutterstock.com; Figure 10.6A   Ari N/Shutterstock.com; Figure 10.6B   Meelena/Shutterstock.com; Figure 10.7   Paul Schlemmer/Shutterstock.com; Lesson 10.2 Warm-Up Activity   Daan Hoffmann/Shutterstock.com; Figure 10.8   Doug Menuez/Photodisc/Thinkstock.com; Figure 10.9   Helder Almeida/Shutterstock.com; Figure 10.10   Arthur Glauberman/Science Source; Figure 10.11   David Pereiras/Shutterstock.com; Figure 10.12   Courtesy of Brookhaven National Laboratory; Lesson 10.3 Warm-Up Activity   Pavel Lysenko/Shutterstock.com; Figure 10.13   dwphotos/Shutterstock.com; Ch 10 Research in Action   Aleksei Potov/Shutterstock.com; Ch 10 Health in the Media   Huntstock/Thinkstock.com; Figure 10.14   Lucky Business/Shutterstock.com; Lesson 10.4 Before You Read   Stuart Jenner/Shutterstock.com; Figure 10.15   milias1987/Shutterstock.com; Figure 10.16   Monkey Business Images/Shutterstock.com; Figure 10.17   CREATISTA/Shutterstock.com; Ch 10 Case Study   ejwhite/Shutterstock.com; Hands-On Activity   Kuzma/iStock/Thinkstock.com

Chapter 11

Figure 11.0   micro10x/Shutterstock.com; Ch 11 Setting Scene Image   jordachelr/iStock/Thinkstock.com; Lesson 11.1 Warm-Up Activity   Joe Belanger/Shutterstock.com, Tyler Olson/Shutterstock.com; Figure 11.1   Thinkstock Images/Stockbyte/Thinkstock.com; Figure 11.2   Anna Khomulo/iStock/Thinkstock.com; Ch 11 Health in the Media   racorn/Shutterstock.com; Figure 11.3   Courtesy of the US Department of Health and Human Services; Figure 11.4   Photodisc/Photodisc/Thinkstock.com; Figure 11.5A   Courtesy of the Drug Enforcement Administration; Figure 11.5B   Courtesy of the Drug Enforcement Administration; Figure 11.6   Courtesy of the Drug Enforcement Administration; Figure 11.7   Courtesy of the Drug Enforcement Administration; Figure 11.9   Courtesy of the US Department of Health and Human Services; Lesson 11.2 Warm-Up Activity   vidguten/Shutterstock.com; Figure 11.10   Courtesy of the Drug Enforcement Administration; Ch 11 Global Health   Hamik/Shutterstock.com; Figure 11.11   Courtesy of the Drug Enforcement Administration; Figure 11.12   Maine Department of Health and Human Services, Center for Disease Control and Prevention, Augusta, ME; Figure 11.13A   Courtesy of the Drug Enforcement Administration; Figure 11.13B   Courtesy of the Drug Enforcement Administration; Figure 11.14   Courtesy of the Drug Enforcement Administration; Figure 11.15   Courtesy of the Drug Enforcement Administration; Ch 11 Case Study   Monkey Business Images/Shutterstock.com; Lesson 11.3 Warm-Up Activity   kubais/Shutterstock.com; Figure 11.17   Adapted from University of Michigan, 2014 Monitoring the Future Study; Ch 11 Research in Action   Thai Soriano/Shutterstock.com; Figure 11.18   Fuse/Thinkstock.com; Figure 11.19   Helder Almeida/Shutterstock.com; Hands-On Activity   ruigsantos/Shutterstock.com; Marjan Apostolovic/Shutterstock.com

Unit 5 Opener   Patrizia Tilly/Shutterstock.com

Unit 5 Video Image   g-stockstudio/Shutterstock.com

Chapter 12

Figure 12.0   Adisa/Shutterstock.com; Ch 12 Setting Scene Image   Courtesy of the Centers for Disease Control and Prevention; Lesson 12.1 Warm-Up Activity   Peeradach Rattanakoses/Shutterstock.com; Ch 12 Global Health   evgenyatamanenko/iStock/Thinkstock.com; Figure 12.2   Courtesy of the Centers for Disease Control and Prevention; Figure 12.4   Courtesy of the Centers for Disease Control and Prevention; Figure 12.5   Courtesy of the Centers for Disease Control and Prevention; Figure 12.6   moreimages/Shutterstock.com; Courtesy of the Centers for Disease Control and Prevention; Lesson 12.2 Warm-Up Activity   Ermolaev Alexander/Shutterstock.com; Figure 12.7A   Andrey_Popov/Shutterstock.com; Figure 12.7B   LeventeGyori/Shutterstock.com; Figure 12.9A   Courtesy of the Centers for Disease Control and Prevention; Figure 12.9B   MikeLane45/iStock/Thinkstock.com; Figure 12.10   Adam Gregor/Shutterstock.com; Figure 12.12   Martin mark Soerensen/Hemera/Thinkstock.com; Figure 12.13   Milos Luzanin/iStock/Thinkstock.com; Ch 12 Case Study   Vanagas/iStock/Thinkstock.com; Ch 12 Research in Action   Courtesy of the Centers for Disease Control and Prevention; Lesson 12.3 Warm-Up Activity   stocksshoppe/Shutterstock.com; Figure 12.14   Courtesy of the Centers for Disease Control and Prevention; Figure 12.15   © Body Scientific International; Figure 12.16   © Body Scientific International; Hands-On Activity   Marcos Mesa Sam Wordley/Shutterstock.com; Math Practice   Courtesy of the Centers for Disease Control and Prevention

Chapter 13

Figure 13.0   Aleksandr Markin/Shutterstock.com; Ch 13 Setting Scene Image   Evgeniya Porechenskaya/Shutterstock.com; Lesson 13.1 Warm-Up Activity   Mega Pixel/Shutterstock.com, monkeybusinessimages/iStock/Thinkstock.com; Figure 13.1   Courtesy of the Centers for Disease Control and Prevention; Figure 13.2   citybrabus/Shutterstock.com; Figure 13.3   Horsche/iStock/Thinkstock.com; Figure 13.6   © Body Scientific International; Ch 13 Research in Action   jarun011/iStock/Thinkstock.com; Figure 13.7A   Courtesy of the Centers for Disease Control and Prevention; Figure 13.7B   Courtesy of the Centers for Disease Control and Prevention; Ch 13 Case Study   Muellek Josef/Shutterstock.com; Figure 13.8   Courtesy of the Centers for Disease Control and Prevention; Lesson 13.3 Warm-Up Activity   Phil Date/Shutterstock.com; Figure 13.11   Courtesy of the Centers for Disease Control and Prevention; Ch 13 Global Health   Hector Conesa/Shutterstock.com; Ch 13 Spotlight on Careers   Jupiterimages/Photos.com/Thinkstock.com; Figure 13.14   Courtesy of the Centers for Disease Control and Prevention; Math Practice   Courtesy of the Centers for Disease Control and Prevention

Chapter 14

Figure 14.0   Stockbyte/Stockbyte/Thinkstock.com; Ch 14 Setting Scene Image   Dragon Images/Shutterstock.com; Lesson 14.1 Warm-Up Activity   sjenner13/iStock/Thinkstock.com; Figure 14.1   BartekSzewczyk/iStock/Thinkstock.com; Figure 14.2   Alexander Raths/Shutterstock.com; Figure 14.3   BlueMoon Stock/BlueMoon Stock/Thinkstock.com; Lesson 14.2 Warm-Up Activity   © Body Scientific International; Lesson 14.2 Before You Read   © Body Scientific International; Figure 14.4   © Body Scientific International; Figure 14.5   Fuse/Thinkstock.com; Figure 14.6   © Body Scientific International; Figure 14.7   © Body Scientific International; Figure 14.8   © Body Scientific International; Figure 14.10   © Body Scientific International; Lesson 14.3 Warm-Up Activity   Ingram Publishing/Thinkstock.com; Figure 14.11   RusN/iStock/Thinkstock.com; Figure 14.14   itsmejust/Shutterstock.com; Figure 14.15   Mark Zelman; Figure 14.18A   Courtesy of Kelly Nelson and the Web site of the National Cancer Institute (http://www.cancer.gov); Figure 14.18B   Courtesy of the Web site of the National Cancer Institute (http://www.cancer.gov); Figure 14.18C   Juan Gaertner/Shutterstock.com; Ch 14 Case Study   Stockbyte/Stockbyte/

Thinkstock.com; Figure 14.19 monkeybusinessimages/iStock/Thinkstock.com; Figure 14.20 Courtesy of the Web site of the National Cancer Institute (http://www.cancer.gov); Lesson 14.4 Warm-Up Activity amanalung/iStock/Thinkstock.com; Figure 14.21 © Body Scientific International; Figure 14.22 wavebreakmedia/Shutterstock.com; Ch 14 Research in Action Courtesy of the National Institute of Diabetes and Digestive and Kidney Diseases, National Institutes of Health; Figure 14.23 © Body Scientific International; Math Practice Courtesy of the Web site of the National Cancer Institute (http://www.cancer.gov)

Unit 6 Opener Arieliona/Shutterstock.com
Unit 6 Video Image g-stockstudio/Shutterstock.com

Chapter 15

Figure 15.0 michaeljung/iStock/Thinkstock.com; Ch 15 Setting Scene Image Digital Vision/Digital Vision/Thinkstock.com; Lesson 15.1 Before You Read Carolyn Franks/Shutterstock.com; Ch 15 Health in the Media Syda Productions/Shutterstock.com; Figure 15.1 Fuse/Thinkstock.com; Ch 15 Research in Action William Perugini/Shutterstock.com; Lesson 15.2 Warm-Up Activity angiolina/Shutterstock.com; Figure 15.2 Miro Kovacevic/Shutterstock.com; Figure 15.3 Purestock/Thinkstock.com; Figure 15.4A dotshock/Shutterstock.com; Figure 15.4B Jupiterimages/Stockbyte/Thinkstock.com; Figure 15.4C Monkey Business Images Ltd/Monkey Business/Thinkstock.com; Figure 15.4D moodboard/moodboard/Thinkstock.com; Figure 15.5 Jupiterimages/Creatas/Thinkstock.com; Lesson 15.3 Warm-Up Activity Phase4Studios/Shutterstock.com; Figure 15.6 Sabphoto/Shutterstock.com; Ch 15 Case Study Jupiterimages/Pixland/Thinkstock.com; Figure 15.7 Goodheart-Willcox Publisher; Lesson 15.4 Warm-Up Activity franz pfluegl/iStock/Thinkstock.com; Figure 15.8 Anthony Ong/Digital Vision/Thinkstock.com; Figure 15.9 pojoslaw/iStock/Thinkstock.com; Figure 15.10 Kirill Linnik/iStock/Thinkstock.com; Figure 15.11 Design Pics/Thinkstock.com; Hands-On Activity oliveromg/Shutterstock.com

Chapter 16

Figure 16.0 George Dolgikh/Shutterstock.com; Ch 16 Setting Scene Image Jupiterimages/Photos.com/Thinkstock.com; Lesson 16.1 Warm-Up Activity George Dolgikh/Shutterstock.com; Figure 16.2 Oleksii Sagitov/Shutterstock.com; Figure 16.3 CREATISTA/Shutterstock.com; Ch 16 Health in the Media Linda Moon/Shutterstock.com; Ch 16 Global Health Hung_Chung_Chih/iStock/Thinkstock.com; Figure 16.4 Fuse/Thinkstock.com; Figure 16.5 OSTILL/iStock/Thinkstock.com; Ch 16 Research in Action DmitriMaruta/Shutterstock.com; Lesson 16.3 Warm-Up Activity Warren Goldswain/Shutterstock.com; Figure 16.6 Warren Goldswain/Shutterstock.com; Figure 16.7 Alexey Stiop/Shutterstock.com; Figure 16.8 auremar/Shutterstock.com; Lesson 16.4 Warm-Up Activity Djomas/Shutterstock.com; Figure 16.9 shironosov/iStock/Thinkstock.com; Figure 16.10 takayuki/Shutterstock.com; Figure 16.11 Monkey Business Images/Shutterstock.com; Ch 16 Case Study pojoslaw/iStock/Thinkstock.com; Figure 16.12 Pete Saloutos/Shutterstock.com; Hands-On Activity Brian A Jackson/Shutterstock.com; Math Practice Courtesy of the US Department of Health and Human Services, Health Resources and Services Administration

Chapter 17

Figure 17.0 Piotr Marcinski/Shutterstock.com; Ch 17 Setting Scene Image Courtesy of Library of Congress, Prints and Photographs Division; Lesson 17.1 Warm-Up Activity Jupiterimages/Stockbyte/Thinkstock.com; Ch 17 Case Study Courtesy of the Centers for Disease Control and Prevention; Figure 17.1 Diego Cervo/Shutterstock.com; Figure 17.2 coldsnowstorm/iStock/Thinkstock.com; Ch 17 Health in the Media Stockbyte/Stockbyte/Thinkstock.com; Figure 17.3 YanLev/Shutterstock.com; Figure 17.4 XiXinXing/Shutterstock.com; Ch 17 Research in Action © Body Scientific International; Figure 17.5 ejwhite/Shutterstock.com; Lesson 17.3 Warm-Up Activity Feverpitched/iStock/Thinkstock.com; Figure 17.7 Twin Design/Shutterstock.com; Figure 17.8 oliveromg/Shutterstock.com; Lesson 17.4 Warm-Up Activity Eimiaj/iStock/Thinkstock.com, ASIFE/iStock/Thinkstock.com; Figure 17.9 Ingram Publishing/Thinkstock.com; Figure 17.10 Rick Becker-Leckrone/Shutterstock.com; Ch 17 Spotlight on Careers 4774344sean/iStock/Thinkstock.com; Hands-On Activity Rob Marmion/Shutterstock.com; Math Practice Courtesy of the Department of Health and Human Services

Unit 7 Opener stokkete/iStock/Thinkstock.com
Unit 7 Video Image g-stockstudio/Shutterstock.com

Chapter 18

Figure 18.0 Samuel Borges Photography/Shutterstock.com; Ch 18 Setting Scene Image Monkey Business Images/Shutterstock.com; Lesson 18.1 Warm-Up Activity Ingram Publishing/Thinkstock.com; Figure 18.1 Rido/Shutterstock.com; Figure 18.2A Pressmaster/Shutterstock.com; Figure 18.2B Monkey Business Images/Shutterstock.com; Figure 18.2C CREATISTA/Shutterstock.com; Figure 18.2D Shvaygert Ekaterina/Shutterstock.com; Figure 18.3 cozyta/Shutterstock.com; Figure 18.4 Lucky Business/Shutterstock.com; Figure 18.5 Joshua Resnick/Shutterstock.com; Figure 18.6 Patricia Marks/Shutterstock.com; Lesson 18.2 Warm-Up Activity Mike Watson Images/moodboard/Thinkstock.com; Lesson 18.2 Before You Read casejustin/Shutterstock.com; Figure 18.7 Petrenko Andriy/Shutterstock.com; Figure 18.8 Michael Blann/Photodisc/Thinkstock.com; Figure 18.9 Jupiterimages/Photos.com/Thinkstock.com; Ch 18 Case Study Paul/Thinkstock.com; Ch 18 Research in Action Doug Menuez/Photodisc/Thinkstock.com; Figure 18.10 shironosov/iStock/Thinkstock.com; Figure 18.11 oliveromg/Shutterstock.com; Ch 18 Health in the Media IPGGutenbergUKLtd/iStock/Thinkstock.com; Figure 18.12 LoloStock/Shutterstock.com; Figure 18.13 Petrenko Andriy/Shutterstock.com; Figure 18.14 Paul Matthew Photography/Shutterstock.com; Hands-On Activity Quang Ho/Shutterstock.com

Chapter 19

Figure 19.0 Kamira/Shutterstock.com; Ch 19 Setting Scene Image Gemenacom/Shutterstock.com; Lesson 19.1 Warm-Up Activity Monkey Business Images/Shutterstock.com; Figure 19.1 savageultralight/Shutterstock.com; Figure 19.2 videnko/Shutterstock.com; Figure 19.3 omgimages/iStock/Thinkstock.com; Lesson 19.2 Warm-Up Activity Artens/Shutterstock.com; Figure 19.4 VBStock/iStock/Thinkstock.com; Ch 19 Research in Action Dikiiy/Shutterstock.com; Figure 19.5 wavebreakmedia/Shutterstock.com; Ch 19 Case Study shironosov/iStock/Thinkstock.com; Lesson 19.3 Warm-Up Activity siamionau pavel/Shutterstock.com; Figure 19.6 Lisa A/Shutterstock.com; Figure 19.7 JPagetRFPhotos/Shutterstock.com; Figure 19.8 Rinky Dink Images/Eyecandy Images/Thinkstock.com; Lesson 19.4 Warm-Up Activity James Pauls/iStock/Thinkstock.com; Figure 19.9 RomanRuzicka/Shutterstock.com; Figure 19.10 Michael Blann/Digital Vision/Thinkstock.com; Figure 19.12 Alexander Raths/Shutterstock.com; Figure 19.13 Bobbie Osborne/iStock/Thinkstock.com; Ch 19 Spotlight on Careers Wavebreakmedia Ltd/Wavebreak Media/Thinkstock.com; Math Practice Courtesy of the Bureau of Justice Statistics

Unit 8 Opener paulprescott72/iStock/Thinkstock.com
Unit 8 Video Image g-stockstudio/Shutterstock.com

Chapter 20

Figure 20.0   Andrey Arkusha/Shutterstock.com; Ch 20 Setting Scene Image   Lana K/Shutterstock.com; Lesson 20.1 Warm-Up Activity   moodboard/moodboard/Thinkstock.com; Figure 20.1   Jane Ades/National Human Genome Research Institute; Figure 20.2   © Body Scientific International; Ch 20 Case Study   Cathy Yeulet/Hemera/Thinkstock.com; Figure 20.3   Mark Zelman; Figure 20.5   © Body Scientific International; Figure 20.6   © Body Scientific International; Figure 20.7   © Body Scientific International; Figure 20.8   © Body Scientific International; Figure 20.10   Lukiyanova Natalia/frenta/Shutterstock.com; Lesson 20.3 Warm-Up Activity   BlueRingMedia/Shutterstock.com; Figure 20.11   © Body Scientific International; Figure 20.12   © Body Scientific International; Lesson 20.4 Warm-Up Activity   chaoss/iStock/Thinkstock.com; Figure 20.14   monkeybusinessimages/iStock/Thinkstock.com; Figure 20.15   Piotr Marcinski/Shutterstock.com; Figure 20.16   Ahturner/Shutterstock.com; Figure 20.17   Karl J Blessing/Shutterstock.com; Lesson 20.5 Warm-Up Activity   amanalang/iStock/Thinkstock.com; Ch 20 Research in Action   medistock/Shutterstock.com; Figure 20.21   © Body Scientific International; Ch 20 Global Health   Alila Medical Media/Shutterstock.com; Math Practice   Courtesy of the Centers for Disease Control and Prevention, National Center for Health Statistics

Chapter 21

Figure 21.0   Zurijeta/iStock/Thinkstock.com; Ch 21 Setting Scene Image   Purestock/Thinkstock.com; Lesson 21.1 Warm-Up Activity   Naypong/Shutterstock.com; Figure 21.1   pojoslaw/iStock/Thinkstock.com; Figure 21.3   © Body Scientific International; Figure 21.5   John Kelly/iStock/Thinkstock.com; Figure 21.6   DNF-Style/iStock/Thinkstock.com; Lesson 21.2 Warm-Up Activity   Marcos Mesa Sam Wordley/Shutterstock.com; Figure 21.7   zer05/iStock/Thinkstock.com; Figure 21.9   Dziurek/iStock/Thinkstock.com; Ch 21 Research in Action   George Doyle/Stockbyte/Thinkstock.com; Figure 21.10   Dr. P. Marazzi/Science Source; Lesson 21.3 Warm-Up Activity   Marlon Lopez MMG1 Design/Shutterstock.com, Flashon Studio/Shutterstock.com; Lesson 21.3 Before You Read   oksun70/iStock/Thinkstock.com; Photodisc/Photodisc/Thinkstock.com; michaeljung/iStock/Thinkstock.com; Figure 21.11   oksun70/iStock/Thinkstock.com; Figure 21.12   Photodisc/Photodisc/Thinkstock.com; Ch 21 Case Study   michaeljung/iStock/Thinkstock.com; Figure 21.13   JGI/Blend Images/Thinkstock.com; Figure 21.14   Vilches/iStock/Thinkstock.com; Figure 21.15   Menna/Shutterstock.com; Lesson 21.5 Warm-Up Activity   brux/Shutterstock.com; Figure 21.16   Mika Heittola/Hemera/Thinkstock.com; Figure 21.18   danr13/iStock/Thinkstock.com; Ch 21 Spotlight on Careers   Jaimie Duplass/iStock/Thinkstock.com; Hands-On Activity   Courtesy of Kathy G. Thacker, Salem Jr. High; Math Practice   Courtesy of the Centers for Disease Control and Prevention

Chapter 22

Figure 22.0   dbdavidova/Shutterstock.com; Ch 22 Setting Scene Image   XiXinXing/Shutterstock.com; Lesson 22.1 Warm-Up Activity   Leremy/Shutterstock.com; Figure 22.1   dotshock/Shutterstock.com; Figure 22.2   AVAVA/Shutterstock.com; Lesson 22.2 Warm-Up Activity   Pixland/Pixland/Thinkstock.com; Figure 22.3A   IuriiSokolov/iStock/Thinkstock.com; Figure 22.3B   Rayes/Digital Vision/Thinkstock.com; Figure 22.3C   Top Photo Corporation/Top Photo Group/Thinkstock.com; Figure 22.4   Julie Campbell/Shutterstock.com; Figure 22.5   Jupiterimages/Creatas/Thinkstock.com; Figure 22.6   Cresta Johnson/Shutterstock.com; Lesson 22.3 Warm-Up Activity   Comstock/Stockbyte/Thinkstock.com; Figure 22.7   LuminaStock/iStock/Thinkstock.com; Figure 22.8   Design Pics/Thinkstock.com; Ch 22 Research in Action   wenht/iStock/Thinkstock.com; Figure 22.9   Digital Vision/Photodisc/Thinkstock.com; Lesson 22.4 Warm-Up Activity   Rawpixel/Shutterstock.com; Figure 22.10   AlexRaths/iStock/Thinkstock.com; Figure 22.11   Blend Images/Shutterstock.com; Figure 22.12   Catherine Yeulet/iStock/Thinkstock.com; Figure 22.13   racorn/Shutterstock.com; Figure 22.14   Lisa F. Young/iStock/Thinkstock.com; Lesson 22.5 Warm-Up Activity   jcjgphotography/Shutterstock.com; Ch 22 Global Health   Jupiterimages/Photos.com/Thinkstock.com; Figure 22.15   Pell Studio/Shutterstock.com; Ch 22 Case Study   Barry Austin Photography/Photodisc/Thinkstock.com; Figure 22.16   Lisa F. Young/Shutterstock.com; Ch 22 Spotlight on Careers   Robert Kneschke/Shutterstock.com; Hands-On Activity   Hurst Photo/Shutterstock.com; Math Practice   Courtesy of the Centers for Disease Control and Prevention

Chapter 23

Figure 23.0   Imazee/iStock/Thinkstock.com; Ch 23 Setting Scene Image   Jack Hollingsworth/Photodisc/Thinkstock.com; Lesson 23.1 Warm-Up Activity   Maridav/iStock/Thinkstock.com; Figure 23.1   orelphoto/iStock/Thinkstock.com; Figure 23.3   Monkey Business Images/Shutterstock.com; Figure 23.4   Andresr/Shutterstock.com; Figure 23.5   kaarsten/Shutterstock.com, Dragan Milovanovic/Shutterstock.com; Figure 23.6   Keith Brofsky/Photodisc/Thinkstock.com; Figure 23.7   Garo/Phanie/Science Source; Figure 23.8   Lalocracio/iStock.com; Figure 23.9   Gary Parker/Science Source; Lesson 23.3 Warm-Up Activity   IT Stock Free/Polka Dot/Thinkstock.com; Figure 23.10   Jacob Kearns/Shutterstock.com; Figure 23.11   Image Point Fr/Shutterstock.com; Figure 23.12   Image Point Fr/Shutterstock.com; Figure 23.14   Image Point Fr/Shutterstock.com; Lesson 23.4 Warm-Up Activity   Huntstock/Thinkstock.com; Figure 23.15   AndreyPopov/iStock/Thinkstock.com; Figure 23.16   Svetlana Larina/Shutterstock.com; Figure 23.18   © Body Scientific International; Figure 23.19   © Body Scientific International; Ch 23 Research in Action   Wavebreakmedia Ltd/Wavebreak Media/Thinkstock.com; Math Practice   Courtesy of the Centers for Disease Control and Prevention

Chapter 24

Figure 24.0   Digital Vision/Photodisc/Thinkstock.com; Ch 24 Setting Scene Image   michaeljung/iStock/Thinkstock.com; Lesson 24.1 Warm-Up Activity   KPG_Payless/Shutterstock.com; Figure 24.1   © Body Scientific International; Figure 24.2   Purestock/Thinkstock.com; Figure 24.3   George Doyle/Stockbyte/Thinkstock.com; Ch 24 Health in the Media   Digital Vision/Photodisc/Thinkstock.com; Figure 24.4   tetmc/iStock/Thinkstock.com; Figure 24.5   Ryan McVay/Photodisc/Thinkstock.com; Ch 24 Case Study   Hemera Technologies/AbleStock.com/Thinkstock.com; Lesson 24.2 Warm-Up Activity   LUNAMARINA/iStock/Thinkstock.com, 4774344sean/iStock/Thinkstock.com; Figure 24.6   Wavebreakmedia Ltd/Wavebreak Media/Thinkstock.com; Ch 24 Global Health   Comstock/Stockbyte/Thinkstock.com; Figure 24.7   Bec Parsons/Digital Vision/Thinkstock.com; Ch 24 Research in Action   Creatas/Creatas/Thinkstock.com; Figure 24.8   BananaStock/BananaStock/Thinkstock.com; Figure 24.9   Dizzy/iStock/Thinkstock.com; Figutre 24.10   Feverpitched/iStock/Thinkstock.com; Figure 24.11   Olga Besnard/Shutterstock.com; Math Practice   Courtesy of the Federal Bureau of Investigation

Background Lessons

Background Lesson Opener Images luminaimages/
Shutterstock.com, Image Point Fr/Shutterstock.com,
Monkey Business Images/Shutterstock.com, Dean Drobot/
Shutterstock.com; Figure BL1.1 © Body Scientific International;
Figure BL1.2 © Body Scientific International;
Background Lesson 2 Images © Body Scientific International;
Background Lesson 3 Images © Body Scientific International;
Background Lesson 4 Images © Body Scientific International;
Background Lesson 5 Images © Body Scientific International;
Background Lesson 6 Images © Body Scientific International;
Background Lesson 7 Images © Body Scientific International;
Background Lesson 8 Images © Body Scientific International;
Background Lesson 9 Images © Body Scientific International;
Background Lesson 10 Images © Body Scientific International;
Background Lesson 11 Images © Body Scientific International;
Figure BL12.1 AntonioGuillem/iStock/
Thinkstock.com; Figure BL13.1 Benjamin Howell/iStock/
Thinkstock.com; Figure BL13.2 Comstock/Stockbyte/
Thinkstock.com; Figure BL13.3 Goodheart-Willcox
Publisher; Figure BL13.4 Igorsky/Shutterstock.com;
Figure BL14.1A Jupiterimages/Stockbyte/Thinkstock.com;
Figure BL14.1B Stockbyte/Stockbyte/Thinkstock.com;
Figure BL14.1C moodboard/moodboard/Thinkstock.com;
Figure BL14.2 Danny Nou, Human Factors Engineer, UC
Davis Occupational Health Services; Figure BL16.1 miriam-
doerr/iStock/Thinkstock.com; Figure BL16.4 StockPhotosArt/
Shutterstock.com; Figure BL16.5 Lisa F. Young/iStock/
Thinkstock.com; Figure BL16.6 Wavebreakmedia Ltd/Wavebreak
Media/Thinkstock.com; Figure BL17.1 American Red Cross;
Figure BL17.2 National Heart, Lung, and Blood Institute
(NHLBI); Figure BL17.3 AlexRaths/iStock/Thinkstock.com;
Figure BL17.4 American Red Cross; Figure BL17.5 Sashkinw/
iStock/Thinkstock.com; Figure BL18.1 Ridofranz/
iStock/Thinkstock.com; Figure BL18.2 Saddako/
iStock/Thinkstock.com; Figure BL18.3 Melodia plus
photos/Shutterstock.com; Figure BL19.1A Suzanne
Tucker/Shutterstock.com; Figure BL19.1B nikkytok/
Shutterstock.com; Figure BL19.1C Naiyyer/
Shutterstock.com; Figure BL19.2A Courtesy of the Centers
for Disease Control and Prevention; Figure BL19.2B Charles
Brutlag/Shutterstock.com; Figure BL19.3 Rob Byron/
Shutterstock.com; Figure BL19.4 Goodheart-
Willcox Publisher; Figure BL20.1 © Body Scientific
International; Figure BL20.2 Ridofranz/iStock/
Thinkstock.com; Figure BL21.1 John Rodriguez/iStock/
Thinkstock.com; Figure BL21.2 Maridav/Shutterstock.com;
Figure BL21.3 Huntstock/Thinkstock.com

Glossary/Glosario

A   English

abortion a surgical procedure that ends a pregnancy

abstinence the decision and practice of refraining from sexual activity

acid reflux disorder a gastrointestinal problem in which acid-containing chyme moves from the lower stomach into the esophagus

acidosis a condition characterized by dangerously high levels of acid in the blood

acne a skin condition in which inflamed, clogged hair follicles cause pimples

acquaintance rape unwanted sexual intercourse that is committed by someone the victim knows

acquaintances individuals with whom you interact regularly but may not consider friends

acquired immunodeficiency syndrome (AIDS) an often fatal disease in which the body's immune system can no longer fight off infections and diseases

active listening the practice of concentrating on what a person is saying

acute diseases diseases that occur and resolve quickly

addiction the physical and psychological need for a substance or behavior

adoption the legal placement of a child with someone other than his or her biological parents

aerobic activity involving the use of oxygen to fuel processes in the body

Affordable Care Act law passed in 2010 to expand access to insurance, address cost reduction and affordability, improve the quality of healthcare, and introduce the Patient's Bill of Rights

Español

aborto un procedimiento quirúrgico que termina un embarazo

abstinencia la decisión y la práctica de abstenerse de la actividad sexual

trastorno de reflujo ácido problema gastrointestinal en el cual quimo que contiene ácido se mueve desde la parte inferior del estómago hacia el esófago

acidosis una condición caracterizada por niveles peligrosamente altos de ácido en la sangre

acné una condición de la piel en la que los folículos pilosos inflamados, obstruidos causan espinillas

violación por un conocido relación sexual no deseada cometida por alguien que la víctima conoce

conocidos individuos con los que interactúa con regularidad, pero puede no considerar amigos

síndrome de inmunodeficiencia adquirida (SIDA) una enfermedad, con frecuencia fatal, en la que el sistema inmunológico del cuerpo ya no puede combatir infecciones y enfermedades

escuchar activamente la práctica de concentrarse en lo que una persona está diciendo

enfermedades agudas enfermedades que se producen y resuelven rápidamente

adicción la necesidad física y psicológica de una sustancia o comportamiento

adopción la colocación legal de un niño con alguien que no sea sus padres biológicos

actividad aeróbica implica el uso de oxígeno para alimentar procesos en el cuerpo

Ley de Cuidado de Salud a Bajo Precio ley aprobada en 2010 para ampliar el acceso a los seguros, tratar con la reducción de costos y la asequibilidad, mejorar la calidad de la atención médica, y la introducción de la Declaración de Derechos del Paciente

aggressive a style of behavior in which you speak or act toward others in a demanding and insulting way

agility the ability to quickly change the body's momentum and direction

airbrush to alter an image using specialized software to conceal imperfections

alcohol a general term used to describe a drink that contains a certain amount of ethanol

alcoholics people who are psychologically and physically addicted to alcohol

alcoholism a disease in which a person is completely dependent on alcohol

alcohol poisoning a medical emergency in which a person has consumed enough alcohol to suppress his or her central nervous system, and which is characterized by unconsciousness, low blood pressure and body temperature, difficulty breathing, and possible death

allergens substances that trigger allergic reactions in the body

allergy an immune response in which the body reacts destructively to a harmless substance

all-or-nothing mindset a way of thinking in which a person has to do it "all" right or he or she has done "nothing" right

amenorrhea a condition in which a female's menstrual cycle is abnormally absent

amino acid a small chemical unit that makes up proteins

amnion a membrane that forms a fluid-filled sac, which cushions and protects a developing fetus

anabolic steroids artificial hormones used to treat muscular disorders; are sometimes illegally used to help people build muscle mass

agresivo un estilo de comportamiento en el que uno habla o actúa hacia los demás de una manera exigente y ofensiva

agilidad la capacidad de cambiar rápidamente el impulso y la dirección del cuerpo

retocar modificar una imagen utilizando un software especializado para ocultar imperfecciones

alcohol un término general utilizado para describir una bebida que contiene una cierta cantidad de etanol

alcohólicos personas que están psicológicamente y físicamente adictas al alcohol

alcoholismo una enfermedad en la cual una persona es completamente dependiente del alcohol

intoxicación por alcohol una emergencia médica en la que una persona ha consumido suficiente alcohol para suprimir su sistema nervioso central, y que se caracteriza por la inconsciencia, baja presión arterial y temperatura corporal, dificultad para respirar, y posible muerte

alérgenos sustancias que desencadenan reacciones alérgicas en el cuerpo

alergia una respuesta inmune en el que el cuerpo reacciona de manera destructiva a una sustancia inofensiva

mentalidad de todo-o-nada una manera de pensar en la que una persona tiene que hacerlo "todo" bien o él o ella no ha hecho "nada" bien

amenorrea una condición en la que el ciclo menstrual de una mujer está anormalmente ausente

aminoácido una unidad química pequeña que compone proteínas

amnios una membrana que forma un saco lleno de líquido, que amortigua y protege al feto en desarrollo

esteroides anabólicos hormonas artificiales utilizadas para tratar trastornos musculares; a veces son utilizadas ilegalmente para ayudar a las personas a construir masa muscular

anaerobic activity occurring in the absence of oxygen

analgesics medications that relieve pain

anaphylaxis an allergic response in which fluid fills the lungs and air passages narrow, restricting breathing

androgynous a term that describes a person who exhibits feminine and masculine traits equally

anemia a condition causing weakness, tiredness, and headaches; results from decrease in red blood cells or insufficient hemoglobin

angina a pressure, squeezing, or pain in the chest that is often a sign of heart disease or a heart attack

anorexia nervosa an eating disorder in which a person has an intense fear of gaining weight, eats too little, and loses far more weight than is healthy for his or her height

antibiotic a substance that targets and kills pathogenic bacteria

antibiotic resistance a pathogen's ability to fight back against an antibiotic; develops over time and as a result of contact with certain antibiotics

antibody a molecule that attaches to and marks a pathogen as foreign, signaling white blood cells to destroy it

antidepressants type of medications that make certain chemicals in the brain more available to combat depression

antiperspirant a product designed to stop or dry up sweat

antipsychotics type of medication used to manage the symptoms of schizophrenia

anti-retroviral therapy (ART) a treatment for HIV/AIDS in which a cocktail of three drugs is given to interfere with HIV reproduction

antisocial personality disorder a common mental illness characterized by disregard for social rules, a tendency for impulsive

actividad anaeróbica ocurre en la ausencia de oxígeno

analgésicos medicamentos que alivian el dolor

anafilaxia una reacción alérgica en la que fluidos llenan los pulmones y las vías aéreas estrechas, restringiendo la respiración

andrógino un término que describe a una persona que exhibe rasgos femeninos y masculinos por igual

anemia una condición que causa debilidad, cansancio y dolores de cabeza; resulta de una disminución de los glóbulos rojos o de hemoglobina insuficiente

angina una presión, compresión, o dolor en el pecho que a menudo es una señal de enfermedad cardiaca o un ataque al corazón

anorexia nerviosa un trastorno alimenticio en el cual una persona tiene un miedo intenso a aumentar de peso, come muy poco, y pierde mucho más peso de lo que es saludable para su estatura

antibiótico una sustancia que ataca y destruye las bacterias patógenas

resistencia a los antibióticos la capacidad de un patógeno para luchar contra un antibiótico; se desarrolla con el tiempo y como resultado del contacto con ciertos antibióticos

anticuerpo una molécula que se adhiere a, y marca a un patógeno como extranjero, señalándolo a las células blancas de la sangre para destruirlo

antidepresivo tipo de medicamentos que hacen que ciertas sustancias químicas en el cerebro estén más disponibles para combatir contra la depresión

antitranspirante un producto diseñado para detener o secar el sudor

antipsicótico tipo de medicamento usado para controlar los síntomas de la esquizofrenia

terapia antirretroviral (TARV) un tratamiento para el VIH/SIDA en el que se administra un cóctel de tres fármacos para interferir en la reproducción del VIH

trastorno de personalidad antisocial una enfermedad mental común caracterizada por el desconsideración de las normas sociales, la

behavior, and indifference toward other people

anxiety disorder a mental illness characterized by extreme or unrealistic worries about daily events, experiences, or objects

aorta the largest artery in the body

Apgar test the measure of a newborn's health and condition through five basic tests

arrhythmias disorders that cause an irregularity in a person's heart rhythm

arteries large, muscular blood vessels that transport blood from the heart to the capillaries

arteriosclerosis a disease of the blood vessels in which arteries harden and become unable to stretch, leading to high blood pressure and heart disease

arthritis a condition in which the joints become inflamed, causing pain and stiffness

asexual reproduction a process that requires only one cell and which produces offspring identical to that cell

assault the threat or use of physical force to injure another person

assertive a style of behavior in which you speak honestly about and act appropriately on your needs, feelings, and goals

asthma a chronic disease characterized by episodes of blocked airflow to the lungs

asymptomatic the quality of exhibiting no recognizable signs or symptoms of disease

atherosclerosis a disease in which fatty substances collect on the walls of the arteries and restrict blood flow

attachment an emotional connection, especially between a baby and his or her caregiver

autoimmune disease a disease in which the immune system attacks and damages healthy body tissues

tendencia al comportamiento impulsivo, y la indiferencia hacia otras personas

trastorno de ansiedad una enfermedad mental caracterizada por preocupaciones extremas o poco realistas acerca de acontecimientos diarios, experiencias, u objetos

aorta la arteria más grande del cuerpo

test de Apgar la medida de la salud y condición de un recién nacido a través de cinco pruebas básicas

arritmias trastornos que causan una irregularidad en el ritmo cardíaco de una persona

arterias grandes vasos sanguíneos musculares que transportan la sangre desde el corazón hacia las capilares

arteriosclerosis una enfermedad de los vasos sanguíneos en la que las arterias se endurecen y se vuelven incapaces de estirar, lo que lleva a la alta presión arterial alta y a las enfermedades del corazón

artritis una condición en la que las articulaciones se inflaman, causando dolor y rigidez

reproducción asexual un proceso que requiere una sola célula y que produce descendencia idéntica a esa célula

asalto la amenaza o al uso de la fuerza física para lesionar a otra persona

firme un estilo de comportamiento en el que uno habla honestamente y actuar apropiadamente en relación a sus necesidades, sentimientos, y objetivos

asma una enfermedad crónica que se caracteriza por episodios de bloqueo de la circulación del aire a los pulmones

asintomático la cualidad de no exhibir señales o síntomas reconocibles de enfermedad

arteriosclerosis una enfermedad en la que sustancias grasas se acumulan en las paredes de las arterias y restringen el flujo sanguíneo

apego una conexión emocional, especialmente entre un bebé y su cuidador

enfermedad autoinmune una enfermedad en la cual el sistema inmunológico ataca y daña los tejidos corporales sanos

autonomy the freedom to direct one's self, independent of other influences

autonomía la libertad para dirigirse uno mismo, independiente de otras influencias

B English

Español

bacteria single-celled organisms that grow and reproduce in and outside of the body, and can be helpful or harmful to body function

bacteria organismos unicelulares que crecen y se reproducen dentro y fuera del cuerpo, y pueden ser útiles o perjudiciales para la función del cuerpo

barrier methods contraceptive methods that physically block fertilization by preventing sperm from reaching the ovum

métodos de barrera métodos anticonceptivos que bloquean físicamente la fertilización mediante la prevención de que los espermatozoides lleguen al óvulo

bath salts manufactured drugs that include the stimulant methylenedioxypyrovalerone (MDPV) and are often found in insect repellent, incense, or plant feeder

sales de baño drogas fabricadas que incluyen el estimulante methylenedioxypyrovalerone (MDPV) y a menudo se encuentran en repelentes de insectos, incienso, o alimentación de plantas

B cell a cell that produces antibodies

célula B una célula que produce anticuerpos

behavioral risk factors choices a person makes that increase his or her chances of developing diseases, disorders, or injuries

factores de riesgo de conducta selecciones que una persona hace que aumentan sus posibilidades de desarrollar enfermedades, trastornos, o lesiones

beneficiaries people or organizations that will receive a person's property and money upon that person's death

beneficiarios personas u organizaciones que recibirán los bienes y el dinero de una persona a la muerte de esa persona

benign tumors masses of abnormal cells that remain in the areas of the body where they first develop

tumores benignos masas de células anormales que permanecen en las áreas del cuerpo donde primero se desarrollan

binge drinking the consumption of a large amount of alcohol in a short period of time

consumo excesivo de alcohol el consumo de una gran cantidad de alcohol en un corto período de tiempo

binge-eating disorder an eating disorder in which a person repeatedly consumes a huge amount of food in a short period of time

trastorno por atracón un trastorno alimenticio en la que una persona consume repetidamente una enorme cantidad de comida en un corto período de tiempo

biological sex a person's sex—male or female—as determined by chromosomes

sexo biológico el sexo de una persona—masculino o femenino—según lo determinado por los cromosomas

biopsy a sample of tissue removed from the body for microscopic study; also the procedure of removing a tissue sample from the body for testing

biopsia una muestra de tejido extraído del cuerpo para estudio microscópico; también el procedimiento de extracción de una muestra de tejido del cuerpo para examinación

bipolar disorder a mental illness characterized by intense periods of depression closely

trastorno bipolar una enfermedad mental caracterizada por intensos períodos de

followed by extreme positive, or manic, feelings

birthing center   a nonmedical facility where a mother can give birth in a homelike environment

birthing room   a private space, often within a hospital, where a mother can give birth surrounded by the familiar comforts of home

birth plan   an outline of a mother's preferences for the birth process

bisexual   the quality of being romantically and physically attracted to members of both genders

blastocyst   a ball of cells formed by the cleaving zygote as it travels into the uterus

blood alcohol concentration (BAC)   the percentage of alcohol that is present in a person's blood

blood cholesterol   a fatty substance that resides in the blood and can block arteries if a healthy level is not maintained

blood pressure   the force that blood exiting the heart exerts on the walls of the arteries

blood vessels   narrow tubes that transport oxygen, blood, and nutrients throughout the whole body; include arteries, capillaries, and veins

body art   permanent decorations that are applied to the body; examples include tattoos and piercings

body composition   the ratio of fat, bone, and muscle that naturally make up a person's body

body image   term that describes a person's thoughts and feelings about how he or she looks

body mass index (BMI)   a number calculated from a person's height and weight; an indicator of excess body fat

BMI =

$$\frac{\text{Weight (lbs.)}}{\text{Height (in.)}^2} \times 703$$

depresión seguidos por sentimientos positivos, o maníacos, extremos

centro de parto   una instalación no médica donde una madre puede parir en un entorno acogedor

sala de parto   un espacio privado, a menudo dentro de un hospital, donde una madre puede dar a luz rodeada de las comodidades del hogar

plan de parto   un resumen de las preferencias de la madre para el parto

bisexual   el atributo de estar atraído románticamente y físicamente a miembros de ambos sexos

blastocito   una bola de células formada por el cigoto escisión a medida que viaja hacia el útero

concentración de alcohol en la sangre (BAC)   el porcentaje de alcohol que está presente en la sangre de una persona

colesterol en la sangre   una sustancia grasa que se encuentra en la sangre y puede bloquear las arterias si no se mantiene un nivel saludable

presión sanguínea   la fuerza que la sangre que sale del corazón ejerce sobre las paredes de las arterias

vasos sanguíneos   tubos estrechos que transportan oxígeno, sangre, y nutrientes a través de todo el cuerpo; incluye las arterias, capilares, y venas

arte corporal   decoraciones permanentes que se aplican al cuerpo; ejemplos incluyen tatuajes y *piercings*

composición corporal   la proporción de grasa, hueso y músculo que forman naturalmente el cuerpo de una persona

imagen corporal   término que describe los pensamientos y sentimientos de una persona sobre cómo él o ella se ve

índice de masa corporal (IMC)   un número calculado de la estatura y el peso de una persona; un indicador de exceso de grasa corporal

IMC =

$$\frac{\text{Peso (libras.)}}{\text{Estatura (pulgadas.)}^2} \times 703$$

bond to form an intimate, emotional attachment

borderline personality disorder a mental illness characterized by a person showing extreme instability in his or her self-concept and relationships

breast cancer a type of cancer that grows in the breasts; the second leading cause of death in women

bruxism a condition in which a person grinds or clenches his or her teeth while sleeping

bulimia nervosa an eating disorder in which a person has recurrent episodes of binge eating followed by purging

bullying aggressive behavior that seeks to injure, frighten, or manipulate another person

vínculo formar un vínculo emocional íntimo

trastorno de personalidad limítrofe una enfermedad mental caracterizada por una persona que muestra extrema inestabilidad en su concepto de sí mismo y de sus relaciones

cáncer de mama un tipo de cáncer que crece en los senos; la segunda causa principal de muerte en las mujeres

bruxismo una condición en la cual una persona muele o aprieta sus dientes mientras se duerme

bulimia nerviosa un trastorno alimenticio en el cual una persona tiene episodios recurrentes de comer en exceso seguido por vómitos o laxantes

intimidación comportamiento agresivo que busca herir, atemorizar, o manipular a otra persona

C English

Español

calorie a unit of measurement for energy provided by food

cancer a disease characterized by a mass of abnormally growing cells that spread and can cause pain, illness, and death

capillaries small, thin blood vessels that carry oxygen and nutrients from the arteries to the body's tissues

carbohydrate a nutrient and major source of energy for the body

carbon monoxide a poisonous gas found in cigarette smoke; negatively affects cells' ability to carry oxygen

carcinogens substances that cause cancer

cardiorespiratory fitness term that describes how efficiently the cardiovascular and respiratory systems deliver oxygen to the muscles during prolonged physical activity

cavities holes in the teeth caused by plaque eating away at tooth enamel

caloría una unidad de medida para la energía proporcionada por los alimentos

cáncer una enfermedad caracterizada por una masa de células que crecen anormalmente que se propagan y pueden causar dolor, enfermedad, y muerte

capilares pequeños vasos sanguíneos, delgados que llevan oxígeno y nutrientes de las arterias a los tejidos del cuerpo

carbohidrato un nutriente y fuente importante de energía para el cuerpo

monóxido de carbono un gas venenoso que se encuentra en el humo del cigarrillo; afecta negativamente la habilidad de células para transportar oxígeno

cancerígenos sustancias que causan cáncer

estado físico cardiorrespiratoria término que describe cuán eficientemente los sistemas cardiovascular y respiratorio entregan oxígeno a los músculos durante la actividad física prolongada

caries orificios en los dientes causados cuando la placa carcome el esmalte de los dientes

cell division the process by which cells multiply

cervical cancer a type of cancer in which the cells of the cervix grow abnormally

cervical cap a flexible, silicone contraceptive product that covers the cervix and prevents sperm from entering the uterus

cesarean section (C-section) delivery of an infant through an incision made in the mother's abdomen and uterus

chemotherapy a treatment in which medicines are administered to kill cancer cells

child abuse any abuse or neglect that harms or seeks to harm a child

child sexual abuse a type of abuse that involves using a child for sexual stimulation

child support the financial contribution legally required of the noncustodial parent

chlamydia an almost asymptomatic STI that may cause pelvic inflammatory disease if not treated

cholesterol a type of fat made by the body that is also present in some foods

chorion a membrane that develops around the implanted embryo

chorionic gonadotropin a hormone that is produced by the chorion; signals pregnancy

chronic bronchitis a condition in which the bronchial tubes swell and become irritated

chronic diseases diseases that occur for many years, even for a lifetime

chronic obstructive pulmonary disease (COPD) term for a group of diseases that cause difficulty breathing; includes chronic bronchitis and emphysema

cilia small, hair-like appendages that move mucus and fluids within the body

división celular el proceso por el cual las células se multiplican

cáncer cervical un tipo de cáncer en el que las células del cérvix crecen de manera anormal

capuchón cervical un producto anticonceptivo de silicona flexible que cubre el cuello uterino y evita que los espermatozoides entren en el útero

cesárea parto de un bebé a través de una incisión en el abdomen y el útero de la madre

quimioterapia un tratamiento en el que se administran medicamentos para destruir células cancerosas

abuso infantil cualquier abuso o negligencia que daña o busca dañar a un niño

abuso sexual infantil un tipo de abuso que implica el uso de niños para la estimulación sexual

manutención infantil la contribución financiera obligada legalmente del padre sin custodia

clamidia una ITS casi asintomática que puede causar enfermedad inflamatoria pélvica si no se trata

colesterol un tipo de grasa producida por el cuerpo que también está presente en algunos alimentos

corión una membrana que se desarrolla alrededor del embrión implantado

gonadotropina coriónica una hormona producida por el corion; señala de embarazo

bronquitis crónica una condición en la que los tubos bronquiales se hinchan y se irritan

enfermedades crónicas enfermedades que se producen por muchos años, incluso toda la vida

enfermedad pulmonar obstructiva crónica (EPOC) término para un grupo de enfermedades que causan dificultad para respirar; incluye la bronquitis crónica y el enfisema

cilio apéndices pequeños, similares a pelos que mueven la mucosidad y los fluidos en el cuerpo

circadian rhythm   physical, behavioral, and mental changes in the body that occur naturally and typically follow the 24-hour cycle of the sun

cirrhosis   a buildup of scar tissue in the liver; often leads to death

citizenship   the legal status of being entitled to the rights and duties of a community

cleavage   the process through which a single-celled zygote divides into many cells

climate   the overall environmental weather pattern of a region

clinical stage   the stage in which the signs and symptoms of a disease arise and are most prominent

clique   a small group of friends who intentionally turn away people who may want to interact with or befriend them

clitoris   an organ filled with erectile tissue and located above the vaginal opening; swells during sexual excitement

club drugs   a category of drugs that are often used at parties, bars, or concerts; include LSD, ecstasy, GHB, and Flunitrazepam (roofies)

cocaine   a stimulant made of white powder that comes from the leaves of coca plants

cochlea   a spiral tube in the inner ear that senses sound vibrations and transmits them to the auditory nerve

cognitive ability   the capacity to think and reason

cognitive-behavioral therapy   a type of therapy that focuses on clarifying patients' distorted thoughts and behaviors

cognitive distortions   unhealthy thinking patterns that people have about the world around them

colonoscopy   a procedure used to examine the colon

ritmo circadiano   cambios físicos, conductuales, y mentales en el cuerpo que ocurren naturalmente y por lo general siguen el ciclo de 24 horas del sol

cirrosis   una acumulación de tejido cicatrizal en el hígado; a menudo conduce a la muerte

ciudadanía   la condición jurídica de tener derecho a los derechos y deberes de una comunidad

escisión   el proceso a través del cual un cigoto unicelular se divide en muchas células

clima   el patrón climático medioambiental global de una región

etapa clínica   la etapa en el que surgen los signos y síntomas de una enfermedad y son más prominentes

camarilla   un pequeño grupo de amigos que intencionalmente dan la espalda a personas que quieran interactuar con o hacerse amigo de ellos

clítoris   un órgano lleno de tejido eréctil y situado encima de la apertura vaginal; se hincha durante la excitación sexual

drogas de club   una categoría de drogas que se utilizan a menudo en fiestas, bares, o conciertos; incluyen el LSD, el éxtasis, el GHB, y Flunitrazepam (rufis)

cocaína   un estimulante hecho de polvo blanco que proviene de las hojas de las plantas de coca

cóclea   un tubo en espiral en el oído interno que detecta las vibraciones del sonido y los transmite al nervio auditivo

capacidad cognitiva   la capacidad de pensar y razonar

terapia conductual-cognitiva   un tipo de terapia que se enfoca en clarificando los pensamientos y comportamientos distorsionados de los pacientes

distorsiones cognitivas   patrones de pensamiento poco saludables que las personas tienen sobre el mundo que les rodea

colonoscopía   un procedimiento usado para examinar el colon

colostrum a protein- and antibody-rich substance secreted in a mother's breasts for a few days after she gives birth

communication process the process by which ideas, thoughts, feelings, and information are exchanged

complication a problem or secondary infection that results from or accompanies a disease

components of fitness different types of fitness, such as strength and flexibility

compromise an arrangement in which each side of a disagreement gives in a little to the other

concussion a brain injury resulting from a severe blow to the head, characterized by nausea, confusion, weakness, memory loss, and unconsciousness

condom a contraceptive product that fits over an erect penis or inside a woman's vagina, where it catches sperm and prevents them from reaching the ovum

conflicts disagreements or problems that result from opposing actions or views

congestive heart failure a condition in which the heart weakens due to strain and becomes unable to successfully pump blood

consent a direct, verbal, non-coerced agreement from someone who is capable of making an informed decision

constipation a condition characterized by infrequent or delayed hard, dry bowel movements

continuous positive airway pressure (CPAP) therapy a type of therapy in which a machine is used to open the airways during sleep; a treatment for sleep apnea

contraception a method or substance that helps to prevent pregnancy; also known as *birth control*

calostro una sustancia rica en proteínas y anticuerpos secretados en los pechos de una madre por unos pocos días después de dar a luz

proceso de comunicación el proceso por el cual las ideas, pensamientos, sentimientos, e información son intercambiados

complicación una infección o problema secundario que resulta o acompaña a una enfermedad

componentes del estado físico diferentes tipos de aptitud, como la fuerza y la flexibilidad

compromiso una disposición en la que cada lado de un desacuerdo da en un poco a la otra

contusión cerebral una lesión cerebral resultado de un fuerte golpe en la cabeza, que se caracteriza por náuseas, confusión, debilidad, pérdida de memoria y pérdida del conocimiento

condón un producto anticonceptivo que se coloca sobre el pene erecto o dentro de la vagina de la mujer, donde atrapa los espermatozoides y les impide alcanzar el óvulo

conflictos desacuerdos o problemas que resultan de acciones u opiniones opuestos

insuficiencia cardíaca congestiva una condición en la que el corazón se debilita debido a la tensión y es incapaz de bombear la sangre correctamente

consentimiento un acuerdo verbal directo, no coaccionado, de alguien que es capaz de tomar una decisión informada

estreñimiento una condición caracterizada por movimientos intestinales infrecuente, retrasados, duros y secos

terapia de presión positiva continua en la vía aérea (CPAP) un tipo de terapia en la que se utiliza una máquina para abrir las vías respiratorias durante el sueño; un tratamiento para la apnea del sueño

anticoncepción un método o sustancia que ayuda a prevenir el embarazo; también conocido como *control de la natalidad*

contraceptive sponge a birth control method that blocks sperm from entering the uterus

convalescent stage the stage during which signs and symptoms of a disease fade and a person is no longer contagious

cornea the clear tissue covering the front of the eye

coronary arteries blood vessels that deliver blood, oxygen, and nutrients to the heart

coronary artery disease a disease in which the arteries that carry blood to the heart become narrow or blocked

creatine an amino acid that helps the body build protein; can be taken as a dietary supplement to help a person build muscle mass

cross training training in different activities to improve performance in a sport and reduce the risk of injury

cryptorchidism a condition in which the testes fail to descend from the abdominal cavity; a common cause of infertility and testicular cancer

crystal meth a manufactured drug that acts as an amphetamine and looks like clear crystal chunks

culture the beliefs, values, customs, and arts of a group of people

cystic acne a severe type of acne that requires medical treatment

esponja anticonceptiva un método de control de natalidad que bloquea que los espermatozoides ingresen al útero

etapa de convalecencia la etapa en la que los signos y síntomas de la enfermedad desaparecen y una persona ya no es contagiosa

córnea el tejido transparente que cubre la parte frontal del ojo

arterias coronarias los vasos sanguíneos que suministran sangre, oxígeno y nutrientes al corazón

enfermedad de la arteria coronaria una enfermedad en la cual las arterias que llevan la sangre al corazón se estrechan o están obstruidas

creatina un aminoácido que ayuda a la proteína de desarrollo corporal; puede ser tomado como un suplemento dietético para ayudar a una persona a desarrollar masa muscular

entrenamiento cruzado capacitación en diferentes actividades para mejorar el rendimiento en un deporte y reducir el riesgo de lesiones

criptorquidia una condición en la que los testículos no descienden de la cavidad abdominal; una causa común de infertilidad y cáncer testicular

cristal una droga fabricada que actúa como una anfetamina y se ve como trozos de cristal claro

cultura las creencias, los valores, las costumbres y las artes de un grupo de personas

acné quístico un tipo de acné severo que requiere tratamiento médico

D English

Español

Daily Values the recommended amounts of nutrients that a person should consume each day

dandruff dead skin that flakes off the scalp due to dryness, infrequent shampooing, or irritation

Valores Diarios las cantidades recomendadas de nutrientes que una persona debe consumir cada día

caspa piel muerta que se desprende del cuero cabelludo debido a la resequedad, el champú poco frecuente, o la irritación

decibels the units by which sound intensity, or loudness, is measured

decision-making skills your ability to make choices about your health and wellness

deductible the amount you pay for healthcare services each year before your insurance company begins to take on the cost

dehydration a condition in which the body's tissues lose too much water

dementia a condition of mental deterioration

deodorant a product designed to cover up body odor

dependence a condition in which a person relies on a given substance to function or feel normal

depressant a substance that slows the central nervous system and causes chemical changes in the brain

depression an emotional state characterized by a feeling of worthlessness and a lack of interest in daily life

dermis the middle layer of skin, which contains hair follicles

detoxification a necessary step in defeating addiction that means complete withdrawal from a substance; may cause intense anxiety, tremors, and hallucinations

diabetes mellitus a disease in which the body is unable to regulate its levels of glucose

diaphragm a flexible, cup-shaped contraceptive product that covers the cervix and blocks sperm from entering the uterus

dietary supplement a product that can be ingested to give a person's body more of a specific nutrient; can be harmful when used in excess

differentiation the process by which embryonic cells develop into cells with specific structures and functions

decibelios las unidades por las cuales la intensidad o el volumen del sonido son medidas

capacidad para tomar decisiones su capacidad para tomar decisiones acerca de su salud y bienestar

deducible la cantidad que uno paga por los servicios de salud todos los años antes de que la compañía de seguros comienza a asumir el costo

deshidratación una condición en la que los tejidos del cuerpo pierden demasiada agua

demencia una condición de deterioro mental

desodorante un producto diseñado para cubrir el olor corporal

dependencia una condición en la cual una persona depende de una sustancia determinada para funcionar o sentirse normal

tranquilizante una sustancia que retrasa el sistema nervioso central y produce cambios químicos en el cerebro

depresión un estado emocional que se caracteriza por una sensación de inutilidad y falta de interés en la vida diaria

dermis la capa intermedia de la piel, que contiene folículos pilosos

detoxificación un paso necesario para derrotar la adicción que significa el rechazo completo de una sustancia; puede causar intensa ansiedad, temblores y alucinaciones

diabetes mellitus a una enfermedad en la cual el cuerpo es incapaz de regular sus niveles de glucosa

diafragma un producto anticonceptivo flexible, en forma de taza, que cubre el cuello del útero y bloquea que los espermatozoides entren en el útero

suplemento dietético un producto que puede ser ingerido para darle al cuerpo de una persona una mayor cantidad de un nutriente específico; puede ser perjudicial cuando se usa en exceso

diferenciación el proceso por el cual las células embrionarias se desarrollan en células con estructuras y funciones específicas

dilation   the widening and thinning of the cervix

disease   a poor state of health and wellness in various areas of your life

disorder   an abnormal physical or mental condition with no single, identifiable cause

distracted driving behaviors   risky driving actions typically taken by teenagers; include texting, talking on the phone, and driving with one or more passengers under 18 years of age

diuretic   a supplement that causes a person to lose fluids

diversity   the wide range of backgrounds, ages, ethnicities, and genders represented in a group of people

domestic violence   physically, mentally, or emotionally abusive behavior that occurs within a romantic relationship

dominant   term used to describe genes that are always expressed in offspring

driving under the influence (DUI)   a legal offense that occurs when a person has driven with a blood alcohol concentration at or over 0.08; a criminal offense in most states; also known as *driving while intoxicated (DWI)*

drug abuse   the act of using drugs excessively or without medical reason

drug addiction   a chronic disease characterized by the continued use of a drug regardless of its harmful consequences

drug overdose   the ingestion of more of a drug than the body can successfully process at one time

drugs   substances that cause physical or psychological changes in the body and brain

dilatación   dilatación el ensanchamiento y adelgazamiento del cérvix

enfermedad   mal estado de salud y bienestar en diversas áreas de la vida

trastorno   una condición física o mental anormal sin ninguna única, causa identificable

comportamientos de conducción distraída   acciones de conducción arriesgadas normalmente realizadas por adolescentes; incluyen los mensajes de texto, hablar por teléfono, y conducir con uno o más pasajeros menores de los 18 años de edad

diurético   un suplemento que hace que una persona pierda líquidos

diversidad   la amplia gama de antecedentes, edades, etnias y géneros representados en un grupo de personas

violencia doméstica   comportamiento abusivo, físico, mental, o emocional, que se produce dentro de una relación romántica

dominante   término utilizado para describir los genes que siempre están expresados en los hijos

conducir bajo la influencia (DUI)   una ofensa legal que se produce cuando una persona ha conducido con una concentración de alcohol en la sangre en o por encima de 0.08; un delito en la mayoría de los estados; también conocido como *conducir en estado de ebriedad (DWI)*

abuso de drogas   el acto de consumir drogas en exceso o sin razón médica

adicción a las drogas   una enfermedad crónica que se caracteriza por el uso continuado de una droga, independientemente de sus consecuencias perjudiciales

sobredosis de drogas   la ingestión de más de una droga de lo que el cuerpo puede procesar con éxito en un momento

drogas   sustancias que causan cambios físicos o psicológicos en el cuerpo y el cerebro

E English

eardrum   the part of the middle ear that vibrates in response to sound

Español

tímpano   la parte del oído medio que vibra en respuesta al sonido

eating disorder   a psychological illness characterized by a serious disturbance in a person's eating behavior

eclampsia   a life-threatening emergency in which a pregnant woman's blood pressure rises, causing seizures

ectopic pregnancy   a condition in which an embryo implants and begins developing in the fallopian tubes

eczema   a chronic skin condition characterized by patches of red, itchy, dry, or swollen skin

edema   the swelling of body tissues during an immune response

ejaculation   a process by which muscular contractions expel semen through the urethral opening in the penis

elder abuse   any abuse or neglect that harms or seeks to harm an older adult

embryo   a ball of cells formed by the cleaving zygote, and which implants in the uterus

emergency contraception   contraceptive method that can be used to prevent pregnancy if other birth control fails or has been used incorrectly

emotional health   a dimension of health that involves your emotions, mood, outlook on life, and beliefs about yourself

emotional intelligence   the skill of identifying one's own emotions and understanding the emotions of others

emotions   moods and feelings that you experience

empathy   the ability to imagine yourself in someone else's place, and to understand someone else's wants, needs, and point of view

emphysema   a disease that permanently enlarges lung airways and destroys lung tissue, making it difficult for a person to breathe

trastorno alimenticio   una enfermedad psicológica que se caracteriza por una grave perturbación en la conducta alimentaria de una persona

eclampsia   una emergencia que amenaza la vida en la que la presión de la sangre de una mujer embarazada aumenta, causando convulsiones

embarazo ectópico   una condición en la que un embrión se implanta y comienza a desarrollar en las trompas de Falopio

eczema   una condición crónica de la piel caracterizada por parches de piel roja, picazón, resequedad, o hinchazón

edema   la hinchazón de los tejidos del cuerpo durante una respuesta inmune

eyaculación   un proceso por el que las contracciones musculares expulsan el semen a través de la apertura uretral en el pene

maltrato de ancianos   cualquier abuso o negligencia que perjudique o busque dañar a un anciano

embrión   una bola de células formadas por el cigoto en clivaje, y que se implanta en el útero

anticoncepción de emergencia   método anticonceptivo que puede ser utilizado para prevenir el embarazo si otro control de la natalidad falla o ha sido utilizado incorrectamente

salud emocional   una dimensión de la salud que consiste de las emociones, el humor, la actitud ante la vida y las creencias sobre uno mismo

inteligencia emocional   la habilidad de identificar sus propias emociones y comprender las emociones de los demás

emociones   estados de ánimo y sentimientos que uno experimenta

empatía   la capacidad de imaginarse a uno mismo en el lugar de otra persona y comprender sus deseos, sus necesidades, y su punto de vista

enfisema   una enfermedad que amplía de forma permanente vías respiratorias pulmonares y destruye el tejido pulmonar, lo que se le hace difícil a una persona a respirar

enabling encouraging an addict's destructive behaviors, either intentionally or unintentionally

endemic a disease that naturally occurs in low numbers in a certain area

endometriosis a condition in which endometrial tissue grows in abnormal places, often leading to pelvic pain and infertility

endorphins chemicals found mainly in the brain that affect emotions and relieve pain

environment the circumstances, objects, and conditions of your surroundings

environmental risk factors characteristics of your surroundings that may expose you to injury or disease

epidemic an outbreak of a disease that occurs in unexpectedly large numbers over a geographic area

epidermis the outermost layer of skin, which protects the body from foreign substances and contains pigment-producing cells

epididymitis inflammation of the epididymis, which leads to pain, swelling, and possible penile discharge

epidural anesthesia pain medication used during childbirth

erectile tissue spongy tissue contained in the penis and clitoris that fills with blood during sexual excitement

estrogens hormones that trigger the development of the ovaries, breasts, and other sexual characteristics in females

ethnicity a person's connection to a cultural or national social group

euphoria a feeling of intense happiness caused by high levels of dopamine in the brain

exclusive term that describes being romantically involved with only one partner

exercise term that describes a type of physical activity that is planned, structured, and purposeful

posibilitar fomentar comportamientos destructivos de un adicto, ya sea con o sin intención

endémico una enfermedad que se produce naturalmente en números bajos en un área determinada

endometriosis una condición en la cual el tejido endometrial crece en lugares anormales, a menudo conduce al dolor pélvico e infertilidad

endorfinas productos químicos que se encuentran principalmente en el cerebro que afectan a las emociones y alivian el dolor

ambiente las circunstancias, objetos, y condiciones de su entorno

factores de riesgo ambiental características de su entorno que puedan exponerlo a una lesión o enfermedad

epidemia brote de una enfermedad que se produce en grandes cantidades de forma inesperada en un área geográfica

epidermis la capa más externa de la piel, que protege al cuerpo de sustancias extrañas y contiene células productoras de pigmento

epididimitis inflamación del epidídimo, que lleva al dolor, la hinchazón y a una posible secreción del pene

anestesia epidural medicamento para el dolor utilizado durante el parto

tejido eréctil tejido esponjoso contenido en el pene y el clítoris que se llena de sangre durante la excitación sexual

estrógenos hormonas que activan el desarrollo de los ovarios, pechos, y otras características sexuales en las mujeres

etnicidad conexión de una persona a un grupo social o cultural nacional

euforia un sentimiento de felicidad intensa causado por altos niveles de dopamina en el cerebro

exclusivo término que describe estar involucrado románticamente con una sola pareja

ejercicio término que describe un tipo de actividad física que se planifica, es estructurada, y con un propósito

F English

fad diet   a diet that is extremely popular for a certain time period; often unhealthy

fallopian tube   a structure that connects the ovaries to the uterus and guides ova out of the ovaries; uterine tube

family-based therapy   a type of therapy that involves parents or guardians, and siblings of patients in treatment

family history   the record of a disease's presence and impact within a family

family planning   the process of making choices about having children, including number of children and spacing between them

family therapy   a method of treatment in which members of a family meet together with a therapist

fasting   the practice of not eating or drinking anything except water for a set period of time

fat   a type of nutrient, composed of fatty acids, that is a valuable source of energy, especially for muscles

fat-soluble vitamin   a type of vitamin that dissolves in the body's fat, where it is stored for later use

feedback   a response that signals a message has been received and understood

female athlete triad   a health problem characterized by three conditions—amenorrhea, disordered eating, and osteoporosis

fertility   the ability to produce children

fertility awareness method (FAM)   a natural birth control method in which couples plan sexual intercourse for times when a woman is least fertile and avoid sexual intercourse during times of high fertility

fertilization   the process by which the sperm and ovum combine to create a zygote

fetal alcohol syndrome (FAS)   term for a group of serious physical and mental birth defects

Español

dieta relámpago   una dieta que es muy popular para un período de tiempo determinado; a menudo poco saludable

trompas de Falopio   una estructura que conecta los ovarios con el útero y guía los óvulos fuera de los ovarios; tubo uterino

terapia basada en la familia   un tipo de terapia que incluye a los padres o tutores, y los hermanos de los pacientes en el tratamiento

historia familiar   el récord de la presencia y el impacto de una enfermedad dentro de una familia

planificación familiar   el proceso de tomar decisiones acerca de tener hijos, incluyendo el número de hijos y la separación entre ellos

terapia familiar   un método de tratamiento en la que los miembros de una familia se reúnen con un terapeuta

ayuno   la práctica de no comer o beber nada excepto agua durante un periodo de tiempo determinado

grasa   un tipo de nutriente, compuesto de ácidos grasos, que es una valiosa fuente de energía, especialmente para los músculos

vitamina liposoluble   un tipo de vitamina que se disuelve en la grasa del cuerpo, donde se almacena para su uso posterior

comentarios   una respuesta que indica que un mensaje ha sido recibido y entendido

tríada de la atleta femenina   un problema de salud que se caracteriza por tres condiciones-amenorrea, trastornos alimentarios, y la osteoporosis

fertilidad   la capacidad de tener hijos

método de conocimiento de la fertilidad (FAM)   un método anticonceptivo natural en el que las parejas planean las relaciones sexuales para los momentos en que una mujer es menos fértil y evitan las relaciones sexuales durante los momentos de alta fertilidad

fertilización   el proceso por el cual el esperma y el óvulo se combinan para crear un cigoto

síndrome de alcoholismo fetal (SAF)   término para una grupo de defectos físicos y mentales

caused by a woman's consumption of alcohol while pregnant

fever a rise in the body's temperature, which stimulates white blood cells and blocks pathogen reproduction

fiber a complex carbohydrate that the body is unable to digest

fibroid a benign tumor that grows in the uterine muscle

fight-or-flight response the body's physiological impulse to either fight off or flee from threatening situations

fine-motor skills movements that use small muscles

fitness the body's ability to meet daily physical demands

flagellum a long, whip-like structure on the sperm that propels the sperm through liquid

flexibility the ability to bend without injury or breakage

fontanel a soft spot on a newborn's skull where the bone has not yet formed

food additives substances added to food products to cause desired changes

food allergy an immune response in which the body reacts to a certain type of food as though the food were a harmful substance; may manifest itself in rashes, swelling, difficulty breathing, indigestion, or dizziness

Food and Drug Administration (FDA) a government agency that regulates medications, biological products, medical devices, food supply, cosmetics, and radiation-emitting products

foodborne illness a disease that is transmitted by food; *food poisoning*

foodborne infection an illness caused by a bacteria, virus, or parasite that has contaminated a food

de nacimiento graves causados por el consumo de alcohol por la mujer durante el embarazo

fiebre un aumento de la temperatura del cuerpo, que estimula las células blancas de la sangre y bloquea la reproducción de patógenos

fibra un carbohidrato complejo que el cuerpo es incapaz de digerir

fibroma un tumor benigno que crece en el músculo uterino

respuesta de lucha o huida impulso fisiológico del cuerpo para ya sea a combatir o huir de situaciones amenazantes

habilidades de motricidad fina movimientos que utilizan músculos pequeños

estado físico la capacidad del cuerpo para satisfacer las demandas físicas diarias

flagelo una estructura larga, en forma de látigo en el esperma que impulsa el esperma a través de líquido

flexibilidad capacidad para doblarse sin lesión o rotura

fontanela un punto débil en el cráneo de un recién nacido donde el hueso aun no se ha formado

aditivos alimenticios sustancias añadidas a los productos alimenticios para provocar los cambios deseados

alergia alimenticia una respuesta inmune en la que el cuerpo reacciona a un cierto tipo de alimentos como si la comida fuera una sustancia dañina; puede manifestarse en erupciones cutáneas, hinchazón, dificultad para respirar, indigestión, o mareos

Administración de Alimentos y Medicamentos (FDA) una agencia gubernamental que regula los medicamentos, productos biológicos, dispositivos médicos, el suministro de alimentos, cosméticos, y los productos que emiten radiación

enfermedad transmitida por los alimentos une enfermedad que es transmitida por los alimentos; *intoxicación alimentaria*

infección transmitida por los alimentos una enfermedad causada por una bacteria, virus o parásito que ha contaminado un alimento

foodborne intoxication an illness caused by toxins that an organism has produced in a food; toxins may also be produced by chemicals, heavy metals, or other substances

food diary a record of what a person eats in each day

food intolerance a condition in which a person cannot properly digest a certain type of food

intoxicación transmitida por los alimentos una enfermedad causada por toxinas que un organismo ha producido en un alimento; las toxinas también pueden ser producidas por productos químicos, metales pesados u otras sustancias

diario de alimentos un registro de lo que una persona come en cada día

intolerancia alimentaria una condición en la cual una persona no puede digerir correctamente un determinado tipo de alimentos

---

G English

Español

gamete a sex cell that contains an individual's genetic material

gender identity a person's biological makeup—male or female—and how a person experiences or expresses that makeup

gender roles attitudes and behaviors that a society considers "appropriate" for males or females

gender stereotypes culturally defined assumptions about what it means to be male or female

generally recognized as safe (GRAS) food additives that have been studied and are considered harmless by the government

generic drug a medication that can be made by many different companies; costs less than brand-name medicines but may be just as effective

genes segments of DNA that determine the structure and function of your cells and affect your development, personality, and health

genetic predisposition a hereditary vulnerability to various diseases and illnesses

genital herpes an STI that infects the genitals, mouth, or rectum, and causes outbreaks of sores sometimes accompanied by fever

gameto una célula sexual que contiene material genético de un individuo

identidad de género constitución biológica de una persona—hombre o mujer—y cómo una persona experimenta o expresa esa constitución

roles de género actitudes y comportamientos que una sociedad considera "apropiado" para hombres o mujeres

estereotipos de género suposiciones culturalmente definidas sobre lo que significa ser hombre o mujer

generalmente reconocido como seguro (GRAS) aditivos alimenticios que han sido estudiados y son considerados inofensivos por el gobierno

medicamento genérico un medicamento que puede ser fabricado por muchas empresas diferentes; cuesta menos que los medicamentos de marca, pero puede ser igual de eficaz

genes segmentos de ADN que determinan la estructura y función de las células y afectan al desarrollo, la personalidad, y la salud

predisposición genética vulnerabilidad hereditaria a diversas enfermedades y enfermedades

herpes genital una ITS que infecta los genitales, la boca o el recto, y causa brotes de llagas a veces acompañada de fiebre

genital warts abnormal growths on the skin and membranes around the genitals and anus

geography the features of the land

germ layers types of embryonic tissues that will eventually constitute the three main types of tissues in the body

germ theory a scientific theory, which states that specific microorganisms cause specific diseases

gestation the period of time between fertilization of an ovum and the birth of a baby

gestational diabetes mellitus a condition in which a woman's body becomes incapable of producing insulin due to the hormones involved in pregnancy

ghrelin a hormone that increases appetite and leads to hunger

gingivitis an inflammation of the gums

glucose a type of carbohydrate and the preferred source of energy for the brain and central nervous system

gluten a protein found in wheat, rye, oats, and barley

glycogen a stored version of glucose located in the muscles and liver; supplies energy between meals

goals a short-term or long-term plan of action that will guide you to the state of wellness you hope to reach

gonorrhea a bacterial STI that causes burning or itching of reproductive parts, and can cause infertility or even death if not treated

gout a type of arthritis characterized by sudden, severe, and painful swelling of a joint

gross-motor skills movements that use large muscles

verrugas genitales masas anormales en la piel y las membranas alrededor de los genitales y el ano

geografía las características de la tierra

capas germinales tipos de tejidos embrionarios que eventualmente constituirán los tres principales tipos de tejidos en el cuerpo

teoría del germen una teoría científica, que establece que microorganismos específicos causan enfermedades específicas

gestación el período de tiempo entre la fertilización de un óvulo y el nacimiento de un bebé

diabetes mellitus gestacional una condición en la que el cuerpo de una mujer se vuelve incapaz de producir insulina debido a las hormonas relacionadas con el embarazo

ghrelina una hormona que aumenta el apetito y provoca el hambre

gingivitis una inflamación de las encías

glucosa un tipo de carbohidrato y la fuente preferida de energía para el cerebro y el sistema nervioso central

gluten una proteína presente en el trigo, el centeno, la avena, y la cebada

glucógeno una versión almacenada de glucosa se encuentra en los músculos y el hígado; suministra energía entre comidas

metas un plan de acción a corto o largo plazo que le guiará al estado de bienestar que espera alcanzar

gonorrea una ITS bacteriana que causa ardor o picazón de los órganos reproductivos, y puede causar infertilidad o incluso la muerte si no se trata

gota un tipo de artritis que se caracteriza por la repentina, severa y dolorosa hinchazón de las articulaciones

habilidades de motricidad gruesa movimientos que utilizan músculos grandes

H English

Español

halitosis the condition of having bad-smelling breath

halitosis la condición de tener mal aliento

hallucinogens drugs that cause hallucinations and alter a person's sense of reality

hangover term for the uncomfortable physical symptoms caused by excessive alcohol consumption

hazard an aspect of your environment that puts you at risk for disease or injury

hazing a humiliating or dangerous activity that someone is required to perform to become part of a group

health literacy the ability to locate, interpret, and apply information pertaining to your health

health promotion a process in which you take charge of your own health and wellness by making responsible and well-informed decisions

health-related fitness type of fitness used to easily perform daily activities

heart attack a medical emergency in which the coronary arteries become blocked and restrict blood flow to the heart, causing the heart to beat irregularly and inefficiently

heroin an opiate drug derived from morphine and often mixed with sugar, powdered milk, or other drugs

heterosexual the quality of being romantically and physically attracted to members of the opposite gender

hippocampus the part of the brain involved in the formation and storage of memory

histamine a substance that causes blood vessels to leak fluids into body tissues, resulting in swelling

HIV-positive a result of laboratory testing that indicates the presence of HIV antibodies in a person's blood

homeostasis the body's internal balance and stability; typically maintained despite changing conditions

alucinógenos drogas que causan alucinaciones y alteran el sentido de la realidad de una persona

resaca término para los síntomas físicos incómodos causados por el consumo excesivo de alcohol

peligro un aspecto de su entorno que le pone a riesgo de una enfermedad o lesión

novatadas una actividad peligrosa o humillante que una persona debe llevar a cabo para formar parte de un grupo

conocimientos de salud la capacidad de localizar, interpretar, y aplicar información relacionada con su salud

promoción de la salud un proceso en el que usted toma las riendas de su propia salud y bienestar al tomar decisiones responsables y bien informadas

condición física relacionada con la salud tipo de gimnasia utilizado para realizar fácilmente las actividades diarias

ataque cardiaco una emergencia médica en la que las arterias coronarias son obstruidas y restringen el flujo de la sangre al corazón, haciendo que el corazón palpite de forma irregular e ineficiente

heroína un fármaco opiáceo derivado de la morfina, a menudo mezclado con azúcar, leche en polvo, u otras drogas

heterosexual la calidad de sentirse atraído románticamente y físicamente a los miembros del sexo opuesto

hipocampo la parte del cerebro involucrada en la formación y el almacenamiento de la memoria

histamina una sustancia que hace que los vasos sanguíneos derramen líquido en los tejidos del cuerpo, resultando en una inflamación

VIH-positivo resultado de pruebas de laboratorio que indican la presencia de anticuerpos del VIH en la sangre de una persona

homeostasis el equilibrio y la estabilidad interna del cuerpo; normalmente mantenido a pesar de condiciones cambiantes

homicide   the killing of one human by another; murder

homophobia   irrational fear, discrimination, and anger that is directed at homosexuality and LGBT individuals

homosexual   the quality of being romantically and physically attracted to members of the same gender

hormone   a chemical substance in your body that influences many basic processes

hospice care   healthcare designed to provide comfort for terminally ill patients and their families

human immunodeficiency virus (HIV)   a virus that infects and kills cells, thus weakening the body's immune system; leads to AIDS

human life cycle   the sequence of developmental stages in a person's life span

human papillomavirus (HPV)   the most common STI, which infects and causes cells to grow abnormally; can result in genital warts, cervical cancer, and oropharyngeal cancer

human sexual response cycle   term for the four phases of physical changes that occur when a person is sexually aroused; includes the excitement phase, plateau phase, orgasmic phase, and resolution phase

human trafficking   a form of modern-day slavery involving the use of force or coercion to make a person perform some type of job or service against his or her will

hyperglycemia   a condition characterized by dangerously high blood glucose levels

hypertension   a condition that is characterized by high blood pressure, which can lead to heart disease or stroke

hypodermis   the innermost layer of skin, which contains fat, blood vessels, and nerve endings; attaches to underlying bone and muscle

homicidio   la muerte de un ser humano por otro; asesinato

homofobia   temor irracional, discriminación, e ira dirigida a la homosexualidad y a los individuos LGBT

homosexual   la calidad de sentirse atraído románticamente y físicamente a miembros del mismo sexo

hormona   una sustancia química en el cuerpo que influye en muchos procesos básicos

cuidado de hospicio   cuidado de la salud diseñado para proveer comodidad para los pacientes con enfermedades terminales y sus familias

virus de la inmunodeficiencia humana (VIH)   un virus que infecta y destruye las células, debilitando así el sistema inmune del cuerpo; lleva al SIDA

ciclo de la vida humana   la secuencia de las etapas de desarrollo durante la vida de una persona

virus del papiloma humano (VPH)   la ITS más común, que infecta y provoca que las células crezcan de manera anormal; puede resultar en verrugas genitales, cáncer cervical, y cáncer de orofarínge

ciclo de respuesta sexual humana   término para las cuatro fases de los cambios físicos que se producen cuando una persona se excita sexualmente; incluye la fase de excitación, la fase meseta, la fase orgásmica, y la fase de resolución

trata de personas   una forma de la esclavitud moderna que implica el uso de la fuerza o la coerción para hacer que una persona desempeñe algún tipo de trabajo o servicio contra de su voluntad

hiperglicemia   una condición caracterizada por niveles de glucosa peligrosamente altos

hipertensión   una condición que se caracteriza por la alta presión arterial, que puede conducir a enfermedades del corazón o un derrame cerebral

hipodermis   la capa más interna de la piel, que contiene grasa, vasos sanguíneos, y terminaciones nerviosas; se une al hueso subyacente y al músculo

hypoglycemia   a deficiency of sugar in the blood; often a result of excessive amounts of insulin being released to lower blood sugar levels

hypothalamus   a part of the brain that regulates appetite and energy consumption

hypoxia   a condition in which cells and tissue are deprived of oxygen; often results in severe cell damage

hipoglicemia   una deficiencia de azúcar en la sangre; a menudo el resultado de cantidades excesivas de insulina siendo liberadas para reducir los niveles de azúcar en la sangre

hipotálamo   una parte del cerebro que regula el apetito y el consumo de energía

hipoxia   una condición en la que las células y tejidos se ven privados de oxígeno; a menudo resulta en daño celular severo

---

I English

Español

idealized image   an image or standard of beauty that does not exist in real life

identity   who you are, which includes your physical traits, activities, social connections, and internal thoughts and feelings

identity theft   the fraudulent act of stealing and using a person's personal information, often for financial gain

immune system   a collection of cells and chemicals that operate together to fight infections and other illnesses in the body

implantation   the process by which an embryo burrows into the endometrial lining of the uterus

incontinence   the inability to prevent urination when urine accumulates in the bladder

incubation period   the time between a pathogen's entrance into the body and the first symptoms of disease

Individualized Education Plan (IEP)   a program that outlines the additional services a child with a developmental delay may require in a classroom setting

Individualized Family Service Plan (IFSP)   an intervention program that outlines the special services a young child with a developmental delay will need

infatuation   term for intense romantic feelings based largely on physical attraction

imagen idealizada   una imagen o un estándar de belleza que no existe en la vida real

identidad   quien eres, que incluye sus características físicas, actividades, relaciones sociales y pensamientos internos y sentimientos

usurpación de identidad   el acto fraudulento de robar y usar la información personal de una persona, a menudo por ganancias financieras

sistema inmune   una colección de células y sustancias químicas que actúan en conjunto para combatir infecciones y otras enfermedades en el cuerpo

implantación   el proceso por el cual un embrión se entierra en el revestimiento endometrial del útero

incontinencia   la incapacidad de prevenir orinar cuando la orina se acumula en la vejiga

periodo de incubación   el tiempo entre la entrada de un patógeno en el cuerpo y los primeros síntomas de una enfermedad

Plan de Educación Individualizado (PEI)   un programa que describe los servicios adicionales que un niño con un retraso en el desarrollo puede requerir en el aula

Plan Individualizado de Servicios para la Familia (PISF)   un programa de intervención que describe los servicios especiales que un niño pequeño con un retraso en el desarrollo necesitará

infatuación   término para intensos sentimientos románticos basado en gran medida en la atracción física

infectious disease a disease caused by microorganisms or pathogens that can be transmitted from one person, animal, or object to another

infertility a condition in which a man or woman is physically unable to reproduce

inflammation increased blood flow to an injured or diseased area of the body, causing redness, hurt, swelling, and pain

inhalants chemicals that people breathe in to experience some type of high

inheritance the transmission of parents' characteristics to their children

inherited disease a disease that is caused by defective genes passed down from an ancestral line

inhibition the psychological restraint that discourages people from engaging in dangerous behaviors

inpatient facility a hospital where patients reside overnight while receiving diagnosis, treatment, surgery, therapy, and rehabilitation

insomnia a condition in which the body is unable to fall asleep or stay asleep

insulin a hormone that is produced in the pancreas and directs cells to consume blood glucose

intellectual health a dimension of health that involves your ability to think clearly and critically, learn, and solve problems

intensity a quality that is measured by how much energy the body uses per minute during physical activity

interdependent the quality of one person or piece of information being reliant on another

interpersonal skills your ability to interact positively with those around you

enfermedad infecciosa una enfermedad causada por microorganismos o agentes patógenos que pueden transmitirse de una persona, animal, u objeto a otro

infertilidad una condición en la que un hombre o una mujer es físicamente incapaz de reproducir

inflamación aumento del flujo sanguíneo a un área lesionada o enferma del cuerpo, causando enrojecimiento, dolor, hinchazón, y dolor

inhalantes productos químicos que las personas inhalan para experimentar algún tipo de dopación

herencia la transmisión de las características de los padres a sus hijos

enfermedad hereditaria una enfermedad que es causada por la transmisión de genes defectuosos de una línea ancestral

inhibición la contención psicológica que desalienta a las personas de incurrir en conductas peligrosas

centro para pacientes hospitalizados un hospital donde residen pacientes durante la noche mientras reciben diagnósticos, tratamientos, cirugías, terapias, y rehabilitación

insomnio una condición en la cual el cuerpo es incapaz de conciliar el sueño o permanecer dormido

insulina una hormona que se produce en el páncreas y dirige a las células para consumir glucosa en la sangre

salud intelectual una dimensión de la salud que implica la capacidad de pensar clara y críticamente, aprender, y resolver problemas

intensidad una calidad que se mide por la cantidad de energía que el cuerpo utiliza por minuto durante la actividad física

interdependiente la calidad de una persona o pieza de información que es dependiente de otra

habilidades interpersonales su capacidad de interactuar positivamente con quienes le rodean

intersex   a condition characterized by ambiguous biological sex at birth

intrauterine device (IUD)   a T-shaped contraceptive product that is inserted into the uterus, where it helps prevent pregnancy

iris   the colored part of the eye that constricts and dilates the pupil

intersexual   una condición caracterizada por el sexo biológico ambiguo al nacer

dispositivo intrauterino (DIU)   un producto anticonceptivo en forma de T que se inserta en el útero, donde ayuda a prevenir el embarazo

iris   la parte coloreada del ojo que se contrae y dilata la pupila

J   English

Español

jet lag   the fatigue that people experience after changing time zones during travel

jet lag   la fatiga que las personas experimentan después de cambiar zonas de tiempo durante un viaje

L   English

Español

labor   the muscle contractions and changes in a woman's body as she gives birth

lactation consultant   a healthcare professional who counsels and assists new mothers as they breast-feed their babies

lanugo   the growth of fine hair all over the body; often a result of anorexia nervosa

laryngectomy   the surgical removal of the larynx

last will and testament   an arrangement outlining how possessions, land, and property are to be divided upon a person's death

latex condom   a birth control device that provides a barrier to semen and microorganisms that cause STIs

laxative   a medication that is used to encourage and aid bowel movements

lens   a clear part of the eye that focuses light on the retina

leptin   a hormone that suppresses appetite and leads to feeling full

leukoplakia   a condition characterized by white, leathery spots inside the mouth; may develop into oral cancer

parto   las contracciones musculares y los cambios en el cuerpo de una mujer mientras ella da a luz

especialista en lactancia   un profesional de salud que asesora y ayuda a las madres mientras amamanten a sus bebés

lanugo   el crecimiento de pelo fino por todo el cuerpo; a menudo el resultado de la anorexia nerviosa

laringectomía   la extirpación quirúrgica de la laringe

última voluntad y testamento   un acuerdo que expone cómo las posesiones, la tierra, y la propiedad se dividirán a la muerte de una persona

condón de látex   un dispositivo de control de la natalidad que proporciona una barrera para el semen y los microorganismos que causan infecciones de transmisión sexual

laxativo   un medicamento que se utiliza para estimular y ayudar los movimientos intestinales

lente   una parte transparente del ojo que enfoca la luz sobre la retina

leptina   una hormona que suprime el apetito y lleva a la sensación de saciedad

leucoplasia   una condición caracterizada por manchas blancas, correosas dentro de la boca; puede convertirse en cáncer oral

lice small insects that attach to hair and feed on human blood

life expectancy an average estimate of how long a person will live

lifelong learning a continuing pursuit of learning and studying that carries through your entire life; a key component of your ability to take charge of your own health

life span the average length of a person's life measured in years

living will an advanced directive that outlines what healthcare a person desires, to be used in the case that he or she is too sick to communicate his or her desires

local allergies allergies that affect a specific part of the body

long-term non-progressors HIV-positive people whose infection progresses to AIDS slowly

lymphocytes white blood cells that eliminate or disable foreign and possibly infected cells

piojos pequeños insectos que se adhieren al pelo y se alimentan de la sangre humana

expectativa de vida una estimación promedio de cuánto tiempo una persona va a vivir

aprendizaje para toda la vida una búsqueda de aprendizaje y estudio continua durante toda su vida; un componente clave de su capacidad para hacerse cargo de su propia salud

periodo de vida a duración promedio de vida de una persona medida en años

documento vital una directiva avanzada que describe el cuidado de salud que una persona desea, que será utilizado en caso de que él o ella esté demasiado enfermo para comunicar sus deseos

alergias locales alergias que afectan a una parte específica del cuerpo

no progresores a largo plazo personas VIH-positivas cuyos infección progresa lentamente al SIDA

linfocitos glóbulos blancos que eliminan o desactivan las células extrañas y posiblemente infectadas

M English

Español

major depression a mental illness characterized by intense and ongoing negative feelings such as hopelessness, sadness, or loneliness; also known as *clinical depression*

malignant tumors masses of abnormal cells that spread and invade other areas of the body

marijuana a drug composed of the dried parts of the Cannabis plant

masturbation self-stimulation of the sex organs in response to sexual excitement

mediation a method of resolving conflict that involves a third, neutral party

mediator a neutral third party who helps resolve conflicts by listening carefully to each perspective

depresión grave una enfermedad mental caracterizada por sentimientos negativos intensos y permanentes, como la desesperanza, la tristeza, o la soledad; también conocida como *depresión clínica*

tumores malignos masas de células anormales que se propagan e invaden otras áreas del cuerpo

marihuana una droga compuesta de las partes secas de la planta Cannabis

masturbación autoestimulación de los órganos sexuales en respuesta a la excitación sexual

mediación a un método de resolución de conflictos que involucra a un tercero neutral

mediador una tercera parte neutral que ayuda a resolver conflictos, escuchando atentamente cada perspectiva

medication   a substance used to treat a disease or relieve pain

medication abuse   the intentional use of medicines for reasons other than the prescribed purpose

medication misuse   any use of medicine that does not follow the medicine's instructions

meditation   the strategy of clearing negative thoughts from your mind and relaxing your body to relieve stress

meiosis   a type of cell division in which a cell splits its own genetic material and then divides into two different cells

melatonin   a hormone released by the pineal gland that increases feelings of relaxation and tiredness

menarche   a girl's first menstrual cycle, which typically occurs between 10 and 15 years of age

menopause   the end of a woman's reproductive years, when her ovaries stop releasing ova

mental illness   a medical condition in which a person experiences mental or emotional problems severe or persistent enough to interfere with daily functioning; also known as *mental disorder*

metabolism   the rate at which the body uses energy

metabolize   term that means to break down ingested substances

metastasis   the spread of abnormal cells from one part of the body (initial site) to another (secondary site)

middle adulthood   a stage of adulthood that occurs from 40 to 65 years of age

milestones   significant events that mark each stage of human development

mineral   inorganic elements found in soil and water; ingested by the body after being absorbed into plants

medicamento   una sustancia utilizada para el tratamiento de una enfermedad o para aliviar el dolor

abuso de medicamentos   el uso intencional de medicamentos por razones distintas a la finalidad prescrita

mal uso de medicamentos   cualquier uso de medicina que no siga las instrucciones del medicamento

meditación   la estrategia de despejar los pensamientos negativos de su mente y relajar su cuerpo para aliviar el estrés

meiosis   un tipo de división celular en el cual una célula se divide su propio material genético y luego se divide en dos células diferentes

melatonina   una hormona liberada por la glándula pineal que aumenta la sensación de relajación y cansancio

menarquía   primer ciclo menstrual de una niña, que normalmente se produce entre los 10 y 15 años de edad

menopausia   el final de los años reproductivos de una mujer, cuando los ovarios dejan de liberar óvulos

enfermedad mental   una condición médica en la que una persona experimenta problemas mentales o emocionales severos o persistentes lo suficiente para interferir con el funcionamiento diario; también conocido como *trastorno mental*

metabolismo   ritmo al que el cuerpo utiliza la energía

metabolizar   término que significa descomponer sustancias ingeridas

metástasis   la propagación de células anormales de una parte del cuerpo (sitio inicial) a otro (sitio secundario)

adultez media   una etapa de la edad adulta que se produce desde los 40 a los 65 años de edad

hitos   eventos significativos que marcan cada etapa del desarrollo humano

mineral   elementos inorgánicos que se encuentran en el suelo y el agua; ingeridos por el cuerpo después de ser absorbido por las plantas

miscarriage a pregnancy that ends before the 20th week

mitosis a type of cell division in which a cell copies its own genetic material and then divides into two identical cells

moderate drinking the consumption of no more than one alcoholic drink per day for women or no more than two alcoholic drinks per day for men

morbidity the prevalence of a disease, disorder, condition, or injury in a population

mortality the number of deaths caused by a disease, disorder, condition, or injury in a population

motor development the increase in a person's coordination and strength of muscles

MRSA (methicillin-resistant Staphylococcus aureus) a strain of *S. aureus* that is resistant to antibiotics

mucous membrane a barrier lining the body cavities and passages that open to the outside world

mucus a thick, watery substance that shields the body from pathogens

muscle dysmorphia a disorder characterized by an extreme concern with becoming more muscular

mutations alterations of a gene's normal structure; can lead to disease

mycosis a fungal infection that usually attacks damaged tissues or weakened people

aborto involuntario un embarazo que termina antes de las 20 semanas

mitosis un tipo de división celular en la cual una célula copia su propio material genético y luego se divide en dos células idénticas

consumo moderado de alcohol el consumo de no más de una bebida alcohólica al día para las mujeres o no más de dos bebidas alcohólicas al día para los hombres

morbidez prevalencia de una enfermedad, trastorno, afección, o lesión en una población

mortalidad el número de muertes causadas por una enfermedad, trastorno, afección, o lesión en una población

desarrollo motor el aumento de la coordinación de una persona y la fuerza de los músculos

SARM (Staphylococcus aureus resistente a la meticilina) una cepa de *S. aureus* que es resistente a los antibióticos

membrana mucosa una barrera que forra las cavidades y vías del cuerpo que están abiertas al mundo exterior

mucosidad una sustancia espesa y acuosa que protege el cuerpo contra los patógenos

dismorfia muscular un trastorno caracterizado por una preocupación extrema con ser más muscular

mutaciones alteraciones de la estructura normal de un gen; puede conducir a la enfermedad

micosis una infección fúngica que normalmente ataca los tejidos dañados o personas debilitadas

N English

Español

narcolepsy a disorder characterized by "sleep attacks" in which a person suddenly falls asleep at various times during the day

neglect a type of abuse that involves caregivers not meeting a dependent person's basic needs

neuron a type of cell that makes up the body's nerve tissues

nicotine an addictive, toxic substance present in tobacco products

narcolepsia un trastorno caracterizado por "ataques de sueño" en el que una persona de repente se queda dormido durante varios momentos durante el día

abandono un tipo de abuso donde los cuidadores no cumplen con las necesidades básicas de una persona dependiente

neurona un tipo de célula que compone los tejidos nerviosos del cuerpo

nicotina una sustancia toxica y adictiva presente en los productos de tabaco

nicotine replacement a method of battling addiction in which tobacco users gradually reduce their nicotine consumption

nocturnal emissions ejaculations of semen while sleeping

noncommunicable diseases diseases that are not caused by a pathogen and cannot be transmitted from one person to another; *noninfectious diseases*

noncustodial parent a parent who does not provide primary care for a child, but has legal rights and responsibilities regarding a child

nonverbal communication the use of body language, tone, volume, and other methods to send messages

nurse-midwife a licensed medical professional who educates women before birth, coaches them through labor and delivery, and aids in routine, uncomplicated births

nutrient a chemical substance that gives your body what it needs to grow and function properly

nutrient-dense food a relatively low-calorie food that provides vitamins, minerals, and other healthful substances

reemplazo de la nicotina un método de combatir contra la adicción en la que los consumidores de tabaco reducen gradualmente su consumo de nicotina

emisiones nocturnas eyaculaciones de semen durante el sueño

enfermedades no transmisibles enfermedades que no son causadas por un patógeno y no pueden ser transmitidas de una persona a otra; *enfermedades no infecciosas*

padre sin custodia un padre que no proporciona atención primaria para un niño, pero tiene derechos y responsabilidades legales respecto al niño

comunicación no verbal el uso del lenguaje corporal, el tono, el volumen, y otros métodos para enviar mensajes

enfermera-partera una profesional médica licenciada que educa a las mujeres antes del nacimiento, las guía durante el parto, y ayudas en partos rutinarios sin complicaciones

nutriente una sustancia química que le da al cuerpo lo que necesita para crecer y funcionar correctamente

alimentos ricos en nutrientes un alimento relativamente bajo en calorías que aporta vitaminas, minerales, y otras sustancias saludables

O   English

Español

obesity a condition characterized by having excess body fat; for adults, a BMI of 30 or higher

object permanence the idea that objects and people are present even when they cannot be seen

obstetrician/gynecologist (OB/GYN) a type of doctor who specializes in the female reproductive system, especially pregnancy, labor, and delivery

older adulthood a stage of adulthood that occurs at 65 years of age and older

obesidad una condición caracterizada por tener exceso de grasa corporal; para los adultos, un IMC de 30 o más

permanencia de los objetos la idea de que los objetos y las personas están presentes incluso cuando no se pueden ver

obstetra/ginecólogo un tipo de médico que se especializa en el sistema reproductor femenino, sobre todo el embarazo y el parto

edad adulta mayor una etapa de la edad adulta que se produce a los 65 años de edad y mayores

opiates   substances that come from the poppy plant

opioids   synthetic opiates that are prescribed for pain relief

opportunistic infection   a disease that takes advantage of a body's weakened immune system

optic nerve   the tissue by which nerve impulses travel from the retina to the brain

optimal health   a state of excellent health and wellness in all areas of your life

optimism   the ability to keep a positive outlook

oral cavity   the area of your mouth that includes the lips, teeth, and tongue

oral contraceptive   a contraceptive substance that contains hormones that thicken cervical mucus and prevent ovulation; also known as the *birth control pill* or the *pill*

orchitis   inflammation of the testes, leading to pain, swelling, and possible penile discharge

organic food   a type of food that is produced without pesticides, bioengineering, or high-energy radiation

organogenesis   the process by which organs belonging to the developing fetus take their familiar locations in the body

orgasm   the climax of sexual excitement, characterized by pleasurable sensations in the genital area

oropharyngeal cancer   a type of cancer in which the cells of the back of the throat, base of the tongue, and tonsils grow abnormally

osteoarthritis   a type of arthritis in which the cartilage in joints wears down so that the bones touch

osteoporosis   a dangerous condition in which bones are fragile and may break easily; can be caused by a lack of calcium during childhood and adolescence

opiáceos   sustancias que provienen de la planta de amapola

opioides   opiáceos sintéticos que son recetados para aliviar el dolor

infección oportunista   una enfermedad que se aprovecha del sistema inmunológico debilitado de un cuerpo

nervio óptico   el tejido por el cual los impulsos nerviosos viajan desde la retina hasta el cerebro

salud óptima   un estado de salud y bienestar excelente en todas las áreas de tu vida

optimismo   la capacidad de mantener una actitud positiva

cavidad oral   el área de su boca que incluye los labios, los dientes, y la lengua

anticonceptivo oral   una sustancia anticonceptiva que contiene hormonas que espesan el moco cervical e impiden la ovulación; también conocida como la *píldora anticonceptiva* o la *píldora*

orquitis   inflamación de los testículos, causando dolor, hinchazón, y posible secreción del pene

alimentos orgánicos   un tipo de alimento que es producido sin pesticidas, bioingeniería, o radiación de alta energía

organogénesis   el proceso por el cual los órganos pertenecientes a los fetos en desarrollo toman sus lugares conocidos en el cuerpo

orgasmo   el clímax de la excitación sexual, caracterizado por sensaciones placenteras en el área genital

cáncer de orofaringe   un tipo de cáncer en el que las células de la parte posterior de la garganta, la base de la lengua, y las amígdalas crecen anormalmente

osteoartritis   un tipo de artritis en la que el cartílago en las articulaciones se desgasta de manera que los huesos se tocan

osteoporosis   una condición peligrosa en la que los huesos son frágiles y pueden romperse con facilidad; puede ser causada por la falta de calcio durante la infancia y la adolescencia

outpatient facility a healthcare establishment where patients receive diagnosis or treatment, but do not reside overnight

ovarian cancer a type of cancer that grows in the ovaries and is often not detected until it has spread elsewhere

ovarian cysts noncancerous tumors on the ovaries, which may need to be removed if they cause pain

ovary a female reproductive organ that contains ova and produces the hormones estrogen and progesterone

overload principle standard which states that gradual increase of a physical demand on the body will improve fitness

overnutrition a condition in which the body takes in too much of some nutrients or too many calories

over-the-counter (OTC) medications medications that are sold without a doctor's prescription

overweight a condition characterized by having excess body weight for a particular height; can be due to fat, bone, muscle, or water

ovulation the release of an ovum from one of the follicles in the ovaries

ovum the female sex cell, which combines with the sperm to create a zygote

oxytocin a hormone that triggers strong uterine contractions to push the baby through the cervix and vagina

centro ambulatorio un establecimiento de atención médica, donde los pacientes reciben un diagnóstico o tratamiento, pero no residen durante la noche

cáncer ovárico un tipo de cáncer que crece en los ovarios y que a menudo no se detecta hasta que se ha extendido a otra parte

quistes ováricos tumores no cancerosos en los ovarios que pueden necesitar ser eliminados si causan dolor

ovario un órgano reproductor femenino que contiene los óvulos y produce las hormonas estrógeno y progesterona

principio de sobrecarga norma que establece que el aumento gradual de la demanda física en el cuerpo va a mejorar la condición física

sobrealimentación una condición en la que el cuerpo recibe demasiado de algunos nutrientes o demasiadas calorías

medicamentos sin receta medicamentos que se venden sin receta médica

con sobrepeso una condición caracterizada por tener exceso de peso corporal para una estatura determinada; puede ser debido a grasa, hueso, músculo, o agua

ovulación la liberación de un óvulo de uno de los folículos en los ovarios

óvulo la célula sexual femenina, que se combina con el esperma para crear un cigoto

oxitocina una hormona que provoca fuertes contracciones uterinas para empujar al bebé a través del cuello uterino y la vagina

P English

Español

palliative care healthcare designed to bring comfort and relief to those being treated for diseases or disorders

pandemic a widespread epidemic that affects an enormous number of people and spreads between countries and across the world

panic attacks episodes of intense fear that are often accompanied by serious physical symptoms

cuidado paliativo cuidado de la salud diseñado para consolar y aliviar a los que están siendo tratados por enfermedades o trastornos

pandemia una epidemia generalizada que afecta a un gran número de personas y se propaga entre los países y en todo el mundo

ataques de pánico episodios de intenso temor que a menudo van acompañados de síntomas físicos graves

parasite   an organism that must live inside or on another living organism to draw upon that organism's strength and energy for survival

parasomnia   a class of sleep disorders in which a person is partially, but not completely, aroused from sleep

pasteurization   the process of heating and then quickly cooling liquids to kill pathogens

pathogens   microscopic living things that may cause infections or other illnesses

Patient's Bill of Rights   summary of a patient's rights regarding fair treatment and appropriate information

pediatrician   a medical professional who specializes in treating infants and children

peer mediation   a method of resolving conflict in which a neutral peer listens to both parties in the disagreement and helps them reach a solution

peer pressure   the internal feeling that one must conform to the wishes of friends to earn their approval

pelvic inflammatory disease   an infection of the fallopian tubes and pelvic cavity, which occurs as the result of an STI and often causes infertility

periodontitis   an infection in which bacteria gets beneath the gums and destroys gum and bone

phagocyte   a white blood cell that engulfs and destroys microorganisms

philanthropists   individuals who make donations to improve others' lives and well-being

physical activity   broad term that describes structured exercise as well as other activities that use energy

Physical Activity Guidelines for Americans   a set of recommendations developed by the government, health professionals, and policymakers to help Americans improve their health through appropriate physical activity

parásito   un organismo que tiene que vivir dentro o sobre otro organismo vivo para utilizar la fuerza y energía de ese organismo para la supervivencia

parasomnia   una clase de trastornos del sueño en el cual una persona está parcialmente, pero no completamente, despierto del sueño

pasteurización   el proceso de calentar y entonces enfriar rápidamente líquidos para matar patógenos

patógenos   seres vivos microscópicos que pueden causar infecciones u otras enfermedades

Declaración de Derechos del Paciente   resumen de los derechos del paciente con respecto al trato justo y la información adecuada

pediatra   un profesional médico que se especializa en el tratamiento de bebés y niños

mediación entre pares   un método de resolución de conflictos en el que un compañero neutral escucha a ambas partes sobre un desacuerdo y les ayuda a llegar a una solución

presión social   la sensación interna de que uno debe cumplir con los deseos de los amigos para ganar su aprobación

enfermedad pélvica inflamatoria   una infección de las trompas de Falopio y la cavidad pélvica, que se produce como resultado de una ITS y a menudo es causa de infertilidad

periodontitis   una infección en la que bacterias se meten debajo de las encías y destruyen las encías y el hueso

fagocito   un glóbulo blanco que envuelve y destruye microorganismos

filántropos   individuos que hacen donaciones para mejorar la vida y el bienestar de los demás

actividad física   término general que describe el ejercicio estructurado, así como otras actividades que utilizan energía

Directrices de Actividad Física para los Americanos   una serie de recomendaciones desarrolladas por el gobierno, profesionales de la salud, y legisladores para ayudar a los norteamericanos a mejorar su salud mediante la actividad física adecuada

physical fitness   the state of being fit; attained by maintaining a healthful diet and exercise regimen

physical health   a dimension of health that involves your body, including physical fitness and the ability to cope with everyday physical tasks

physiological need   the body's requirement for something; necessary

placenta   the merged chorion and endometrial tissue that surrounds, protects, and nurtures a developing fetus

plaque   a sticky, colorless substance formed by bacteria in the mouth; coats the teeth and slowly dissolves enamel

pores   hair follicles underneath your skin that contain oil-producing glands

portion size   the amount of food served for a single person

positive reappraisal   the strategy of focusing on the positive aspects of a stressful event

post-traumatic stress disorder (PTSD)   a mental disorder that results from an extremely stressful event, and which is characterized by flashbacks to the event, feelings of numbness and guilt, and difficulty sleeping

preeclampsia   a condition in which the mother experiences high blood pressure

premenstrual dysphoric disorder (PMDD)   a condition in which the symptoms of PMS become severe enough to interfere with a woman's day-to-day living

premenstrual syndrome (PMS)   a collection of symptoms that occur before menstruation, including cramps, mood changes, and physical changes such as bloating and acne

premium   a regular fee paid in exchange for insurance services

prenatal care   medical care provided to the mother and fetus before birth

buen estado físico   el estado de estar en forma; alcanzado por el mantenimiento de un régimen de dieta y ejercicio saludable

salud física   una dimensión de la salud que involucra a su cuerpo, incluyendo la aptitud física y la capacidad para hacer frente a tareas físicas cotidianas

necesidad fisiológica   requerimiento del cuerpo por algo; necesario

placenta   el corion fusionado y el tejido endometrial que rodea, protege, y nutre al feto en desarrollo

placa   una sustancia pegajosa, incolora formada por bacterias en la boca; cubre los dientes y disuelve lentamente el esmalte

poros   folículos pilosos debajo de la piel que contienen glándulas productoras de aceite

tamaño de la porción   la cantidad de comida que se sirve para una sola persona

reevaluación positiva   la estrategia de concentrarse en los aspectos positivos de un evento estresante

trastorno por estrés postraumático (TEPT)   un trastorno mental que resulta de un acontecimiento extremadamente estresante, y que se caracteriza por recuerdos del evento, sensaciones de entumecimiento y culpa, y dificultad para dormir

pre-eclampsia   una condición en la que la madre sufre de alta presión arterial

trastorno disfórico premenstrual (TDPM)   una condición en la que los síntomas del síndrome premenstrual se vuelven lo suficientemente grave como para interferir con la vida diaria de una mujer

síndrome premenstrual (SPM)   un conjunto de síntomas que se producen antes de la menstruación, incluyendo calambres y cambios de humor, y cambios de físicos como la hinchazón y el acné

prima   un cargo fijo pagado a cambio de servicios de seguros

cuidado prenatal   la atención médica proporcionada a la madre y el feto antes del nacimiento

prescription medications medication that can only be sold to a person with a prescription from a doctor or other licensed healthcare professional

primary care physician a regular doctor who provides checkups, screenings, treatments, and prescriptions

primary sexual characteristics physical features that are directly involved in sexual reproduction; penis, testes, ovaries, vagina

problem drinking the consumption of enough alcohol that a person experiences problems in his or her daily life; often characterized by psychological but not physical dependence on alcohol

prognosis the probable consequence of a disease (death or recovery, for example)

progression principle standard which states that FITT factors should be increased over time to improve fitness

progressive muscle relaxation the strategy of tensing and then relaxing each part of your body and breathing deeply to relieve stress

prostate a male reproductive gland that secretes fluid to mix with sperm and create semen

prostate cancer a type of cancer that grows in the prostate; the second most common cancer in the world

prostatitis inflammation or infection of the prostate gland, leading to pain and blood in the urine

protein a nutrient the body uses to build and maintain all types of cells; can provide energy in the absence of fat and carbohydrates

proto-oncogenes genes that trigger division in cells

protozoa single-celled organisms that are larger and more complex than bacteria, and which may cause disease

pseudoscience theories and health claims that are described as being based in science when they are not

medicamentos con receta medicamento que sólo pueden ser vendidos a una persona con una receta de un médico u otro profesional de la salud autorizado

médico de atención primaria un médico de cabecera que ofrece chequeos, proyecciones, tratamientos y recetas

características sexuales primarias características físicas que están directamente involucradas con la reproducción sexual; el pene, los testículos, los ovarios, la vagina

problemas con el alcohol el consumo de suficiente alcohol que una persona experimenta problemas en su vida diaria; a menudo caracterizado por la dependencia psicológica pero no física en el alcohol

prognosis la consecuencia probable de una enfermedad (por ejemplo, la muerte o la recuperación)

principio de progresión norma que establece que los factores FITT deben incrementarse con el tiempo para mejorar la condición física

relajación muscular progresiva la estrategia de tensar y luego relajar cada parte de su cuerpo y respirar profundamente para aliviar el estrés

próstata una glándula reproductiva masculina que secreta líquido para mezclar con el esperma y crear esperma

cáncer del próstata un tipo de cáncer que se desarrolla en la próstata; el segundo tipo de cáncer más común en el mundo

prostatitis inflamación o infección de la glándula prostática, lo que lleva al dolor y sangre en la orina

proteína un nutriente que el cuerpo utiliza para construir y mantener todo tipo de células; puede proporcionar energía en la ausencia de grasa y carbohidratos

protooncogenes genes que activan la división en las células

protozoo organismos unicelulares que son más grandes y más complejos que las bacterias, y que pueden ocasionar enfermedades

pseudociencia teorías y alegaciones sobre la salud que son descritas como que están basadas en la ciencia cuando no lo están

psychological desire   the body's yearning for something; something wanted but not needed

puberty   the period during which levels of sex hormones increase and primary and secondary sexual characteristics develop

pupil   the black opening in the middle of the iris through which light passes

deseo psicológico   el anhelo del cuerpo para algo; algo deseado pero no necesario

pubertad   el período durante el cual los niveles de hormonas sexuales aumentan y las características sexuales primarias y secundarias se desarrollan

pupila   la apertura negra en el centro del iris través de la cual pasa la luz

---

Q   English

quality of life   a person's level of satisfaction with his or her life

Español

calidad de vida   nivel de satisfacción de una persona con su vida

---

R   English

range of motion   a measure of flexibility that tells how far a joint or body part can be moved

rape   sexual intercourse to which one party did not consent

receptive language   term for the understanding and processing of speech

recessive   term used to describe genes that are not always expressed in offspring

reflex   automatic muscle movement in response to stimulus

refusal skills   your ability to stand up to pressures and influences that hinder your progress toward wellness

relapse   the recurrence of a disease, in which signs and symptoms return after a period of remission

remission   a period of time in which the signs and symptoms of a disease subside

resilience   the ability to recover from traumatic or stressful events

respiratory etiquette   the practice of covering your mouth and nose with a tissue while coughing or sneezing, or sneezing into your sleeve

Español

amplitud de movimiento   una medida de flexibilidad que indica qué tan lejos una articulación o parte del cuerpo se puede mover

violación   relaciones sexuales a las que una de las partes no consintió

lenguaje receptivo   término para el entendimiento y el procesamiento del habla

recesivo   término utilizado para describir los genes que no siempre se expresan en la descendencia

reflejo   movimiento muscular automático en respuesta al estímulo

habilidades de rechazo   su capacidad para enfrentarse a presiones e influencias que dificultan su progreso hacia el bienestar

relapso   la recurrencia de una enfermedad, en el que las señales y los síntomas reaparecen después de un periodo de remisión

remisión   un período de tiempo en el que las señales y síntomas de una enfermedad desaparecen

resistencia   la capacidad de recuperarse de eventos traumáticos o estresantes

etiqueta respiratoria   la práctica de cubrirse la boca y la nariz con un pañuelo desechable al toser o estornudar, o estornudar en la manga

response substitution a technique in which people train themselves to respond to stress with healthy methods of coping and relaxation, rather than smoking

restless legs syndrome (RLS) a disorder in which people experience prickling, tingling, or other irresistible urges to move their legs

retina the innermost, light-sensitive area of the eye, composed of photoreceptors that convert light into nerve impulses and electrical signals

rheumatoid arthritis a type of arthritis in which the body's immune system attacks, damages, and eventually immobilizes the joints

risk factors aspects of a person's life that increase the likelihood he or she will develop a disease or infection, or experience an injury

rooting reflex an automatic muscle movement in which an infant turns his or her head and tries to suck when hungry

rumination the act of thinking repeatedly about something for a long period of time

sustitución de respuesta una técnica en la el que las personas se entrenan para responder al estrés con métodos saludables de afrontamiento y relajación, en lugar de fumar

síndrome de piernas inquietas (SPI) un trastorno en el cual las personas experimentan picazón, hormigueo, u otros impulsos irresistibles para mover sus piernas

retina el área más interno, sensible a la luz del ojo, compuesto de los fotoreceptores que convierten la luz en impulsos nerviosos y señales eléctricas

artritis reumatoide un tipo de artritis en la que el sistema inmunológico del cuerpo ataca, daña, y, finalmente, inmoviliza las articulaciones

factores de riesgo aspectos de la vida de una persona que aumentan la probabilidad de que él o ella desarrollarán una enfermedad o infección, o sufrirán una lesión

reflejo de búsqueda un movimiento muscular automático en el cual un bebé gira su cabeza e intenta succionar cuando tiene hambre

rumiación el acto de pensar sobre algo repetidamente durante un largo periodo de tiempo

---

S English

Español

safe haven laws laws that allow parents to leave their infant at designated locations if they wish to give up their child for adoption; age restrictions for the child vary by state; *safe surrender laws*

saliva a substance produced in the mouth, which contains enzymes that break down food

sandwich generation term that describes adults who care for their parents as well as their children

saturated fat a type of fat found primarily in animal-based foods that is solid at room temperature

schizophrenia a mental illness characterized by delusions, hallucinations, and irregular thought patterns

leyes de refugio seguro leyes que permiten a los padres dejar a sus bebés en lugares designados si desean renunciar a su hijo en adopción; restricciones de edad para el niño varían según el estado; *leyes de rendición segura*

saliva una sustancia producida en la boca, que contiene enzimas que descomponen los alimentos

generación sándwich término que describe a los adultos que cuidan de sus padres, así como a sus hijos

grasa saturada un tipo de grasa que se encuentra principalmente en alimentos de origen animal que es sólida a temperatura ambiente

esquizofrenia una enfermedad mental caracterizada por delirios, alucinaciones y patrones de pensamiento irregulares

school violence violent behavior that occurs on school property or at school events

science a collection of and the pursuit of knowledge about the natural world drawn from observation and experimentation

scientific knowledge conclusions about the natural world that have been obtained through peer-reviewed, repeatable observation and experimentation

secondary sexual characteristics physical features that correspond with sexual development but are not directly involved in reproduction; pubic hair, breasts

secondhand smoke tobacco smoke in the environment that may affect a person even if he or she does not smoke

sedentary behavior activities such as sitting or lying down that use very little energy

self-actualization the feeling that you are striving toward and becoming the best person you can be

self-esteem your feelings of self-worth

self-image your mental picture of yourself

self-medication the use of drugs to treat symptoms that have not been diagnosed by a medical professional

semen a substance secreted during ejaculation, which contains sperm and other fluid

sensory input the information that the brain receives related to sight, hearing, touch, and smell

separation anxiety fear of being away from caregivers

sexual activity behavior related to sexual intercourse; considered a risk factor for teenagers

sexual assault the act of forcing someone into sexual activity that he or she does not want

sexual harassment any unwanted sexual attention

violencia escolar comportamiento violento que ocurre en la escuela o en eventos escolares

ciencia una colección de y la búsqueda de conocimientos sobre el mundo natural extraída de la observación y la experimentación

conocimiento científico conclusiones sobre el mundo natural que han sido obtenidas a través de la observación y la experimentación repetible, y revisada por expertos

características sexuales secundarias características físicas que corresponden al desarrollo sexual, pero no están directamente involucrados en la reproducción; vello púbico, los senos

humo de segunda mano humo de tabaco en el medio ambiente que puede afectar a una persona, aun si él o ella no fuma

comportamiento sedentario actividades como sentarse o acostarse que utilizan muy poca energía

autorrealización la sensación de que te estás esforzando para ser y convirtiéndote en la mejor persona que puedes ser

autoestima sus sentimientos de autovaloración

imagen de sí mismo su imagen mental de sí mismo

automedicación el uso de medicamentos para tratar síntomas que no han sido diagnosticados por un profesional médico

semen una sustancia secretada durante la eyaculación, que contiene espermatozoides y otro fluido

información sensorial la información que el cerebro recibe relacionada con la vista, el oído, el tacto y el olfato

ansiedad de separación miedo de estar lejos de los cuidadores

actividad sexual comportamiento relacionado con las relaciones sexuales; considerado un factor de riesgo para los adolescentes

asalto sexual el acto de forzar a alguien a la actividad sexual que él o ella no quiere

acoso sexual cualquier atención sexual no deseada

sexuality the expression of a person's gender through behavior and mature anatomy and physiology

sexually transmitted infections (STIs) infections that are transmitted by sexual contact, and are caused by bacteria, viruses, or protozoa that live in and on reproductive organs

sexual orientation term that describes which gender a person is attracted to

sexual reproduction the process by which the genetic material of two organisms—one male and one female—combine to create offspring

sexual violence any sexual activity to which one party did not consent

shaken baby syndrome trauma and brain damage caused by an infant being jostled or handled roughly

short sleepers people who can function well on less sleep than others

sibling rivalry competitive feelings and behaviors that exist between siblings; may include competing for attention, praise, or material objects

skill-related fitness type of fitness that improves a person's performance in a particular sport

skinfold test a method of measuring body composition in which a person uses a skinfold caliper to measure the thickness of a fold of fat

sleep apnea a serious disorder in which a person stops breathing during sleep

sleep deficit a shortage of sleep that leads to tiredness and to other health problems

smokeless tobacco a tobacco-related product that does not require burning; includes chewing tobacco and electronic nicotine delivery systems (ENDS)

social health a dimension of health that involves your communication skills, relationships, and ability to interact with others

sexualidad la expresión de género de una persona a través del comportamiento y la anatomía y fisiología madura

infecciones de transmisión sexual (ITS) infecciones que son transmitidas por contacto sexual, y son causadas por bacterias, virus, o protozoos que viven en y sobre los órganos reproductores

orientación sexual término que describe a cual género una persona se siente atraída

reproducción sexual el proceso por el cual el material genético de dos organismos: uno masculino y otro femenino, se combinan para crear descendencia

violencia sexual cualquier actividad sexual a la que una de las partes no dio su consentimiento

síndrome del bebé sacudido trauma y daño cerebral causado por un bebé que es sacudido o maltratado

personas que duermes poco personas que pueden funcionar bien con dormir menos que otros

rivalidad entre hermanos sentimientos y comportamientos competitivos que existen entre hermanos; puede incluir competir por la atención, elogios, u objetos materiales

condición física relacionada con la habilidad tipo de gimnasia que mejora el rendimiento de una persona en un deporte en particular

prueba del pliegue cutáneo un método para medir la composición del cuerpo en el que una persona utiliza un calibrador del pliegue cutáneo para medir el espesor de un pliegue de grasa

apnea del sueño un trastorno grave en el que una persona deja de respirar durante el sueño

déficit de sueño la falta de sueño que lleva al cansancio y otros problemas de salud

tabaco sin humo un producto relacionado con el tabaco que no requiere de quemar; incluye masticar tabaco y los sistemas de entrega de nicotina electrónica (ENDS)

salud social una dimensión de la salud que consiste de su capacidad de comunicación, las relaciones, y su capacidad de interactuar con los demás

socioeconomic risk factors   characteristics of your status in society that may expose you to injury or disease

specialist   medical providers who are extensively trained in one or two areas of health; a physician may refer you to a specialist to seek specific treatments

specificity principle   standard which states that exercising a particular component leads to improvements in the fitness of only that component

sperm   the male sex cell, which combines with the ovum to create a zygote

spermicide   a substance that inactivates sperm; often applied to condoms and other contraceptive products

statutory rape   sexual activity that occurs between an adult and an adolescent

stent   a circular, hollow, wire mesh tube

sterilization   a surgical contraceptive method in which a person is rendered permanently unable to conceive children

stigma   a negative or unfair belief circulated within society

stillbirth   the birth of a dead fetus

stimulant   a substance that increases the body's activity and makes it more difficult to sleep

stimulus control   the technique of avoiding situations that may lead to drug use

stranger anxiety   fear of unfamiliar people or situations

stress   term for the body's physical and psychological response to traumatic or challenging situations

stress hormones   hormones that trigger the body's physiological response to stress; epinephrine and norepinephrine

stressor   any factor that causes stress

stroke   an interruption of the blood flow to a section of the brain

factores de riesgo socioeconómicos   características de su estatus en la sociedad que pueden exponerlo a una lesión o enfermedad

especialista   proveedores de servicios médicos que están ampliamente capacitados en una o dos áreas de salud; un médico puede referirlo a un especialista para buscar tratamientos específicos

principio de especificidad   norma que establece que el ejercicio de un componente en particular conduce a mejoras en la aptitud de solamente ese componente

esperma   la célula sexual masculina, que se combina con el óvulo para crear un cigoto

espermicida   una sustancia que inactiva los espermatozoides; a menudo se aplica a los preservativos y otros productos anticonceptivos

corrupción de menores   actividad sexual que se produce entre un adulto y un adolescente

estent   un tubo circular, hueco, de malla alámbrica

esterilización   un método anticonceptivo quirúrgico en el que una persona se vuelve permanentemente incapaz de concebir hijos

estigma   una creencia negativa o injusta que circula dentro de la sociedad

muerte fetal   el nacimiento de un feto muerto

estimulante   una sustancia que aumenta la actividad del cuerpo y hace más difícil dormir

control de estímulos   la técnica de evitar situaciones que puedan conducir al consumo de drogas

ansiedad ante desconocidos   temor a personas desconocidas o situaciones

estrés   término para la respuesta física y psicológica del cuerpo a situaciones traumáticas o difíciles

hormonas del estrés   hormonas que desencadenan la respuesta fisiológica del organismo al estrés; epinefrina y norepinefrina

estresor   cualquier factor que causa el estrés

derrame cerebral   una interrupción del flujo sanguíneo a una sección del cerebro

substance abuse   the use of a drug (nicotine, alcohol, or illegal drugs) or intentional misuse of medication

sudden infant death syndrome (SIDS)   the death of a healthy baby while sleeping; while the cause is unknown, it may be due to difficulty breathing

suicide clusters   a series of suicides in a community over a relatively short period of time

suicide contagion   term for the copying of suicide attempts after exposure to another person's suicide

sunscreen   a product that protects the skin by absorbing and scattering UV rays

support groups   groups of people who communicate about their struggles and progress in battling a shared problem

suprachiasmatic nucleus (SCN)   a cluster of nerve cells in the hypothalamus that controls sleep, body temperature, hormone levels, and brain activity

survivors   people who lose a loved one to suicide

syphilis   a bacterial infection that causes a sore (or chancre), rashes, and internal infection in later stages, and can be fatal if untreated

systemic allergies   allergies that affect the entire body

abuso de sustancias   el uso de una droga (nicotina, alcohol, o drogas ilegales) o mal uso intencional de medicamentos

síndrome de muerte súbita del lactante (SMSL)   la muerte de un bebé sano mientras duerme; aunque se desconoce la causa, puede ser debido a dificultad respiratoria

grupos de suicidios   una serie de suicidios en una comunidad durante un período relativamente corto de tiempo

contagio de suicidio   término para la copia de los intentos de suicidio después de estar expuesto al suicidio de otra persona

protector solar   un producto que protege la piel mediante la absorción y dispersión de los rayos UV

grupos de apoyo   grupos de personas que se comunican sobre sus luchas y avances en la lucha contra un problema compartido

núcleo supraquiasmático   un grupo de células nerviosas en el hipotálamo que controla el sueño, la temperatura corporal, los niveles hormonales, y la actividad cerebral

sobrevivientes   las personas que pierden un ser querido por suicidio

sífilis   una infección bacterial que causa dolor (o chancro), erupciones, e infección interna en las etapas posteriores, y puede ser mortal si no es tratada

alergias sistémicas   alergias que afectan a todo el cuerpo

T   English

Español

tar   a thick, sticky substance produced by burning tobacco; can disrupt the respiratory systems of smokers

target heart rate   the heart rate to aim for while performing aerobic exercise that leads to optimal cardiorespiratory fitness; varies by age

T cell   a cell that coordinates the body's immune response and attacks cells that have been infected by a virus

alquitrán   una sustancia espesa, pegajosa producida por la combustión del tabaco; puede perturbar los sistemas respiratorios de los fumadores

meta de ritmo cardíaco   la frecuencia cardíaca deseada para el desempeño de ejercicio aeróbico que conduce a la aptitud cardiorrespiratoria óptima; varía según la edad

célula T   una célula que coordina las células de respuesta y ataques inmunes del cuerpo que han sido infectados por un virus

temper tantrum a frustrated or angry reaction that includes crying, yelling, or mild physical violence

testes male reproductive organs that produce sperm and the hormone testosterone

testicular cancer a type of cancer that grows in one or both of the testes; treatable if detected early

therapist a professional who is trained to diagnose and treat people with mental illnesses and disorders

tobacco a plant that is used to produce cigarettes and other products; contains nicotine

tolerance a condition in which the body adjusts to a given substance, requiring increased amounts of the substance to feel its effect

trans fat a type of fat that is created by hydrogenation; poses health risks acknowledged by the FDA

transgender term that describes a person who identifies with the gender opposite his or her biological sex

traumatic brain injury (TBI) damage caused by a severe blow or jolt to the head, which may alter mental functioning

trichomoniasis a curable STI, caused by a protozoan, which may cause burning or itching, but is usually asymptomatic

tryptophan an amino acid that aids the body in producing chemicals that cause sleep

tubal ligation a sterilization surgery in which a woman's fallopian tubes are cut, making it impossible for sperm to reach the ova

tumor a growth of abnormal cells in the body's tissues

tumor-suppressor genes genes that stop cell division when it is no longer necessary

rabieta una reacción frustrada o enojada que incluye el llanto, los gritos, o la violencia física leve

testículos órganos reproductores masculinos que producen los espermatozoides y la hormona testosterona

cáncer testicular un tipo de cáncer que crece en uno o ambos de los testículos; tratable si se detecta a tiempo

terapeuta un profesional que está capacitado para diagnosticar y tratar a las personas con enfermedades mentales y trastornos

tabaco una planta que se utiliza para producir cigarrillos y otros productos; contiene nicotina

tolerancia una condición en la que el cuerpo se ajusta a una determinada sustancia, lo que requiere una mayor cantidad de la sustancia para sentirse su efecto

grasas saturadas un tipo de grasa que se crea mediante la hidrogenación; plantea riesgos para la salud reconocidos por la FDA

transgénero término que describe a una persona que se identifica con el género opuesto de su sexo biológico

lesión cerebral traumática los daños causados por un severo golpe o sacudida en la cabeza, que puede alterar el funcionamiento mental

tricomoniasis una ITS curable, causada por un protozoo, que puede causar ardor o picazón, pero suele ser asintomática

triptófano un aminoácido que ayuda al cuerpo a producir los químicos que causan el sueño

ligadura de trompas una cirugía de esterilización en la que se cortan las trompas de Falopio de una mujer, lo que hace imposible que los espermatozoides lleguen a los óvulos

tumor un crecimiento de células anormales en los tejidos del cuerpo

genes supresores de tumores genes que detienen la división celular cuando ya no es necesario

type 1 diabetes mellitus a disorder in which the body cannot process glucose properly due to a lack of insulin-producing cells

type 2 diabetes mellitus a disorder in which the body cannot process glucose properly due to the body developing insulin resistance

diabetes mellitus tipo 1 un trastorno en el cual el cuerpo no puede procesar la glucosa adecuadamente debido a la falta de células productoras de insulina

diabetes mellitus tipo 2 un trastorno en el cual el cuerpo no puede procesar la glucosa adecuadamente debido a que el cuerpo desarrolla resistencia a la insulina

U English

Español

ultraviolet (UV) light an invisible type of radiation that emanates from the sun, tanning beds, and sunlamps

umbilical cord a structure that connects the developing fetus to the placenta to provide the fetus with nutrients required for growth

undernutrition a condition in which the body takes in too few nutrients for health and growth

underweight a condition characterized by having too little body weight for a particular height

unsaturated fat a type of fat that is liquid at room temperature and is found in plant-based foods

uterine cancer a type of cancer that grows in the endometrium; the most common cancer of the female reproductive organs

uterus a hollow organ of the female reproductive system that is lined with endometrial tissue and which houses and nurtures a developing fetus

luz ultravioleta (UV) un tipo de radiación invisible que emana del sol, las camas de bronceado, y las lámparas solares

cordón umbilical una estructura que conecta al feto en desarrollo a la placenta para proporcionarle al feto con nutrientes requeridos para el crecimiento

desnutrición una condición en la que el cuerpo toma muy pocos nutrientes para la salud y el crecimiento

bajo peso una condición que se caracteriza por tener muy poco peso corporal para una estatura determinada

grasa insaturada un tipo de grasa que es líquida a temperatura ambiente y se encuentra en alimentos de origen vegetal

cáncer uterino un tipo de cáncer que crece en el endometrio; el cáncer más común de los órganos reproductivos femeninos

útero un órgano hueco del sistema reproductor femenino que está forrado de tejido endometrial y que alberga y nutre al feto en desarrollo

V English

Español

vaccine a dead or nontoxic part of a pathogen that is injected into a person to train his or her immune system to eliminate the live pathogen

vagina a tube-like structure that extends from the external vaginal opening to the cervix, which leads into the uterus

vacuna una parte muerta o no tóxica de un patógeno que se inyecta en una persona para entrenar a su sistema inmunológico a eliminar el patógeno vivo

vagina una estructura similar a un tubo que se extiende desde la abertura vaginal externa al cérvix, lo que conduce al útero

valves flaps of tissue that control blood flow in the heart

vas deferens a tube in the male reproductive system that carries sperm from the testes to the penis

vasectomy a sterilization surgery in which a man's vas deferens is cut, preventing sperm from leaving the testes

vector an animal that transmits a disease from one living thing to another

veins blood vessels that carry blood from the capillaries back to the heart

verbal communication the use of spoken or written words to send messages

vernix a temporary, white protective coating that may cover a newborn at birth

virus a pathogen that infects cells and uses their energy because it cannot reproduce or grow on its own

visualization the strategy of imagining a pleasant environment when faced with stress

vitamins organic substances derived from plants or animals, which are necessary for normal growth and development

voyeurism looking at someone for sexual pleasure

válvulas colgajos de tejido que controlan el flujo sanguíneo en el corazón

conducto deferente un tubo en el sistema reproductivo masculino que lleva el esperma desde los testículos al pene

vasectomía una cirugía de esterilización en la que el conducto deferente de un hombre es cortado, impidiendo que los espermatozoides salgan de los testículos

portador un animal que transmite una enfermedad de un ser vivo a otro

venas los vasos sanguíneos que llevan la sangre desde los capilares hacia el corazón

comunicación verbal el uso de palabras habladas y escritos para enviar mensajes

vérnix una capa protectora temporal, blanca, que puede cubrir al recién nacido al nacer

virus un patógeno que infecta las células y utiliza su energía porque no puede reproducirse o crecer por sí mismo

visualización la estrategia de imaginarse un ambiente agradable cuando se enfrentan con el estrés

vitaminas sustancias orgánicas derivadas de plantas o animales, que son necesarias para el crecimiento y desarrollo normal

voyerismo mirar a una persona para obtener placer sexual

W English

water-soluble vitamin a type of vitamin that dissolves in water and passes into the bloodstream

well-being a state of health and wellness in which one feels safe, fulfilled, and productive, and looks forward to enjoying a long life

wellness a healthy balance of physical, emotional, intellectual, and social health

withdrawal (1) the unpleasant physical or psychological symptoms associated with attempting to stop using a substance; (2) an unreliable birth control method in which a man pulls his penis out of a woman's vagina before he ejaculates; also known as *pulling out*

Español

vitamina soluble en agua un tipo de vitamina que se disuelve en agua y pasa al flujo sanguíneo

bienestar un estado de salud y bienestar en el que uno se siente seguro, satisfecho, y productivo, y espera disfrutar de una larga vida

bienestar un sano equilibrio de bienestar físico, emocional, intelectual, y social

abstinencia (1) los desagradables síntomas físicos o psicológicos asociados con el intento de dejar de usar una sustancia; (2) un método anticonceptivo poco confiable en el que un hombre saca su pene de la vagina de una mujer antes de eyacular

Y English

young adulthood   a stage of adulthood that occurs from 20 to 40 years of age

Español

adultez joven   una etapa de la edad adulta que ocurre entre los 20 a 40 años de edad

Z English

zoonosis   an infection transferred from an animal to a human

zygote   an ovum that has been fertilized by a sperm and which contains half of a mother's genes and half of a father's genes

Español

zoonosis   una infección transferida de un animal a un ser humano

cigoto (zigoto)   un óvulo que ha sido fecundado por un espermatozoide y que contiene la mitad de los genes de la madre y la mitad de los genes del padre

Index

A

Ablation, 420
Abortion, 727
Abstinence, 23–24, 48, 385–386, 425, 702–703, 716, 742–743, 744
    challenges, 385
    definition, 385
    developing refusal skills, 23–24, 385–386
Accident. *See* Unintended injuries
Acid reflux disorder, 145
Acidosis, 431
Acne, 234–235, 618, 676
Acquaintance rape, 578
Acquaintances, 539
Acquired immunodeficiency syndrome (AIDS), 40, 398
Active listening, 533
Acute diseases, 11, 412
Addiction, 267–269, 507
    alcoholism, 301–302
    definition, 267
    dependency and addiction, 268–269
    drugs, 337–343
    experimentation, 268
    exploring a new identity, 270
    nicotine, 272–279
    regular use, 268
    tolerance, 268
    withdrawal symptoms, 269
Adolescent years, 675–679
    emotional and social development, 678
    health and wellness issues, 679
    intellectual development, 677–678
    physical development and puberty, 676–677
Adoption, 636, 655
Adulthood, 680–686
    adaptations to aging, 686
    health changes, 683–686
    mature adult, 681
    stages, 681–683
Adult-onset diabetes, 54, 432
Aerobic, 170
Aerobic endurance, 174–175
Affordable Care Act, 29–30
    cost reduction and affordability, 29–30
    definition, 29
    expanded access to insurance, 29
    improved healthcare, 30
Age spots, 683
Aggressive, 560–561
Agility, 178

Aging, 687–693
    caring for older adults, 688
    financial and medical issues at end of life, 690–691
    grief and loss, 691–693
    health changes, 683–686
    hospice and palliative care, 689–690
    housing options, 689
    stages of grief, 691–693
    transportation options, 689
AIDS. *See* Acquired immunodeficiency syndrome
Airbrush, 150
Alcohol abuse. *See* Alcoholism
Alcohol, 284–311
    alcohol poisoning, 295–296
    binge drinking, 295
    blood alcohol concentration, 288
    definition, 287
    effects on brain, 287–288
    effects on health, 293–299
    hangover, 291–292
    impact on body, 286–292
    long-term health consequences, 296–298
    motor vehicle accidents, 294
    pregnancy, 297–298
    problem drinking, 301
    strategies for preventing and treating alcohol abuse, 306–311
    underage drinking, 298–299
    use and abuse, 300–305
    use, accidents, and violence, 294–295
Alcoholics, 301
Alcoholism,
    definition, 301
    factors affecting, 302–305
    prevention, 307–308
    strategies for treating, 308–311
Alcohol poisoning, 295
Allergens, 99, 433
Allergies, 99, 433–434
All-or-nothing mindset, 122
Amenorrhea, 190, 618
Americans with Disabilities Act (ADA) of 1990, 402
Amino acid, 72, 137, 219
Amnion, 607
Amphetamines, 323
Anabolic steroids, 137, 333
Anaerobic, 170
Analgesics, 319
Anaphylaxis, 434
Androgynous, 453
Anemia, 77, 144, 615
Angina, 417